MEDICAL SECRETS

Second Edition

ANTHONY J. ZOLLO, JR., MD

Assistant Professor
Department of Internal Medicine
Baylor College of Medicine
Ambulatory Care Service
Houston VA Medical Center
Houston, Texas

HANLEY & BELFUS, INC./ Philadelphia

Publisher: HANLEY & BELFUS, INC.
                Medical Publishers
                210 South 13th Street
                Philadelphia, PA 19107
                (215) 546-7293; 800-962-1892
                FAX (215) 790-9330

Library of Congress Cataloging-in-Publication Data

Medical Secrets / [edited by] Anthony J. Zollo, Jr. – 2nd ed.
     p.   cm. – (The Secrets Series®)
  Includes bibliographical references and index.
  ISBN 1-56053-172-X (alk. paper)
  1. Internal Medicine–Examinations, questions, etc. I. Zollo, Anthony J., 1954-
II. Series.
  [DNLM: 1. Internal Medicine–examination questions. WB 18.2 M4855 1997]
RC58.M43 1997
616' .0076–dc21
DNLM/DLC
for Library of Congress   96-47625
                                                   CIP

MEDICAL SECRETS, 2nd edition   ISBN 1-56053-172-X

Last digit is the print number: 9 8 7 6 5 4 3

DEDICATION

To my wife, Mary, without whose help and support
this book, and many other things, would not be possible.

CONTENTS

CONTRIBUTORS

Carol M. Ashton, M.D., M.P.H.
Associate Professor, Department of Internal Medicine, Baylor College of Medicine; Director, General Medicine Consultation Service, Department of Veterans Affairs Medical Center, Houston, Texas

Douglas W. Axelrod, M.D., Ph.D.
Medical Director, Bone and Mineral Research, Procter & Gamble Pharmaceuticals, Cincinnati, Ohio

Rhonda A. Cole, M.D.
Assistant Professor, Department of Internal Medicine, Baylor College of Medicine; Chief, Gastrointestinal Endoscopy, Digestive Disease Section, Department of Veterans Affairs Medical Center, Houston, Texas

Charlene M. Dewey, M.D.
Assistant Professor, Section of General Internal Medicine, Department of Internal Medicine, Baylor College of Medicine; Medicine Service, Ben Taub General Hospital, Houston, Texas

Mary Anne Doherty, M.D.
Associate Clinical Professor, Section of Oncology, Department of Internal Medicine, Boston University School of Medicine, Boston; Associate Chief of Staff for Ambulatory Care, Edith Nourse Rogers Memorial Veterans' Hospital, Bedford, Massachusetts

Sheila Goodnight-White, M.D.
Associate Professor of Medicine, Section of Pulmonary Medicine, Department of Internal Medicine, Baylor College of Medicine; Staff Physician, Pulmonary Section, Department of Veterans Affairs Medical Center, Houston, Texas

Gabriel B. Habib, M.D.
Assistant Professor, Section of Cardiology, Department of Internal Medicine, Baylor College of Medicine; Director, Coronary Care Unit, Department of Veterans Affairs Medical Center, Houston, Texas

Richard J. Hamill, M.D.
Associate Professor, Departments of Internal Medicine and Microbiology & Immunology, Baylor College of Medicine; Section of Infectious Diseases, Department of Veterans Affairs Medical Center, Houston, Texas

Mary P. Harward, M.D.
Associate Professor, Department of Internal Medicine, University of Florida Health Sciences Center, Gainesville, Florida

Teresa G. Hayes, M.D., Ph.D.
Assistant Professor, Department of Internal Medicine, Baylor College of Medicine; Director, Oncology Clinic, Department of Veterans Affairs Medical Center, Houston, Texas

Christopher J. Lahart, M.D.
Assistant Professor of Medicine, Department of Internal Medicine, Baylor College of Medicine; Chief, AIDS Unit, Department of Veterans Affairs Medical Center, Houston, Texas

Sharma S. Prabhakar, M.D.
Director of Dialysis and Staff Nephrologist, Department of Veterans Affairs Medical Center, Bronx, New York; Assistant Professor, Department of Medicine, Mount Sinai School of Medicine, New York, New York

Wayne J. Riley, M.D.
Instructor, Section of General Internal Medicine, Department of Internal Medicine, Baylor College of Medicine, Houston, Texas

Loren A. Rolak, M.D.
Department of Neurosciences, Marshfield Clinic, Marshfield, Wisconsin; Clinical Associate Professor, Department of Neurology, University of Wisconsin, Madison, Wisconsin

Richard A. Rubin, M.D.
Clinical Instructor, Section of Rheumatology, Department of Internal Medicine, Baylor College of Medicine, Houston, Texas

George E. Taffet, M.D.
Assistant Professor, Department of Internal Medicine, Baylor College of Medicine; Staff Physician, Huffington Center on Aging, Houston, Texas

Mark M. Udden, M.D.
Associate Professor, Section of Hematology/Oncology, Department of Internal Medicine, Baylor College of Medicine, Houston, Texas

Anthony P. Weiss, M.D.
Department of Psychiatry, Harvard Medical School, Massachusetts General Hospital, Boston, Massachusetts

Nelda P. Wray, M.D., M.P.H.
Professor, Department of Internal Medicine, Baylor College of Medicine; Chief, General Medicine Section, Department of Veterans Affairs Medical Center, Houston, Texas

Anthony J. Zollo, Jr., M.D.
Assistant Professor, Department of Internal Medicine, Baylor College of Medicine, Houston; Chief Medical Officer, Lufkin Department of Veterans Affairs Outpatient Clinic, Lufkin, Texas

PREFACE TO THE FIRST EDITION

The art of Internal Medicine involves questions. It involves questions asked when taking a medical history, when forming a differential diagnosis, or when planning a diagnostic and therapeutic plan. Students of Internal Medicine, regardless of their level of training, are constantly confronted with questions posed from patients, from mentors, and from within themselves. The time-honored, question-based, Socratic approach to teaching is alive and well in the academic and clinical world of Internal Medicine. This book is intended to provide the reader with many of the questions (and answers) commonly encountered in training.

The knowledge base of Internal Medicine is substantial, probably more than any other specialty. Its acquisition is the goal of medical students, house officers, and all others who endeavor to learn and practice the discipline. There are many formal textbooks of internal medicine that provide complete coverage of all topics within the field. This work is not meant to replace the use of those texts. Rather, it is intended to focus on the lead-in questions and topics commonly encountered on teaching rounds, in clinical situations, and in examinations.

In preparing this text, we have attempted to take a middle ground between over-simplification and over-complication. We have included questions on common subjects and on "zebras," which, owing to their academic interest, are frequently discussed. We are grateful to our patients, our teachers, and our students for these questions and answers. As editor, I am indebted to my contributors on the faculty of Baylor College of Medicine for their assistance in this enjoyable and educational undertaking.

PREFACE TO THE SECOND EDITION

The editing of the first edition of this book was an act of love. The tasks of assembling a team of contributors, collecting suggestions for question and answer sets, developing the final list of Q&A sets for each chapter, writing my share of those sets, and editing the overall manuscript was thoroughly enjoyable, albeit very time-consuming. This has been true for the second edition as well. I would like to acknowledge again the hard work and dedication of all the contributors to this book. Only by utilizing the talents of experts in various subspecialties, with up-to-date knowledge of current developments, was it possible to complete the revision. Although many questions are the same, the answers often required revision. We are all proud of the finished product.

I would like to thank Linda Belfus, President of Hanley & Belfus, Inc., and her entire staff for their assistance and support. I would like to thank the readers of the first edition for their positive response to our work. After the countless hours spent producing the manuscript, one loses the ability to view the final result objectively. The success of the first edition was a validation of our hard work. I am confident you will receive the second edition with equal enthusiasm.

Anthony J. Zollo, Jr., M.D.

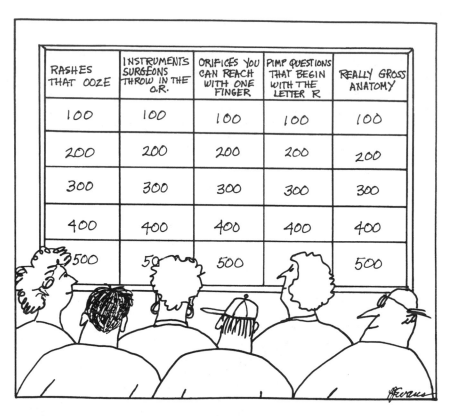

Medical School Jeopardy

Reprinted with permission from Bennett HA (ed): The Best of Medical Humor, 2nd ed. Philadelphia, Hanley & Belfus, 1997. Cartoon by Phyllis J. Evans.

1. GENERAL MEDICINE

Charlene M. Dewey, M.D., Wayne J. Riley, M.D., MPH., and Anthony J. Zollo, M.D.

The extraordinary development of modern science may be her undoing. Specialism, now a necessity, has fragmented the specialties themselves in a way that makes the outlook hazardous. The workers lose all sense of proportion in a maze of minutiae.
Sir William Osler (1849–1919)
Address, Classical Association, Oxford, May 16, 1910

To my sons: Whatever specialty they follow, may they never forget to be doctors.
Harry E. Mock
Dedication to Skull Fractures and Brain Injuries

1. What are Loeb's Laws of Medicine?
1. If what you're doing is working, keep doing it.
2. If what you're doing is not working, stop doing it.
3. If you don't know what to do, don't do anything.
4. Above all, never let a surgeon get your patient.

Matz R: Principles of medicine. NY State J Med 77:99–101, 1977.

2. What are the predominant organisms constituting the normal flora of the human body?

Oropharynx
Viridans
  (α-hemolytic)
  streptococci
Staphylococci
Str. pyogenes
Str. pneumoniae
Moraxella catarrhalis
Neisseria sp.
Lactobacilli
Corynebacteria
Haemophilus sp.
Obligate anaerobes (not
  Bacteroides fragilis)
Candida albicans
Various protozoa

Upper intestine
Streptococci
Lactobacilli
Candida sp.

Lower genitourinary tract
Staphylococci
Streptococci (incl. enterococci)
Lactobacilli (vaginal)
Corynebacteria
Neisseria sp.
Obligate anaerobes
Aerobic gram-negative bacilli
C. albicans
Trichomonas vaginalis

Conjunctiva
Staphylococci
Corynebacteria
Haemophilus sp.

Nasopharynx
Staphylococci (incl. *S. aureus*)
Streptococci (incl.
  S. pneumoniae)
M. catarrhalis
Neisseria sp.
Haemophilus sp.

Skin
Staphylococci (incl. *S. aureus*)
Corynebacteria
Propionibacteria
Candida sp.
Malassezia furur
Dermatophytic fungi

Large intestine and feces
Obligate anaerobes
  (incl. *B. fragilis*)
Aerobic gram-negative
  bacilli
Streptococci (incl.
  enterococci)
C. albicans
Various protozoa

Adapted from Rosebury T: Microorganisms Indigenous to Man. New York, McGraw-Hill, 1962, pp 310–384.
Mackowiak PA: The normal microbial flora. N Engl J Med 307:83–93, 1982.

3. What are the principles of "diagnostic roundsmanship"?

1. Common things occur commonly.

2. The race may not always be to the swift nor the battle to the strong, but it's a good idea to bet that way.

3. When you hear hoofbeats think of horses, not zebras.

4. Place your bets on uncommon manifestations of common conditions rather than common manifestations of uncommon conditions.

Matz R: Principles of medicine. NY State J Med 77:99–101, 1977.

4. List the risk factors for thromboembolism.

1. Heart disease, especially:
   a. Myocardial infarction (MI)
   b. Atrial fibrillation
   c. Cardiomyopathy
   d. Congestive heart failure (CHF)
2. Postoperative states, especially following abdominal or pelvic operations, splenectomy, and orthopedic procedures on the lower extremities.
3. Pregnancy and parturition
4. Neoplastic disease
5. Polycythemia
6. Prolonged immobilization
7. Hemorrhage
8. Fractures, especially of the hip
9. Obesity
10. Varicose veins
11. Prior history of thromboembolic disease
12. Drugs, especially oral contraceptives and estrogens
13. Following cerebrovascular accidents
14. Abnormal blood flow
15. Myeloproliferative disorders with thrombocytosis
16. Antithrombin III deficiency
17. Protein C deficiency, protein S deficiency
18. Abnormal fibrinolysis

From Greenberger NF, et al: The Medical Book of Lists, 4th ed. Chicago, Year Book Medical Publishers, 1990, p 29; with permission.

5. How are prothrombin times (PT) standardized for monitoring patients on anticoagulant therapy with warfarin?

The International Normalization Ratio (INR) system standardizes the (PT) for different thromboplastin reagents, thus providing a universal standard by which to compare any given laboratory's results with that of the World Health Organization standard. The INR is calculated as follows:

$$INR = (patient\ PT/normal\ PT)^{ISI}$$

where normal PT = mean PT of the target population (in sec) and ISI = International Sensitivity Index (provided with each batch of thromboplastin reagent).

Nichols WL, Bowie EJ: Standardization of the prothrombin time for monitoring orally administered anticoagulant therapy with use of the International Normalization Ratio system. Mayo Clin Proc 68:897–898, 1993.

6. What are the advantages of using the INR system?

1. Easier, smoother regulation of anticoagulation.

2. Traveling patients will have a standard regardless of the laboratory used.

3. Standardization for research and publication efforts.

4. Reduced risks of complications associated with higher doses of oral anticoagulants.

7. Compare the sensitivity, specificity, benefits, and shortcomings of the various tests used in the diagnosis of deep venous thrombosis.

Objective Diagnostic Tests for Deep Vein Thrombosis

TEST	BASIS OF TEST	SENSITIVITY (%)	SPECIFICITY (%)	CLINICAL SITUATIONS PRODUCING FALSE-POSITIVE RESULTS OR PREVENTING TESTING	COMMENTS
Contrast venography	Presence of thrombus (filling defect) Evidence of occlusion (cut-off) and evidence of collateral circulation	Standard against which other tests have been compared		Inadequate venous access for injection of contrast	Highly specific, painful, invasive, expensive
Doppler ultrasound	Obstruction Evidence of collateral circulation	84*	88*	False-positive due to external compression	Sensitive and specific for proximal vein thrombosis; insensitive to calf vein thrombosis; requires skilled examiner
Impedance plethysmography	Obstruction	93*	94*	False-positive may occur—cardiac failure, constrictive pericarditis, severe arterial insufficiency, external venous compression Cannot be performed for technical reasons (leg amputation, leg surgery or trauma)	Sensitive and specific for proximal vein thrombosis; insensitive to calf vein thrombosis Excellent screening test when combined with 125I-labeled fibrinogen scan
125I-labeled fibrinogen Prospective screening Symptomatic patients Hip surgery	Active thrombus formation	90† 56† 75†	96† 84† 70†	False-positive may occur—torn or contused muscle, leg trauma or surgery, cellulitis, ruptured Baker's cyst, severe edema Cannot be performed for technical reasons (leg cast or bandages, pregnancy, interference with other isotopes)	Sensitive to calf and distal thigh vein thrombi; insensitive to proximal thigh and iliac vein thrombi May not become positive for 72 hr
Ultrasonic compression	Presence of thrombus	89	100	—	Early reports excellent for sensitivity to proximal thrombi; noninvasive

*Correlations based on popliteal, femoral, and iliac thrombi.
†Correlations based on thrombi but mostly calf thrombi.

From Kelley WN (ed): Essentials of Internal Medicine. Philadelphia, J.B. Lippincott, 1994, 409; with permission.

8. What is a Baker's cyst? What condition can its rupture simulate?

Baker's cysts result from the build-up of synovial fluid in the knee. Also called popliteal bursitis, it is most common in males 15–30 years of age. Symptoms consist of local pain, limitation of knee extension, and symptoms related to compression of adjacent structures (i.e., popliteal artery, deep veins, and tibial nerve). The cyst can be felt as a swelling in the popliteal space. When a nonruptured cyst softens with knee flexion, it is known as Foucher's sign.

Rupture of a Baker's cyst, usually due to trauma, can cause acute inflammation, pain, and swelling that can extend down into the posterior calf. This presentation can be confused with **venous thrombophlebitis.**

9. When is anticoagulation contraindicated?

Absolute Contraindications	Relative Contraindications
Subarachnoid or cerebral hemorrhage	Active GI hemorrhage
Serious active bleeding (postoperative, spontaneous, or trauma-associated)	Hemorrhagic diathesis
	Recent stroke
Recent brain, eye, or spinal cord surgery	Recent major surgery
Malignant hypertension	Severe hypertension
	Bacterial endocarditis
	Severe renal or hepatic failure

Kelley, WN (ed): Textbook of Internal Medicine, 2nd ed. Philadelphia, J. B. Lippincott, 1992, p 1780.

10. How do you convert deciliters to milliliters? Grains to milligrams? Teaspoons to milliliters?

Useful Calculations and Conversions

- Swallow, avg (not a mouthful)
  Adult ≈ 10 ml
  Child ≈ 5 ml
- 1 teaspoon (tsp) = 5 ml
  1 tablespoon (tbsp) = 15 ml
- Grain   = 64.8 mg
  1/65 grain   = 0.015 grain   = 1 mg
  1/150 grain   = 0.0067 grain   = 0.3 mg
  1/400 grain   = 0.0025 grain   = 0.15 mg

- Percent solution   1% solution   = 1 gm/100 ml
                      = 10 mg/1 ml
                      = 10 mg/liter

- Milligram percent (mg%) 1 mg%   = mg/100 ml
                                   = 10 μg/ml
                                   = 1 mg/dl
                                   = 10 mg/liter

- Deciliter (dl) = 100 ml
  1 mg/dl = 1 mg/100 ml
         = 1 mg%
         = 10 μg/ml
- Part per million (ppm) = 1 part in a million
  1 ppm = 1 mg/liter
        = 0.1 mg%
        = 1 μg/ml

- Milligram (mg)   = 0.001 gm
  1 mg   = 1000 μg
                       = 0.015 grain

- Microgram (μg)   = 0.001 mg
  1 μg/ml   = 0.1 mg%
                       = 0.1 mg/dl
                       = 1 mg/liter

- Nanogram (ng)   = 0.001 μg
  1 ng/ml   = 0.001 μg/ml
                       = 0.1 μg
                       = 0.1 μg/dl
                       = 1 μg/liter

                       = 0.001 mg%

- Milliequivalent (meq)
  1 meq $= \dfrac{MW\ gm}{valence \times 1000}$

  1 meq/L $= \dfrac{mg/L \times valence}{MW}$

  mg/100 ml $= \dfrac{meq/L \times MW}{10 \times valence}$

Flomenbaum NE, Roberts JR: Emergency Department Reference Guide, 2nd ed. New York, Cahners Publishing, 1989, p 20.

11. Who was Baron von Münchausen? Why is a syndrome named after him?

Baron von Münchausen, an 18th century German soldier/storyteller, is reputed to have been prone to wild exaggeration. Patients with a history of repeated factitious symptoms, illnesses, and accidents, usually of a dramatic or emergency nature, are said to have Münchausen's syndrome. The history often includes multiple invasive procedures with negative findings. Münchausen's syndrome is seen in women more frequently than men. It is considered to be a psychiatric condition and must be separated from malingering, which involves a conscious intent to deceive.

12. What criteria should be used to evaluate any preventive health care intervention?

Frame proposed the following six criteria:

1. The condition must have a significant effect on the quantity or quality of life.

2. Acceptable methods of treatment must be available.

3. The condition must have an asymptomatic period during which detection and treatment can significantly reduce the morbidity or mortality.

4. Treatment during the early asymptomatic period must yield a therapeutic result superior to that obtained if treatment is delayed until symptoms appear.

5. Tests to detect the condition in the asymptomatic period must be acceptable to patients and available at a reasonable cost.

6. The incidence of the condition must be sufficient to justify the cost of a screening program.

Frame PS: A critical review of adult health maintenance (pts 1–4). J Fam Pract 22:341, 417, 511, 1985; 23:29, 1986.

13. Define sensitivity, specificity, and predictive value of a test. How are they calculated?

These terms are frequently used in the assessment of a test and its ability to rule in or rule out a given condition (also called the **accuracy** of the test). To use these values, you must understand how they are derived. Since a test can be positive or negative (if we disregard inconclusive results) and a patient either has or does not have a condition, there are four possible outcomes in any test situation:

Disease:

	Present	Absent	
+	a	b	a = True positive b = False positive
–	c	d	c = False negative d = True negative

Test result

$$\text{Sensitivity} = \frac{a}{a+c} = \text{Percentage of patients who have the disease and test positive}$$

$$\text{Specificity} = \frac{d}{b+d} = \text{Percentage of persons who do not have the disease and test negative (True-Negative).}$$

$$\text{Positive predictive value} = \frac{a}{a+b} = \text{Percentage of patients who test positive and actually do have the disease.}$$

$$\text{Negative predictive value} = \frac{d}{c+d} = \text{Percentage of patients who test negative and really do not have the disease.}$$

Last JM: A Dictionary of Epidemiology, 2nd ed. New York, Oxford University Press, 1988.

14. What is the pneumococcal polysaccharide vaccine (Pneumovax 23, Pneu-Imune 23)?

This vaccine is composed of 25 μg of purified capsular polysaccharide antigens from 23 types of *Streptococcus pneumoniae*. When introduced in 1983, this vaccine replaced the older 14-valent type (released in 1977). These 23-capsular types represent 88% of the causes of bacteremic pneumococcal disease in the U.S. Cross-reactivity with other capsular types may increase this coverage by another 8%. In healthy adults, antibody levels remain elevated for at least 5 years but then may fall to prevaccination levels within 10 years in some patients. Revaccination is recommended if more than 5 years have elapsed since the previous dose. The overall protective efficacy of the vaccine against pneumococcal bacteremia is approx. 60%.

15. Who should get this vaccine?

The U.S. Public Health Service's Immunization Practices Advisory Committee recommends that the pneumococcal polysaccharide vaccine be administered to the following groups:

1. Adults aged 65 years or older.

2. Adults with chronic illnesses who are at increased risk for pneumococcal disease or its complications (e.g., cardiovascular disease, pulmonary disease, diabetes mellitus, alcoholism, cirrhosis, cerebrospinal fluid [CSF] leaks).

3. Immunocompromised adults at increased risk for pneumococcal disease or its complications (e.g., splenic dysfunction or anatomic asplenia, Hodgkin's disease, lymphoma, multiple myeloma, chronic renal failure, nephrotic syndrome, organ transplantation).

4. Adults or children (age ≥2) with asymptomatic or symptomatic HIV infection.

5. Children (age ≥2) with chronic illnesses associated with increased risk for pneumococcal disease or its complications (e.g., anatomic or functional asplenia [including sickle cell disease], nephrotic syndrome, CSF leaks, and conditions associated with immunosuppression).

6. Persons living in special environments or social settings associated with an increased risk for pneumococcal disease or its complications (e.g., certain Native American populations, nursing home inhabitants, prisoners).

Note: The vaccine is *not* recommended for patients with only recurrent upper respiratory tract disease, including otitis media and sinusitis.

CDC: Pneumococcal polysaccharide vaccine. MMWR 38(5):64–68, 73–76, 1989.

16. Are routine, periodic chest x-rays recommended as screening for lung cancer?

No. Most lung cancers are already systemic diseases at the time of earliest possible detection by chest x-rays, and the outcome as a result of screening by routine chest x-rays is not changed.

17. Outline the current recommendations by the various organizations for colorectal cancer screening in patients who are asymptomatic and not members of a high-risk group.

Recommendations for Colon Cancer Screening in Persons at Average Risk

	DIGITAL RECTAL EXAM	STOOL FOR OCCULT BLOOD	SIGMOIDOSCOPY	COLONOSCOPY
American Cancer Society	Annually starting at age >40	Annually starting at age 50	Annually for 2 yrs, then every 3–5 yrs starting at age 50	N/A
Canadian Task Force	No	Annually for those over age 46	No recommendation	No
U.S. Preventive Services Task Force	No	No	No	No
American College of Physicians	No	Annually starting at age 50	Every 3–5 yrs starting at age 50	No
World Health Organization	Every 3–5 yrs starting at age 50	Annually starting at age 50	Every 3–5 yrs starting at age 50	No
National Cancer Institute	No	Annually for "case finding" asymptomatic patients	Every 3–5 yrs for "case finding" asymptomatic patients	No

Sox H: Preventive health care services in adults. N Engl J Med 330:1589–1595, 1994.
DeCosse, et al: Colorectal cancer: Detection, treatment, and rehabilitation. CA 44(1):27–42, 1994.
Eddy D: Screening for colorectal cancer: Diagnosis and treatment. Ann of Intern Med 113:373–384, 1990.
Winawer, et al: Prevention of colorectal cancer: Guidelines based on new data. Bull WHO 73(1):7–10, 1995.

18. What conditions can lead to false-positive or false-negative results with the HemOccult Slide Test?

The HemOccult Slide Test (Smith-Kline Diagnostics) detects the presence of hemoglobin in feces. **False-negative** results are obtained in patients with colonic neoplasms that are not bleeding (lesions < 1–2 cm, nonulcerated lesions), that bleed intermittently, or that are not producing the 20 ml of blood per day required for a reliably positive result. Stool that is stored prior to testing and large doses of ascorbic acid may also lead to false-negative results.

False-positive results can be produced by the dietary intake of rare beef or fruits and vegetables that contain peroxidases. This effect is seen mainly in tests performed on rehydrated stool specimens. Oral iron preparations also have been implicated in some studies but not in others. **False-positive** results can occur due to blood from sources other than colorectal carcinoma, such as gastric blood loss caused by nonsteroidal anti-inflammatory drugs (NSAIDs).

Fleischer DE, et al: Detection and surveillance of colorectal cancer. JAMA 261:580–586, 1989.

19. What screening programs for colorectal cancer are recommended for patients in high-risk groups?

Recommended Surveillance Programs for Patients
at High Risk for Colorectal Cancer

PATIENT GROUP AND RISK	SURVEILLANCE PROGRAM*
Markedly increased risk	
Familial polyposis coli and associated syndromes	FS every 6–12 mo from teens to age 40 yr; colectomy if multiple polyps found
Cancer family syndrome	Annual FOBT and colonoscopy every 2–3 yr, beginning at age 20 yr
Universal ulcerative colitis for 8–10 yr	Annual colonoscopy with multiple biopsies; colectomy if severe dysplasia is found and confirmed
Moderately increased risk	
Previous colon cancer or previous adenoma(s)	Colonoscopy 1 yr after resection and then every 3 yr if findings are normal; annual FOBT
Left-sided ulcerative colitis for 15–20 yr	Colonoscopy every 1–2 yr with multiple biopsies; colectomy if severe dysplasia found and confirmed
First-degree relative(s) with history of colon cancer	Annual FOBT and FS every 3–5 yr beginning at age 35–40 yr; if ≥ 2 relatives, colonoscopy every 3–5 yr
Woman undergoing irradiation for gynecologic cancer	Annual FOBT and FS every 3 yr after diagnosis and radiation therapy
Probable increased risk	
Previous gynecologic or breast cancer or ureterosigmoidoscopy	Institution of usual screening tests or annual rectal exam and FOBT and FS every 3–5 yr after diagnosis of underlying associated disease
Other GI tract polyposis syndromes	Periodic exam of upper and/or lower GI tract, depending on cancer risk in specific syndrome

*FS indicates flexible sigmoidoscopy, either 60 or 35 cm, which is preferred to rigid sigmoidoscopy; FOBT, fecal occult blood test. Colonoscopy refers to total colonoscopy to the cecum; in some cases, double-contrast barium enema exam plus flexible sigmoidoscopy may be substituted.

From Fleischer DE, et al: Detection and surveillance of colorectal cancer.
JAMA 261:580–586, 1989; with permission.

20. What is the erythrocyte sedimentation rate (ESR)? What causes it to be increased or decreased?

The ESR is a nonspecific index of inflammation. The normal values for patients under age 50 are 0–15 mm/hr in men and 0–20 mm/hr in women. The normal values increase with age and may be higher in individuals over age 60, even in the absence of disease.

Whether the ESR is normal, increased, or decreased depends on the sum of forces acting on the erythrocytes (RBCs). These include the downward force of gravity (dependent on the mass of the RBC), upward buoyant forces (dependent on the density [mass/volume] of the RBC), and bulk plasma flow (created by the downward-moving RBCs).

Conditions that Increase and Decrease the ESR

INCREASE	DECREASE
Inflammatory disorders	Increased serum viscosity
Hyperfibrinogenemia	Hypofibrinogenemia
Rouleaux formation	Sickle cell disease
Anemia (hypochromic, microcytic)	Leukemoid reaction
Pregnancy	Polycythemia
Hyperglobulinemia	Spherocytosis
Hypercholesterolemia	Anisocytosis
	High-dose corticosteroids
	CHF
	Cachexia

21. Is the ESR useful in screening for any conditions?

The ESR is of little value in screening asymptomatic patients. It also is of little value in screening for malignancy, since it is often normal in patients with cancer. It is indicated in the diagnosis and monitoring of temporal arteritis and polymyalgia rheumatica. It may also be of value in monitoring the course and therapy of rheumatoid arthritis, Hodgkin's disease, other malignancies, and other inflammatory disorders.

22. Which disease is associated with pagophagia (ice-eating)?

Iron-deficiency anemia (IDA). Patients with IDA may also crave other food and nonfood substances (**pica**). Although this behavior is rarely volunteered, it is found in approx. 50% of such patients. The pica of IDA responds to iron-repletion therapy.

Rector WG: Pica: Its frequency and significance in patients with iron-deficiency anemia due to chronic gastrointestinal blood loss. J Gen Intern Med 4:512–513, 1989.

23. Describe the four stages of alcohol withdrawal.

1. **Tremulousness** occurs 8–12 hours after cessation of drinking. The tremor is aggravated by intention or agitation and may be accompanied by nausea and vomiting, insomnia, headache, diaphoresis, tachycardia, and anxiety. The symptoms usually subside within 24 hours, unless the patient progresses to the next stage.

2. **Alcoholic hallucinosis** usually occurs 12–24 hours after the cessation of drinking but may take 6–8 days to develop. Auditory or visual hallucinations alternate with periods of lucidity. The symptoms of the first stage continue and worsen.

3. **Grand mal seizures** ("rum fits") occur in 90% of cases between 6–48 hours after cessation of drinking. The seizures are generalized and usually multiple. This stage occurs in 3–4% of untreated patients.

4. **Delirium tremens** usually occurs 3–4 days after the cessation of drinking but may not develop for up to 2 weeks. It manifests as confusion, hallucinations, tremors, and signs of autonomic hyperactivity (fever, tachycardia, dilated pupils, diaphoresis). It is a *medical emergency* and carries a mortality of 5–15% despite treatment. Death is usually due to cardiovascular collapse.

24. What is the LD_{50} for ethanol?

500 mg/dl is the serum level that will be lethal in 50% of patients who ingest a sufficient quantity of ethanol to achieve such a serum level. The amount of orally ingested ethanol needed to produce this serum level (LD_{50}) varies with the size of the person, rates of ingestion, absorption, hepatic metabolism, and other factors.

25. Which organs are directly affected by chronic alcohol abuse?

Alcohol has pathologic effects in nearly every organ system:

CNS	Alcohol withdrawal "blackouts"	Hallucinations
	Dementia	Seizures
	Wernicke-Korsakoff syndrome	Peripheral neuropathy
Gastrointestinal	Esophageal varices	Neoplasm
	Esophagitis, gastritis	Cirrhosis
	Vitamin deficiencies (niacin, B_{12}, thiamine)	Chronic pancreatitis
Cardiovascular	Arrhythmias	Cardiomyopathy
	Congestive heart failure	Hypertension
Pulmonary	Pneumonia (aspiration)	Tuberculosis
Genitourinary	Impaired spermatogenesis	Testicular atrophy
	Impotence/infertility	Amenorrhea
Musculoskeletal	Myopathy	Rhabdomyolysis
	Higher incidence of gout	Osteonecrosis
Endocrine	Increased cortisol	Hyperglycemia
	Decreased T4 and T3	
Hematopoietic	Impaired granulocyte function	Anemia (iron, B_{12}, and folate deficiency, sideroblastic)
	Thrombocytopenia	

26. How quickly can a healthy person clear ethanol from his or her body?

A normal person can metabolize 150 mg of ethanol/kg body weight/hr. In a normal 70-kg person, this leads to a decrease in blood ethanol level of approx. 20 mg/dl/hr.

27. What laboratory data support a diagnosis of liver disease due to chronic alcohol abuse?

- Elevated gamma-glutamyl transpeptidase (GGT)
- AST:ALT (SGOT:SGPT) ratio $\geq$ 2:1
- Hypoalbuminemia
- Prolonged prothrombin time (PT)
- Low blood urea nitrogen (BUN)
- Low glucose
- Thrombocytopenia
- Macrocytosis of RBCs

28. What constellation of symptoms comprise the Wernicke-Korsakoff syndrome?

This syndrome most commonly occurs in the malnourished, alcoholic patient and includes the following symptoms:

Symptoms of the Wernicke-Korsakoff Syndrome

Ocular	**Altered mental status**
Horizontal/vertical nystagmus	Alcohol withdrawal
Paralysis of conjugate gaze	Global confusion (apathetic, inattentive, lethargic,
External rectus muscle paralysis	slurred speech, irrational)
	Korsakoff's amnesic psychosis
Ataxia	Anterograde amnesia (impairment of learning new
Stance and gait affected	ideas)
Cannot walk without assistance	Past memory disturbances (confabulation)

29. Which laboratory tests should be done when evaluating a person with altered mental status?

Complete blood count (CBC)	Erythrocyte sedimentation rate (ESR)
Full chemistry panel	Serologic test for syphilis (VDRL)

Vitamin B_{12}
Serum folate
Urinalysis
Urine toxicology screen
ECG
CT scan (in selected patients)
EEG (in selected patients)

Thyroid function tests (TSH, FT4)
Arterial blood gas
HIV test
Lumbar puncture (in selected patients)
Chest x-ray
MRI scan (in selected patients)

30. What are the causes of dementia?

Causes of Dementia

METABOLIC-TOXIC	STRUCTURAL	INFECTIOUS
Anoxia	Alzheimer's disease	Neurosyphilis (general paresis)
Pernicious anemia	Vascular disease	Tuberculous and fungal meningitis
Pellagra	Multi-infarct dementia	Viral encephalitis
Folic acid deficiency	Binswanger's dementia	HIV–related disorders
Hypothyroidism	Huntington's chorea	Gerstmann-Sträussler syndrome
Bromide intoxication	Multiple sclerosis	
Hypoglycemia	Pick's disease	
Hypercalcemia associated	Cerebellar degeneration	
with hyperparathyroidism	Wilson's disease	
Organ system failure	Amyotrophic lateral sclerosis	
Hepatic encephalopathy	Progressive multifocal	
Uremic encephalopathy	leukoencephalopathy	
Respiratory encephalopathy	Progressive supranuclear palsy	
Chronic drug-alcohol-nutritional	Brain tumor	
abuse	Irradiation to frontal lobes	
	Surgery	
	Normal-pressure hydrocephalus	
	Brain trauma	
	Chronic subdural hematoma	
	Dementia pugilistica	

31. Which etiologies of dementia can be treated?

Treatable Causes of Dementia

Medications
Psychoactive agents
  Tricyclic antidepressants
  Tranquilizers
  Lithium carbonate
  Sedatives
Methyldopa
Clonidine
Propranolol
Phenytoin
Barbiturates
Corticosteroids
Digitalis
Quinidine
NSAIDs
Cimetidine
Diuretics

Metabolic derangements
Hepatic encephalopathy
Hypercalcemia
Hyponatremia
Uremia

Chemical intoxication
Alcohol
Carbon monoxide
Lead
Arsenic
Mercury
Organophosphates
Trichloroethylene

Endocrinopathies
Hypo- or hyperthyroidism
Addison's disease
Cushing's disease
Hypoglycemia
Panhypopituitarism

Intracranial lesions
Subdural hematomas
Cerebrovascular disease
Brain tumor
Brain abscess
Multiple sclerosis
Hydrocephalus

Infections
Neurosyphilis
Meningitis
Abscess

Miscellaneous
Depression
Pellagra
Wernicke-Korsakoff syndrome
Schizophrenia
Changes in environment
  Nursing home placement
  Hospitalization

32. What is the risk of recurrence after a first unprovoked seizure?

In a study of 224 patients with a first unprovoked seizure, the overall recurrence rate was 16% at 12 months, 21% at 24 months, and 27% at 36 months. Patients with a history of prior neurologic insult had a higher rate of recurrence (34%), all of which occurred within 20 months. Among those without a history of neurologic insult ("idiopathic"), patients free of recurrence at 36 months did not have a subsequent seizure. Among the idiopathic cases, recurrence risk was higher in those with generalized spikewave EEGs (50% at 18 months) and in those who had a sibling with seizures.

Hauser WA, et al: Seizure recurrence after a first unprovoked seizure. N Engl J Med 307:522–527, 1982.

33. What are the causes of delirium?

Differential Diagnosis of the Acute Confusional State (Delirium)

NEUROLOGIC

Trauma
  Concussion
  Intracranial hematoma
  Subdural hematoma
Vascular disorders
  Multiple infarcts
  Right hemisphere or posterior circulation infarcts
  Hypertensive encephalopathy
  Vasculitis (e.g., SLE, polyarteritis nodosa,
    giant-cell arteritis)
  Air and fat embolism
  Subarachnoid hemorrhage

Neoplasia
  Multiple parenchymal metastases
  Meningeal carcinomatosis
  Midline brain tumors
  Brain tumors causing brainstem compression,
    edema, or hydrocephalus
  Paraneoplastic syndromes (limbic encephalitis)
Infections
  Meningitis and encephalitis (viral, bacterial, fungal,
    protozoal)
  Multiple abscesses
  Progressive multifocal leukoencephalopathy
Inflammations
  Acute disseminated encephalomyelitis
  Postinfectious encephalitis
Epilepsy
  Postictal state
  Temporal lobe status (complex partial status)

SYSTEMIC

Substrate depletion
  Hypoglycemia
  Diffuse hypoxia (pulmonary, cardiac, CO
    poisoning)
Metabolic encephalopathy
  Diabetic ketoacidosis
  Renal failure
  Liver failure
  Electrolyte, fluid, and acid-base imbalance
    (esp. Na^+, Ca^{2+}, Mg^{2+})
  Hereditary metabolic disease (e.g., porphyria,
    metachromatic leukodystrophy, mitochon-
    drial cytopathy)
Vitamin deficiency
  Thiamine (Wernicke's encephalopathy)
  Nicotinic acid (pellagra)
  B_{12}

Endocrine, over- or underactivity
  Thyroid
  Parathyroid
  Adrenal
Infection
  Septicemia
  Malaria
  Subacute bacterial endocarditis
  Focal infection (e.g., pneumonia)
Thermal injuries
  Hypothermia
  Heat stroke
Hematologic disorders
  Hyperviscosity syndrome
  Severe anemia
Toxic causes
  Drug and alcohol intoxication (therapeutic, social,
    illegal)
  Drug withdrawal (e.g., alcohol, barbiturates, narcotics)
  Chemical toxins (e.g., heavy metals, organic toxins)

PSYCHIATRIC

Acute mania
Depression or extreme anxiety

Schizophrenia
Hysterical fugue states

From Brown MM, Hachinski VC: Acute confusional states, amnesia, and dementia. In Isselbacher KJ, et al: Harrison's Principles of Internal Medicine, 13th ed. New York, McGraw-Hill, 1994, p 140; with permission.

34. What is St. Anthony's dance? St. Guy's dance? St. Vitus' dance?

They are all chorea. The following is a list of diseases and syndromes named after the saints:

Saint Syndromes

PATRONYMIC NAME	DISEASE OR SYNDROME
St. Agatha's	Mastopathic inflammatory disease
St. Aignan's or Agnan's	Favus ringworm, tinea
St. Arman's	Pellagra
St. Anthony's	
St. Anthony's dance	Chorea (see also St. Vitus)
St. Anthony's fire	Ergotism (epidemic gangrene and psychotic alterations)
St. Anthony's fire	Erysipelas
St. Apollonia's	Toothache
St. Avertin's	Epilepsy
St. Avidus'	Deafness
St. Blasius'	Quinsy (peritonsillar abscess)
St. Dymphna's	Mental derangements
St. Erasmus'	Colic pain
St. Fiacre's or Flacre's	Hemorrhoids
St. Francis'	Erysipelas
St. Gervasius'	Juvenile or adult rheumatic pains
St. Gete's	Carcinoma
St. Giles'	Leprosy
St. Gothard's	Ancylostomiasis (hookworm)
St. Guy's dance	Chorea
St. Hubert's	Rabies
St. Ignatius'	Pellagra
St. Kilda's	Colds, infections
St. Louis	Encephalitis
St. Main's	Scabies
St. Martin's	Alcoholism
St. Mathurin's	Idiocy
St. Modestus'	Chorea
St. Roch's or Roche's	Plague
St. Sebastian's	Plague
St. Valentine's	Epilepsy
St. Vitus' dance	Chorea
St. Zachary's	Mutism

From Magalini SI, Euclide S: Dictionary of Medical Syndromes, 2nd ed. Philadelphia, J.B. Lippincott, 1981, p 728; with permission.

35. What is Bell's palsy?

Bell's palsy is a demyelinating viral inflammatory disease that is the most common ailment of the facial nerve (cranial nerve [CN] VII). It is characterized by the following:

Bell's Palsy

Onset	Usually preceded by viral prodrome
	Onset is acute
Duration	Approx 5 days
	Peak symptoms at 48 hrs
Findings	Unilateral
	Loss of facial expression
	Widened palpebral fissure
	Diminished taste
	Difficulty in chewing (food collects between lips and teeth)
	Hypesthesia in $\geq$ 1 branches of CN V
	Hyperacusis
Treatment	Protect the affected eye
	Prednisone (if patient presents within first 2 days)
	Symptoms are self-limited

Adam KK: Current concepts in neurology: Diagnosis and management of facial paralysis. N Engl J Med 307:348–351, 1982.

36. Which organisms are implicated in meningitis of the adult?

Streptococcus pneumoniae is the most common cause of bacterial meningitis in the adult, followed by *Neisseria meningitidis* and *Haemophilus influenzae*. The proportion of disease caused by other gram-negative bacilli has been increasing in recent years, whereas that due to staphylococci and other streptococci has been decreasing. In adults over age 60, *Listeria monocytogenes* becomes the second or third most common cause of meningitis.

Organisms Implicated in Adult Meningitis

Bacterial
  H. influenzae
  N. meningitidis
  S. pneumoniae
  Group A streptococci
  Staphylococcus aureus
  Enterobacteriaceae
  Klebsiella sp.
  Pseudomonas sp.
  Proteus sp.
  L. monocytogenes
  Neisseria gonorrhoeae
  Clostridium sp.
  Myobacterium tuberculosis

Spirochetal
  Treponema pallidum
  Borrelia burgdorferi (Lyme disease)
  Leptospira sp.

Viral
  Nonparalytic poliomyelitis
  Mumps
  Enterovirus
  Echovirus
  Coxsackievirus
  Adenovirus
  Lymphocytic choriomeningitis

Other considerations
  Neoplastic disease
  Toxoplasma sp.
  Cryptococcus sp.

Bensan CA, et al: Acute neurological infection. Med Clin North Am 70:987, 1986.

37. Do the cerebrospinal fluid (CSF) findings differ among bacterial, tuberculous, fungal, and viral meningitis?

CSF Findings in Bacterial and Nonbacterial Meningitis

	BACTERIAL	VIRAL	MYCOBACTERIAL OR FUNGAL
Total cells (per μl)	Usually >500	Usually <500	Usually <500
WBCs	Predominantly PMN	Predominantly mononuclear	Predominantly mononuclear
Glucose (% of blood)	≤40%	>40%	≤40%
Protein (mg/dl)	>50	>50	>50
Gram stain	Positive (65–95%)	Negative	Negative

Differential Diagnosis of CSF Pleocytosis

Predominantly Polymorphonuclear (>90%)
  Bacterial meningitis
  Early viral meningitis
  Early tuberculous or fungal meningitis
  Brain abscess or subdural empyma with rupture
    into subarachnoid space
  Chemical arachnoiditis

Predominantly Mononuclear (< 90% PMNs)
  Viral meningitis or encephalitis
  Tuberculous or fungal meningitis
  Partially treated bacterial meningitis
  Brain abscess or subdural emphyema
  Listeriosis (variable)
  Neurosyphilis
  Neuroborreliosis (Lyme disease)
  Neurocysticercosis
  Neurosarcoidosis
  Primary amebic meningoencephalitis
  Guillain-Barré syndrome
  CNS vasculitis, tumor, hemorrhage
  Multiple sclerosis
  Others

From Kelly WN (ed): Textbook of Internal Medicine, 2nd ed. Philadelphia, J.B. Lippincott, 1992, p 2329; with permission.

38. Name the five leading etiologies of cerebrovascular disease (stroke).
- Embolism
- Atherosclerotic disease
- Lacunar infarcts
- Hypertensive hemorrhage
- Ruptured aneurysms/AV malformation

Cerebrovascular disease is the third leading cause of adult deaths. The major risk factors include hypertension, hypercholesterolemia, smoking, and cardiovascular disease (particularly atrial fibrillation and recent MI). Other causes include advanced age, diabetes mellitus, migraine headaches, and the use of oral contraceptive agents.

39. What are the types and causes of peripheral neuropathies in the adult?

Motor	Sensory	Sensorimotor	
Guillain-Barré syndrome	Alcohol	Diabetes mellitus	Alcohol
Porphyria	Diabetes mellitus	Uremia	Inherited neuropathies
Lead poisoning	Vascular disease	Chronic inflammatory polyradiculopathy	Metronidazole
Sulfonamides	Neoplasm	Clofibrate	Colchicine
Amphotericin B	Uremia	Chlorpropamide	Chlorambucil
Dapsone	Arsenic	Phenytoin	Tolbutamide
Imipramine		Nitrofurantoin	Ergotamine
Amitriptyline		Ethambutol	Streptomycin
Gold		Penicillamine	Ethionamide
		Indomethacin	Gold
			Phenylbutazone

Farrante JA: Focusing on peripheral neuropathies. Emerg Med 22:57–62, 1990.

40. Which cranial nerves (CN) are commonly affected in tuberculous meningitis?
These CN palsies may be either unilateral or bilateral and most commonly occur in CN VI (abducens, usually bilateral). Palsies may also develop in CN III (oculomotor) > CN IV (trochlear) > CN II (optic).

Johnson JL, Ellner JJ: Tuberculous meningitis. In Evans RW, Baskins DS, Yatsu FM: Prognosis of Neurological Disorders. Oxford, Oxford University Press, 1992.

41. Which common viral illnesses are frequently seen in adults?

Influenza A > influenza B
Epstein-Barr virus
Herpes simplex virus I and II
Varicella-zoster virus
Cytomegalovirus

Respiratory viruses
Rhinoviruses
Coronaviruses
Respiratory syncytial virus
Parainfluenza virus
Adenoviruses

42. Which groups are most susceptible to infection by the herpes zoster virus?

Elderly (age >60)
Patients with Hodgkin's and non-Hodgkin's lymphoma
Immunocompromised patients
    Cancer
    Organ transplant
    AIDS and HIV infection
Patients on high-dose steroid therapy

43. Which organism is responsible for the cellulitis of marine workers and fisherman?
Vibrio vulnificus is an ubiquitous, invasive, gram-negative rod found in warm, salty, coastal waters. It is found in zooplankton and shellfish and has been associated with two disease syn-

dromes: (1) sepsis in alcoholics and persons with liver disease, and (2) wound infections from minor abrasions and/or lacerations. Advanced cases can result in necrotizing vasculitis and gangrene.

44. What are the common etiologies of pneumonia?

Common Etiologies of Pneumonia

Bacterial	Viral
Streptococcus pneumoniae	Influenza A or B
Haemophilus influenzae type B	Parainfluenza virus
Gram-negative bacilli	Adenovirus
Klebsiella	Cytomegalovirus
Pseudomonas	
Escherichia coli	**Fungal**
Proteus	*Cryptococcus*
Mixed flora	*Aspergillus*
Anaerobic bacteria (aspiration)	*Histoplasma*
Staphylococcus aureus	*Candida*
	Coccidioides
Atypical	
Mycoplasma	
TWAR *chlamydia (Chlamydia pneumoniae)*	
Legionnaire's disease	

45. What factors predispose to acquiring the toxic shock syndrome (TSS)?

TSS is secondary to infection caused by *Staphylococcus aureus*. It should be considered in any patient presenting with fever, rash, and hypotension. Risk factors include:
- Use of high-absorbency tampons
- Diaphragm placement for contraception
- Postoperative wounds (breast augmentation, cesarean section, indwelling catheters)
- Cutaneous infections (esp. in the axillary or perianal areas)

Cellulitis	Insect bites
Burns	Abscess

Cunha BA: Case studies in infectious diseases: Toxic shock syndrome. Emery Med 21:119–126, 1989.

46. Which organisms are commonly implicated in infective endocaditis?

Incidence of Microbial Pathogens in Infective Endocarditis

ORGANISMS	NATIVE VALVE (%)		PROSTHETIC VALVE (%)	
	NONADDICTS	ADDICTS	EARLY (<2 MOS)	LATE (>2 MOS)
Streptococci	50–70	20	5–10	25–30
Enterococci	10	8	<1	5–10
Staphylococci	25	60	45–50	30–40
(*S. aureus*)	(90)	(99)	(15–20)	(10–12)
(*S. epidermidis*)	(10)	(1)	(25–30)	(23–28)
Gram negative bacilli	<1	10	20	10–12
Fungi	<1	5	10–12	5–8
Diphtheroids	<1	2	5–10	4–5
Miscellaneous organisms	5–10	1–5	1–5	1–5
Multiple	<1	5	8	8
Culture negative	5–10	10–20	5–10	5–10

From Gorbach, et al (eds): Infectious Diseases. Philadelphia, W.B. Saunders, 1992, 549; with permission.

47. What is the differential diagnosis of generalized lymphadenopathy?

Causes of Generalized Lymphadenopathy*

INFECTIONS		NEOPLASMS
Bacterial		Lymphoma
Scarlet fever	Tuberculosis	Acute lymphocytic leukemia
Syphilis	Atypical mycobacteria	Chronic lymphocytic leukemia
Brucellosis	(Melioidosis)	Other lymphoproliferative disorders
Leptospirosis	(Glanders)	Immunoblastic lymphadenopathy
Viral		Reticuloendothelioses
HIV/(AIDS)	Rubella	**MISCELLANEOUS**
Epstein-Barr virus	(Dengue fever)	Sarcoidosis
Cytomegalovirus	(West Nile fever)	Other chronic granulomatous
Hepatitis B	(Epidemic hemorrhagic fever)	disorders
Measles	(Lassa fever)	Systemic lupus erythematosus
Parasitic		Rheumatoid arthritis
Toxoplasmosis	(African trypanosomiasis)	Hyperthyroidism
(Kala azar)	(Filariasis)	Lipid storage diseases
(Chagas' disease)		Generalized dermatitis
Rickettsial	**Fungal**	Serum sickness
(Scrub typhus)	Histoplasmosis	Phenytoin

*Parentheses indicate infections that are uncommon or not reported in the United States. Other infections that characteristically may produce regional lymphadenopathy (e.g., tularemia, Lyme disease, lymphogranuloma venereum) rarely cause generalized lymphadenopathy.

Adapted from Libman H: Generalized lymphadenopathy. J Gen Intern Med 2:48–58, 1987.

48. Describe the clinical features of cat scratch fever.

Who:	Children represent 75% of the cases
When:	Following a cat scratch, bite, or close contact with a cat (in 93% of cases). Usually occurs in fall or winter.
What:	Pleomorphic, gram negative, bacillary organism (*Rochalimaea henselae*)
Symptoms:	Primary lesion is raised, slightly tender papule or pustule that:
	may be single or multiple.
	appears 3–10 days after contact with cat
	Regional lymphadenopathy including axillary (most common), cervical, preauricular, submandibular, inguinal, femoral, and epitrochlear nodes
	Other symptoms and signs: Fever, headache, malaise, rash, anorexia, emesis, splenomegaly, sore throat
Diagnosis:	Exclude other possibilities
	History of contact with a cat
	Primary lesion on skin
	Regional lymphadenopathy
	Positive intradermal skin test
	Skin or lymph node biopsy demonstrating the bacillus
Therapy:	Penicillin, erythromycin, cephalosporins, or clindamycin
	Disease is usually self-limited and resolves spontaneously in 1–2 mos

49. What is the classic pentad seen in Lyme disease?

Lyme disease, named after a town on the Connecticut shoreline where the disease was first identified in 1975, is a tick-borne spirochetal infection caused by the fastidious, microphilic bacterium *Borrelia burgdorferi*. Occurrences are more common in the summer and fall. The incidence of Lyme disease corresponds to the habitat of the *Ixodid tick*.

Clinical Pentad of Lyme Disease

Rash (erythema migrans)	Myalgias
Chills	Fever
Headache	

50. How many clinical stages are observed in Lyme disease?

Clinical Stages of Lyme Disease

STAGE	TIMING	SYMPTOMS
Stage 1	3–20 days after tick bite	Erythema migrans (EM), headache, lerthargy, malaise, fever, chills
Stage 2	2–3 mos after tick bite	**Cardiac symptoms:** prolonged PR interval, AV block, palpitations, syncope. These symptoms can last 6 mos or more.
		Neurologic symptoms: usually occur while EM is still present. Include headache, stiff neck, photophobia, CN palsies (Bell's palsy), radiculoneuritis, encephalitis.
Stage 3	1–22 wks after tick bite	Arthritis: asymmetric mono- or oligoarticular pattern. May have several recurrences of short (1–6 wks) duration that primarily affect the large joints (e.g., knees).

Steere AC, et al: The early clinical manifestations of Lyme disease. Ann Intern Med 99:76–82, 1983.

51. How is spontaneous bacterial peritonitis (SBP) diagnosed?

SBP is an infection of preexisting ascites without an obvious cause for peritoneal contamination (such as trauma or perforation) and has an incidence of 10–25% among patients with liver disease and ascites. It occurs most frequently in patients with Laennec's cirrhosis but also has been described in patients with other types of liver disease, such as chronic active hepatitis, acute viral hepatitis, and metastatic disease. Children with ascites due to nephrosis are also at risk.

SBP usually presents as fever, chills, and abdominal pain or tenderness, but it may be asymptomatic and should be looked for in any patient with ascites who presents with a sudden onset of hypotension or hepatic encephalopathy. It can be diagnosed by demonstrating an ascitic fluid leukocyte count of >1000/μl or an absolute PMN cell concentration of >250 μl.

52. Which bacteria are most commonly involved in SBP?

The infecting organism can be identified in approx. 10–50% of cases by Gram stain and culture of the ascitic fluid.

Bacteriology in 253 Cases of Spontaneous Bacterial Peritonitis

CAUSATIVE BACTERIA	CASES (%)
Gram-negative bacilli	175 (69)
Escherichia coli	119 (47)
Klebsiella sp.	28 (11)
Other	28 (11)
Gram-positive cocci	76 (30)
Streptococci (all species)	65 (26)
Strep. pneumoniae	21 (8)
Enterococci	13 (5)
Other	31 (12)
Staphylococci	11 (4)
Anaerobes/microaerophils	13 (5)
Miscellaneous	3 (1)
Polymicrobial	20 (8)

From Wilcox CM, Dismukes WE: Spontaneous bacterial peritonitis: A review of pathogenesis, diagnosis, and treatment. Medicine 66:447–456, 1987, with permission.

53. Which areas of the GI tract can be involved in Crohn's disease?

Crohn's disease had been reported to affect all areas from the mouth to the anus. The major site of involvement is the **colon.**

54. What is the most common cause of infectious diarrhea?

Enterotoxigenic *Escherichia coli* is the most frequently documented pathogen and the most likely cause of "traveler's diarrhea." There are also a host of viral, bacterial, protozoal, and parasitic causes.

55. What is the significance of projectile emesis?

Projectile emesis is characterized by the forceful expulsion of material from the mouth. It is most commonly observed in gastric outlet obstruction but may also occur in persons with increased intracranial pressure.

56. Name the common etiologies of GI hemorrhage.

Upper GI hemorrhage	Lower GI hemorrhage
Peptic ulcer disease	Hemorrhoids
Varices	Angiodysplasia
Esophagitis	Diverticulosis
Mallory-Weiss tear	Carcinoma
Erosive gastritis	Inflammatory bowel disease (Crohn's and
Carcinoma	ulcerative colitis)
AV malformation	Polyps
	Ischemic colitis

The first four conditions listed in each column are the most common causes, in order of frequency.

57. What are the symptoms suggestive of peptic ulcer disease?

Epigastric pain that is described as deep, aching, or gnawing; is relieved with food or antacids; and awakens the patient at night.

58. What conditions precipitate hepatic encephalopathy?

Hepatic encephalopathy is a syndrome comprised of altered mentation (lethargy, obtundation), fetor hepaticus (peculiar odor of the breath in patients with liver disease), and asterixis ("wrist-flapping" tremor) occurring in the patient with underlying hepatic insufficiency. The causes are multifactorial and include:

Factors causing increased blood ammonia:

GI hemorrhage	Increased dietary protein
Constipation	Metabolic alkalosis
Onset of renal insufficiency (dehydration,	Insufficient treatment with laxatives and
diuretics, or acute tubular necrosis)	lactulose

Factors leading to worsened hepatic insufficiency:

Sedatives and tranquilizers	Hepatorenal syndrome
Analgesics	Progressive hepatocellular dysfunction
Viral hepatitis	
Ethanol use	

Systemic factors:

Infections	Hypercarbia
Electrolyte abnormalities	Hypokalemia
Hypoxemia	

Fraser CL: Hepatic encephalopathy. N Engl J Med 313:865–873, 1985.

59. Which hepatic disorders are associated with pregnancy? How are they diagnosed and treated?

Hepatic Disorders during Pregnancy

DIAGNOSIS	SYMPTOMS	LABORATORY FINDINGS	TREATMENT
Viral hepatitis	Most common etiology of jaundice during pregnancy Symptoms same as nonpregnant	Marked transaminase elevation Serologic markers Ultrasound normal	Newborn immuno- prophylaxis at time of delivery
Intrahepatic cholestasis of pregnancy	Third-trimester pruritus without other symptoms	Bilirubin usually <6 mg/dl Alkaline phosphatase 4–8 times normal Mild transaminase elevation Ultrasound normal	Cholestyramine, 4–24 gm/day Vitamin K
Preeclampsia	Second to third trimester	Hypertension, edema Bilirubin usually <6 mg/dl Transaminase 5 times normal Microangiopathic hemolytic anemia, thrombocytopenia Ultrasound normal; subcapsular hemorrhage	Delivery
Acute fatty liver	Third trimester	Abdominal pain, nausea, vomiting, hypertension Moderate transaminase increase PT prolonged Hypoglycemia Leukocytosis, thrombocytopenia Ultrasound: increased echogenicity	Delivery

From Carson JL, Elliot DL: Care of the pregnant patient with medical illness. J Gen Intern Med 3:577–588, 1988; with permission.

60. What are the common etiologies of acute pancreatitis?

Alcoholism and gallstones are the most common causes, accounting for 60–80% of cases, and idiopathic acute pancreatitis is the third leading etiology, representing up to 15% of cases.

Etiologies of Acute Pancreatitis

Obstruction
  Choledocholithiasis
  Ampullary/pancreatic tumors
  Choledochocele
  Worms/foreign body obstruction
  Periampullary duodenal diverticula
  Hypertensive sphincter of Oddi
  Pancreas divisum with accessory-duct
    obstruction
Infection
  Parasitic (ascariasis, clonorchiasis)
  Viral (i.e. hepatitis, mumps, EBV, HIV,
    echo, adeno)
  Bacterial (*mycoplasma, Mycobacterium avium*
    complex, campylobacter, legionella,
    M. tuberculosis)
Vascular abnormalities
  Ischemia (hypoperfusion)
  Atherosclerotic emboli
  Vasculitis (SLE, polyarteritis nodosa, ma-
    lignant hypertension)
Miscellaneous
  Penetrating peptic ulcer
  Crohn's disease
  Reye's syndrome
  Cystic fibrosis
  Hypothermia

Toxins or drugs
  Toxins (ethyl alcohol, organophosphates, scorpion
    venom)
  Drugs (azathioprine, mercaptopurine, thiazides, sul-
    fonamides, metronidazole, estrogens, cimetidine,
    sulindac, acetaminophen, erythromycin, furosemide,
    salicylates)

Trauma
  Accidental (blunt trauma to abdomen)
  Iatrogenic (i.e., postoperative trauma, ERCP)

Metabolic
  Hypertriglyceridemia
  Hypercalcemia

Inherited conditions

Idiopathic causes

Steinberg W, Tenner S: Acute pancreatitis. N Engl J Med 330:1198–1210, 1994.

61. What are common causes of jaundice in adults?

Biliary tract obstruction   Hepatocellular dysfunction
   Gallstones   Hepatitis
   Tumor   Viral
   Pancreatic neoplasm   Alcohol-induced
Congestive heart failure   Drug-induced
Hepatocellular carcinoma   Cirrhosis

62. What is the carcinoid syndrome?

The carcinoid syndrome is a symptom complex caused by carcinoid tumors, which are the commonest endocrine tumors of the digestive tract. These tumors arise from enterochromaffin cells and have the ability to produce a wide variety of biologically active amines and peptides, including serotonin, bradykinin, histamine, ACTH, prostaglandins, and others. Because the liver, via the portal circulation, receives blood from the digestive tract and clears these products from the blood prior to their entry into the systemic circulation, most patients do not manifest symptoms until hepatic metastases occur.

Patients usually present with "cutaneous flushing" episodes, which typically are red in the beginning and then become purple, start on the face and then spread to the trunk, and last several minutes. These episodes are often accompanied by tachycardia and hypotension. Symptoms are paroxysmal in character and provoked by alcohol, stress, or palpation of the liver or may be triggered by the administration of catecholamines, pentagastrin, or reserpine. The tumors can also cause diarrhea, crampy abdominal pain, obstruction, GI bleeding, and malabsorption.

63. Discuss the two theories of site-specific tumor metastases.

Certain tumors exhibit site-specific metastases, indicating a tendency of these tumors to spread preferentially to specific sites. The two theories proposed to explain this phenomenon, both of which are valid in selected cases, are:

1. The **seed & soil hypothesis** was proposed by Stephen Paget in 1889 and hypothesizes that certain tumors tend to spread to tissues that have the ability to support the tumor's growth.

2. The **mechanical hypothesis,** proposed by James Ewing in 1928, theorizes that certain tumors spread to specific tissues because these tissues lie in the path of blood flow that carries tumor cells away from the primary site.

Zetter BR: The cellular basis of site-specific tumor metastases. N Engl J Med 322:605–612, 1990.

64. Which drugs can cause gingival hyperplasia?

Phenytoin, cyclosporine, and nifedipine.

Butler RT, et al: Drug-induced gingival hyperplasia: Phenytoin, cyclosporine and nifedipine. J Am Dent Assoc 114:56–60, 1987.

65. Which drugs are frequently abused in the U.S.?

   Alcohol
   Marijuana
   Cocaine/crack
   PCP (phencyclidine)
   Prescription medications
      Tricyclic antidepressants   Sedative-hypnotics
      Narcotic analgesics   Anxiolytic agents
      Diet aids (amphetamines)
   Heroin

Polydrug abuse is common among all individuals who abuse drugs, regardless of socioeconomic levels.

66. How do overdoses of tricyclic antidepressant (TCA) medications cause death?

TCAs are the third most frequent cause of drug-related deaths. More than two-thirds of deaths occur in women. The agents most commonly implicated are amitriptyline, desipramine, and nortriptyline. The pathogenetic mechanisms of death include:

Cardiovascular arrhythmias	Respiratory arrest
Ventricular fibrillation	Intractable seizures
Prolonged QRS	CNS depression/coma
Asystole	

67. What antidotes are available for common drug and chemical overdoses?

Antidotes Available for Specific Drugs

DRUG	ANTIDOTE AND DOSAGE
Acetaminophen	*N*-acetylcysteine: 140 mg/kg initially, followed by 70 mg/kg every 8 hrs for 17 doses.
Narcotics	Naloxone (Narcan): 0.4–2.0 mg IV. Can be repeated at 2–3-min intervals.
Benzodiazepines	Flumazenil (Romazicon): 0.3 mg IV. Additional doses of 0.5 mg over 30 sec at 1-min intervals to a cumulative dose of 3 mg.
Anticholinergic agents	Physostigmine: 2 mg by slow IV. Repeat in 20 min if no improvement, followed by 1–2 mg IV for recurrent symptoms.
Methanol, ethylene glycol	Ethanol (absolute): 1 ml/kg in D5W IV over 15 min. Maintenance dose: 125 mg/kg/hr IV in D5W.
Phenothiazines, haloperidol, loxitane	Diphenhydramine: 25–50 mg; or benztropine: 1–2 mg (may be given IV or IM).
Cyanide	Sodium nitrite: 300 mg IV; or sodium thiosulfate: 12.5 gm
Organophosphates (insecticides)	Atropine sulfate: 2–5 mg IV. Repeat every 10–30 min to maintain a decrease in bronchial secretions. After atropine, pralidoxime: 1 mg IV for 2 doses. Repeat every 8–12 hrs for 3 doses if muscle weakness is not relieved.

Guzzardi LJ: Role of the emergency physician in poisoning. Med Clin North Am 2: 10–11, 1982.
Physican's Desk Reference, 49th ed. Oradell, NJ, Medical Economics, 1995.

68. A 19-year-old girl is admitted with salicylate poisoning. What acid-base disturbances are seen in this condition on serial blood gas monitoring?

Acute salicylate intoxication is characterized by profound effects on acid-base balance. Early in the course of intoxication, there is a primary **respiratory alkalosis** resulting from direct stimulation of the respiratory center in the medulla by salicylates. This causes an increase in pH and fall in $PaCO_2$. A compensatory **metabolic acidosis** due to renal excretion of bicarbonate may be seen, which tends to bring the pH back toward normal. In young adults and children (especially with toxic doses), a primary metabolic acidosis ensues due to:

1. Impaired hepatic carbohydrate metabolism leading to accumulation of ketones and lactate in plasma.

2. Accumulated salicylic acid itself, which displaces several meq of bicarbonate.

3. Dehydration and hypotension impair renal excretion of inorganic acids and cause further metabolic acidosis.

The resulting primary metabolic acidosis is normochloremic and associated with a high anion gap. The continuation of primary respiratory alkalosis and metabolic acidosis should give a clue to the diagnosis of acute salicylate intoxication. In more severe cases, primary respiratory acidosis occurs due to the depression of the respiratory center at very high salicylate levels.

69. What are the initial steps in the assessment and treatment of a patient with a suspected drug overdose?

- Control airway.
- Check vital signs (blood pressure, respiration, pulse, temperature).
- Stabilize any abnormalities in vital signs.
- Check mental status/level of consciousness.
- Obtain blood for laboratory studies (chemistries, arterial blood gases, toxicology screen).
- IV fluid: D5W with thiamine ± naloxone.
- Quick physical exam (heart, lungs, abdomen, neurologic).

Goldfrank LJR, et al: Management of overdose with psychoactive medications. Med Clin North Am 2:65, 1982.

70. Which organs are frequently damaged by intravenous drug abuse (IVDA)?
In descending order of frequency, the lung, heart, and kidneys.

71. Which infectious diseases are commonly observed among IVDAs?
Persons who are IVDAs run a high risk of acquiring serious infections from all classes of pathogens, and any organ system may be affected.

Common Infections in IVDA

CNS	LUNGS	HEART
Meningitis	Pneumonia	Endocarditis
Abscess	*S. aureus*	*S. aureus* (>50% of cases)
	Aspiration (anaerobes)	Gram-negative bacilli
Eye	Gram negative bacilli	*Enterococcus*
Endophthalmitis	Abscess	*Candida* sp.
	Septic pulmonary emboli	Polymicrobial
	Empyema	
	Tuberculosis	
Abdomen	**Muscle**	**HIV Infection**
Hepatitis B	Necrotizing fasciitis	(most common infection in IVDAs)
	Pyomyositis	AIDS, ARC, etc.
		AIDS-related
		Pneumocystis carinii
Skin	**Joints**	pneumonia
Cellulitis	Osteomyelitis	Cytomegalovirus
S. aureus	Septic arthritis	Toxoplasmosis
Streptococci		Cryptococcal meningitis
Gram negative bacilli	**Genitourinary**	*Mycobacterium avium* complex
Suppurative phlebitis	Sexually transmitted diseases	
	Renal abscesses	

Levine DP, Sobel JD: Infections in intravenous drug abusers. In Mandell GL, Bennett JE, Dolin R (eds): Principles and Practice of Infectious Disease, 4th ed. New York, Churchill Livingstone, 1995, pp 2696–277.

72. What factors indicate a poor prognosis in hypertension?

1. Black race
2. Youth
3. Male sex
4. Persistent diastolic pressure >115 mm Hg
5. Smoking
6. Diabetes mellitus
7. Hypercholesterolemia
8. Obesity
9. Excessive alcohol intake
10. Evidence of end-organ damage
   a. Cardiac (cardiac enlargement, ECG changes of ischemia or left ventricular strain, MI, CHF)
   b. Eyes (retinal exudates, hemorrhages, and papilledema)
   c. Renal (impaired renal function)
   d. Nervous system (cerebrovascular accident)

Isselbacher KJ, et al (eds): Harrison's Principles of Internal Medicine, 13th ed. New York, McGraw-Hill, 1994, p 1119.

73. Which valves are most frequently affected in rheumatic heart disease?
In order of frequency, mitral > aortic > tricuspid > pulmonary.

74. What are the etiologies of the common cardiac arrhythmias seen in adults?

Arrhythmia	Rate (bpm)	Etiologies
Sinus tachycardia	100–200	Fever, pain, drugs, hyperthyroidism, hypotension
Paroxysmal supraventricular tachycardia (PSVT)	130–220 (usually 160)	Pre-excitation syndrome (Wolff-Parkinson-White syndrome), AV nodal re-entry, congenital abnormalities, atrial septal defect, concealed accessory bypass tracts
Atrial flutter	Atrial, 250–350 Ventricular, 140–160	Mitral valve disease, COPD, pulmonary embolus, alcohol abuse, organic heart disease, MI, cardiac surgery
Atrial fibrillation	Atrial, 350–500 Ventricular, 100–160	Myocardial ischemia, MI, organic heart disease, rheumatic heart disease, alcohol abuse, CHF, elderly patients, febrile illness, hyperthyroidism, chest surgery
Ventricular tachycardia	100–230	Ischemic heart disease, MI, mitral valve prolapse, cardiomyopathy, hypercalcemia, hypokalemia, hypomagnesemia, hypoxemia

75. How do you differentiate the common tachyarrhythmias?

	Sinus Tachycardia	Paroxysmal Atrial Tachycardia	Atrial Fibrillation	Atrial Flutter	Ventricular Tachycardia
Rate	100–200	169–190	160–190	140–160	100–230
Rhythm	Regular	Regular	Irregular	Regular	Slightly irregular
QRS shape	Normal*	Normal*	Normal*	Normal*	Abnormal
Atrial activity	Sinus P wave†	Absent or nonsinus P wave†	Absent	Flutter waves	Sinus P waves†
P-QRS relation	Yes	May be masked by rapid ventricular rate	No	May be masked by rapid ventricular rate	No
Carotid massage	Slows	No response, or converts to sinus rhythm	No response	Increased block	No response

*Unless intraventricular conduction disturbance.
†Sinus P waves are upright in lead II and occur at least 0.12 sec before the QRS complex begins.
    From Gottlieb AJ, et al: The Whole Internist Catalog. Philadelphia, W.B. Saunders, 1980, p 158, with permission.

76. Discuss the mechanism of Cheyne-Stokes breathing in patients with severe CHF.
    In the patient with left ventricular failure, the circulation time between the lungs and respiratory center of the brain is slowed. This delay causes the system to respond sluggishly, leading to the oscillations in breathing patterns observed in Cheyne-Stokes respiration. Cheyne-Stokes breathing, also known as periodic or cyclic breathing, is characterized by periods of apnea alternating with hyperpnea. During apnea, the PCO_2 rises and PO_2 falls, causing stimulation of the brain center. The end result is hyperventilation. This results in a fall in the PCO_2, which results in suppression of the respiratory drive, and another period of apnea ensues.

77. Which classes of medications should be given cautiously to persons with a prolonged QT interval?
    Antiarrhythmics:

Class IA	Class IC	Class III
Quinidine	Flecainide	Amiodarone
Procainamide	Lorcainide	
Disopyramide		

Others:
Phenothiazines
Tricyclic antidepressants

78. What are the manifestations of digitalis toxicity?

1. **Arrhythmias:** the most dangerous and, unfortunately, often the first manifestation. Many different brady- and tachyarrhythmias have been described. The more common include supraventricular tachycardia with AV block, ventricular ectopy, all degrees of AV block, and sinoatrial or AV nodal exit block.

2. **Neurologic:** headache, fatigue, lethargy, confusion, delirium, seizures, and malaise

3. **Gastrointestinal:** nausea, vomiting, diarrhea, anorexia

4. **Visual:** disturbed color vision (greenish or yellow tinting, halos around objects), blurred vision, photophobia

5. **Endocrine:** gynecomastia in males

79. What special management does a non-Q-wave MI require?

A non-Q-wave MI (NQWMI) has a better short-term prognosis, but these patients are at higher risk of reinfarction or extension of the infarct area, early onset of postinfarction pain, and an overall higher late mortality rate.

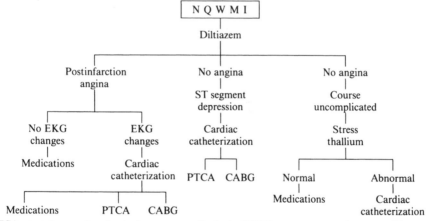

PTCA=percutaneous transluminal coronary agntioplasty; CABG=coronary artery bypass grafting.

80. Which symptoms indicate the need for corrective surgery in a patient with aortic stenosis?

In order of decreasing severity, heart failure, angina, and syncope.

81. When do ventricular premature depolarizations (VPDs) warrant medical therapy?

VPDs, or premature ventricular contractions (PVCs), are usually not associated with an increased risk of sudden death. Although they occur in persons with otherwise normal hearts, they are more common in those with ischemic heart disease or cardiomyopathies and in the elderly. Treatment is advised in cases of:

- Frequent, repetitive ventricular ectopy
- Coronary artery disease: angina, post-MI
- Clinically significant valvular disease
- Mitral valve prolapse associated with syncope and/or ventricular tachycardia
- Cardiomyopathies
- Severe associated symptoms
- Syncope

82. What is torsade de pointes?

Torsade de pointes (pronounced *tōr-sahd' dĕ pwahnt*), or "twisting of the points," is a polymorphic ventricular tachycardia characterized by QRS complexes that change in amplitude and electrical polarity, appearing to "twist" around the isoelectric line. A prolonged QT interval must be present. There may also be U waves.

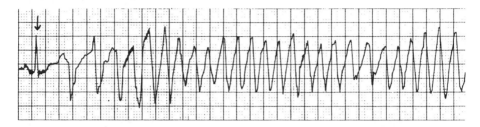

Torsade de pointes. A single sinus beat (arrow) is followed by ventricular tachycardia with an oscillating or swinging pattern of the QRS complexes. (From Seelig CB: Simplified EKG Analysis. Philadelphia, Hanley & Belfus, 1992, p 75, with permission.)

83. What are the etiologies of torsades de pointes?

Quinidine

Amiodarone

Disopyramide

Procainamide

Third-degree heart block

Psychotropic drugs

   Phenothiazines

   Tricyclic antidepressants

   Lithium

Hypokalemia

Hypomagnesemia

Myocardial ischemia

Myocarditis

CNS lesions

Trauma

Tumors

Subarachnoid hemorrhage

Severe bradycardia

Saffer J, et al: Polymorphous ventricular tachycardia associated with normal and long Q T intervals. Am J Cardiol 49:2021–2029, 1982.

84. Name the risk factors for the development of coronary artery disease (CAD).

Positive Risk Factors (increase risk)

Age

   Male ≥ 45 yrs

   Female ≥ 55 yrs or premature menopause without estrogen replacement therapy

Family history of premature CAD (definite MI or sudden death before age 55 years in father or other male first-degree relative, or before age 65 in mother or other female first degree relative)

Current cigarette smoking

Hypertension (BP ≥ 140/90 mm Hg confirmed by several measurements or taking antihypertensive medication)

Elevated LDL cholesterol

Low HDL cholesterol (< 35 mg/dl or 0.9 mmol/l confirmed by several measurements)

Diabetes mellitus

Negative Risk Factor: (decrease risk)

High HDL cholesterol (≥ 60 mg/dl or 1.6 mmol/l])

Summary of the second report of the National Cholesterol Education Program (NCEP) ex-pert panel on detection, evaluation, and treatment of high blood cholesterol in adults (Adult Treatment Panel II). JAMA 269:3015–3023, 1993.

85. What hormonal change in women increases their risk of CAD?

Menopause. The risk of CAD, while lower in premenopausal females than in age-matched males, rapidly increases in postmenopausal females.

86. A 35-year-old black man with a past history of nephrotic syndrome is admitted for elective knee surgery. He has been taking ibuprofen for 3 weeks. His admission serum creatinine is 3 mg/dl. What points help you to differentiate acute renal failure (ARF) from chronic renal failure (CRF)?

This patient with a previous history of nephrotic illness has been taking an NSAID and has a moderate degree of renal insufficiency. This could be ARF induced by the NSAID or could be an unrecognized progressive CRF. Urinary sediment can be useful in this situation. Acute interstitial nephritis is associated with red and white blood cell casts, whereas CRF is associated with broad casts (usually two to three times the diameter of a WBC). The presence of significant anemia, hyperphosphatemia, hypocalcemia, and changes of renal osteodystrophy is suggestive of advanced CRF. The most important confirmation of chronicity is demonstration of shrunken or small kidneys by ultrasound or CT scanning.

87. How do NSAIDs cause acute renal failure?

The NSAIDs inhibit cyclooxygenase, an enzyme responsible for synthesizing prostaglandins from arachidonic acid. The intrarenal production of prostaglandins, especially PGE_2, contributes significantly to the maintenance of renal blood flow (RBF) and glomerular filtration rate (GFR) in states of diminished effective arterial blood volume. In any of the prerenal states, angiotensin II and norepinephrine production is increased, which in turn increases renal vasodilator prostaglandin synthesis and thus leads to improvement of renal ischemia. The NSAIDs have the potential to significantly lower RBF and GFR in certain disease states (such as hypovolemia, CHF, nephrotic syndrome, and lupus nephritis) and to produce ARF. An acute interstitial nephritis associated with nephrotic syndrome may also occur, particularly after the use of fenoprofen.

88. Who is at highest risk for NSAID-induced renal failure?

The elderly

Diabetic

Patients on angiotensin-converting enzyme inhibitors and/or beta-blockers

Patients receiving >1 NSAIDs (i.e., aspirin *and* indomethacin)

Patients on diuretics or who are dehydrated

Patients with underlying CHF

89. Which conditions related to pregnancy predispose to ARF?

Although its incidence has declined markedly with control of septic abortions and antenatal care, ARF is not uncommon in pregnancy. Toxemia of pregnancy, antepartum hemorrhage, and postpartum hemorrhage are associated with an increased risk of ARF. Other predisposing factors include postpartum sepsis, abortion, postpartum hemolytic uremia syndrome, and amniotic fluid embolism. In addition, acute fatty liver and urinary tract obstruction are occasionally associated with ARF during pregnancy.

90. Describe the physiologic changes in the kidney during pregnancy.

Pregnancy is associated with an increase in GFR of about 50% and a mild decrease in plasma creatinine and BUN. There is a slight increase in kidney size (about 1 cm) and dilation and tortuosity of the ureters. These changes were believed secondary to pressure by the gravid uterus, but it is now known that these changes can be related to increased progesterone levels. Other physiologic changes include increased uric acid clearance, resulting in slight hypouricemia.

91. How does aging affect the kidney?

1. Diminished (GFR)
2. Decreased creatinine production (due to decreased muscle mass)
3. Obstructive uropathy (due to benign prostatic hypertrophy)
4. Urinary incontinence

92. List the most common etiologies of ARF in hospitalized patients.
- Hypoperfusion (approx. 50%)

  Dehydration   Sepsis

  CHF   Arrhythmia
- Postoperative renal failure
- IV contrast dye
- Drugs (especially aminoglycosides)
- Obstruction
- Hepatorenal syndrome

93. Which class of antihypertensive agents is contraindicated in patients with bilateral renal artery stenosis?

Angiotensin-converting enzyme (ACE) inhibitors. In bilateral renal artery stenosis or stenosis to a solitary kidney, the renal perfusion pressure (and thus GFR) depends on the local renin-angiotensin system. When the system is blocked by an ACE inhibitor, a marked decrease in the efferent arterial pressure with subsequent decrease in renal perfusion pressure results, causing a diminished GFR.

94. What does the presence of eosinophils in urine denote?

Normal urine does not contain eosinophils, so their presence in a urine sample points to renal disease. The contribution of eosinophils to the immune response is not clearly known, but they are activated by antigens and antigen-induced hypersensitivity reactions. Eosinophils in the urine are characteristic of tubulo-interstitial disease (i.e., interstitial nephritis), especially if they comprise >5% of the total number of WBCs in the sample. Eosinophils in the urine are seen in:

Interstitial nephritis   Acute tubular necrosis

Urinary tract infections   Hepatorenal syndrome

Kidney transplant rejection

Carwin HL, et al: Clinical correlates of eosinophiluria. Arch Intern Med 145:1097–1099, 1985.

95. What three findings comprise the hyporeninemic-hypoaldosteronism syndrome?
1. Low serum aldosterone levels (due to impaired secretion)
2. Low serum renin levels
3. Hyperkalemia (which is more severe than expected by the degree of renal insufficiency)

Clinical Characteristics in Patients with Hyporeninemic-Hypoaldosteronism

Mean age	65 yrs
Asymptomatic hyperkalemia	75%
Chronic renal insufficiency	70%
Diabetes mellitus	50%
Cardiac arrhythmias	25%
Normal aldosterone response to ACTH	25%

96. In CRF patients, what is the importance of the $Ca^{++} \times PO_4^-$ product (calcium-phosphate product)?

When the product of the serum concentrations of calcium and phosphate exceeds 70, metastatic calcifications are more likely to occur. Calcium phosphate ($CaPO_4$) may precipitate out of the plasma and deposit in arteries, soft tissues, peri-articular areas, and viscera.

97. Which organisms typically colonize the bronchioles of smokers?

Haemophilus influenzae

Streptococcus pneumoniae

Moraxella catarrhalis

A variety of respiratory viruses

98. What are the common etiologies of diffuse bilateral interstitial lung infiltrates?

Pulmonary edema
Miliary tuberculosis
Pneumocystis carinii pneumonia
Lymphangitic spread of carcinoma
  (breast, gastric)
Sarcoidosis
Lymphoma
Idiopathic

Drugs/toxins
Nitrofurantoin
Amiodarone
Sulfonamides
Zidovudine
Bleomycin
Methotrexate
Cyclophosphamide
Chlorambucil

Crystal RG, et at: Interstitial lung disease of unknown cause. N Engl J Med 310:154–166, 235–244, 1984.

99. Where do you find Hampton's hump?

Hampton's hump, named after Aubrey Otis Hampton (1900–1955), a U.S. radiologist, is a radiographic finding that is highly suggestive of a pulmonary infarction. It is a dense, homogeneous, wedge-shaped consolidation occurring in the middle and lower lobes. The base is contiguous with the pleura, but the apex points, in a convex fashion, toward the hilum. This gives the appearance of a hump.

100. Which lung neoplasm is most prevalent among nonsmokers?

Adenocarcinoma. It usually originates in the periphery of the lung and characteristically metastasizes to the contralateral lung, adrenal glands, liver, and brain. However, 90% of all persons who develop lung cancer smoke.

101. Which skin cancer is most common in adults?

Basal cell carcinoma. It occurs 4–10 times as frequently as squamous cell carcinoma. The primary risk factor is excessive sun exposure, especially in fair-skinned individuals, and 90% of tumors occur in sun-exposed areas of the skin. Metastasis is very rare, and the prognosis is usually excellent, although deaths from local extension do occur. Therapy is based on location and extent of the tumor. Removal of the tumor, by a variety of means, is curative in 90% of the cases.

Kurban RS, Kurban AK: Common skin disorders of aging: Diagnosis and treatment. Geriatrics 48(4):30–42, 1993.

102. Which skin cancer is associated with the highest mortality? What are its risk factors?

Melanoma causes the largest number of deaths related to skin cancer.

Risk Factors for Cutaneous Melanoma

High risk (>50-fold increased risk)
Persistently changing mole
Atypical moles in patients with 2 family members with melanoma
Adulthood >childhood
> 50 nevi ≥ 2 mm
Intermediate risk (approx. 10-fold increased risk)
Family history of melanoma
Sporadic atypical moles
Congenital nevi (?)
Whites > African-Americans or Asians
Prior history of melanoma
Low risk (2–4-fold increasd risk)
Immunosuppression
Sun sensitivity or excess exposure

Washington CV: Skin cancer. In Isselbacher KJ, et al (eds): Harrison's Principles of Internal Medicine, 13th ed. New York, McGraw Hill, 1994, p 1867.

103. What criteria should be remembered when evaluating a lesion suspicious for a melanoma?

The **ABCD rule** lists the key criteria for evaluating these lesions:

A = Asymmetry
B = Border irregularity
C = Color variation (usually purple/black)
D = Diameter ≥ 6 mm

Kurban RS, Kurban AK: Common skin disorders of the aging: Diagnosis and treatment. Geriatrics 48(4):30–42, 1993.

104. What are actinic keratoses? In whom do they occur?

What:	Benign dysplasia of the epidermis. Multiple erythematous or tan plaques with an adherent scaly surface.
Whom:	Most common in elderly patients
Where:	Sun-exposed areas: face, dorsal surface of hands, forearms, balding scalp
Risk:	<1% risk of developing squamous cell carcinoma in early lesions and up to 20% in late lesions.
Treatment:	Primary prevention: use of sunscreens and protective clothing and prophylaxis (topical vitamin C)
	Medical: 2–5% topical 5-fluorouracil twice daily × 3–6 wks
	Surgical: excision

105. Are tinea versicolor and vitiligo manifestations of the same disease?

No. The differences are shown in the following table:

	Vitiligo	*Tinea*
Etiology	? Autoimmune	Fungal infection
Pathology	Destruction of melanocytes	Decreased melanosomes in the stratum corneum
Incidence	1%	Common
Age of onset	Young adults	Young adults
Description	Macular depigmented areas. Absence of melanin	Small hypopigmented-to-tan macules with a bran-like scale
Associated conditions	Graves' disease, pernicious anemia, diabetes mellitus, Addison's disease	Seborrhea
Diagnosis	Chalk-white under Wood's lamp Absence of melanocytes on skin biopsy	Gold fluorescence on Wood's lamp Spores/hyphae on skin biopsy KOH=positive, "spaghetti and meatballs" appearance
Therapy	Trioxsalen with sun exposure at least two times a week	Selenium sulfide, sulfur ointments, ketoconazole, salicylic acid

106. How do a chancre and a chancroid ulcer differ?

	Chancre	*Chancroid Ulcer*
Disease	Syphilis	Chancroid (a disease in itself)
Organism	*Treponema pallidum*	*Haemophilus ducreyi*
Description	Painless papule that rapidly erodes. Edge feels cartilaginous. Indurated.	Painful, superficial ulcer with ragged edges. Base is covered by necrotic exudate. More often multiple.
Location	Penis, cervix/labia, and anus/rectum/mouth in homosexuals	Males: Preputial orifice, prepuce, frenulum Females: labia, clitoris, vestibule
Treatment	Penicillin G, tetracycline	Trimethoprim/sulfamethoxazole, erythromycin

107. What are petechiae?

Small, 1–3 mm, round, reddish or brown lesions that do not blanch. They are caused by hemorrhage into the skin. They are commonly seen in platelet disorders and vasculitic processes.

108. When should a mole be removed?

Indications for Removal of a Mole

Change in size or diameter	Onset of bleeding, itching, or pain
Color becomes darker or lighter	Increase in height
Development of irregular borders	Congenital moles after one reaches adulthood
Elevation of the surface	(>50 ys)

Rhodes AR, et al: Risk factors for cutaneous melanoma. JAMA 258:3146–3154, 1987.

109. What are cutaneous manifestations of hyperthyroidism?

Warm, moist, "velvety" texture of skin	Vitiligo
Increased palmar/dorsal sweating	Altered hair texture
Facial flushing	Alopecia
Palmar erythema	Pretibial myxedema

110. Which cardiac abnormality is a common cause of CHF in the elderly hypertensive patient?

Hypertensive hypertrophic cardiomyopathy. The disease is characterized by:
1. Severe concentric cardiac hypertrophy
2. Small left ventricular cavity
3. Elevated left ventricular ejection fraction

Tapale J, et al: Hypertensive hypertrophic cardiomyopathy of the elderly. N Engl J Med 312: 277–283, 1985.

111. What is the frequency of asymptomatic bacteriuria in patients over age 65? Is treatment necessary?

Asymptomatic bacteriuria is present in at least 20% of women and 10% of men over age 65. Treatment is not necessary unless it is associatd with an obstructive uropathy.

Boscia JA, et al: Asymptomatic bacteriuria in the elderly. Infect Dis Clin North Am 1:893–905, 1987.

112. Headaches in an elderly patient should always alert one to the possibility of which illness?

Temporal (giant cell) arteritis should be considered in any patient over age 50 with a headache. Untreated temporal arteritis can result in irreversible monocular blindness. Symptoms include:

- Continuous, throbbing, unilateral "temporal" headache
- Claudication of jaw when chewing and/or talking
- Transient loss of vision (amaurosis fugax), visual-field deficits, diploplia, sudden visual loss
- Symptoms of polymyalgia rheumatica (girdle-hip pain) seen in 50%
- Tender, swollen, red, nodular temporal artery with decrease pulsation on palpation seen in two-thirds
- Fever
- Weight loss

113. What are the leading causes of blindness in the elderly?

- Cataracts
- Glaucoma
- Retinopathies
- Temporal arteritis
- Diabetes mellitus

114. What are the common presentations of insulin-dependent diabetes mellitus (IDDM) versus non-insulin-dependent diabetes mellitus (NIDDM)?

	IDDM	*NIDDM*
Age	<40 years	>40 years, elderly
Onset	Short period	Insidious, found incidentally on lab tests
Complications	Diabetic ketoacidosis	Hyperosmolar coma
Body habitus	Normal, thin	Obese
Pathology	Islet cells destroyed	Insulin resistance, low insulin secretion, islet cells intact
Ketosis prone	Yes	No
Therapy	Insulin	Weight loss, balanced diet, oral hypoglycemic agents, perhaps insulin

115. List the contraindications to sulfonylurea (hypoglycemic) drugs.
1. Type I diabetes or pancreatic diabetes
2. Pregnancy
3. Major surgery
4. Severe infections, stress, or trauma
5. History of severe adverse reaction to sulfonylurea or similar compound (sulfa drug)
6. Predisposition to severe hypoglycemia (e.g., patients with significant liver or kidney disease)

Lebovitz HE, et al: Therapy for Diabetes Mellitus and Related Disorders, 2nd ed. Alexandria, VA, American Diabetes Association, 1994, p 120.

116. What are the proposed mechanisms of action and the advantages of metformin in diabetes therapy?

Proposed Mechanisms for Antidiabetic Action of Metformin

Increase insulin receptors on cell surface or insulin-sensitive tissues
Increase glucose-transport units in insulin-sensitive cells
Increase glucose uptake of muscle and adipose tissue
Decrease hepatic glucose production
Potentiate insulin action
Decrease GI absorption of glucose
Cause anorexia

Advantages of Metformin Therapy in Type II Diabetes

Usually modest weight loss
No hypoglycemia
Decreased plasma VLDL cholesterol and increased HDL cholesterol
Unchanged or slightly decreased plasma insulin levels

Lebovitz HE, et al: Therapy for Diabetes Mellitus and Related Disorders, 2nd ed. Alexandria, VA, American Diabetes Association, 1994, pp 125–126.

117. Why are oral agents useful in the treatment of NIDDM?
Patients with NIDDM still have functioning beta cells in the islets of Langerhans of the pancreas. Therefore, some endogenous insulin production remains. The oral hypoglycemic agents' primary mechanism of action is thought to include:
- Stimulation of insulin release from islet cells
- Increased insulin receptors in target tissues
- Improved action of insulin
- Decrease in the previously increased rates of hepatic glucose production

118. What are the end-organ effects of chronically elevated blood glucose?

Skin
Dermopathy
Diabetic foot ulcers
Lower susceptibility to skin infections

Eyes
Cataracts
Retinopathy

Peripheral nerves
Peripheral neuropathy
Mononeuropathy (median nerve)

Genitourinary
Impotence
Retrograde ejaculation

Kidneys
Renal insufficiency
End-stage renal disease
Nephrotic syndrome
Repeated urinary tract infections

CNS
Coma (due to diabetic ketoacidosis or
   hyperosmolar coma)
Personality changes
Autonomic insufficiency

Cardiovascular
Increased risk of CAD
Silent MI
Cardiomyopathy
Hypertriglyceridemia
Elevated total cholesterol
Lowered HDL cholesterol
Hypertension
Peripheral vascular disease

119. What recommendations on foot care should the diabetic receive?
1. Check feet daily.
2. Wear cushioned shoes that fit properly. (Jogging shoes are great!)
3. Always turn shoes over and shake them out before putting them on.
4. Never go barefoot.
5. Use cotton socks and cornstarch powder to reduce moisture in shoes.
6. Report redness, skin breakdown, or trauma to a physician immediately.
7. Soak feet in warm water 15–20 minutes daily, followed by lubrication with lotion.
8. Test bath water temperature with hands, not feet.
9. Calluses should be treated by a physician, nurse, or podiatrist (no bathroom surgery!).
10. Trim nails squarely (do not round edges).

120. What is the strict definition of hypoglycemia?
Documented low blood sugar accompanied by symptoms that resolve with the ingestion of glucose or food. Symptoms include:

Anxiety
Nervousness
Headache
Tachycardia

Trembling
Difficulty thinking
Sweating
Confusion

Kahn CR (ed): Joslin's Diabetes Mellitus, 13th ed. Philadelphia, Lea & Febiger, 1994.

121. What are consistent laboratory findings in adrenal insufficiency?
Hyponatremia (rarely <120 meq/l)
Hyperkalemia (rarely >7 meq/l)
Hypocarbia (HCO_3 ~15–20 meq/l)
Hypoglycemia
Elevated BUN
Elevated eosinophils
Elevated lymphocytes

122. Which hormonal imbalance can cause obstructive sleep apnea?
Severe hypothyroidism associated with myxedema. The upper airway constriction is caused by myxedematous swelling of the face, tongue, and pharyngeal structures.
Brown LK: Sleep apnea syndromes: Overview and diagnostic approach. Mt Sinai Med 61(2):99–112, 1994.

123. What complaints in elderly hypothyroid patients most commonly bring them to medical attention?

Constipation   Lethargy, easy fatigability
Difficulty in thinking   Cold intolerance

Bartuska DG: Thyroid disease in the news. Contemp Intern Med (Jun):23–32, 1989.

124. What protection is afforded to patients with the heterozygous sickle cell gene?
The high frequency of the sickle cell gene in areas endemic for malaria is an example of **balanced polymorphism.** The sickle cell gene protects the host from lethal *Plasmadium falciparum* malaria. The actual mechanism is not fully understood, but it is postulated that the entry of the parasite into the host cell lowers RBC oxygen saturation. This desaturation leads to sickling and arrests the maturation of the parasite. The sickled cells are cleared by the phagocytic system.
Luzzatto L: Genetics of red cells susceptibility to malaria. Blood 54:961–976, 1979.

125. Name the five types of crises in sickle cell disease.
1. **Vaso-occlusive** (painful): The typical "sickle crisis" whose symptoms depend on the location of occlusion.
2. **Aplastic:** Bone marrow suppression due to infection.
3. **Sequestration:** Seen in younger patients (aged 1–5 yrs.) while the spleen is still intact.
4. **Hemolytic:** Look for G6PD deficiency or malaria.
5. **Megaloblastic:** Seen in conditions of increased folate requirements (as in pregnancy).

126. How quickly does a megaloblastic bone marrow recover after the deficient vitamins are added to the patient's diet?
Within 6–8 hours after ingestion of even small amounts of vitamin B_{12} or folate, the bone marrow begins to normalize.

127. Which drugs are most commonly implicated in drug-induced immune thrombocytopenia?

Antibacterials:
Sulfonamides
Rifampin
Trimethoprim
Ampicillin
Cephalosporins
p-Aminosalicylate
Nitrofurantoin
Isoniazid

NSAIDs:
Aspirin
Indomethacin
Phenylbutazone
Sulindac

Anticonvulsants:
Carbamazepine
Phenytoin
Sodium valproate
Diphenylhydantoin
Phthalazinol

Antihypertensives:
Methyldopa
Chlorothiazide
Hydrochlorothiazide
Diazoxide
Furosemide

Cinchona alkaloids:
Quinine
Quinidine

Miscellaneous:
Heroin
Chlorpropamide
Bleomycin
Desipramine
Gold
Heparin
Cimetidine
Digitoxin
Acetaminophen

128. What are the differential diagnoses of macrocytic and microcytic anemias?

Macrocytic Anemia	Microcytic Anemia
Liver disease	Iron deficiency (most common type of
Vitamin B_{12} deficiency	anemia worldwide)
Folate deficiency	Hemoglobinopathies
Myelodysplastic syndrome	Thalassemia
Drugs that impair DNA synthesis	Sickle cell
6-Mercaptopurine	SC disease
Zidovudine	Sideroblastic anemias
5-Fluorouracil	Anemia of chronic disease
Hydroxyurea	

129. What are the characteristics of anemia of chronic disease?

Hemoglobin 7–10%	Reticulocyte count <2%
RBC normochromic/normocytic	Saturated Fe-binding capacity <20%
Total Fe-binding capacity ↓	Tissue storage Fe: ↑ bone marrow Fe
In hospital, without renal failure	Mild hypochromia and microcytosis
Serum Fe < 60 μg/100 mL	
Ferritin > 100 ng/ml	

130. What criteria must be met to make the diagnosis of systemic lupus erythematosus (SLE)?

SLE is a chronic, inflammatory disease that results from an immunoregulatory disturbance and is characterized by an exaggerated production of autoantibodies. There is a marked female predominance of the disease, with a female:male ratio of 9:1. For a definitive diagnosis, 4 of the following 11 criteria must be met:

1982 Revised Criteria for Classification of SLE

CRITERION	DEFINITION
1. Malar rash	Fixed erythema, flat or raised, over the malar eminences, tending to spare the nasolabial folds
2. Discoid rash	Erythematous raised patches with adherent keratotic scaling and follicular plugging; atrophic scarring may occur in older lesions
3. Photosensitivity	Skin rash as a result of unusual reaction to sunlight, by patient history or physician observation
4. Oral ulcers	Oral or nasopharyngeal ulceration, usually painless, observed by a physician
5. Arthritis	Nonerosive arthritis involving 2 or more peripheral joints, characterized by tenderness, swelling, or effusion
6. Serositis	Pleuritis—convincing history of pleuritic pain or rub heard by a physician or evidence of pleural effusion, *or*
	Pericarditis—documented by ECG or rub or evidence of pericardial effusion
7. Renal disorder	Persistent proteinuria >0.5 gm/day or >3+ if quantitation not performed, *or*
	Cellular casts—may be red cell, hemoglobin, granular, tubular, or mixed
8. Neurologic disorder	Seizures—in the absence of offending drugs or known metabolic derangements (e.g., uremia, ketoacidosis, or electrolyte imbalance), *or*
	Psychosis—in the absence of offending drugs or known metabolic derangements (e.g., uremia, ketoacidosis, or electrolyte imbalance)
9. Hematologic disorder	Hemolytic anemia—with reticulocytosis, *or*
	Leukopenia—<4,000/mm³ total on two or more occasions, *or*
	Lymphopenia—<1,500/mm³ on two or more occasions, *or*
	Thrombocytopenia—<100,000/mm³ in the absence of offending drugs
10. Immunologic disorder	Positive LE cell preparation, *or*
	Anti-DNA: antibody to native DNA in abnormal titer, *or*
	Anti-Sm: presence of antibody to Sm nuclear antigen, or
	False-positive serologic test for syphillis known to be positive for at least 6 months and confirmed by *Treponema pallidum* immobilization or FTA-ABS test
11. Antinuclear antibody (ANA)	Abnormal titer of ANA by immunofluorescence or equivalent assay at any time and in the absence of drugs known to be associated with "drug-induced lupus"

Tan EM, Cohen AS, Fries JF, et al: The 1982 revised criteria for the classification of systemic lupus erythematosus (SLE). Arthritis Rheum 25:1271–1277, 1982.

131. Which enzyme is usually elevated in lymphoma?

Lactate dehydrogenase (LDH) is elevated in many lymphomas and other lymphoproliferative disorders. The source is believed to be tumor cells, and LDH is used as a measurement of disease activity.

132. Neutropenia is most commonly observed in which peoples?

Africans, West Indian blacks, and African-Americans. This is not a genetic trait but rather an acquired one. The neutropenia probably results from an abnormal release of neutrophils by the bone marrow. The WBC count ranges from 3,000–4,000 in African-Americans. There is a normal response to infections, steroids, and pregnancy.

133. What causes the hyperpigmentation of chronic venous stasis?

The breakdown of RBCs as they pass through small blood vessels in the dermis, over a long period of time, leads to the hyperpigmentation.

134. What is the classic tetrad in Henoch-Schönlein purpura?

Palpable purpura, arthralgia or arthritis, abdominal pain, and hematuria.

135. Name the three phases of discoloration in Raynaud's phenomenon.

Pallor (white)—Vasospasm
Cyanosis (blue)—Digital ischemia
Rubor (red)—Reperfusion

136. What criteria must be met to diagnose rheumatoid arthritis (RA)?

RA affects 0.3–1.5% of the U.S. population, most commonly women in the fourth to sixth decades. For a definitive diagnosis, at least 4 of the following 7 criteria must be met:

American Rheumatism Association 1987 Revised Criteria for the Classification of Rheumatoid Arthritis

CRITERION	DEFINITION
1. Morning stiffness	Morning stiffness in and around the joints, lasting at least 1 hr before maximal improvement
2. Arthritis of ≥3 joint areas	At least 3 joint areas simultaneously have had soft tissue swelling or fluid (not bony overgrowth alone) observed by a physician. The 14 possible areas are right or left PIP, MCP, wrist, elbow, knee, ankle, and MTP joints.
3. Arthritis of hand joints	At least 1 area swollen (as defined above) in a wrist, MCP, or PIP joint
4. Symmetric arthritis	Simultaneous involvement of the same joint areas (as defined in 2) on both sides of the body (bilateral involvement of PIPs, MCPs, or MTPs is acceptable without absolute symmetry)
5. Rheumatoid nodules	Subcutaneous nodules, over bony prominences, extensor surfaces, or in juxtaarticular regions, observed by a physician
6. Serum rheumatoid factor (RF)	Demonstration of abnormal amounts of serum RF by any method for which the result has been positive in <5% of normal control subjects
7. Radiographic changes	Radiographic changes typical of RA on posteroanterior hand and wrist radiographs, which must include erosions or unequivocal bony decalcification localized in or most marked adjacent to the involved joints (osteoarthritis changes alone do not quality)

Criteria 1–4 must have been present for at least 6 weeks.

Schumacher HR (ed): Primer on the Rheumatic Diseases, 10th ed. Atlanta, The Arthritis Foundation, 1993, p 328.

BIBLIOGRAPHY

1. Hurst JW (ed): Medicine for the Practicing Physician, 3rd ed. Boston, Butterworth, 1992.
2. Kelley WN, et al (eds): Textbook of Internal Medicine, 2nd ed. Philadelphia, J.B. Lippincott, 1991.
3. Conn RB (ed): Current Diagnosis, 8th ed. Philadelphia, W.B. Saunders, 1991.
4. Dale D, Federman D (eds): Scientific American Medicine. New York, Scientific American, 1996.
5. Tierney LM, et al (eds): Current Medical Diagnosis & Treatment, 36th ed. Norwalk, CT, Appleton & Lange, 1997.
6. Stein JH (ed): Internal Medicine, 4th ed. St. Louis, Mosby, 1995.
7. Isselbacher KJ, et al (eds): Harrison's Principles of Internal Medicine, 13th ed. New York, McGraw-Hill, 1994.
8. Bennett JC, et al (eds): Cecil Textbook of Medicine, 20th ed. Philadelphia, W.B. Saunders, 1996.
9. Kelley WN, et al (eds): Essentials of Internal Medicine. Philadelphia, J.B. Lippincott, 1994.

2. ENDOCRINOLOGY

Douglas W. Axelrod, M.D., Ph.D.

It would indeed be rash for a mere pathologist to venture forth on the uncharted sea of the endocrines, strewn as it is with the wrecks of shattered hypotheses, where even the most wary mariner may easily lose his way as he seeks to steer his bark amid the glandular temptations whose siren voices have proved the downfall of many who have gone before.

William Boyd (1885–1972)
Pathology for the Surgeon, 7th edition, Ch. 32

1. Who was William of Ockham (or Occam)? What was his razor? How did he die?

William of Ockham, known as Doctor Invincibilis, was a 14th century philosopher. His "razor," a philosophical means of choosing doctrinal postulates, was *"Essentia non sunt multiplicanda praetor necessitatum,"* or "Entities [or postulates] are not to be multiplied without necessity." We use Occam's razor to choose the fewest etiologies to explain multiple problems. Ironically, William of Ockham died of multiple causes (Axelrod's corollary to Occam's razor).

2. What is the most important thing in approaching a patient (according to Zen master Ikkyu)?

Attention. Before one takes the history or does the physical, one should attend fully to the patient and thereby maximize the appreciation of the sensory data that are incoming. Failure to do so leads to the prejudicial selection of data and may bring about an erroneous or incomplete diagnosis.

DIABETES AND METABOLISM

3. How does one calculate caloric needs in prescribing a diet?

Make an initial estimate of caloric needs by multiplying the patient's weight by the energy use per kilogram based on activity level. Bedrest is estimated to use 20–25 cal/kg/day; desk work uses 30; work including walking uses up to 35; very active physical labor uses 40–50. These estimates may be used as a first approximation but should be adjusted as the patient demonstrates his or her own caloric needs.

4. How many calories must one lack each day to lose 1 lb a week?

One pound of fat stores approx. 3,500 cal. Thus, one must establish a deficit of 500 cal each day to lose 1 lb of fat each week. Of course, overall weight loss entails a day-to-day balance of salt, water, and muscle, as well as fat, so that this calculation may not match changes in the actual measured body weight.

5. What are the current recommendations for the distribution of dietary nutrients?

Protein	20%
Fat	30%
Carbohydrate*	45–50%

The carbohydrate portion is preferably made up of complex carbohydrates.

6. What is C-peptide?

C-peptide is the fragment that is clipped out of the center of the original insulin polypeptide after sulfhydryl bonding has connected what will become the α and β chains. It is secreted from

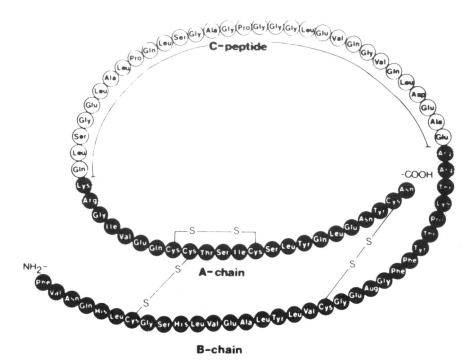

Amino acid sequence and covalent structure of human proinsulin. (From Skyler JS: Insulin dependent diabetes mellitus. In Kohler PO (ed): Clinical Endocrinology. New York, Churchill Livingstone, 1986, p 505; with permission.)

the pancreatic β-cells with insulin on an equimolar basis and may be used in assessing endogenous insulin secretion.

7. What factors influence glucose control? Which factors may be modulated?

Glucose control is an overall result of the balance between glucose production and disposal. Glucose production is controlled by gluconeogenic substrate supply and the hormonal environment, including insulin, growth hormone, cortical, glucagon, and catecholamines.

Glucose disposal may be divided into two processes. The first is cellular uptake, governed by actual caloric needs created by exercise and by circulating insulin. Second, disposal is controlled in part by renal losses when the circulating glucose concentration exceeds the maximum renal threshold (T_{max}).

In the diabetic patient, production may be modulated by diet, exercise, insulin, or hypoglycemic agent selection and by the avoidance of stressors.

8. What is the average hepatic glucose production per day? What does this suggest about hyperglycemia attributed to routine intravenous fluids?

Within the first 24 hours of fasting, the liver generates roughly 180 gm of glucose for metabolic support. The usual regimen of 125 ml/hr of 5% dextrose would provide 150 gm of glucose per day. Obviously this amount should be easily tolerated, so hyperglycemia cannot be attributed to the IV fluids used.

9. Where does the major clearance of insulin occur?

Insulin has approx. 50% clearance on first pass through the liver. Once in the periphery, roughly 30% of the remainder is cleared by the kidney.

10. What is the difference between Type I and Type II diabetes?

Type I diabetes is defined as that form of glucose intolerance in which diabetic ketoacidosis (DKA) will ensue without exogenous insulin. **Type II** diabetes is glucose intolerance in which DKA does not occur (barring extraordinary stress). These two forms have similarities to the former designations juvenile-onset and adult-onset diabetes, respectively. Note that the type of diabetes is not dependent on whether or not the patient uses insulin.

11. What are some causes of secondary diabetes?

Causes of Secondary Diabetes

Processes causing reduced insulin secretion:

Pancreatitis or pancreatectomy	Somatostatinoma
Cystic fibrosis	Aldosteronoma
Hemochromatosis	Hypokalemia
Pheochromocytoma	

Processes producing impairment of insulin action:

Insulin receptor defects	Diseases producing excess anti-insulin hormones
With acanthosis nigricans	Pheochromocytoma
Insulin receptor antibodies	Cushing's syndrome
Anti-insulin antibodies	Acromegaly
	Glucagonoma
	Thyrotoxicosis

Diseases producing secondary diabetes by unknown mechanism:

Muscular dystrophy	Friedreich's ataxia	Chromosomal abnormalities
Myotonic dystrophy	Lawrence-Moon-Biedl syndrome	Klinefelter's syndrome
Acute intermittent porphyria	Progeria	Turner's syndrome
Glycogen storage disease, type I	Prader-Willi syndrome	Down's syndrome
Hyperlipidemia		Sexual ateliotic dwarfism

From Garber AJ: Diabetes mellitus. In Stein JH (ed): Internal Medicine, 3rd ed. Boston, Little, Brown, 1990, p 2244, with permission.

12. How is type II diabetes diagnosed?

The diagnosis is made by demonstrating one of the following diagnostic criteria:

1. Classic symptoms of uncontrolled diabetes (polydypsia, polyuria, rapid weight loss) along with unequivocal elevation of random blood sugar (>200 mg/dl).

2. Fasting venous plasma glucose > 140 mg/dl on > 1 occasion.

3. Fasting venous plasma glucose > 115 mg/dl.

and

4. Oral glucose tolerance test with 2-hour value and one other value both at least 200 mg/dl.

13. What do the terms insulin-dependent, insulin-requiring, and insulin-using mean?

You must bear in mind the definitions of type I and II diabetes. A person using the terms **insulin-dependent** and **insulin-requiring** may mean that the patient lapses into DKA without insulin, indicating type I diabetes. Alternatively, however, the person may mean that the patient cannot be rendered euglycemic without the use of insulin. **Insulin-using** is a helpful term when used to describe a type II diabetic, suggesting that the patient has failed control on diet and/or oral agents and has therefore been placed on insulin therapy. These descriptions are prone to misinterpretation and should not be used as diagnostic terms.

14. In diabetic ketoacidosis, what are the usual deficits of sodium, potassium, and water?

	Total	*Per Kg Body Weight*
Water	5–11 liters	100 ml
Sodium	300–700 meq	7 meq
Chloride	350–500 meq	5 meq
Potassium	200–700 meq	5 meq
Phosphate	70–100 mmole	1 mmole

15. Continuous IV insulin is the usual means of insulin administration. What dose should be used?

After an IV bolus of 0.1 U/kg, infusion should begin at 0.1 U/kg/hr. After this rate is initiated, blood glucose should be carefully followed and insulin administration tailored to the individual patient.

16. How does one convert to intermittent insulin after IV therapy?

Begin a regimen of intermediate and short-acting insulins, starting with 75% of the IV dose administered over the previous 24 hours. On discontinuing IV insulin, be sure to give the subcutaneous (SC) insulin for a long enough period before stopping the IV insulin to allow the SCQ insulin to act.

17. When would one choose human insulin over another source?

Patients started on insulin should be started on human insulin. Patients experiencing lipodystrophy or in whom insulin resistance becomes problematic may benefit from switching to human insulin. Otherwise, there is no pressing reason to change insulin species in a well-controlled diabetic.

18. Why is there a high frequency of recurrent DKA in the alcoholic or malnourished patient? How can this complication be avoided?

Such patients are often depleted of potential glucogenic substrates, with low liver glycogen stores and even frank muscle wasting. If adequate glucose is not administered during the first 24–48 hours of therapy, there will be a tendency for recrudescence of the ketosis, burning adipose tissue because of the lack of gluconeogenic substrate. This may be prevented by glucose loading during this period, using insulin to ensure repletion of glycogen. Also, you should avoid cutting back on glucose therapy in an attempt to modulate circulating glucose levels. This should be accomplished by using insulin.

19. How is the management of hypertension different in the diabetic? Why?

Hypertension is implicated in accelerating the microangiopathy of diabetes, particularly the retinopathy and nephropathy. Therapy should be more aggressive, initiated at a blood pressure 5–10 mm Hg less than conventional therapeutic guidelines indicate.

20. What are the antihypertensives of choice for diabetics? Which ones should be avoided and why?

In the diabetic, the antihypertensives chosen should not worsen glucose or lipid control; they should not block normal "alerting" or counter-regulatory mechanisms if hypoglycemia should occur; and finally, they should not antagonize common neurologic defects in diabetes, such as autonomic insufficiency and impotency. Among the most-used agents in hypertensive diabetics, angiotensin-converting enzyme (ACE) inhibitors have been shown to slow the progression of diabetic nephropathy. Calcium-channel blocking agents provide pressure reduction without adverse effects on lipids, glucose control, or autonomic interference. Alpha-blocking agents may also provide smoother control and an improved lipid profile.

Beta-blocking agents should be used with extreme care because of their blockade of hypoglycemic responses, degraded lipid profile, and incidence of impotence. Thiazide diuretics may also create worsened glucose and lipid profiles.

21. What are the kinetics of action of regular, NPH, and Ultralente insulin?

Type	Onset (hr)	Peak (hr)	Duration (hr)
Regular	1/4–1	2–5	4–8
NPH	1–4	4–12	12–24
Ultralente	3–5	10–30	24–36

NPH=neutral protamine Hagedorn.

22. What steps can be taken to avoid or slow the progression of diabetic nephropathy?
Excellent glucose control
Excellent blood pressure control
ACE inhibitors
Protein restriction

23. How often should diabetics see an ophthalmologist?
Type I diabetics—After 5 years of disease and at least yearly thereafter.
Type II diabetics—start yearly check-ups at diagnosis.

24. To which type of ear infection is the diabetic predisposed? How is it treated?
Malignant otitis externa, an infection of the external auditory canal due to *Pseudomonas aeruginosa,* is mainly seen in elderly diabetic patients. It is an invasive and necrotizing infection with a high mortality, mainly due to meningitis. The typical clinical presentation consists of pain in the ear with or without a purulent drainage, swelling of the parotid gland, trismus, and paralysis of the 6th through 12th cranial nerves. Treatment consists of antipseudomonal antibiotics with or without surgical debridement.

25. Why might a diabetic's insulin requirement drop?
Success in weight control
Improved exercise program
Change in type or brand of insulin
Decrease in renal function (lessened insulin clearance)

26. What is a reliable sign that the house officer has done a good job in seeing a diabetic patient in clinic?
The patient has his or her shoes off. A careful examination of the feet of a diabetic is a necessary part of comprehensive care. The patient must be taught to self-examine the feet and to administer proper foot care.

27. When are multiple injection regimens indicated for diabetes?
Inability to maintain pre- and postprandial glucose levels to near-normal on single-dose regimens.

28. When is an insulin pump indicated?
Patient and physician preference may lead a patient to use a pump instead of an intensive regimen (preprandial regular insulin plus intermediate or long-acting insulin). Failure of a well-monitored and executed intensive SC regimen is a reasonable indication for a pump. Pregnant patients often do well with insulin pumps.

29. What are the complications of multiple-injection regimens as compared to an insulin pump?
"Tight" glucose control may lead to loss of autonomic and cognitive appreciation of hypoglycemia (hypoglycemic unawareness). The lack of a depot of SC insulin leads to rapid loss of control in the event of pump failure. This carries the potential for rapid hyperglycemia.

30. What is the Somogyi phenomenon? What are its signs and symptoms?
This process is hyperglycemia following hypoglycemia, known parochially as "the bounce." The overuse of insulin with attendant hypoglycemia causes counter-regulatory stress-hormone secretion, most notably glucagon, growth hormone, cortisol, and catecholamines. These agents lead to a rebound hyperglycemia, which may be confused with under-insulinization and result in mistaken therapy with larger doses of insulin.
This hypoglycemia and rebound hyperglycemia phenomenon often occurs at night, with high glucose on awakening. The symptoms include poor sleep, nightmares, nighttime diaphoresis, and

morning headache. The signs include hyperglycemia with positive urine ketones, the latter related to the hypoglycemia and fatty acid released. Early-morning home blood glucose surveillance may document the hypoglycemic pattern.

31. How may type II diabetics be treated?
Diet, exercise, oral agents, and insulin can be used.

32. What hypoglycemic agents are currently most useful?
Glipizide and **glyburide** are both sulfonylureas and are the most commonly used oral agents. They are true "hypoglycemic" agents in that their major action is to lower blood glucose through increased insulin release.

Although used widely in Europe, **metformin** was recently introduced into the United States. It is one of the biguanide class, which increases glucose utilization primarily through increasing glucose transport. It does not lower glucose in normal subjects and leads to lower insulin levels and improved lipid profiles, particularly in obese patients. It may also minimize weight gain. Metformin may be added to a sulfonylurea as a secondary agent or may be considered as primary therapy in the obese Type II diabetic.

Oral Agents for Diabetes Therapy

GENERIC NAME	BRAND NAMES	STRENGTH (MG)	DOSAGE RANGE (MG)	MAJOR TOXICITIES
Glyburide	Micronase, DiaBeta, Glynase	1.25, 2.5, 5	2.5–20	Hypoglycemia
Glipizide	Glucotrol	5, 10	5–40	Hypoglycemia
Metformin	Glucophage	500, 850		Lactic Acidosis

U.K. Prospective Diabetes Study Group. BMJ 310:83–88, 1995.

33. What factor may lead you to choose one hypoglycemic agent over another?
Both metformin and another member of the biguanide class, phenformin, have been associated with the development of lactic acidosis, particularly in the presence of renal or hepatic insufficiency or in circumstances of poor tissue perfusion. Metformin appears to have considerably less tendency toward this complication, but care should be used to avoid its use in renal or hepatic insufficiency and in the setting of vascular insufficiency.

34. How do fasting and reactive hypoglycemia differ? What are the types of reactive hypoglycemia?
Fasting hypoglycemia develops in the absence of substrate intake and is aggravated by prolonged fasting. **Reactive** hypoglycemia occurs within a characteristic time after eating. Three forms of reactive hypoglycemia have been described:

1. The alimentary form, most often seen in dumping syndrome, shows a rapid increase in blood glucose followed by a rapid decrease.

2. Early type II diabetes often shows a slower-than-normal rise in blood glucose, which rises to supranormal levels, followed by an exaggerated drop in glucose at 3–5 hours.

3. The idiopathic form does not show the exaggerated increase in blood glucose prior to a late fall to subnormal levels. This group may contain defects in gluconeogenic enzymes as well as in insulin and other gut hormone release.

35. How is C-peptide useful in assessing the etiology of fasting hypoglycemia?
C-peptide is absent in commercial insulin preparations. High endogenous insulin levels should be accompanied by high C-peptide levels. High insulin levels with low C-peptide levels are strongly suggestive of exogenous insulin use.

36. Describe the biochemical mechanism for alcohol-induced hypoglycemia.
The oxidation of alcohol to acetaldehyde increases the NADH:NAD ratio, which in turn pushes the lactate:pyruvate redox pair toward lactate. Low pyruvate levels slow gluconeogenesis, and this can lead to hypoglycemia.

37. What is hemoglobin A1-C? What does it reflect?

Hemoglobin Al-C (glycohemoglobin) is hemoglobin glycosylated by nonenzymatic means. The percentage of glycohemoglobin in the circulation is indicative of the average ambient glucose concentration over the prior 4–8 weeks. The measurement of hemoglobin Al-C can be used as an indicator of the degree of glucose control over that time period.

PITUITARY

38. How is prolactin secretion regulated, and how is it different from the other anterior pituitary hormones? And while you're at it, name them.

Prolactin is primarily controlled by negative feedback from the hypothalamus via the portal system. Prolactin inhibitory factor (PIF) has been identified as dopamine, so that dopamine and dopamine agonists suppress the secretion of prolactin. Thyrotropin releasing hormone (TRH) is a mild positive modulator of prolactin secretion. However, the major control is exerted by negative feedback.

The other anterior pituitary hormones are positively stimulated by hypothalamic-releasing hormones: **luteinizing** (LH) and **follicle-stimulating hormones** (FSH) by gonadotropin-releasing hormone (GnRH), **thyrotropin** by thyrotropin-releasing hormone (TRH), **growth hormone** (GH) by growth-hormone-releasing hormone (GH-RH) (and negatively by somatostatin), and **ACTH** by corticotropin-releasing hormone (CRH).

39. How does prolactinoma usually present in women? In men?

Women usually present with interference of the menstrual cycle and galactorrhea (amenorrhea-galactorrhea syndrome). These changes are effected by relatively low prolactin levels, characteristically seen with very small prolactinomas.

Men usually present with impotence or with effects from the tumor mass. These changes are seen much later than those seen in women and therefore are associated with larger tumors.

40. What are the therapeutic options for prolactinomas?

Bromocriptine, a dopamine agonist, is very effective in shrinking prolactinomas, even those of very large size. **Surgery** is usually reserved for women wishing pregnancy and in whom the tumor is large enough to cause concern should it expand during pregnancy. Larger tumors have a high recurrence rate after surgery.

41. What medical therapies may be used in acromegaly?

Transsphenoidal surgery and irradiation, of course, are the primary therapeutic modalities in acromegaly, but dopamine agonists (bromocriptine) are the medication of choice when surgery is contraindicated or fails. Octreotide, a somatostatin analogue, reduces tumor size in about 50% of patients but produces only a 25–50% reduction in tumor size.

42. How is IGF-1 (somatomedin C) used in the management of acromegaly?

Monitoring IGF-1 (insulin-like growth factor-1) levels allows assessment of the efficacy of initial therapy and follow-up in the posttherapeutic period.

43. Which circulating protein may help in diagnosing a gonadotropin-secreting pituitary tumor?

The α subunit, which is common to the glycoprotein hormones LH, FSH, and TSH, is elevated in many of these cases.

44. Why would a woman with hypothyroidism have galactorrhea?

If her hypothyroidism is primary (i.e., due to thyroid gland dysfunction), the lack of feedback at the hypothalamus leads to an elevation of TRH, which is also a positive modulator of prolactin release.

45. What causes panhypopituitarism?

Etiologies of Hypopituitarism

Tumors	Infarction (cont.)	Infiltrative disease (cont.)
Pituitary adenomas	Diabetes necrosis	Lymphoma
Craniopharyngiomas	Trauma with stalk section	Lymphocytic hypophysitis
Metastatic carcinoma	Epidemic hemorrhagic fever	Hemochromatosis
Primary pituitary carcinoma	Malaria	
Meningioma	Arteritis	**Miscellaneous causes**
	Sickle cell anemia (crisis)	Pituitary abscess
Infarction		Aneurysm
Pituitary adenomas (pituitary	**Infiltrative disease**	Radiation therapy
apoplexy)	Sarcoidosis	Congenital absence of pituitary
Postpartum pituitary necrosis	Eosinophilic granuloma	Therapeutic ablation
(Sheehan's syndrome)	Leukemia	Hypothalamic disease

Boyd, et al: Disorders of the hypothalamus and anterior pituitary. In Kohler PO (ed): Clinical Endocrinology. New York, John Wiley, 1986, p 44.

46. How closely is antidiuretic hormone (ADH) release related to osmolarity? How much volume must one lose to trigger ADH release?

An osmolarity change of < 1% will produce changes in ADH secretion. A loss of 10–15% of circulating volume will trigger ADH secretion.

47. Why is cortisol deficiency associated with hyponatremia?

It appears that cortisol negatively modulates the release of ADH and that its deficiency is associated with a syndrome of inappropriate antidiuretic hormone-like (SIADH-like) physiology.

This is to be distinguished from the hyponatremia and hyperkalemia seen in primary adrenal deficiency with both cortisol and aldosterone deficiency. In that setting, aldosterone deficiency leads to potassium retention and sodium loss. The loss of sodium and volume contributes to an appropriate increase in ADH.

48. What is DDAVP? How is it used?

DDAVP, or desmopressin, is 1-desamino-8-D-arginine vasopressin, a long-acting ADH analogue, which may be administered intranasally, IV, or subQ. Its long action allows it to be used intranasally on a once- or twice-daily basis for diabetes insipidus.

ADRENAL

49. How much cortisol can the normal adrenal axis make during stress in one day? How, then, should "stress steroids" be administered for patients adrenally insufficient for surgery or in sepsis?

Estimates of maximal adrenal output range from 125–300 mg cortisol/24 hrs. The usual approach for treatment of a high-stress period in a patient deemed adrenally insufficient is to administer 100 mg of hydrocortisone IV every 6–8 hrs. The use of amounts greater than this is not directed to physiologic adrenal replacement but rather for pharmacologic effects.

50. What is the distinction between Cushing's syndrome and Cushing's disease?

Cushing's syndrome is the symptom complex produced by an excess of adrenal corticosteroids. **Cushing's disease** is the most common cause of Cushing's syndrome, accounting for about two-thirds of all cases. It is caused by pituitary overproduction of ACTH, leading to bilateral adrenal hyperplasia. Other causes of Cushing's syndrome include excess cortisol production originating in the adrenal gland (adrenal adenoma or carcinoma), excess production of ACTH from a nonpituitary source (ectopic ACTH syndrome), and iatrogenic or factitious ingestion of excess exogenous corticosteroids.

51. Is there an indication for a random cortisol or ACTH measurement in the diagnosis of Cushing's disease?

No. These tests are not reliable in screening for Cushing's disease.

52. What are the signs and symptoms of Cushing's disease?

Skin	Endocrine	Adipose tissue
Atrophic, thin skin	Amenorrhea	Weight gain
Easy bruising	Diabetes	Truncal obesity
Broad, purple striae on hips, abdomen, axillae	Hypertension	Fat deposition in supraclavicular area and dorsum of back (buffalo hump)
Hair loss	**Immune system**	Moon facies
Tinea versicolor	Susceptible to infections	
	Poor wound healing	

Muscles	Skeleton	Psychiatric	Sexual characteristics (women)
Muscle wasting	Osteoporosis	Psychosis	Hirsutism
Decreased strength	Chronic backache	Paranoia	Deepened voice
	Bone pain	Mood swings	Clitoral enlargement

53. Which are the most reliable physical findings in Cushing's syndrome?

Purple striae and thinning of the skin. Proximal muscle weakness may also be striking and unexpected until tested.

54. How should one screen for Cushing's syndrome?

a. Low-dose dexamethasone suppression test: 1 mg of dexamethasone at midnight should suppress 8 A.M. cortisol to < 5 µg/dl, *or*

b. Collection of a 24-hr urine for urinary free cortisol: should be < 100 µg/24 hr.

The dexamethasone suppression test may yield false positive results in depression, obesity, or in patients taking phenobarbital.

55. What is Addison's disease? What causes it?

Addison's disease is primary adrenal insufficiency. It is due to a failure of the adrenals to produce sufficient amounts of adrenal corticosteroids. Autoimmune destruction is responsible in approx. 80% of cases, and adrenal destruction by tuberculosis (TB) in approx. 20% of cases. Other rare causes include adrenal destruction by bilateral hemorrhage or infarction, tumor, infections (other than TB), surgery, radiation, drugs, amyloidosis, sarcoidosis, hyporesponsiveness to ACTH, and congenital abnormalities. Symptoms of adrenal insufficiency require loss of >90% of both adrenal cortices.

56. What are the major symptoms and signs of Addison's disease?

Symptoms	Signs
Hyperpigmentation	Hyperpigmentation (most prominent on
Weakness	skinfolds, extensor surfaces, pressure points,
Fatigue	buccal mucosa and gums, nipples, areolae,
Anorexia	perivaginal and perianal mucosa, and newly
Weight loss	formed scars)
Salt craving	Hyperkalemia (usually mild)
Nausea	Weight loss
Diarrhea	Orthostatic hypotension
Postural dizziness	Adrenal calcifications
	Vitiligo

57. How do primary and secondary adrenal insufficiency differ in their presentation? Why?

Primary adrenal insufficiency (Addison's disease) is caused by failure or destruction of the adrenal glands, leading to underproduction of glucocorticoids and mineralocorticoids. This results in an increase in ACTH production by the pituitary. Its signs and symptoms are described in Question 56. **Secondary** adrenal insufficiency (SAI) is caused by deficient production of ACTH, leading to underproduction of glucocorticoids. The manifestations are the same as those of Addison's disease, except for the following:

1. Hyperpigmentation is not seen. This is a product of the hypersecretion of ACTH and its related peptides (including melanocyte-stimulating hormone), which is not present in SAI.

2. Signs and symptoms due to a deficiency of mineralocorticoids are not seen. Since mineralocorticoid activity is largely regulated by the renin-angiotensin system and not ACTH, these manifestations of Addison's disease are lacking in SAI.

3. Other manifestations of hypopituitarism may be seen with SAI.

4. Hypoglycemia is more commonly seen with SAI due to the presence of combined ACTH and growth hormone deficiency.

58. How is adrenal axis reserve tested?

An insulin tolerance test (ITT) provokes hyperfunction of the entire axis by inducing hypoglycemia. If adequate hypoglycemia is produced, the test has some predictive capacity for subsequent stress. Patients with seizure disorders or cardiac disease may not be candidates for ITT-induced hypoglycemia, but in them, metyrapone may be used.

59. What does metyrapone do? How is it used?

Metyrapone inhibits the 11-hydroxylase step of cortisol synthesis, causing accumulation of 11-deoxycortisol, which does not provide feedback inhibition at the hypothalamus. The administration of metyrapone therefore causes an intact axis to hyperfunction, with accumulation of 11-deoxycortisol, which may then be measured.

It is also important to measure cortisol, which should be low. If cortisol is not low, there has been inadequate enzyme inhibition, and the test is not adequate.

60. How do you wean a patient off corticosteroids?

First, place the patient on a short-acting corticosteroid, such as prednisone or hydrocortisone, on a twice daily basis. Next, the evening dose should be weaned down, leaving a solitary morning dose. By this time, hydrocortisone should be substituted for prednisone. As the morning dose is weaned toward a physiologic level (20 mg), the next morning's cortisol may be measured. When a normal AM cortisol is attained, daily supplementation may be stopped. However, the patient should still use supplements for stress until an insulin tolerance test or metyrapone test documents adequate hypothalamic-pituitary-adrenal axis response to stress.

61. How should an incidentally found adrenal mass be evaluated? What parameters are of importance?

Because roughly 2% of patients demonstrate an incidental adrenal tumor by CT, screening should be thoughtful. Tumors > 3 cm are most likely to be primary or metastatic carcinomas and CT-guided biopsy should be considered. The most common functioning adrenal tumor secretes corticosteroids. Therefore, low-dose dexamethasone screening may be appropriate.

In the absence of family history, hypertension, or symptoms, pheochromocytoma is unlikely. Otherwise, urinary metanephrines and catecholamines may be obtained. In the presence of isolated hypertension with or without attendant hypokalemia, a single aldosterone and plasma renin activity (PRA) may be used to test for an aldosterone-secreting tumor, looking for an aldosterone:PRA ratio ≥ 25.

62. What are the differences among the ACTH stimulation test, insulin tolerance test (ITT), and metyrapone tests? What are the appropriate settings for their use?

ITT and metyrapone tests evaluate the response of the entire adrenal axis. The ACTH stimulation test stimulates only the adrenal glands. This test will suggest adrenal insufficiency when there had been prolonged defect anywhere in the adrenal axis or when there had been direct adrenal damage.

63. What is the rapid ACTH stimulation test?

This test is used to assess adrenal function; 250 μg of synthetic ACTH (cosyntropin, Cortrosyn) is administered to the patient, and cortisol levels are measured at 0 and 60 min. A normal cortisol response to the ACTH rules out primary adrenal insufficiency. Lack of a normal response indicates decreased adrenal reserve but does not differentiate between primary and secondary adrenal insufficiency.

64. How do you differentiate primary and secondary adrenal insufficiency?

Plasma ACTH levels can be used in this differentiation. In the face of adrenal insufficiency, ACTH levels > 250 pg/ml are associated with primary adrenal insufficiency (usually 400–2000 pg/ml) and ACTH levels of 0–50 pg/ml are associated with pituitary ACTH deficiency (secondary adrenal insufficiency) (usually < 20 pg/ml).

65. Which aspect of the hypothalamic-pituitary-adrenal axis is last to return after suppression by exogenous corticosteroids?

Corticotropin-releasing hormone from the hypothalamus.

66. How does partial 17-hydroxylase deficiency present? How is it diagnosed?

This presents as hirsutism in the female. ACTH-stimulated 17-OH-progesterone levels will be elevated.

67. What gene do familial Hirschsprung's disease and multiple endocrine neoplasia (MEN) type 2B have in common?

The *ret* proto-oncogene is mutated in both conditions. Familial Hirschsprung's disease has a mutation that causes nonexpression with resultant disordered neuronal development of the colon. An activating mutation results in MEN 2B.

68. Categorize the MEN syndromes.

MEN 1	**Variants of MEN 2A**
Parathyroid neoplasia	Familial medullary thyroid carcinoma only
Pituitary neoplasia	MEN 2A with Hirschsprung's disease
Pancreatic islet-cell tumors	MEN 2A with cutaneous lichen amyloidosis
Other manifestations	
Carcinoid	**MEN 2B**
Lipomas	Medullary thyroid carcinoma
	Pheochromocytoma
MEN 2A	Mucosal and alimentary tract ganglioneuromatosis
Medullary thyroid carcinoma	Marfanoid features
Pheochromocytoma	Absence of parathyroid neoplasia
Parathyroid neoplasia	

Gagel RF: Multiple endocrine neoplasia. Endocrinol Metabol Clin North Am 23: 1994.

69. Why is β-blockade of a pheochromocytoma a bad idea as initial therapy?

Pheochromocytomas may secrete epinephrine, norepinephrine, or both. Because β-adrenergic activity dilates peripheral blood vessels, β-adrenergic blockade in the presence of unopposed α-agonists may lead to net peripheral vasoconstriction and an exacerbation of the patient's hypertension.

70. What are the organs of Zuckerkandl?

These are rests of chromaffin tissue located in the para-aortic sympathetic chain in which extra-adrenal pheochromocytomas may arise.

71. What is the best screening test for primary hyperaldosteronism? How should a positive test be followed up?

An upright plasma aldosterone concentration and plasma renin activity (PRA), taken in the absence of drugs that alter the renin-aldosterone axis (such as most antihypertensives and diuretics). A ratio of aldosterone (ng/dl) to PRA (ng/ml/hr) of ≥ 25 is nearly 100% sensitive but has inadequate specificity (75–80%) for a definitive diagnosis. Confirmation requires a high 24-hour urine aldosterone level in the presence of normokalemia and adequate volume status.

72. How do you decide whether to treat hyperaldosteronism medically or surgically? What is the drug of choice?

Patients with unilateral aldosteronomas are best treated surgically. Patients who are poor operative risks or who have bilateral hyperplasia are best treated with a specific aldosterone receptor antagonist, spironolactone.

73. What are the most common settings for hyporeninemic hypoaldosteronism?

Type II diabetes
Interstitial nephritis
AIDS

THYROID

74. How much does the normal adult thyroid gland weigh?

15–20 grams

75. What are the goals and limitations of the various tests of the thyroid gland?

Comparison of Thyroid Tests

TEST	GOAL	COMMENTS
Total T_4	T_4 level	Detects 90% of hyperthyroid cases; affected by alterations of TBG and can be misleadingly high or low; FT_4 is only a fraction of the total T_4.
Free T_4 (FT_4)	Assessment of FT_4	Directly measures FT_4; independent of TBG levels.
Serum T_3	T_3 level	Used to detect hyperthyroidism; misleadingly low in patients with non-thyroidal illness (i.e., low value does not usually indicate hypothyroidism). Do not confuse with RT_3U.
RT_3U	Assessment of FT_4	Clarifies whether alterations in T_4 are due to thyroid disease or alteration in T_4 binding proteins. Does *not* measure T_3.
Radioactive iodine uptake (RAIU)	Extent of thyroid function	Normal range must be determined for each population district. Difficult to distinguish low from low-normal values when dietary iodine is high. Hyperthyroidism does not always cause high iodine uptake.
TSH level	Index of thyroid status	Most sensitive test for primary hyperthyroidism (TSH high before other tests show low T_4).
Thyroid scan	Functional status of nodular goiter	Often not needed in other types of thyroid disease.
Ultrasound	Status of single nodule	Reliably discriminates between cystic and solid nodules in 90% of cases.

TBG=Thyroxine-binding globulin; RT_3U=resin T_3 uptake test; TSH=thyroid-stimulating hormone.
Rubenstein E, et al (eds): Scientific American Medicine. New York, Scientific American, 1989.

76. What causes hyperthyroidism?

Hyperthyroidism is a syndrome resulting from the response to excess thyroid hormone levels. The excess thyroid hormone can come from hyperfunction of the thyroid gland, inflammation, destruction of all or part of the gland with resultant release of stored hormone, or from a source outside the thyroid. Separation of the causes by a low or high RAIU can help narrow the differential diagnosis:

Normal or High RAIU	**Low RAIU**
Graves' disease	Subacute thyroiditis
Toxic multinodular goiter	Hyperthyroiditis
Solitary toxic nodule	Factitious thyrotoxicosis
Hypothalamic-pituitary disease	Jod-Basedow phenomenon (iodine-induced
Choriocarcinoma or hydatidiform mole	thyrotoxicosis)
Tumor metastases to the thyroid	Metastatic thyroid carcinoma
	Struma ovarii (teratoma)

Kohler PO (ed): Clinical Endocrinology. New York, John Wiley, 1986, p 90.

77. Name the major signs and symptoms of hyperthyroidism.

Signs and Symptoms of Hyperthyroidism

SYSTEM	SYMPTOMS	SIGNS
↑ metabolic rate	Heat intolerance, increased appetite, weight loss	Sweating, ↓ muscle mass and fat; rarely fever
Cardiovascular	Palpitation; may have symptoms of heart failure	Tachycardia; hypertension (esp. systolic); arrhythmia (esp. atrial fibrillation); heart murmur or rub
Neuromuscular	Fatigue, muscular weakness	Tremor; ↑ deep tendon reflexes; proximal muscle weakness; rarely paralysis
Neuropsychiatric	Nervousness, irritability, depression, difficulty sleeping	Emotional lability, frank psychosis
Ophthalmologic	Eye irritation and stare,* photophobia,* diplopia,* brittle nails	Stare, lid retraction, lid lag, Graves' ophthalmopathy (proptosis, extra-ocular muscle dysfunction, optic neuropathy, chemosis)*
Skin, hair, nails	Alopecia, rash of pretibial myxedema,* ankle swelling,	Smooth, soft, warm skin; hair of fine texture and easily removable; edema; pretibial myxedema in Graves' disease*; onycholysis
Respiratory	Dyspnea	↑ respiratory rate
Gastrointestinal	↑ frequency and softening of stools	Usually normal; may be splenomegaly*
Reproductive	Oligomenorrhea, impotence	Gynecomastia
Other	Anorexia, constipation	Lymphadenopathy*

*These findings are not manifestations of increased circulating thyroid hormone levels but are related to the disturbance in the immune system that occurs in Graves' disease.

From Kohler PO (ed): Clinical Endocrinology. New York, John Wiley, 1986, p 93, with permission.

78. What is a thyroid storm?

Thyroid storm is a dramatic, life-threatening exacerbation of **thyrotoxicosis.** It is characterized by severe signs and symptoms of exaggerated thyrotoxicosis, with hypermetabolism, excessive adrenergic response, diaphoresis, and fever that, if untreated, can lead to death from cardiovascular collapse. There is usually marked tachycardia, widened pulse pressure, agitation, and delirium (or coma).

Thyroid storm is usually not associated with T_4 and T_3 levels markedly higher than the "pre-storm" values, and so its diagnosis must be made on clinical grounds. Thyroid storm can be initiated by another acute illness, such as infection, surgery, trauma to the thyroid, or withdrawal of partially effective antithyroid therapy.

79. How do you treat thyroid storm?

Treatment involves the use of propranolol to control the cardiovascular manifestations, IV saturated solution of potassium iodide (SSKI) to block the release of thyroid hormone, and propylthiouracil (PTU) to block thyroid hormone synthesis. The peripheral conversion of T_4 to T_3 is partially blocked by PTU, propranolol, and hydrocortisone. Supportive therapy, IV fluids, antipyretics, cooling blankets, and sedatives also play a role. In extreme cases, plasmapheresis or peritoneal dialysis have been used to remove thyroid hormone. In all cases, search for and treatment of the initiating condition should be undertaken.

80. Name the four basic mechanisms that lead to hypothyroidism.

Hypothyroidism is a clinical syndrome caused by the cellular responses to a deficiency of thyroid hormone. It can be produced by the following four mechanisms:

1. **Primary:** due to a pathologic process intrinsic to the thyroid gland, leading to defective production of thyroid hormone or destruction of the gland

2. **Secondary:** due to a deficiency of TSH stimulation of a normal thyroid gland

3. **Tertiary:** due to a deficiency of thyrotropin-releasing hormone (TRH) from the hypothalamus

4. **Peripheral resistance to the action of thyroid hormone:** a rare cause of hypothyroidism (Refetoff syndrome)

81. What are the causes of hypothyroidism?

Causes of Hypothyroidism

CLASSIFICATION	SPECIAL FEATURES
Primary	
Autoimmune (chronic thyroiditis, idiopathic, "burnt out" Graves' disease)	Thyroid antibodies positive in most cases; pernicious anemia and other primary endocrine deficiencies may coexist
Postablative	After radioactive iodine or surgery
Subacute thyroiditis	Transient phase, usually preceded by sore neck and thyrotoxicosis with low ^{131}I uptake
Drugs (iodines, lithium, thionamides)	Coexistent thyroiditis (autoimmune) prior to ablative therapy; recent history of drug administration
Thyroid agenesis	Most common cause in neonates
Thyroid dysgenesis	May cause juvenile hypothyroidism
Dyshormonogenesis	Goiter, family history
Head and neck irradiation	History of treatment with radiation
Neoplasia	Primary or metastatic tumor (rare)
Secondary	Associated with low TSH; impaired TSH response to TRH, when present, is helpful in diagnosis. Requires thorough evaluation for underlying cause of pituitary failure
Tertiary	Same as secondary, except TSH response to TRH is usually preserved
Peripheral resistance	Raised levels of thyroid hormone and TSH

From Kohler PO (ed): Clinical Endocrinology. New York, John Wiley, 1986, p 105, with permission.

82. What are the major signs and symptoms of hypothyroidism?

Signs and Symptoms of Hypothyroidism

SYSTEM	SYMPTOMS	SIGNS
↓ Metabolic rate	Cold intolerance, ↓ appetite, weight gain	Obesity, hypothermia
Neuromuscular	Muscle cramps, joint stiffness, paresthesias, weakness	Delayed deep tendon reflexes, ↑ muscle mass and rigidity, myotonia, joint effusions, carpal tunnel syndrome
		In infants: mental retardation, short stature
Neuropsychiatric	Lethargy, ↓ energy, ↑ sleeping	Delirium, dementia, frank psychosis
Skin, hair, and nails	Dry skin, hair loss, straightened hair, brittle nails, edema	Cool, thin, scaling skin; alopecia; coarse hair; myxedema (esp. face and periorbital tissues)
Cardiovascular	Angina	Bradycardia, hypertension, cardiomegaly with effusion ("myxedema heart")
Ear, nose and throat	Hoarseness, hearing loss, altered taste/smell, vertigo	Deep voice, slow speech, conductive hearing loss, enlarged tongue
Respiratory	Dyspnea	Reduced inspiratory effort, pleural effusion
Gastrointestinal	Epigastric pain, constipation	Abdominal distention rarely toxic megacolon
Reproductive	Infertility, impotence In children: Precocious puberty, delayed puberty	Galactorrhea

From Kohler PO (ed): Clinical Endocrinology. New York, John Wiley, 1986, p 109, with permission.

83. Describe the pathogenesis of Graves' disease.

Graves' disease is an autoimmune disease in which T lymphocytes produce antibodies to certain thyroid antigens. Thyroid-stimulating immunoglobulin (TSI) is an antibody to the TSH receptor on the thyroid cells, which results in stimulation of growth and function. The cause of the autoimmune process is not known.

84. What is the NO-SPECS classification for Graves' ophthalmopathy?

CHANGE	CLASS
N—No signs or symptoms	0
O—Only signs	1
S—Soft tissue involvement	2
P—Proptosis	3
E—Extraocular muscle involvement	4
C—Corneal involvement	5
S—Sight loss in visual acuity	6

Graves' ophthalmopathy does not necessarily progress in order of the NO-SPECS classes.

85. Which antithyroid drugs are used for hyperthyroidism? Which is unsafe in pregnancy?
Methimazole (Tapazole) and propylthiouracil (PTU). Methimazole has been associated with aphasia cutis in the newborn and is therefore not used in pregnancy in the U.S.

86. Which characteristics are predictive of spontaneous remission in Graves' disease?
Small thyroid gland
Young age
Female sex
Acute onset of disease
Low antithyroid antibody titers

87. What therapies are available for Graves' ophthalmopathy? What are their indications?
Medical therapy may include the use of corticosteroids and/or cyclosporine. Steroids may be useful in moderate-to-severe disease. Cyclosporine may be useful as an adjunct in therapeutic failure.

Nonmedical therapy includes radiotherapy to the orbit and surgical decompression. These methods are usually reserved for the more severe complications, such as corneal involvement or visual compromise.

88. How do the antibody profiles differ in Graves' disease, Hashimoto's thyroiditis, and subacute thyroiditis?
Hashimoto's thyroiditis has an increased prevalence of high titers of antimicrosomal and antithyroid antibodies. Graves' patients often have high titers of antithyroid antibodies and thyroid-stimulating immunoglobulin. Subacute thyroiditis is rarely associated with short-lived elevations of antithyroid antibodies, usually in low titers.

89. What is hashitoxicosis?
This term is used when Hashimoto's thyroiditis is associated with hyperthyroidism secondary to uncontrolled release of thyroid hormone.

90. What is Jod-Basedow phenomenon? What is its mechanism of occurrence?
Jod-Basedow phenomenon is hyperthyroidism resulting from an iodine load. It is usually seen in the setting of endemic goiter, multinodular goiter, or Graves' disease previously treated with antithyroid drugs. Any source of iodine, including contrast media, iodine-containing expectorants, or kelp, may induce this process.

91. Discuss the natural history and treatment of subacute thyroiditis.
Usually a prodromal viral-like syndrome is followed 2–3 weeks later by thyroid or ear pain, sometimes with dysphagia. The thyroid gland is slightly enlarged, firm, and tender. The patient may range from euthyroid to thyrotoxic. The active phase lasts from days to months and may recur before final resolution.

Nonsteroidal anti-inflammatory drugs are usually sufficient to relieve the pain. Hyperthyroidism is usually treated with β-blockers. Antithyroid medications are poorly effective. More severe pain or active thyroiditis may be treated with a tapering dose of corticosteroids.

92. What historical and physical findings are suggestive of malignancy in a thyroid nodule?
Risk factors include positive family history and head or neck irradiation. Multinodular goiter or longstanding thyroiditis may also increase risk. A single node, fixation of the node, local lymphadenopathy, and involvement of the recurrent laryngeal nerve suggest malignancy.

93. How is papillary carcinoma of the thyroid staged and treated?
Stage I: Single or multiple intrathyroidal nodules. Treatment may involve simple lobectomy followed by suppressive thyroxine therapy or, alternatively, lobectomy with near-total contralateral lobectomy followed by ablative radioiodine (particularly in multicentric disease or patients >40).
Stage II: Cervical metastasis, nonfixed, and without invasion. Treatment consists of near-total or total thyroidectomy, followed by radioiodine ablation and thyroid replacement with follow-up iodine scanning.
Stage III: Local cervical invasion or fixed cervical metastases. Treatment consists of near-total thyroidectomy with resection of available neoplastic tissue, followed by radioiodine ablation and thyroid replacement with follow-up iodine scanning.
Stage IV: Metastases outside the neck. Treatment is as per Stage III, with body scanning after ablation to assess metastases outside the neck and with follow-up higher-dose radioiodine therapy as indicated.

94. How should you follow up thyroid carcinoma?
Physical examination, thyroid function tests, thyroglobulin levels, and whole-body radioiodine scanning at 6–9 months, 1 year, 3 years, and then at 5-year intervals thereafter.

95. What is struma ovarii?
Ectopic thyroid tissue in an ovarian teratoma producing a hyperthyroid state. It is one of the rare causes of low-uptake hyperthyroidism. Other causes of low-uptake hyperthyroidism are thyroiditis, Jod-Basedow phenomenon, and exogenous thyroxine.

96. What is Reidel's thyroiditis?
A rare thyroiditis in which the gland has extensive fibrosis with adherence to adjacent structures, producing a characteristic "woody" consistency.

97. How is the TRH stimulation test useful in hyperthyroidism and hypothyroidism?
The pituitary gland is less responsive to TRH in the presence of high circulating levels of T_4. A "flat" TRH stimulation test suggests that the patient's axis is suppressed. On the other hand, the pituitary will be hyperresponsive to TRH with low circulating T_4, allowing the assessment of subtle hypothyroidism or in interpreting an axis with altered binding proteins or T_4 metabolism, such as in phenytoin or amiodarone use.

98. What does "euthyroid sick" mean? What are the usual findings?
Euthyroid sick designates the changes in thyroid hormone levels in patients with severe systemic illness. T_4 and T_3 will decrease, with increased reverse T_3. Despite maintenance of a functional euthyroid state, T_4 to T_3 conversion is decreased, with shunting to reverse T_3. TSH is normal or at the upper limit of normal. Recovery may be associated with a self-limited rise in TSH.

99. What is the earliest means of detecting medullary carcinoma of the thyroid (MCT)? What is the best therapy?
Pentagastrin stimulation testing. This test provokes an exaggerated rise in calcitonin, even in very early MCT. Surgery is the best therapy and should seek for cure.

GONADS

100. Discuss the differential diagnosis for impotence in the male.
Impotence may have circulatory, neurogenic, hormonal, pharmacologic, and psychiatric components. A drug history, particularly noting antihypertensives and alcohol, may be key in evaluat-

ing the source. Studies on REM-associated erections may help differentiate between psychogenic causes and other reasons. Barring patients with drug-induced impotence or those with normal nocturnal erections, further evaluation of penile circulation and neurologic integrity may be indicated.

101. What is nocturnal penile tumescence?

This describes erections associated with REM sleep. This phenomenon is detected using penile strain gauges and EEG in a sleep lab.

102. What does the Lyon hypothesis have to do with a buccal mucosal scraping in a man with long arms and infertility?

The Lyon hypothesis predicts random inactivation of an X chromosome in XX women, producing the distinctive Barr body in somatic cells. Men should not have Barr bodies, but men with Klinefelter's syndrome, XXY, will have them on a smear of buccal cells.

103. What does obesity have to do with a hypogonadal male who can't smell well?

These findings suggest Kallmann's syndrome, a defect in midline hypothalamic development that produces obesity, hypogonadotropic hypogonadism, and disordered smell.

104. What is the difference between hirsutism and virilization?

Hirsutism is excess hair only. Virilization includes increased androgen response, including increased muscle mass, lowered voice, clitoral enlargement, and behavioral changes.

105. What is the differential diagnosis for hirsutism in a woman?

Racial or familial predilection	Polycystic ovarian syndrome
Ovarian or adrenal neoplasm	Partial adrenal hyperplasia syndrome

BONE

106. List the mediators of humoral hypercalcemia of malignancy.

Interleukin 1	Tumor necrosis factor
Lymphotoxin	Parathyroid hormone-related protein
Prostaglandins	

107. What are bisphosphonates?

Bisphosphonates are a class of compounds whose backbone is modeled on pyrophosphate in which the bridge oxygen is replaced by carbon. These compounds generally inhibit bone resorption through multiple mechanisms and differ in potency and side effect profiles. They are generally useful in conditions of high bone turnover, such as humoral hypercalcemia and Paget's disease, and are now seeing use in osteoporosis.

108. When is medical therapy indicated for Paget's disease of bone? What medicines are available?

Pain, deformity, nerve entrapment, and cranial involvement indicate the need for medical therapy. Calcitonin and bisphosphonates are indicated for suppression of disease activity.

109. How may bone density be measured and why? Isn't there anything easier?

Bone density is now most commonly measured by dual-energy x-ray absorptiometry (DXA) scanning, although quantitative CT may also be used. Bone mass has been shown prospectively to correlate with skeletal fragility and fracture risk. Typically, bone mass is compared to the "peak" bone mass achieved in a person's second and third decade, with deviations from peak described in standard deviations (SD). Responses to therapy may also be followed by bone densitometry.

Bone ultrasound is now being evaluated as another means of assessing bone quality. Prospective studies have shown a correlation between bone ultrasound attenuation and subsequent fracture risk. This technology will likely become more used in the future.

110. What are the indications for bone biopsy?

Bone biopsy is best used for evaluation of bone disorders of unknown etiology. Direct sampling of bone allows assessment of bone architecture and qualitative disorders of formation. The use of timed fluorescent labels allows kinetic parameters to be assessed, including turnover rate and bone formation rate. Special stains can detect aluminum and other heavy metals.

Indications for Bone Biopsy in the Clinical Setting

Suspected osteomalacia
Diagnostic classification of renal osteodystrophy
Osteopenia in young individuals (< 50 yrs)
Osteopenia in individuals with abnormal calcium metabolism
Hereditary childhood bone diseases that are classification problems
Evaluation of treatment in certain diseases (e.g., osteomalacia, hypophospatasia)

Eriksen EF, Axelrod DW, Melsen F: Bone Histomorphometry. New York, Raven Press, 1994, p 35.

111. How do osteopenia and osteoporosis differ?

Osteopenia only denotes loss of bone mass. This may or may not be accompanied by an increase in fragility. For example, hyperparathyroidism is accompanied by some degree of osteopenia, but is not associated with increased fragility, probably because of maintained microarchitecture.

In **osteoporosis,** bone mass and architecture are progressively lost with a resultant increase in susceptibility to fracture. According to the WHO nomenclature, *osteoporosis* denotes a loss of bone mass > 2.5 SD from the peak achieved earlier in life, and *established* or *severe osteoporosis* denotes the additional presence of osteoporotic (fragility) fracture.

Assessment of Fracture Risk and Its Application to Screening for Postmenopausal Osteoporosis: Report of a WHO Study Group. Geneva, World Health Organization, 1994.

112. What is the differential diagnosis of osteoporosis?

	Primary Osteoporosis	
Juvenile	Idiopathic (young adults)	Involutional
	Secondary Osteoporosis	
Endocrine diseases		
Hypogonadism	Hyperadrenocorticism	Hyperthyroidism
Hyperparathyroidism	Diabetes mellitus	
Gastrointestinal diseases		
Subtotal gastrectomy	Malabsorption syndromes	Chronic obstructive jaundice
Primary biliary cirrhosis	Severe malnutrition	Anorexia nervosa
Bone marrow disorders		
Multiple myeloma	Mastocytosis	Metastatic carcinoma
Connective tissue diseases		
Osteogenesis imperfecta	Homocystinuria	Ehlers-Danlos syndrome
Marfan's syndrome		
Miscellaneous causes		
Immobilization	Rheumatoid arthritis	Chronic alcoholism
Chronic heparinization	Chronic obstructive pulmonary disease	

Riggs BL: Osteoporosis. In DeGroot LJ (ed): Endocrinology, 2nd ed. Philadelphia, W.B. Saunders, 1989, p 1196.

113. Why are women more prone to osteoporosis than men?

They aren't. Men are equally prone to osteoporosis, just later in life. Men develop the classical fractures of osteoporosis (Colles', vertebral, and hip) later in life than do women.

In women, the loss of sex steroids at menopause or through medical or surgical causes leads to an increase in bone turnover through activation of bone remodeling. This itself causes an overall loss of bone and loss of cancellous (trabecular) bone. Further, with loss of estrogen, the amount of bone resorbed is greater than that replaced, leading to a continuing decline in overall bone mass and worsening microarchitecture.

114. What is the principle of the intact parathyroid hormone (PTH) assay? Why is it particularly useful in renal failure?

Antibodies to one end of the PTH molecule are attached to a solid phase, such as beads or the inside of the test tube. The patient's serum is then added, incubated, and washed out, leaving PTH attached to the solid phase. A radiolabeled antibody to the other end of the PTH molecule is then added. This antibody only binds to intact PTH, the other end of which is attached to the solid phase. Any fragments bound to the solid phase will not be recognized by the second antibody. In this manner, only "intact" PTH produces a signal. Renal failure causes poor clearance of PTH fragments, which produce large signals on one-site PTH assays, but which do not interfere with the two-site assay.

115. How does magnesium deficiency cause hypocalcemia?

Magnesium deficiency inhibits PTH release from the parathyroid glands, as well as interferes with its action at bone and kidney.

116. How should surgery for sporadic primary hyperparathyroidism differ from surgery for MEN syndrome?

Sporadic hyperparathyroidism is almost always secondary to an isolated parathyroid adenoma, which leads to cure on its resection. MEN is associated with diffuse parathyroid hyperplasia and hyperfunction. The therapy of choice is resection of 3½ glands, usually with implantation of the remaining ½ gland in the sternomastoid muscle or forearm.

117. What is familial hypocalciuric hypercalcemia (FHH)? How can it be differentiated from hyperparathyroidism?

FHH is a familial-dominant disorder in which the calcium level is set higher than normal in the face of high-normal PTH levels. Urine calcium levels are remarkably low, in contrast to those seen in hyperparathyroidism. No long-term morbidity is associated with FHH. All patients with suspected hyperparathyroidism should be checked for FHH by urine calcium determination.

118. How does sarcoidosis cause hypercalcemia?

Sarcoid tissue is able to hydroxylate 25-hydroxyvitamin D to the active 1,25-dihydroxy form and produce an endogenous hypervitaminosis D.

LIPIDS

119. What are the major lipoproteins and their compositions?

Lipoproteins are composed of nonpolar (and therefore water-insoluble) cholesterol esters and triglycerides (TG), surrounded by a layer of polar (and therefore water-soluble) proteins and lipids (unesterified cholesterol and phospholipids). This structure allows the entire particle to remain miscible in serum. The major lipoproteins are:

Composition (%)

TYPE	DIAMETER Å	ELECTRO-PHORETIC MOBILITY	PROTEIN	TG	CHOLESTEROL FREE	ESTER	PHOSPHO-LIPID
Chylomicrons	5000	Origin	1–2	85–95	1–3	2–4	3–6
VLDL	2000	Pre-β	6–10	50–65	4–8	16–22	15–20
LDL	250	β	18–22	4–8	6–8	45–50	18–24
HDL	80	α	45–55	2–7	3–5	15–20	26–32

120. Compare familial hypercholesterolemia (FHC) and primary moderate (polygenic) hypercholesterolemia (PHC). How does the latter contrast with primary (familial) combined hyperlipidemia (PCHL)?

FHC stems from a LDL receptor defect, leading to diminished LDL-cholesterol uptake at the liver and increased cholesterol synthesis. Homozygotes have extremely elevated cholesterol levels and accelerated atherosclerosis in childhood. Heterozygotes show LDL-cholesterol levels of about twice normal.

PHC is much more common, presenting with LDL-cholesterol levels of 160–220 mg/dl. This syndrome probably represents several defects in LDL receptors, receptor binding, or intracellular cholesterol metabolism. It may be differentiated from **PCHL** syndrome in that the latter also incorporates elevated triglycerides, through elevated LDL and/or VLDL levels.

121. Which apolipoprotein directs LDL binding to its receptor?

Apolipoprotein B-100 directs LDL binding to its cellular receptor and its subsequent uptake into the cell.

122. What is the chylomicronemia syndrome and its differential diagnosis?

The syndrome is characterized by markedly elevated triglyceride levels (often > 1,000 mg/dl), eruptive xanthomas, and pancreatitis. It may be a primary disease caused by deficiency of lipoprotein lipase or apoprotein C-II, but is more commonly seen in the setting of excessive alcohol intake, uncontrolled diabetes, or use of oral contraceptives.

123. What are the noncholesterol risk factors used in assessing treatment modalities for hypercholesterolemia?

Atherosclerotic disease in the patient
    Definitive coronary artery disease (CAD)
    Peripheral vascular disease
Positive risk factors (increase risk of morbidity/mortality)
    Men > 45 yrs old
    Women > 55 or premature menopause without estrogen replacement
    Premature CAD in first-degree relatives (males < 55, females < 65 yrs)
    Current cigarette smoking
    Hypertension
    Low HDL-cholesterol (< 35 mg/dl)
Negative risk factors (decrease risk of morbidity/mortality)
    High HDL-cholesterol (> 60 mg/dl)

Summary of the second report of the National Cholesterol Education Program (NCEP) expert panel on detection, evaluation, and treatment of high blood cholesterol in adults (Adult Treatment Panel II). JAMA 269:3015–3023, 1993.

124. At what LDL levels should dietary and pharmacologic treatments for hyperlipidemia be initiated? What are the treatment goals?

Risk Factors and Treatment of Hyperlipidemia

	INITIATION LEVEL	LDL-C GOAL
Diet and Exercise		
No CAD and < 2 CAD risk factors	≥ 160 mg/dl	≤ 160 mg/dl
No CAD and ≥ 2 CAD risk factors	≥ 130 mg/dl	≤ 130 mg/dl
CAD present	≥ 100 mg/dl	≤ 100 mg/dl
Pharmacologic		
No CAD and < 2 CAD risk factors	≥ 190 mg/dl	≤ 160 mg/dl
No CAD and ≥ 2 CAD risk factors	≥ 160 mg/dl	≤ 130 mg/dl
CAD Present	≥ 130 mg/dl	≤ 100 mg/dl

125. How can you estimate a patient's LDL from measurements of total cholesterol, HDL, and triglyceride?

$$\text{Serum LDL} = (\text{total cholesterol} - \text{HDL}) - (\text{TG/5})$$

126. Who should have their cholesterol measured? How often?

All adults aged 20 and older should have their total and LDL cholesterol tested at least once every 5 years. These may be tested in a nonfasting state.

The Expert Panel: Report of the National Cholesterol Education Program (NCED) expert panel on detection, evaluation and treatment of high blood cholesterol in adults. JAMA 269:3015–3023, 1993.

127. List the currently available lipid-lowering agents, their mechanism of action, and their side effects.

Summary of Lipid-Lowering Agents

CLASS	AGENT(S)	MECHANISM	ACTIONS	SIDE-EFFECTS & CONSIDERATIONS
Bile-acid resins	Cholestyramine Colestipol	Bind bile acids in gut, with resultant ↑ cholesterol utilization, ↑ LDL receptor activity, and ↑ LDL clearance from circulation	LDL ↓ VLDL, TG↑ HDL ↔	Constipation Bloating Impaired absorption of some medications
Nicotinic acid (Niacin)	Nicotinoic acid (slow-release forms available)	Inhibits hepatic secretion of VLDL and FFA release from fat	LDL↓ TG ↓ HDL ↑	Flushing (suppressed with with low-dose aspirin) Worsening of glucose tolerance Elevated LFTs
HMG-CoA reductase inhibitors	Lovastatin Pravastatin Simvastatin Fluvastatin	Inhibit cholesterol formation through inhibition of HMG CoA reductase, with ↑ LDL receptor activity.	LDL ↓ TG ↓ (small) HDL ↑	Myositis Elevated LFTs
Gemfibrozil	Gemfibrozil	↑ activity of lipoprotein lipase, may inhibit hepatic secretion of VLDL	TG ↓↓ HDL ↓ (variable) LDL ↓	Myositis, diarrhea Nausea, skin rash (rare)

LFT, liver function tests; FFA, free fatty acids

128. What effect does alcohol use have on lipids?

Alcohol causes an increase in triglyceride levels but does not affect LDL levels. It does cause an increase in HDL levels through an unknown mechanism. This may lead to a reduction of the risk of CAD, although use of alcohol is not specifically recommended for this purpose.

The Expert Panel: Report of the National Cholesterol Education Program Expert Panel on detection, evaluation and treatment of high blood cholesterol in adults. Arch Intern Med 148:36–69, 1988.

129. Can other factors increase HDL levels?

The following have been found to elevate HDL levels:
1. Weight loss
2. Aerobic exercise (however, mild to moderate exercise may have little effect)
3. Discontinuation of cigarette smoking
4. Drugs (nicotinic acid, gemfibrozil)

130. What are prostaglandins (PG)?

PGs are oxygenation products of 20-carbon (eicosanoic) fatty acids that produce a wide variety of biologic effects. They are part of a group of compounds derived from eicosanoic fatty acids (called eicosanoids) that also includes thromboxanes and leukotrienes. PGs are produced by many different tissues and have regulatory actions throughout the body. They are produced and exert their effects locally rather than systemically.

131. What are the causes of gynecomastia?

1. Idiopathic
2. Physiologic
   Puberty
   Aging
   Newborn
3. Drugs
   Drugs with estrogen activity: conjugated or synthetic estrogens, oral contraceptives, digitalis (digitoxin only, not digoxin)
   Drugs that stimulate estrogen synthesis or effect: clomiphene citrate, HCG, LHRH
   Drugs that decrease testosterone synthesis or effect: cimetidine, spironolactone, ketoconazole, cancer chemotherapeutic agents
   Unknown mechanisms: methyldopa, marijuana, testosterone, isoniazid, diazepam, ethionamide, tricyclic antidepressants, D-penicillamine, ?heroin, ?phenothiazines, ?amphetamines
4. Tumors with increased HCG or estrogen formation
   Choriocarcinoma (testicular or teratoma)
   Other testicular tumors
   Bronchogenic carcinoma
   Adrenal carcinoma
5. Increased estrogen synthesis
   Liver disease (may be combined with decreased androgens)
   Thyrotoxicosis
   Obesity (presumed)
   True hermaphroditism
   Familial
6. Decreased androgen synthesis or androgen resistance
   Testicular failure: orchitis, trauma or castration, granulomatous disease, myotonic dystrophy, neurologic disorders
   Klinefelter's syndrome
   Defects in testosterone synthesis
   Congenital anorchism
   Androgen resistance syndromes
   Renal failure
7. Altered testosterone and estrogen binding
   Thyrotoxicosis
8. Unknown mechanism
   Starvation-refeeding

HCG = human chorionic gonadotropin; LHRH = luteinizing hormone-releasing hormone.
From: Kohler PO (ed): Clinical Endocrinology. New York, John Wiley, 1986, p 373, with permission.

BIBLIOGRAPHY

1. DeGroot LJ (ed): Endocrinology, 3rd ed. Philadelphia, W.B. Saunders, 1995.
2. Eriksen EF, Axelrod DW, Melsen F: Bone Histomorphometry. New York, Raven Press, 1994.
3. Kohler PO (ed): Clinical Endocrinology. New York, John Wiley, 1986.
4. Stein JH (ed): Internal Medicine, 4th ed. St. Louis, Mosby, 1994.
5. Wilson JD, et al: Textbook of Endocrinology, 8th ed. Philadelphia, W.B. Saunders, 1992.

3. CARDIOLOGY

Gabriel B. Habib, M.D., and Anthony J. Zollo, Jr., M.D.

Of all the ailments which may blow out life's little candle, heart disease is the chief.

William Boyd
Pathology for the Surgeon

*Art is long and Time is fleeting
And our hearts, though stout and brave,
Still, like muffled drums are beating
Funeral marches to the grave.*

Henry Wadsworth Longfellow
A Psalm of Life

PHYSICAL EXAM

1. What are the cardiac physical examination findings in cardiac tamponade?

When the clinical triad of cardiac tamponade was first described by Beck in 1935, it consisted of hypotension, elevated systemic venous pressure, and a small quiet heart and was commonly due to penetrating cardiac injuries, aortic dissection, or intrapericardial rupture of an aortic or cardiac aneurysm. Today, the most common causes are neoplastic disease, idiopathic pericarditis, acute myocardial infarction (MI), and uremia. The physical findings are:

1. Jugular venous distension. It is almost universally present except in patients with severe hypovolemia.

2. Pulsus paradoxus, defined as a decrease in systolic BP of > 10 mm Hg excess of 10 mmHg during quiet inspiration. Pulsus paradoxus is difficult to elicit in volume-depleted patients.

3. Tachycardia, with a thready peripheral pulse. Sometimes, severe cardiac tamponade may restrict LV and RV filling enough to cause hypotension, but a thready and rapid pulse is almost invariably present.

Kussmaul's sign, an inspiratory increase in systemic venous pressure, is commonly present in chronic constrictive pericarditis but is rarely detected in acute cardiac tamponade.

2. What is the third heart sound (S_3)? What is a physiologic S_3?

An S_3 (or ventricular gallop) is a low-frequency sound that is heard just after the second heart sound (S_2). It is found in normal young patients (called a **physiologic S_3**) and also in a variety of pathologic conditions (**pathologic S_3**), including congestive heart failure (CHF), mitral valve prolapse, thyrotoxicosis, coronary artery disease (CAD), cardiomyopathies, pericardial constriction, mitral or aortic insufficiency, and left-to-right shunts.

The mechanism behind an S_3 is controversial. It may be due to an increase in the velocity of blood entering the ventricles (rapid ventricular filling). It usually represents myocardial decompensation when associated with heart disease.

3. What is an S_4?

An S_4, or atrial gallop, occurs just before S_1 and reflects decreased ventricular compliance (a stiff ventricle). It is associated with CAD, pulmonic or aortic valvular stenosis, hypertension, and ventricular hypertrophy from any cause.

4. How are heart murmurs graded?

Grading System for Heart Murmurs

GRADE	PHYSICAL EXAMINATION FINDINGS
1	Barely audible intensity (only a cardiologist can hear it!)
2	Low-intensity murmur (the upper-level resident can hear it)
3	Loud murmur (everyone can hear it)
4	Loud murmur with palpable thrill
5	Loudest murmur audible (still requires a stethoscope placed on the chest)
6	Murmur loud enough to be heard with the stethoscope off the chest

5. What is paradoxical splitting of S_2? What are its causes?

S_2 is normally split into an aortic (A_2) and pulmonic components (P_2) caused by the closing of the two respective valves. The degree of splitting varies with the respiratory cycle (physiologic splitting). With inspiration, the negative intrathoracic pressure leads to increased venous return to the right side of the heart and a decrease to the left side; this causes P_2 to occur slightly later and A_2 to occur slightly earlier, which leads to a widening of the splitting of S_2. With expiration, the negative intrathoracic pressure is eliminated and A_2 and P_2 occur almost simultaneously. **Paradoxical splitting** of S_2 refers to the situation in which the split of A_2 and P_2 seems to widen with expiration and shorten with inspiration (the opposite of normal). This is caused by P_2 preceding A_2 during expiration and is usually due to conditions that delay A_2 by delaying ejection of blood from the left ventricle (LV) and therefore closure of the aortic valve. Causes include aortic insufficiency, aortic stenosis, hypertrophic obstructive cardiomyopathy, myocardial ischemia, left bundle branch block, or a right ventricular (RV) pacemaker.

6. What causes fixed splitting of S_2?

In fixed splitting of S_2, the interval between A_2 and P_2 does not change with the respiratory cycle. It is typically associated with atrial septal defects or RV dysfunction.

7. How do you measure the jugular venous pulse at the bedside?

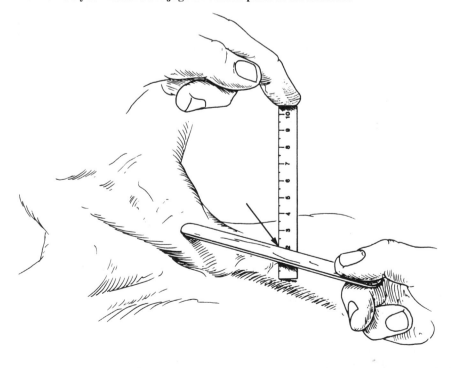

The patient's chest should be elevated to the point where the pulsations are maximally visualized (usually 30–45° of elevation). The height of this oscillating venous column above the sternal angle (angle of Louis) can then be measured. Since the sternal angle is about 5 cm from the right atrium (regardless of elevation angle), central venous pressure can be estimated by adding 5 cm to the measurement. Normal central venous pressure is 5–9 cm H_2O.

From Adair OV, Havranek EP: Cardiology Secrets. Philadelphia, Hanley & Belfus, 1995, p 6; with permission.

8. Name the three waves comprising the jugular venous pulse.

1. **a-wave,** produced by right atrial contraction, occurs just before S_1.

2. **c-wave** is caused by bulging upward of the closed tricuspid valve during RV contraction. (Often difficult to see.)

3. **v-wave** is caused by right atrial filling just before opening of the tricuspid valve.

9. What are "cannon" a-waves?

These very large and prominent a-waves occur when the atria contract against a closed tricuspid valve. Irregular "cannon" a-waves are seen in AV dissociation or ectopic atrial beats. Regular "cannon" a-waves are seen in a junctional or ventricular rhythm in which the atria are depolarized by retrograde conduction.

10. What is the likely cause of a systolic ejection murmur, best heard at the second right intercostal space, in an 82-year-old symptomatic man?

By far, the most common cause in this situation is **aortic sclerosis.** This valvular abnormality is characterized by thickening and/or calcification of the aortic valve, and unlike valvular aortic stenosis, it is typically *not* associated with any significant transvalvular systolic pressure gradient. On physical examination, aortic sclerosis can be differentiated from aortic stenosis as follows:

	AORTIC STENOSIS	*AORTIC SCLEROSIS*
Diminished carotid upstroke	+	−
Diminished peripheral pulses	+	−
Late peaking of systolic murmur	+	−
Loud S_4	+	−
Syncope, angina, or heart failure	+	−
Loud systolic murmur and thrill	+	−

11. How do standing, squatting, and leg-raising affect the intensity and duration of the systolic murmur heard on dynamic auscultation in a patient with idiopathic hypertrophic subaortic stenosis (IHSS)?

In IHSS, a decrease in the size of the LV increases the dynamic LV outflow obstruction, leading to an increased intensity of the murmur. A decrease in LV volume occurs on standing. In contrast, leg-raising and squatting increase venous return and thereby increase LV volume, decreasing the dynamic LV obstruction and the murmur intensity.

12. What is the mechanism of pulsus paradoxus? What medical diseases can present with pulsus paradoxus?

Pulsus paradoxus was first described by Kussmaul in 1873 as the apparent disappearance of the pulse during inspiration despite persistence of the heartbeat. In fact, pulsus paradoxus is an exaggeration of the normal decline in systolic BP and LV stroke volume on inspiration. The fall in intrathoracic pressure is rapidly transmitted through the pericardial effusion and results in an exaggerated increase in venous return to the right side of the heart. This, in turn, causes bulging of the interventricular septum toward the LV, thereby resulting in a smaller LV volume and LV stroke volume during inspiration.

Pulsus paradoxus is **not** a *sine qua non* of cardiac tamponade. It may also occur in patients with severe chronic obstructive pulmonary disease complicated by the need for large negative intrathoracic pressures on inspiration. Interestingly, pulsus paradoxus is usually absent in chronic constrictive pericarditis.

ELECTROCARDIOGRAPHY

13. Describe the sequence of ECG changes in an acute transmural MI. What is their timing in relation to the onset of symptoms?

The evolution of an acute MI consists of three phases on ECG:

1. **Abnormal T wave,** which is tall, prolonged, inverted, or upright. Hyperacute tall T waves are typically seen in the first hour or two of MI evolution. The T wave usually becomes inverted *after* ST-segment elevation has occurred and may remain inverted for days, weeks, or years.

2. **ST-segment elevations** in leads facing the infarcted myocardial wall and **reciprocal ST depressions** in opposite leads. ST-segment changes are the most common ECG signs of acute MI. ST-segment elevations rarely persist > 2 weeks except in patients with a ventricular aneurysm.

3. Appearance of **new Q waves,** often several hours or days after the onset of MI symptoms. Alternatively, the amplitude of the QRS complex is decreased. Q waves may develop earlier when thrombolytic therapy is administered.

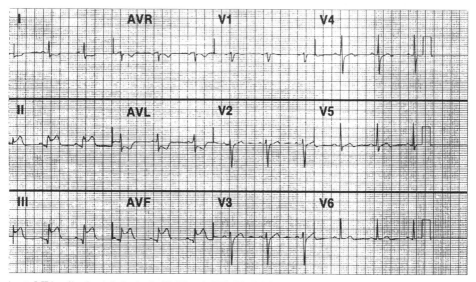

Acute MI localized to inferior leads (II, III, and aVF). The ECG shows ST elevation with hyperacute peaked T waves and the early development of significant Q waves. Reciprocal ST depression is also seen (leads I and aVL). (From Seelig CB: Simplified EKG Analysis. Philadelphia, Hanley & Belfus, 1992, p 13; with permission.)

14. What are the ECG manifestations of atrial infarction?

1. Depressed or elevated PR segment
2. Atrial arrhythmias:
    a. Atrial flutter
    b. Atrial fibrillation
    c. AV nodal rhythms

15. Where does an S_3 occur in relation to the QRS complex? Where does the venous a-wave appear in the cardiac cycle?

During the course of one cardiac cycle, note that the electrical events (ECG) initiate and therefore precede the mechanical (pressure) events and that the latter precede the auscultatory events (heart sounds) they produce. Shortly after the P wave, the atria contract to produce the a-

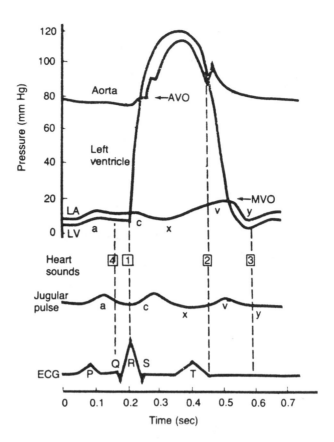

wave; S_4 may succeed the latter. The QRS complex initiates ventricular systole, followed shortly by LV contraction and the rapid build-up of LV pressure. Almost immediately, LV pressure exceeds left atrial (LA) pressure to close the mitral valve and produces S_1. When LV pressure exceeds aortic pressure, the aortic valve opens (AVO), and when aortic pressure is once again greater than LV pressure, the aortic valve closes to produce S_2 and terminate ventricular ejection. The decreasing LV pressure drops below LA pressure to open the mitral valve (MVO), and a period of rapid ventricular filling commences. During this time, an S_3 may be heard. (For simplification, right-sided heart pressures have been omitted.)

From Andreoli TE, et al (eds): Cecil Essentials of Medicine, 2nd ed. Philadelphia, W.B. Saunders, 1990, p 8; with permission.

16. Which arrhythmias can be detected in young patients without apparent heart disease?

In a study of 24-hour continuous ECG monitoring performed on 50 male medical students, severe sinus bradycardia (40 bpm or fewer), sinus pauses of up to 2 sec, and nocturnal AV nodal block were frequently found. Frequent premature atrial or ventricular beats were not commonly found.

Brodsky M, et al: Arrhythmias documented by 24-hour continuous electrocardiographic monitoring in 50 male medical students without apparent heart disease. Am J Cardiol 39:390–395, 1977.

17. How do you differentiate between the various types of supraventricular tachycardias (SVTs)?

Atrial fibrillation (AF) differs from all other SVTs by having totally disorganized atrial depolarizations without effective atrial contraction. An ECG may occasionally show small, irregular waves of variable amplitude and morphology, occurring at a rate of 350–600/min, but these are often difficult to recognize on a routine 12-lead ECG.

Atrial tachycardia (or paroxysmal atrial tachycardia) and **atrial flutter,** unlike AF, demonstrate a regular ventricular rhythm and are characterized by regular and slower atrial rhythms. The flutter rate (i.e., the atrial rate) in atrial flutter ranges between 250–350 bpm. The most common flutter rate is 300 bpm, and the most common ventricular rates are 150 and 75 bpm, respectively. Atrial tachycardias have slower atrial rates, ranging from 150–250 bpm. The most common cause of atrial tachycardia with block is digitalis toxicity.

Comparison of Supraventricular Tachycardias

	ATRIAL FIBRILLATION	ATRIAL FLUTTER	ATRIAL TACHYCARDIA
Atrial rate	>400	240–350	100–240
Atrial rhythm	Irregular	Regular	Regular
AV block	Variable	2:1, 4:1, 3:1, or variable	2:1, 4:1, 3:1, or variable
Ventricular rate	Variable	150, 75, 100, or variable	Variable

18. What is the significance of capture and fusion beats on ECG in differentiating between ventricular tachycardia (VT) and SVT with aberrancy?

Distinguishing Features of Wide-Complex VT and SVT

	VT	SVT
History of MI	+	−
Ventricular aneurysm	+	−
Fusion beats	+	−
Capture beats	+	−
Complete AV dissociation	+	−
Similar QRS when in sinus rhythm	−	+
RBBB + QRS > 0.14 sec	+	−
LBBB + QRS > 0.16 sec	+	−
Positive concordance in V_1–V_6	+	−
LBBB + right QRS axis	+	−
Intermittent cannon waves	+	−

LBBB = left bundle branch block; RBBB = right bundle branch block.

Three ECG findings are virtually pathognomonic of VT: AV dissociation, capture beats, and fusion beats. A capture beat is a normally conducted sinus beat interrupting a wide-complex tachycardia. A fusion beat has a QRS morphology intermediate between a normally conducted narrow beat and a wide-complex ventricular beat. The clinical hallmark of AV dissociation is the presence of intermittent cannon waves in the jugular neck veins.

19. Give the medical contraindications to exercise ECG testing.

Exercise stress testing is widely used to detect and assess the functional significance of CAD. It also has been shown to predict survival in patients recovering from an acute MI. Because exercise stress testing is commonly requested, its contraindications should be widely known and clearly understood so that use of this test is appropriate and safe. Contraindications include:

1. Myocardial infarction acute or pending
2. Unstable angina
3. Acute myocarditis or pericarditis
4. Left main coronary artery disease
5. Severe aortic stenosis
6. Uncontrolled hypertension
7. Uncontrolled cardiac arrhythmias
8. Second- or third-degree AV block
9. Acute noncardiac illness

20. What are the types of AV block?

1. **First-degree AV block:** Prolongation of the PR interval due to a conduction delay at the AV node.

2. **Second-degree AV block:** Manifested by dropped beats in which a P wave is not followed by a QRS complex (no ventricular depolarization and therefore no ventricular contraction). It is divided into two types:

    a. **Type I:** (Wenckebach phenomenon): The PR interval lengthens with each successive beat until a beat is dropped and the cycle repeats itself.

    b. **Type II:** The PR intervals are prolonged but do not gradually lengthen until a beat is suddenly dropped. The dropped beat may occur regularly, with a fixed number (X) of beats for each dropped beat (called an X:1 block). Type II is much less common than Type I and is commonly associated with bundle branch blocks.

3. **Third-degree AV block** (complete heart block): The atria and ventricles are controlled by separate pacemakers. It is associated with widening of the QRS complex and a ventricular rate of 35–50 bpm.

21. What ECG changes are seen in hyperkalemia?

A tall, peaked, symmetrical T wave with a narrow base (so-called tented T wave) is the earliest ECG abnormality and is usually present in leads II, III, V_2, V_3, and V_4. This is followed by shortening of the QT interval, widening of the QRS interval, ST-segment depression, flattening of the P wave, and PR-interval prolongation. Eventually, the P waves disappear and the QRS complexes assume a configuration similar to a sine wave, eventually degenerating into ventricular fibrillation (VF). Widening of the QRS complex can assume a configuration consistent with atypical RBBB or LBBB, making the recognition of hyperkalemia more difficult. Unlike typical RBBB, hyperkalemia often causes prolongation of the entire QRS complex.

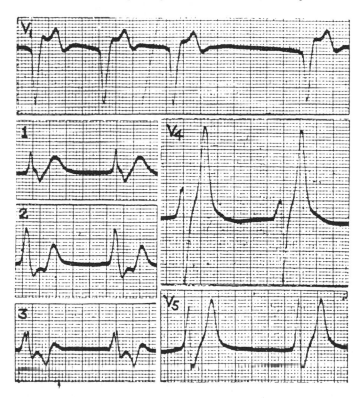

Hyperkalemia. This ECG shows evidence of advanced potassium intoxication: tall peaked T waves, absent P waves, widened QRS complexes, and irregular rhythm. The patient's serum K^+ level was 8.1 meq/liter. (From: Marriott HJL: Practical Electrocardiography, 9th ed. Baltimore, Williams & Wilkins, 1994, p 183; with permission.)

Sequence of ECG Changes in Experimental Hyperkalemia

Tall, symmetrical T waves	$K^+ > 5.7$ meq/l
Reduced P wave amplitude	$K^+ > 7.0$ meq/l
Prolongation of PR interval	$K^+ > 7.0$ meq/l
Disappearance of P waves	$K^+ > 8.4$ meq/l
Widening of QRS interval	$K^+ = 9–11$ meq/l
Ventricular fibrillation (VF)	$K^+ > 12$ meq/l

22. What ECG signs suggest hypercalcemia? Are similar changes seen in other conditions?

Hypercalcemia shortens the QT interval, particularly the interval between the beginning of the QRS complex and the peak of the T wave. The abrupt slope to the peak of the T wave is most characteristic of hypercalcemia. Another cause of shortened QT interval is digitalis toxicity.

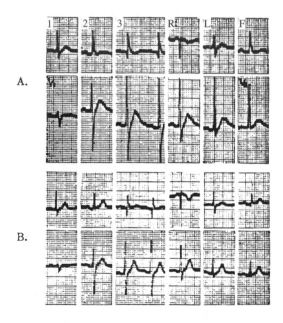

Hypercalcemia in a patient with hyperparathyroidism. *A*, Before parathyroidectomy (serum calcium, 15 mg/dl). Note virtual absence of ST segment, early peak of T wave, and relatively gradual downslope of descending limb of T wave. *B*, After parathyroidectomy (serum calcium, 10.7 mg/dl). Note normal contour of ST-T pattern. (From Marriott HJL: Practical Electrocardiography, 9th ed. Baltimore, Williams & Wilkins, 1994, p 185; with permission.)

23. What is the normal range for PR and QT intervals on a 12-lead ECG? Do these intervals vary with heart rate, sex, or age?

The normal range for the **PR interval** is 0.12–0.20 sec. It is not significantly related to age, sex, or heart rate.

The normal range for the **QT interval** also is unrelated to age, but it does vary with heart rate. As the heart rate increases, the QT interval shortens. To help evaluate a QT interval independent of heart rate, the corrected QT interval (QTc) can be calculated:

$$\text{QTc (in sec)} = \text{measured QT (in sec)} / \sqrt{\text{RR interval (in sec)}}$$

The normal range for the **QTc** is 0.36–0.44 sec. A prolonged QTc is defined as QTc > 0.39 sec in men or > 0.44 sec in women.

24. In the frontal plane, is a QRS axis of +120° compatible with a diagnosis of left anterior hemiblock?

This diagnosis requires the presence of a QRS of −60° to −90° in the frontal plane. A frontal plane QRS axis of +120° degrees is consistent with right axis deviation and is therefore not compatible with a diagnosis of left anterior hemiblock (left anterior fascicular block).

Diagnostic Criteria for Left Anterior Fascicular Block

1. QRS axis −60° to −90°
2. Small q-wave in lead I
3. Small r-wave in lead III

25. Describe the ECG manifestations of RV hypertrophy.

1. R wave > S wave in V_1 or V_2
2. R wave > 5 mm in V_1 or V_2
3. Right axis deviation
4. Persistent rS pattern (V_1–V_6)
5. Normal QRS duration

26. What are the causes of a prolonged QT interval?
Congenital

1. With deafness: Jervell syndrome
2. Without deafness: Romano-Ward syndrome

Acquired

1. Drugs: Class IA/IC antiarrhythmics
2. Electrolyte abnormalities: low K^+, Ca^{2+}, Mg^{2+}
3. Hypothermia
4. CNS injury (least common cause)
5. Liquid diets
6. CAD
7. Cardiomyopathy
8. Mitral valve prolapse

Prolongation of the QT interval is associated in certain patients with a definite increase in risk of VF and death.

DIAGNOSIS

27. How are cardiac and noncardiac causes of chest pain differentiated?

Cardiac Causes of Chest Pain

CONDITION	LOCATION	QUALITY	DURATION	AGGRAVATING/ RELIEVING FACTORS	ASSOCIATED SIGNS AND SYMPTOMS
Angina	Retrosternal, radiates to neck, left	Pressure, burning, squeezing	< 10 min	Aggravated by exercise, cold, emotional stress, after meals. Relieved by rest, nitroglycerin	S_4, paradoxically split S_2, murmur of papillary muscle
Rest or crescendo angina	Same as angina	Same as angina	> 10 min	Same as angina with gradually decreasing tolerance for exertion	Same as angina
Myocardial infarction	Substernal; may radiate like angina	Heaviness, pressure, burning, constriction	30 min or longer, variable	Unrelieved	Shortness of breath, diaphoresis, nausea, vomiting, weakness, anxiety
Pericarditis	Substernal or cardiac apex; may radiate to left arm	Sharp, stabbing, knifelike	Hours to days	Aggravated by deep breathing, rotating chest, or supine position. Relieved by sitting up and leaning forward.	Pericardial friction rub, cardiac tamponade, pulsus paradoxus
Dissecting aortic aneurysm	Anterior chest, back, abdominal	Excruciating, tearing, knifelike	Sudden onset, lasts for hours	Unrelated to anything	Lower BP in one arm, absent pulses, murmur of aortic insufficiency, paralysis, pulsus paradoxus

Noncardiac Causes of Chest Pain

CONDITION	LOCATION	QUALITY	DURATION	AGGRAVATING/ RELIEVING FACTORS	ASSOCIATED SIGNS AND SYMPTOMS
Pulmonary embolism	Substernal or over area of pulmonary infarction	Pleuritic or like angina	Sudden onset, min to > 1 hr	May be aggravated by breathing	Dyspnea, tachypnea, tachycardia, hypotension, signs of right-sided (CHF, rales, pleural rub, hemoptysis (with infarction)
Pulmonary hypertension	Substernal	Pressure	—	Aggravated by effort	Dyspnea, signs of pulmonary hypertension
Pneumonia with pleuritis	Over area of consolidation	Pleuritic, well-localized	—	Aggravated by breathing	Dyspnea, cough, fever, dull to percussion, bronchial breath sounds, pleural rub
Spontaneous pneumothorax	Unilateral	Sharp, well-localized	Sudden onset, hours	Painful breathing	Dyspnea, hyperresonance, and decreased breath and voice sounds
Musculoskeletal	Variable	Aching	Short or long	Aggravated by movement, history of muscle exertion	Tender to pressure or movement
Herpes zoster	Dermatomal distribution	—	Prolonged	None	Rash appears in area of discomfort
GI disorders (esophageal reflux, ulcer)	Lower substernal, epigastric	Burning, colicky, aching	—	Precipitated by recumbency or meals, partial relief with antacids	Nausea, vomiting, food intolerance, melena, hematemesis, jaundice
Anxiety	Often localized to a point, moves	Sharp, burning, variable	Variable	Situational anger, usually brief	Sighing respirations, often chest wall tenderness

From Andreoli TE, et al (eds): Cecil Essentials of Medicine, 2nd ed. Philadelphia, W.B. Saunders, 1990, pp 12–13; with permission.

28. A 31-year-old man complains of a sudden onset of sharp left chest pain, increased by deep inspiration and coughing. Physical findings, chest x-ray, and the ECG are all normal. What is your differential diagnosis?

Differential Diagnosis of Pleuritic Chest Pain

1. Acute pleuritis (coxsackievirus A, B)
2. Acute pericarditis (coxsackievirus B)
3. Pneumonia (viral, bacterial)
4. Pulmonary embolus or infarction
5. Pneumothorax

In this patient, the most likely clinical diagnosis causing pleuritic chest pain in the presence of a normal physical, chest x-ray, and ECG findings is acute viral pleuritis or pericarditis.

29. A 56-year-old man presents to the emergency center with acute onset of squeezing, diffuse, anterior chest pain associated with diaphoresis and dyspnea. What is your differential diagnosis? Which tests will help confirm your clinical suspicions?

The differential diagnosis consists of the following:

1. Acute MI
2. Angina pectoris
3. Acute aortic dissection
4. Acute pericarditis
5. Acute pulmonary embolus
6. Acute pneumothorax

Among these diagnoses, the first three are most common and should be carefully considered in the diagnostic work-up of this patient. A **12-lead ECG** is done to look for ST-segment elevations (evidence of acute myocardial injury due to infarction or pericarditis), ST-segment depressions (evidence of subendocardial ischemia), or T-wave changes. Determination of **serial cardiac enzymes** (creatine kinase and MB isoenzyme) over the first 24–48 hours of hospitalization will help to confirm a diagnosis of acute MI. The absence of any ECG changes of acute MI or ischemia in a patient with severe anterior chest pain radiating to the back should suggest the clinical diagnosis of acute aortic dissection. Finally, a **chest x-ray** is helpful in the work-up of patients with acute chest pain to look for evidence of pneumothorax, cardiac enlargement suggestive of cardiac failure, or wedge-shaped pulmonary consolidation suggestive of acute pulmonary embolus.

30. Identify the types of shock and their causes.

Classification of Shock States

TYPE	PRIMARY MECHANISM	CLINICAL CAUSES
Hypovolemic	Volume loss	Exogenous Blood loss due to hemorrhage Plasma loss due to burn, inflammation Fluid/electrolyte loss due to vomiting, diarrhea, dehydration, osmotic diuresis (diabetes) Endogenous Extravasation due to inflammation, trauma, tourniquet, anaphylaxis, snake venom, and adrenergic stimulation (pheochromocytoma)
Cardiogenic	Pump failure	MI, CHF, cardiac arrhythmias, intracardiac obstruction (incl. valvular stenosis)
Distributive (vasomotor dysfunction)		
1. High or normal resistance	Expanded venous capacitance	Hypodynamic septic shock due to gram-negative enteric bacillemia; autonomic blockade; spinal shock; tranquilizer, sedative, or narcotic overdose
2. Low resistance	AV shunting	Pneumonia, peritonitis, abscess, reactive hyperemia
Obstructive	Extracardiac obstruction of main blood flow channels	Vena caval obstruction (supine hypotensive syndrome), pericarditis (tamponade), pulmonary embolism, dissecting aortic aneurysm, aortic compression.

From: Weil MH, et al: Acute circulatory failure (shock). In Braunwald E (ed): Heart Disease: A Textbook of Cardiovascular Medicine, 3rd ed. Philadelphia, W.B. Saunders, 1988, p 569; with permission.

31. What is a pseudoinfarction? What is its differential diagnosis?

Some patients exhibit ECG changes similar to those of MI but do not have any other definitive evidence of an MI. These patients are said to have ECG evidence of "pseudoinfarction." Causes include:

1. LV or RV hypertrophy
2. Left bundle branch block
3. Wolff-Parkinson-White syndrome
4. Hypertrophic cardiomyopathy
5. Hyperkalemia
6. Early repolarization
7. Cardiac sarcoid or amyloid
8. Intracranial hemorrhage

32. A patient presents to the cardiac care unit with clinical signs and symptoms suggestive of acute right ventricular MI. How would an ECG help to confirm this clinical diagnosis?

About one-third of patients with acute inferior wall MI develop an RV infarction. The clinical syndrome of RV MI should be suspected when the following clinical triad is present in a patient suffering from an inferior wall MI:

(1) Hypotension
(2) Elevated jugular veins
(3) Clear lungs.

The clinical recognition of RV infarction is important. The clinical suspicion can be confirmed by performing a right-sided ECG. The presence of at least 1 mm of ST-segment elevation in lead V_3R or V_4R is characteristically present in RV MI. Further confirmation can be derived from noninvasive assessment of RV systolic function using radionuclide techniques or two-dimensional echocardiography.

33. Name the three types of cardiomyopathies. How are they distinguished?

Classification of Cardiomyopathy

TYPE	CHARACTERISTICS	SYMPTOMS AND SIGNS	LABORATORY DIAGNOSIS
Dilated (congestive)	Cardiac dilation, generalized hypocontractility	LV and RV failure	X-ray: cardiomegaly with pulmonary congestion ECG: sinus tachycardia, nonspecific ST-T changes, arrhythmias, conduction disturbances, Q waves Echo: dilated LV, generalized decreased wall motion, mitral valve motion consistent with low flow Catheterization: dilated hypocontractile ventricle, mitral regurgitation
Hypertrophic	Ventricular hypertrophy, esp. of the septum, with or without outflow tract obstruction Typically good systolic but poor diastolic (compliance) ventricular function	Dyspnea, angina, presyncope, syncope, palpitations Large jugular a-wave, bifid carotid pulse, palpable S_4 gallop, prominent apical impulse, "dynamic" systolic murmur and thrill, mitral regurgitation murmur	X-ray: LV predominance, dilated left atrium ECG: LV hypertrophy, Q waves, nonspecific ST-T waves; ventricular arrhythmias Echo: hypertrophy, usually asymmetric (septum > free wall); systolic anterior motion of mitral valve; midsystolic closure of aortic valve Catheterization: provokable outflow tract gradient; hypertrophy with vigorous systolic function and cavity obliteration; mitral regurgitation
Restrictive	Reduced diastolic compliance impeding ventricular filling; normal systolic function	Dyspnea, exercise intolerance, weakness Elevated jugular venous pressure, edema, hepatomegaly, ascites, S_4 and S_3 gallops, Kussmaul's sign	X-ray: mild cardiomegaly, pulmonary congestion ECG: low voltage, conduction disturbances, Q waves Echo: characteristic myocardial texture in amyloidosis with thickening of all cardiac structures Catheterization: square root sign, M-shaped atrial waveform, elevated left and right filling pressures

From Andreoli TE, et al (eds): Cecil Essentials of Medicine, 2nd ed. Philadelphia, W.B. Saunders, 1990, p 106; with permission.

34. An 89-year-old woman was found unconscious in her backyard. She "woke up" a few minutes after arrival to the EC. Physical, neurologic, ECG, and chest x-ray findings are all normal. She feels fine and demands to be released. Would you admit her to the hospital?

Syncope, defined as a transient loss or impairment of consciousness, can be due to a wide variety of etiologies, both cardiovascular and noncardiovascular. Patients most likely to have cardiovascular syncope are older and may or may not have a prior history of documented cardiac disease (manifested by angina pectoris, MI, or sudden cardiac death). Common cardiovascular causes of syncope include:

1. **Tachyarrhythmias,** such as VT or SVT (AF, atrial flutter, or paroxysmal SVT).

2. **Bradyarrhythmias,** such as second- or third-degree AV block, AF with a slow ventricular response rate, or sinus bradycardia due to sick sinus syndrome.

3. **LV outflow obstruction** due to fixed lesions (valvular, subvalvular, or supravalvular aortic stenosis) or dynamic obstruction such as hypertrophic cardiomyopathy. Characteristically, these patients present with syncope during or immediately after exercise.

4. **LV inflow obstruction** due to severe mitral stenosis or a large left atrial myxoma.

5. **Primary pulmonary hypertension**

It is desirable to hospitalize patients who are at high risk for cardiovascular syncope, since they have a much worse prognosis and may have potentially life-threatening complications of their underlying cardiovascular disease. This elderly woman should be hospitalized since she is at high risk for cardiovascular syncope.

35. Should a thorough work-up be done on all patients with syncope?

No. The routine use of expensive or invasive studies into the cause of syncope is not warranted. The etiology of syncope will be undetermined in 30–50% of cases even after a thorough (and expensive) work-up. In up to 85% of cases in which an etiology is identifiable, it will be identified or at least suggested by the initial history, physical exam, and ECG. Further studies should be ordered on the basis of the results of this initial evaluation.

36. A 68-year-old man with hypertension presents with a 2-week history of progressive exertional dyspnea, orthopnea, and paroxysmal nocturnal dyspnea. What is the differential diagnosis?

Differential Diagnosis of CHF in Hypertensive Patients

1. Coronary artery disease
2. Diastolic dysfunction associated with hypertension
3. Dilated cardiomyopathy (idiopathic or alcoholic)
4. Valvular heart disease (mitral regurgitation, aortic stenosis, aortic insufficiency)
5. Restrictive heart disease (amyloidosis)
6. Hypertrophic cardiomyopathy (idiopathic hypertrophic subaortic stenosis)

37. What is a hyperdynamic precordial impulse?

It is a thrust of exaggerated height that falls away immediately from the palpating fingers. It is typically found in patients with a large stroke volume. The clinical conditions include thyrotoxicosis, anemia, beriberi, AV shunts or grafts, exercise, or mitral regurgitation. A hyperdynamic precordial impulse should be differentiated from the sustained apical impulse, a graphic equivalent of a heave, detected in the presence of LV hypertrophy due to hypertension or aortic stenosis.

38. What is the differential diagnosis of an abnormal early diastolic sound heard at the apex and lower left sternal border?

1. Loud P_2
2. S_3 gallop
3. Opening snap
4. Pericardial knock
5. Tumor plop (atrial myxoma)

An early diastolic sound may be due to wide splitting of S_2, with or without a loud pulmonic closure sound. An atrial septal defect (ASD) causes wide and fixed splitting of S_2.

A **loud P_2** usually indicates the presence of pulmonary hypertension, whether primary or secondary to chronic pulmonary disease.

Unlike other causes of an early diastolic sound, a **third heart sound** (S_3) can best be heard using the bell of the stethoscope. Unlike a physiologically split A_2-P_2, the A_2-S_3 interval does not change during respiration. Associated physical findings of CHF, such as pulmonary rales, distended neck veins, or edema are usually present along with an S_3.

An **opening snap** may be the only finding in a patient with a mild noncalcified and pliable mitral valve. In such a patient, a loud S_1 is also commonly present. A diastolic rumble at the apex confirms the physical diagnosis of mitral stenosis.

In patients with chronic constrictive pericarditis, the sudden slowing of LV filling in early diastole associated with the restriction of a rigid pericardium acting as "a rigid shell" causes the **pericardial knock**.

In some patients with large atrial myxomas protruding through the mitral valve during diastole, the sudden cessation of LV filling, caused by the tumor's obstruction to the flow of blood, creates an audible tumor plop. Cardiac auscultation in various positions helps to detect a tumor plop. Likewise, cardiac symptoms in these patients are often related to body position.

39. In patients with mitral stenosis, what are the pathophysiology and significance of an opening snap? Does its presence imply a more severe degree of stenosis?

An opening snap is typically present only when the mitral valve leaflets are pliable, and it is therefore usually accompanied by an accentuated S_1. Diffuse calcification of the mitral valve can be expected when an opening snap is absent. If calcification is confined to the tip of the mitral valve, an opening snap is still commonly present.

The interval between the aortic closure sound and opening snap (A_2–OS) is inversely related to the mean left atrial pressure. A short A_2–OS interval is a reliable indicator of severe mitral stenosis; however, the converse is not necessarily true.

40. What is the "figure 3" sign? What congenital cardiac disease does it most likely suggest?

A routine chest x-ray may reveal a characteristic "3" sign. This is the result of poststenotic dilatation of the descending aorta and the dilated left subclavian artery. A barium swallow may reveal a reverse "3" sign. Along with rib-notching, the presence of the "3" sign is almost pathognomonic for **aortic coarctation.**

41. What are the major and minor Jones criteria for diagnosing acute rheumatic fever?

Major Jones Criteria	Minor Jones Criteria
Carditis	Fever
Polyarthritis	Arthralgia
Chorea	Prolonged PR internal
Erythema marginatum	Elevated ESR or positive C-reactive protein
Subcutaneous nodules	Previous rheumatic fever or rheumatic heart disease

The clinical diagnosis of acute rheumatic fever is made if two major criteria or one major and two minor criteria are present in a patient with a preceding streptococcal infection (as evidenced by recent scarlet fever, positive throat culture for group A **Streptococcus,** or increased ASO or other streptococcal antibody titer).

CORONARY ARTERY DISEASE

42. Is aspirin effective in the treatment of unstable angina pectoris?

There is unequivocal evidence from two clinical trials, the VA and Canadian cooperative trials, that aspirin reduces subsequent MI and mortality in unstable angina patients. Both mortality and MI are reduced by about 50% in aspirin-treated patients. On the other hand, there is less evidence to suggest a beneficial effect of aspirin in chronic stable angina pectoris.

Lewis HD, et al: Protective effects of aspirin against acute myocardial infarction and death in men with unstable angina: Results of a Veterans Administration Cooperative Study. N Engl J Med 309: 396–403, 1983.

Cairns JA, et al: Aspirin, sulfinpyrazone, or both in unstable angina: Results of a Canadian multicenter trial. N Engl J Med 313:1369–1375, 1985.

43. Which coronary artery is most often involved in patients with Prinzmetal's angina?

The clinical diagnosis of variant (Prinzmetal's) angina should be confirmed by obtaining a 12-lead ECG during episodes of angina. Characteristically, the ECG shows transient ST-segment elevations during episodes of chest discomfort or pain. These ECG changes are due to transient epicardial coronary spasm and are often complicated by arrhythmias or conduction disturbances. The ST-segment elevation is most commonly present in inferior leads, reflecting the frequency of involvement of the **right coronary artery.**

44. What are the common precipitating factors for variant angina?

In patients with Prinzmetal's angina, attacks do not typically occur following physical activity. More likely, anginal episodes occur at rest, at night, after emotional upsets, on exposure to cold weather, or during or after meals. It is hypothesized that cold-induced angina may be due to coronary vasoconstriction, and that a rapid rise in heart rate and BP accompanying meals may increase myocardial O_2 consumption, thus causing an imbalance between oxygen supply and demand in the myocardium.

45. Which test should you perform in a patient presenting with recurrent oppressive chest pains at rest with associated ST-segment elevations?

This patient's symptoms should suggest Prinzmetal's angina. Of all available provocative tests, the **ergonovine test** is the most sensitive and specific for provoking coronary artery spasm. A positive test is defined by the induction of severe *focal* spasm in response to low doses (0.05–0.40 mg, IV) of ergonovine administered by experienced personnel.

Winniford MD, et al: Ergonovine provocation to assess efficacy of long-term therapy with calcium antagonists in Prinzmetal's variant angina. Am J Cardiol 51:684, 1983.

46. Do the various classes of antianginal drugs differ in their efficacy and safety when used in the management of vasospastic angina as compared to classic effort angina?

Patients with both forms of angina respond promptly to **nitrates.**

Although the response of patients with effort angina to **β-blockers** is uniformly good, the response of patients with Prinzmetal's angina is variable. In some patients, the duration of episodes of angina pectoris may be prolonged during therapy with propranolol, a noncardioselective β-blocker. In others, especially those with associated fixed atherosclerotic lesions, β-blockers may reduce the frequency of anginal episodes. Noncardioselective β-blockers may, in some patients with variant angina, leave α-receptor-mediated coronary arterial vasoconstriction unopposed and thereby worsen anginal symptoms.

In contrast to β-blockers, **calcium blockers** are quite effective in reducing the frequency and duration of episodes of variant angina. Along with nitrates, calcium blockers are the mainstay of treatment of Prinzmetal's angina because of their proven efficacy and safety.

47. Is treadmill exercise ECG testing helpful in confirming the diagnosis of variant angina?

Exercise testing is the most common provocative test used by clinicians to confirm the clinical diagnosis of exertional angina pectoris. An exercise ECG test is considered positive for CAD if it shows at least a 1-mm ST-segment depression during exercise. Myocardial ischemia is induced in these patients by an increase in myocardial O_2 demand, primarily due to the increase in heart rate with exercise.

In patients with variant angina, myocardial ischemia is primarily due to a decrease in O_2 supply rather than to an increase in O_2 demand. Exercise testing is thus of limited diagnostic value in these patients. It may show ST-segment elevation, ST-segment depression, or no change in ST segments during exercise.

48. A 78-year-old asthmatic man has stable exertional angina of 3 years' duration. His past medical history reveals intermittent claudication after walking 50 yards. What is your approach to managing this patient's anginal symptoms?

This elderly man has three medical problems: asthma, intermittent claudication, and chronic stable angina.

Of the available antianginal drugs, β-blockers are contraindicated because of the presence of asthma. Cardioselective β-blockers, such as metoprolol (Lopressor) or atenolol (Tenormin), may be used cautiously in low doses in asthma, but noncardioselective β-blockers are not safe in this patient. However, the presence of peripheral vascular disease manifested by intermittent claudication also is a contraindication for the use of any β-blocker. Calcium antagonists or nitrates are thus the antianginal drugs of choice in this patient.

49. Based on clinical history, physical examination, and initial admission ECG, which patients with unstable angina are at highest risk for death or acute MI?

Unstable angina is a common potentially life-threatening medical condition. In 1991, it accounted for 570,000 hospital admissions in the U.S. The risk of death or nonfatal MI is highest in patients with unstable angina complicated by any of the following features:

1. Ongoing prolonged chest pain > 20 min in duration
2. Acute pulmonary edema (by physical exam or chest x-ray)
3. New or worsening mitral regurgitation murmurs
4. Rest angina with dynamic ST-segment changes ≥ 1 mm
5. S_3 gallop or lung rales
6. Hypotension

Patients with one or more of these high-risk indicators should generally be admitted to the coronary care unit for ECG monitoring and intensive medical therapy with IV nitrates, heparin, aspirin, and calcium and/or β-blockers.

Braunwald E, et al: Diagnosing and managing unstable angina. Circulation 90:613–622, 1994.

50. Which patients with unstable angina should undergo cardiac catheterization?

Cardiac cath should be entertained in patients with unstable angina refractory to medical management or with any of the following features:

1. Prior revascularization
2. Depressed LV function (LV ejection fraction <50%)
3. Life-threatening "malignant" ventricular arrhythmias
4. Persistent or recurrent angina/ischemia
5. Inducible myocardial ischemia (provoked by exercise, dobutamine, adenosine, or dipyridamole)

Braunwald E, et al: Diagnosing and managing unstable angina. Circulation 90:613–622, 1994.

51. A 48-year-old man presents with acute severe epigastric pain, anorexia, nausea, vomiting, and diaphoresis. Which myocardial wall is likely affected? Explain the rationale for such an unusual clinical presentation.

Patients with an **acute inferior wall MI** sometimes present with epigastric pain associated with gastrointestinal symptoms, as in this patient, or less commonly hiccupping, which may at times be intractable. These unique clinical manifestations are thought to be related to increased vagal tone and irritation of the diaphragm by the adjacent infarcted inferior wall.

52. Does early administration of thrombolytic therapy after MI decrease mortality?

The effect of IV thrombolytic therapy on MI mortality is well-established. In the GISSI trial, 11,806 patients with acute MI presenting within 12 hours of symptom onset were given IV streptokinase or placebo. The hospital mortality was significantly reduced in patients treated with streptokinase within the first 6 hours. Most importantly, there was a remarkable 50% reduction in hospital mortality in patients treated within 1 hour of symptom onset.

Present standards of care for patients with acute transmural MI include administration of IV thrombolytic therapy in all patients admitted within 6 hours of symptom onset (in the absence of contraindications). Contraindications include bleeding disorders, severe uncontrolled hypertension, recent history of cerebrovascular accident, prolonged cardiopulmonary resuscitation (over 10 min), or active bleeding from a peptic ulcer or other source.

GISSI Trial: Effect of time to treatment on reduction in hospital mortality observed in streptokinase-treated patients. Lancet i:397–401,1986.

53. Which drug is more effective in achieving successful recanalization of a thrombosed coronary artery: tissue plasminogen activator (tPA) or streptokinase?

In the multicenter phase I TIMI trial, tPA was shown to result in about twice as many successful reperfusions (due to clot lysis) as streptokinase. In the recent GUSTO trial, consisting of about 40,000 patients with acute MI, tPA was more effective than streptokinase in opening coronary arteries and in preventing death in the first 30 days after acute MI. An open coronary artery (normal coronary flow in the infarct-related artery) is an excellent predictor of short-term (hospital) and long-term (1 year post-discharge) survival, regardless of which thrombolytic drug is used.

GUSTO Angiographic Investigators: The effects of tissue plasminogen activator, streptokinase, or both on coronary-artery patency, ventricular function and survival after acute myocardial infarction. N Engl J Med 329:1615–1622, 1993.

54. Should oral nitrates be administered routinely to all patients with uncomplicated MI?

IV, transdermal, and/or oral nitrates have traditionally been used routinely in all patients admitted with suspected acute MI. However, despite the encouraging results of early small clinical studies, two recent large clinical trials, ISIS-4 and GISSI-3, consisting of about 78,000 patients, showed no significant benefit of early oral nitrates on survival, infarct size, or ventricular function. Their routine administration should thus be limited to patients with well-established indications for nitrates, such as postinfarction angina pectoris or CHF.

Gruppo Italiano per lo Studio della Sopravivenza nell' Infarto Miocardio (GISSI-3): Effects of lisinopril and transdermal glyceryltrinitrate singly and together on 6-week mortality and ventricular function after acute myocardial infarction. Lancet 343:1115–1122, 1994.

ISIS-4: A randomized factorial trial assessing early oral captopril, oral mononitrate, and intravenous magnesium sulphate in 58,050 patients with suspected acute myocardial infarction. Lancet 345:669–685, 1995.

Morris JL, et al: Nitrates in myocardial infarction: Influence on infarct size, reperfusion, and ventricular remodeling. Br Heart J 73:319–319, 1995.

55. What is the most common cause of death in the first 48 hours after an acute MI?

Ventricular fibrillation (VF). Other causes of death include cardiac rupture, pump failure due to massive infarction, acute mechanical complication such as ventricular septal rupture or acute mitral regurgitation, and cardiogenic shock.

56. Which calcium antagonist, if any, reduces the risk of reinfarction during hospitalization for a non-Q-wave MI?

Non-Q-wave MI is more likely than Q-wave MI to be complicated by early recurrent infarction. The recently completed Diltiazem Reinfarction Study revealed a 50% reduction in recurrent infarction during hospitalization of patients with non-Q-wave MI treated with the calcium antagonist diltiazem compared to placebo. No published clinical trial has shown a reduction in reinfarction after non-Q-wave MI using any other calcium antagonist. Based on the results of this study, administration of diltiazem, in doses of 60–90 mg orally every 6 hours, is recommended for patients admitted with a non-Q-wave MI.

57. Cardiac rupture is almost always a fatal complication of acute MI. What are three risk factors for its development, and what are its clinical features?

RISK FACTORS	CLINICAL FEATURES
1. Female sex	1. LV to RV infarction ratio is 7:1
2. Hypertension	2. Seen in anterior or lateral wall MI
3. First MI	3. Usually with large MI (>20%)
	4. Usually 3–6 days post-MI
	5. Rare with LV hypertrophy or good collateral vessels

58. What complication of acute inferior wall MI typically presents with hypotension, elevated neck veins, clear lungs, and a normal cardiac silhouette on chest x-ray?

This is the classic triad of right ventricular MI. The diagnosis can be confirmed by demonstrating at least 1-mm ST elevation in right-sided chest leads V_3R or V_4R. Clinical management consists of volume expansion in combination with IV dopamine. In these patients, avoid giving any diuretics or preload-reducing drugs such as nitrates, as these would further worsen the low cardiac output state.

59. What is the single most important predictor of prognosis after acute MI?

The LV ejection fraction. This is a more powerful predictor of 1- and 2-year survival after hospital discharge than frequency or complexity of ventricular premature beats detected by ambulatory monitoring.

60. Do angiotension-converting enzyme (ACE) inhibitors improve survival in patients recovering from acute MI?

Long-term oral ACE inhibitors started 3–16 days after acute MI and maintained for about 3 years reduce mortality by about 19% in patients with asymptomatic LV systolic dysfunction (LVEF < 40%). Even a short 1-month course of an ACE inhibitor started within 24 hours of infarct onset decreases 5–6-week mortality by 7–12%, corresponding to 5 deaths prevented for every 1,000 treated patients. However, IV ACE inhibitors should be avoided in the first 24 hours of acute MI evolution since they may cause a potentially harmful acute decrease in BP with a resultant reduction in coronary blood flow.

ISIS-4: A randomized factorial trial assessing early oral captopril, oral mononitrate, and intravenous magnesium sulphate in 58,050 patients with suspected acute myocardial infarction. Lancet 345:669–685, 1995.

Gruppo Italiano per lo Studio della Sopravvivenza nell' Infarto Miocardio (GISSI-3): Effects of lisinopril and transdermal glyceryltrinitrate singly and together on 6-week mortality and ventricular function after acute myocardial infarction. Lancet 343:1115–1122, 1994.

Swedberg K, et al: Effects of the early administration of enalapril on mortality in patients with acute myocardial infarction: Results of the cooperative New Scandinavian Enalapril Survival Study II (CONSENSUS-II). N Engl J Med 327:678–684, 1992.

61. What is the differential diagnosis of a new systolic murmur and acute pulmonary edema appearing 3 days after an acute anterior wall MI?

(1) Acute mitral regurgitation due to papillary muscle rupture, and (2) interventricular septal rupture. Both are potentially fatal complications and are most common 3–6 days postinfarction.

Rupture of the posteromedial papillary muscle, associated with inferior wall MI, is more common than that of the anterolateral papillary muscle. Unlike rupture of the interventricular septum, which occurs with large infarcts, papillary muscle rupture occurs with a small infarction in about 50% of cases.

Differentiation between acute mitral regurgitation and ventricular septal rupture is difficult at the bedside. Two-dimensional and Doppler echocardiography at the bedside can demonstrate the presence and severity of mitral regurgitation and localize the site of a ventricular septal defect (VSD). Further confirmation of the presence of a left-to-right shunt across a VSD can be obtained by a step-up in blood oxygen saturation from the right atrium to the pulmonary artery, documented by blood sampling using a Swan-Ganz catheter.

62. What is the most likely cause of a persistent ST-segment elevation several weeks after recovery from a large transmural anterolateral wall MI?

Persistent ST-segment elevation is not an uncommon complication of a large anterolateral transmural MI. It may be a manifestation of dyskinesis of the thinned-out infarcted myocardium. However, persistent ST-segment elevations should suggest the presence of an **LV aneurysm,** and noninvasive confirmation of this diagnosis by two-dimensional echocardiography or radionuclide ventriculography should be sought.

63. Which MIs are most commonly complicated by LV aneurysms?

A ventricular aneurysm develops in 12–15% of survivors of an **acute transmural MI.** Aneurysms range from 1–8 cm in diameter. They are four times more common at the apex and anterior wall than in the inferoposterior wall, and they are more common in patients with larger infarcts. The mortality is about six times higher in patients with an LV aneurysm than in those with comparable global LV function. Death is often sudden, suggesting an increased risk of sustained VT and VF in these patients.

64. How do β-blockers reduce cardiovascular mortality in survivors of acute MI?

There is a reduction in sudden cardiac deaths due to VF. Thus, the protective effect of oral β-blockers in post-MI patients is primarily due to their "anti-fibrillatory" effects.

65. β-Blockers are effective in the treatment of stable exertional angina pectoris. Would you recommend routine administration of oral β-blockers in MI survivors who are angina-free?

Several large-scale, multicenter clinical trials conducted in the U.S. and abroad have shown a consistent reduction in total and cardiovascular mortality in survivors of acute transmural MI treated with oral β-blockers for 1–3 years. The largest published U.S. trial is the β-Blocker Heart Attack Trial, which randomized 3,837 MI survivors to either propranolol (180 or 240 mg/day) or placebo. At 3 years of follow-up, a 26% reduction in mortality was found in those patients treated with propranolol compared to placebo-treated patients. Thus, regardless of the presence or absence of angina, the routine administration of oral β-blockers—propranolol (180–240 mg), timolol (10 mg bid), or metoprolol (100 mg bid), to be started 5–21 days post-MI and continued for up to 3 years—is recommended in survivors of transmural MI.

Beta-Blocker Heart Attack Trial Research Group: A randomized trial of propranolol in patients with acute myocardial Infarction: 1. Mortality results. JAMA 247:1707–1714, 1982.

66. A 67-year-old man has stayed in bed for the last 3 days with flu-like symptoms. A 12-lead ECG reveals new Q waves in leads V_1 to V_6 and ST-segment elevation of 3 mm in leads V_2–V_5, I, and aVL. What do you suspect in this patient? Is plasma creatinine kinase (CK) likely to be high in this patient?

This patient has ECG changes of the recent evolution of an extensive anterolateral MI, as evidenced by:

1. 3-mm ST-segment elevations in anterolateral leads V_2–V_5, I, and aVL
2. New Q waves in all anterolateral chest leads

The most likely clinical diagnosis is an acute, extensive anterolateral MI that occurred 3–4 days ago, when he first complained of flu-like symptoms.

The laboratory confirmation of this clinical diagnosis is routinely done by measuring serum CK levels at 6-hour intervals for 24–48 hours. Serum CK levels are elevated starting at 4–8 hours after symptom onset, reach a peak at 18–24 hours, and normalize within 3–4 days. Thus, serum CK levels in this patient are likely to be normal.

In these late-comers, a measurement of lactate dehydrogenase-1 (LDH-1) isoenzyme or LDH-1/LDH-2 ratio is recommended. An LDH-1/LDH-2 ratio > 1.0 supports the clinical diagnosis of acute MI. Unlike serum CK, LDH is elevated at 1–2 days, reaches a peak at 3–6 days, and returns to normal 8–14 days after an acute MI. Newer, more specific enzymatic cardiac markers, such as cardiac troponins I or T, may also help.

67. What is Dressler's syndrome?

Dressler's syndrome, first described in 1854, is post-MI chest pain not due to coronary insufficiency. Its exact etiology is unclear, but it is characterized by inflammation of the pericardium and surrounding tissues. It occurs 2–10 weeks post-MI in 3–4% of cases and can be treated with corticosteroids and nonsteroidal anti-inflammatory agents.

68. How does Bayes' theorem help determine the value of exercise ECG testing in the detection of CAD?

Bayes' theorem allows prediction of the presence or absence of CAD in a patient, given the prevalence of CAD in the population and the sensitivity and specificity of the diagnostic test used in that patient. In general, the ability of noninvasive stress tests (treadmill exercise ECG test, treadmill thallium myocardial scintigraphy, or bicycle exercise radionuclide ventriculography) to predict the presence or absence of CAD in patients with a very low or very high pretest probability of CAD is poor. Thus, at both ends of the spectrum of pretest probability, noninvasive testing does not help the clinician decide whether to perform or not perform a definitive diagnostic test, such as coronary arteriography. On the other hand, patients with a reasonable pretest probability of CAD (30–70%) are good candidates for noninvasive stress testing.

Probability of Coronary Artery Disease

PRETEST PROBABILITY	AFTER TREADMILL ECG		AFTER TREADMILL THALLIUM
80%	Positive test: 95%	→	Positive test: 99%
		→	Negative test: 85%
	Negative test: 60%	→	Positive test: 90%
		→	Negative test: 30%

In the patient with typical exertional angina pectoris (associated with an 80% pretest probability of CAD), a negative treadmill ECG and thallium myocardial scintigram predict only a 30% probability of CAD. However, a positive treadmill thallium test in the same patient predicts a 90% probability of CAD. In such patients, coronary angiography is recommended in the latter case (positive treadmill thallium test) but not in the former.

HYPERTENSION

69. A 45-year-old hypertensive woman has been treated with nifedipine, 30 mg po qid, for chronic stable angina pectoris. She complains of ankle edema that worsened after her dose of nifedipine was recently increased. Are diuretics indicated in this patient?

Edema is a common side effect of chronic nifedipine treatment, occuring in 10–30% of patients treated with oral nifedipine in daily doses of 30–120 mg. Unlike other side effects of nifedipine, edema is dose-dependent and commonly responds to decreasing the nifedipine dose. Characteristically, edema secondary to nifedipine is not associated with volume expansion and does not respond to diuretics.

70. Are there different types of hypertension?

1. **Idiopathic** or **essential HTN** is the most common, affecting approx. 40 million American adults. Men are more frequently affected than women (until the postmenopausal age); black and Hispanic men and women are more commonly affected than whites.

2. **Labile** or **intermittent HTN** occurs only in certain circumstances, such as visits to the physician, stress, or exercise. These patients are at increased risk for the development of chronic HTN.

3. In **isolated systolic HTN**, systolic BP is elevated but diastolic BP is < 90 mm Hg. This type occurs typically in the elderly, in whom large-vessel compliance is decreased secondary to atherosclerosis and age. Systolic BP is usually > 160 mm Hg.

4. **Borderline HTN** is defined as elevated BP (120–140/80–90) but not in the hypertensive range. Usually, these patients are in transition from the normotensive to the hypertensive state and are at increased risk for the development of chronic HTN. Typically they have a family history of essential HTN.

5. **Malignant HTN** is a medical emergency requiring immediate therapy. It is characterized by marked elevation in BP, usually > 180/120 mm Hg, and is associated with evidence of acute end-organ damage, profound intravascular volume loss, and activation of the renin-angiotensin-aldosterone axis.

6. **Accelerated, urgent, or emergent HTN** is a milder form of malignant HTN in which the patient may be symptomatic but papilledema or evidence or renal injury is not present. However, due to the explosive nature of this disorder, these patients should be treated emergently.

71. Describe your approach to the initial evaluation of a patient with possible secondary causes of hypertension (HTN)? What is the value of such findings as postural HTN, paroxysmal HTN, and hypokalemia in the workup of these patients?

The initial evaluation of the hypertensive patient should be focused on historical or physical clues to the various causes of secondary HTN, including:

Alcohol consumption	Dietary salt intake
Muscle weakness	Paroxysmal episodes of palpitation
Headache	Sweating
Nervousness	Nausea or vomiting

History of renal parenchymal disease   Concomitant history of generalized
Documented postural hypotension   atherosclerotic vascular disease

A careful history (including age at onset of HTN, and family history of HTN), physical examination, and laboratory panel consisting of urinalysis, microscopy, CBC, blood electrolytes, serum creatinine, chest x-ray, and 12-lead ECG should be obtained in all patients evaluated for HTN.

Paroxysmal HTN and postural HTN suggest pheochromocytoma. The presence of generalized atherosclerosis and abdominal or flank bruits suggest renal artery stenosis. Muscle weakness and unexplained hypokalemia suggest aldosteronism. Prior history of renal parenchymal disease and the presence of an abnormal urine sediment suggest secondary HTN due to parenchymal renal disease.

72. It is generally accepted that antihypertensive therapy lowers the risk of stroke, but does it have any effect on risk of CAD (MI and angina)?

The Systolic HTN in the Elderly Program (SHEP) demonstrated that a thiazide-based antihypertensive regimen (chlorthalidone, 12.5–25 mg/day, alone or combined with atenolol, 25–50 mg/day) reduces stroke risk by 36% and nonfatal MI plus coronary death by 27% in *older* (> 60 yrs) patients with isolated systolic HTN (systolic BP > 160 mm Hg/diastolic BP < 90 mm Hg). Major cardiovascular events are reduced by 32%. As a result, overall all-cause mortality is 13% lower. Similar studies in younger hypertensive patients have shown a smaller beneficial effect or no effect of antihypertensive drug therapy on CAD events.

SHEP Cooperative Research Group: Prevention of stroke by antihypertensive drug treatment in older persons with isolated systolic hypertension. Final results of the Systolic Hypertension in the Elderly Program (SHEP). JAMA 265:3255–3264, 1991.

73. A 42-year-old woman has an office BP reading of 150/90 mm Hg. Would you initiate antihypertensive therapy in this patient?

Initiation of chronic antihypertensive drug therapy in a patient with a single office BP measurement of 150/90 mm Hg is *not* recommended. Unlike diastolic BP, systolic BP is subject to wider variations between office visits and even between examiners during a single office visit. Among the factors that may affect systolic BP measurement and thus result in the erroneous diagnosis of systemic hypertension are:
- Patient's anxiety level
- Ambient temperature at the doctor's office
- Examiner (physician or nurse)
- Time of day
- Physical activity preceding BP measurements
- Size of cuff used
- Patient's posture (supine, sitting, or standing)
- Presence of coexistent medical problems, such as fever, thyrotoxicosis, anemia, AV fistula, etc.

Drug therapy for hypertension is recommended for sustained elevations of sitting BP exceeding 140/90 mm Hg on > 2 clinic visits.

74. Which antihypertensive drug classes are currently recommended as "preferred" first-line drugs in the treatment of hypertension?

In the last 3 decades, several clinical trials have conclusively demonstrated that antihypertensive drugs improve survival and reduce the risk of stroke, heart failure, and renal failure in severe, moderate, and mild HTN. All of these studies used a treatment strategy consisting of a **thiazide diuretic** or **β-adrenergic blocker** alone or in combination with other drugs if necessary. There are no published clinical trials demonstrating a favorable effect of newer antihypertensive drugs, such as ACE inhibitors, calcium antagonists, or α-adrenergic blockers, on fatal or morbid complications of HTN. The Fifth Report of the Joint National Committee on Detection, Evaluation and Treatment of HTN, published in 1993, recommends diuretics and β-adrenergic blockers as "preferred" first-line antihypertensive drugs. Pharmacologic therapy

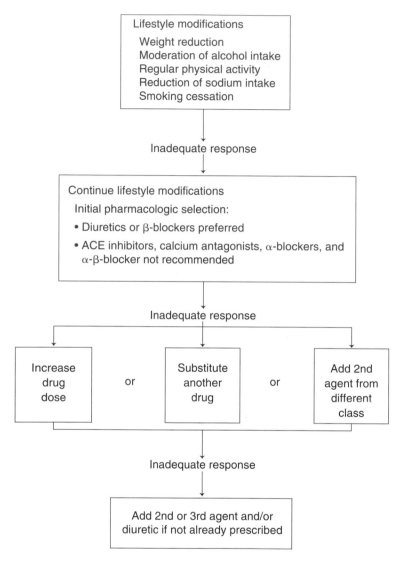

Treatment algorithm for HTN. (Adapted from Joint National Committee on Detection, Evaluation, and Treatment of High Blood Pressure: The fifth report of the Joint National Committee on Detection, Evaluation, and Treatment of High Blood Pressure (JNCV). Arch Intern Med 153:154–83, 1993.)

should be considered after life-style modifications have failed to achieve a reduction of BP to < 140/90 mm Hg.

75. What classes of antihypertensive drugs are preferred for use in a patient with a known history of CHF? Which drugs should you avoid?

The following classes of antihypertensive drugs are *desirable* in patients with CHF:

Vasodilators, such as direct vascular smooth-muscle-relaxing drugs (hydralazine and minoxidil), or **angiotensin-converting enzyme inhibitors** (captopril, enalapril, lisinopril)

Diuretics, such as thiazides

Drugs to *avoid* in these patients are ones with negative inotropic properties:

Calcium channel blockers (verapamil or diltiazem)

β-blockers (propranolol, metoprolol, atenolol, etc.)

76. Discuss the effect of alcohol consumption on hypertension.

Alcohol intake is one of the most common causes of secondary HTN. A linear relationship between alcohol consumption and BP has been described, with even small quantities of alcohol sometimes raising BP. A threshold effect has also been described, with a lower BP observed in patients who consume 1–2 oz of alcohol a day, compared to those who do not drink any alcohol. It is likely that alcohol causes HTN by raising cardiac output and heart rate. The mechanism is probably a rapid rise in plasma epinephrine and cortisol levels.

Klatsky AL, et al: The relationship between alcoholic beverage use and other traits to blood pressure: A new Kaiser-Permanente study. Circulation 73:628, 1986.

77. Among the nonpharmacologic interventions for HTN, many popular beliefs such as dietary garlic or onion intake and dietary magnesium or calcium in excess of RDA levels have not withstood careful evaluation in controlled clinical trials. Which lifestyle modifications have proven to benefit hypertensive patients?

Lifestyle Modifications for Hypertension Control and Overall Cardiovascular Health

- Lose weight if overweight
- Limit alcohol intake to 1 oz/day of ethanol (24 oz of beer, 8 oz of wine, or 2 oz of 100 proof whiskey)
- Exercise (aerobic) regularly
- Reduce sodium intake to < 100 mmol/day (< 2.3 gm of sodium or approx. < 6 gm of NaCl)
- Maintain adequate dietary potassium, calcium, and magnesium intake
- Stop smoking and reduce dietary saturated fat and cholesterol intake for overall cardiovascular health (reducing fat intake also helps reduce caloric intake, which is important for control of weight and Type II diabetes)

Joint National Committee on Detection, Evaluation and Treatment of High Blood Pressure. The fifth report of the Joint National Committee on Detection, Evaluation and Treatment of High Blood Pressure (JNCV). Arch Intern Med 153:154–183, 1993.

CONGESTIVE HEART FAILURE

78. What are some common signs and symptoms of CHF?

Listed in order of decreasing specificity:

Right Heart Failure	*Left Heart Failure*
Jugular vein distension	Chest x-ray with redistribution of perfusion or interstitial edema
Hepatomegaly	
Increased PT	Third heart sound (S_3)
Peripheral edema	Cardiomegaly
Increased AST/SGOT, bilirubin	Pulmonary rales
Pleural effusion	Paroxysmal nocturnal dyspnea, orthopnea
Decreased albumin	Dyspnea on exertion
Abdominal discomfort	
Anorexia	
Proteinuria	

79. What is the differential diagnosis of CHF?

Isolated Right Heart Failure	*Left or Biventricular Failure*
Pulmonary embolus	Aortic stenosis
Tricuspid stenosis	Aortic insufficiency
Tricuspid regurgitation	Mitral stenosis
Right atrial tumor	Mitral regurgitation
Cardiac tamponade	Most cardiomyopathies
Constrictive pericarditis	Acute MI
Pulmonic insufficiency	Myxoma
Right ventricular (RV) infarction	Hypertensive heart disease
Intrinsic lung disease	

Ebstein's anomaly
High cardiac output states (anemia,
    systemic fistulae, beriberi, Paget's
    disease, carcinoid, thyrotoxicosis, etc.)

Myocarditis
Supraventricular arrhythmias
Left ventricular (LV) aneurysm
Cardiac shunts
High cardiac output states

80. What factors can precipitate an exacerbation of formerly well-controlled chronic CHF?

When patients with well-controlled chronic CHF experience sudden exacerbations, in addition to consideration of worsening of the underlying condition(s) that led to CHF in this patient, a precipitating factor must be searched for and corrected. These factors include:

Increased consumption of salt
Fluid overload
Pulmonary emboli
Fever, infection
Anemia
Renal failure
Pregnancy

Paget's disease
Poor compliance with medications
Arrhythmias
Elevated BP
High environmental temperature
Cardiac ischemia or MI
Thyrotoxicosis

81. A 78-year-old man with a longstanding history of CHF presents with weakness, anorexia, nausea, and dizziness. He has been receiving digoxin, 0.5 mg po daily, and furosemide, 120 mg po twice a day. What specific tests would you request in your evaluation?

Any patient receiving digitalis who presents with GI symptoms, such as anorexia, nausea, or vomiting, should be suspected of having digitalis toxicity. The nausea and vomiting are thought to be mediated by stimulation of the area postrema in the medulla oblongata of the brainstem, rather than by any direct effects of digitalis on the GI mucosa. These GI manifestations may also occur in patients receiving excessive parenteral doses of digitalis.

Not uncommonly, patients with chronic CHF complain of similar GI symptoms due to passive hepatic congestion or ascites. Differentiation of the various causes of nausea and vomiting in such patients, on clinical grounds alone, can be difficult. Other manifestations of digitalis toxicity include:

1. **Neurologic symptoms:** headache, neuralgia, confusion, delirium and seizures
2. **Visual symptoms:** scotomata, halos, altered color perception
3. **Cardiac toxicity:**
    a. Ventricular or junctional tachyarrhythmias
    b. AV block
4. **Other manifestations:** gynecomastia, skin rash

The single most useful laboratory test to confirm the clinical suspicion of digitalis intoxication is a **serum digoxin level.** However, even serum digoxin levels in the "therapeutic range" may be toxic in elderly patients or in patients with hypokalemia, hypercalcemia, acid-base disorders, or thyroid disorders.

82. Describe the cardiac complications of digitalis intoxication.

Cardiac manifestations are by far the most life-threatening complications of digitalis intoxication. Almost any arrhythmia can be a manifestation of digitalis intoxication. Common ones include paroxysmal atrial tachycardia with AV block, junctional tachycardia with or without AV block, and first-degree or Mobitz I second-degree AV block. The coexistence of increased automaticity of ectopic pacemakers with impaired AV conduction is also very suggestive of digitalis intoxication.

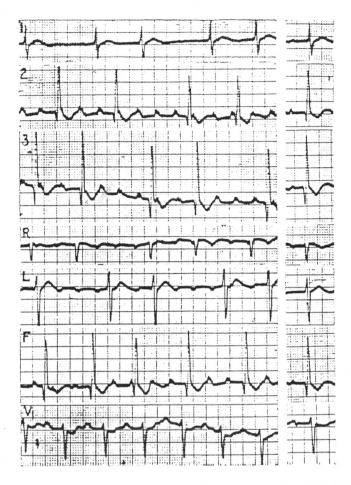

Digitalis intoxication presenting with paroxysmal atrial tachycardia with varying AV block. Note that the P waves are almost normally directed (axis +90°), the AV conduction ratio varies, and the atrial rhythm is not precisely regular. The single column of complexes on the right shows the form and direction of P waves (axis +60°) once sinus rhythm was restored. (From Marriott HJL: Practical Electrocardiography, 8th ed. Baltimore, Williams & Wilkins, 1988, p 488; with permission.)

83. A large variety of cardiac drugs is presently available for use in the treatment of CHF. Which one(s) have been proven to decrease mortality?

The drugs used to treat CHF include various classes of vasodilators (nitrates, hydralazine, prazosin, ACE inhibitors), digitalis, and diuretics. Unlike digitalis or diuretics, some **vasodila-tors** have been shown to reduce mortality in patients with CHF. **Enalapril,** an ACE inhibitor, re-duces mortality in patients with moderate or severe CHF (NYHA Class II, III, or IV). A combi-nation of **isosorbide dinitrate,** a predominant venous vasodilator, and **hydralazine,** an arteriolar vasodilator, reduces mortality in mildly to moderately severe CHF (NYHA Class II or III). Inter-estingly, not all vasodilators decrease mortality in patients with CHF. Prazosin, a postsynaptic α-1-receptor blocker, did not alter mortality when compared to placebo.

The Consensus Trial Study Group: Effects of enalapril on mortality in severe congestive heart failure: Results of the Cooperative North Scandinavian Enalapril Survival Study (CONSENSUS). N Engl J Med 316:1429–1435, 1987.

Cohn JN, et al: Effect of vasodilator therapy on mortality in chronic congestive heart failure: Results of a Veterans Administration Cooperative Study. N Engl J Med 314:1547–1552, 1986.

INFECTIONS

84. When is surgical intervention generally indicated in infectious endocarditis?

1. Heart failure refractory to adequate medical therapy
2. More than one major systemic embolic episode
3. Persistent bacteremia despite appropriate antibiotics
4. Severe valvular dysfunction by echocardiography
5. Ineffective antimicrobial therapy (e.g., fungal endocarditis)
6. Resection of mycotic aneurysm
7. Many cases of prosthetic valve endocarditis, especially with dehiscence or obstruction
8. Development of persistent heart block or bundle branch block, usually seen in aortic valve involvement and unrelated to drug therapy or ischemic heart disease
9. Extravalvular myocardial invasion, such as myocardial abscess or purulent pericarditis

85. What infectious pathogens may produce culture-negative endocarditis?

There are many potential reasons why blood cultures may be negative in the presence of infective endocarditis. They include prior administration of antibiotics, presence of uremia, and infection by fastidious organisms. Nutritionally deficient streptococci, *Brucella* sp., intracellular organisms (rickettsia and chlamydia), fungi, anaerobes, and the HACEK group of organisms (*Haemophilus* sp., *Actinobacillus actinomycetemcomitans, Cardiobacterium hominis, Eikenella corrodens,* and *Kingella kingae*) must also be considered when cultures are negative.

86. What does the new onset of conduction system abnormalities in the setting of endocarditis imply?

Perivalvular and/or myocardial abscesses. Surgical drainage and valve replacement are usually necessary.

87. What are the so-called immunologic manifestations of subacute bacterial endocarditis (SBE)?

Immunologic manifestations of infective endocarditis are thought to be mediated by the deposition of immune complexes within extracardiac structures, such as the retina, joints, fingertips, pericardium, skin, and kidney, rather than direct bacterial invasion. Interestingly, these immunologic manifestations of endocarditis are reported almost exclusively in patients with a prolonged course of SBE. They include:

1. **Roth spots:** cytoid bodies in the retina
2. **Osler nodes:** tender nodular lesions in the terminal phalanges
3. **Janeway lesions:** painless macular lesions on palms and soles
4. **Petechiae** and purpuric lesions
5. **Proliferative glomerulonephritis**

88. What are the most common causes of acute pericarditis?

In the **outpatient setting,** pericarditis is usually idiopathic. Many of these cases are probably due to viral infections. The coxsackie A and B viruses are highly cardiotropic and are two of the most common viruses to lead to pericarditis and myocarditis. Other responsible viruses include mumps, varicella-zoster, influenza, Epstein-Barr, and HIV.

In the **inpatient setting,** some of the more common etiologies can be recalled with the mnemonic **TUMOR.** "Tumor" also serves to remind that metastatic cancer is a frequent cause of pericarditis and pericardial effusion in hospitalized patients:

T = Trauma

U = Uremia

M = **M**yocardial infarction (acute and post), **M**edications (e.g., hydralazine and procainamide)

O = **O**ther infections (bacterial, fungal, tuberculous)

R = **R**heumatoid arthritis and other autoimmune disorders, **R**adiation

89. What is the major cardiac finding in Lyme disease?

Lyme disease is caused by the tick-borne spirochete, *Borrelia burgdorferi*. The initial infection is often marked by a rash, followed in weeks to months by involvement of other organ systems, including the heart, neurologic system, and joints. About 1 in 10 patients manifest cardiac involvement, usually with severe AV block which is often associated with syncope, since there is concomitant depression of ventricular escape rhythms. Temporary pacing is indicated (the AV block usually resolves), as is antibiotic treatment with high-dose IV penicillin or oral tetracycline.

CONGENITAL HEART DISEASE

90. Which congenital cardiac lesions most often present in adulthood?

Bicuspid aortic valve and atrial septal defect (ASD). Congenital cyanotic cardiac lesions are distinctly uncommon. ASDs alone account for about 30% of all congenital heart disease in adults.

Types and Frequencies of ASDs

1. Ostium secundum	70%
2. Ostium primum	15%
3. Sinus venosus	15%

91. *Coeur-en-sabot* is a term coined in 1888 by a French scientist in his first report of a congenital cardiac disease. Which congenital heart disease is it?

Coeur-en-sabot (wooden-shoe heart) was coined by E.L. Fallot in a report of tetralogy of Fallot. It describes the typical configuration of the cardiac silhouette on chest x-ray in these patients. The four components of this malformation are:

1. Ventricular septal defect
2. Obstruction to RV outflow
3. Overriding of the aorta
4. RV hypertrophy

The most distinctive radiographic finding in tetralogy of Fallot is RV hypertrophy. This results in a fairly classic boot-shaped (or wooden shoe-shaped) configuration of the cardiac silhouette, with prominence of the RV and a concavity in the region of the underdeveloped RV outflow tract and main pulmonary artery.

92. Which cardiac disease most commonly presents in adulthood with right bundle branch block (RBBB), first-degree AV block, and left axis deviation on ECG? Discuss the mechanism of these ECG findings.

The presence of complete or incomplete RBBB is an ECG hallmark of RV volume overload, often accompanied by rightward deviation of the QRS axis, except in patients with ostium primum ASD. Because of hypoplastic changes in the left anterior fascicle, patients with ostium primum ASD have left axis QRS deviation. Thus, the combination of RBBB and left axis QRS deviation is a fairly distinctive feature of **ostium primum ASD**, and it is often accompanied by first-degree AV block.

CARDIAC SYNDROMES AND OTHER ENTITIES

93. What are the cardiac manifestations of ankylosing spondylitis? What valvular dysfunction is commonly encountered in this syndrome?

The incidence of cardiovascular involvement in ankylosing spondylitis ranges from 3–10%, depending on the duration of the disease. The characteristic cardiac involvement consists of dilatation of the aortic valve ring and the sinuses of Valsalva, as well as inflammatory changes in the aortic valve ring. The resultant clinical hallmark is aortic root dilatation and aortic regurgitation, often rapidly progressive and ultimately requiring aortic valve replacement. Echocardiography is the diagnostic technique of choice in the evaluation and follow-up of these patients.

94. What is the ECG triad of Wolff-Parkinson-White (WPW) syndrome?
1. Short PR interval (<0.12 sec)
2. Wide QRS complex (>0.12 sec)
3. Delta wave or slurred upstroke of QRS complex

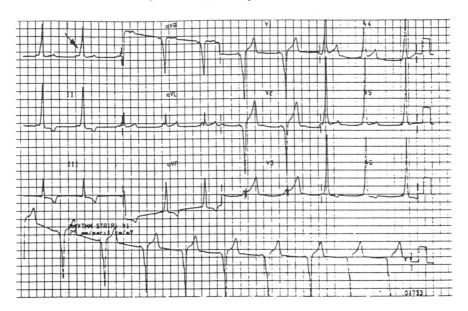

Right anteroseptal accessory pathway in WPW. The 12-lead ECG characteristically exhibits a normal to inferior axis. The delta wave is negative in V_1 and V_2, upright in lead I, II, AVL, and AVF; isoelectric in lead III, and negative in AVR. The arrow indicates delta wave (lead 1). (From Braunwald E [ed]: Heart Disease: A Textbook of Cardiovascular Medicine, 3rd ed. Philadelphia, W.B. Saunders, 1988, p 686; with permission.)

95. Discuss the mechanism underlying sudden cardiac death in patients with WPW syndrome.

Patients with a pre-excitation syndrome such as WPW are at risk for developing AF with antegrade conduction along the accessory pathway. This tachycardia presents a serious risk because of its propensity to degenerate into VF due to very rapid conduction over the accessory pathway.

Patients with accessory pathways and *short refractory periods* (<200 msec) are at highest risk for this antegrade conduction AF and therefore sudden cardiac death. Intermittent pre-excitation during sinus rhythm and loss of conduction along the accessory pathway during exercise or during administration of ajmaline or procainamide suggest that the refractory period of the accessory pathway is long (>250 msec). These patients are *not* at risk of developing very rapid ventricular rates when AF or atrial flutter occurs and are therefore not at risk for sudden cardiac death.

96. How does Marfan's syndrome affect the heart?

Marfan's syndrome is a generalized disorder of connective tissue that is inherited as an autosomal dominant trait. Cardiac abnormalities occur in over 60% of these patients and are almost always responsible for early death when it occurs. The most common cardiac lesion is dilatation of the aortic ring, sinuses of Valsalva, and ascending aorta. This dilatation leads to progressive aortic regurgitation and may be complicated by acute aortic dissection. The risk of dissection is markedly increased during pregnancy.

Another common valvular dysfunction in Marfan's syndrome is mitral regurgitation due to a redundant myxomatous mitral valve (called "floppy" prolapsed mitral valve). In contrast to adults, children with Marfan's are much more likely to have severe isolated mitral regurgitation than aortic root or aortic valve disease.

97. To what does the term Marfan's syndrome-forme fruste refer?

Mitral valve prolapse (MVP) in the absence of other systemic manifestations of Marfan's syndrome has been referred to as Marfan's syndrome–forme fruste, in view of the similar pathologic appearance of the myxomatous mitral valve in both disorders. Isolated MVP is more common than Marfan's syndrome.

98. What are the three types of Takayasu's arteritis?

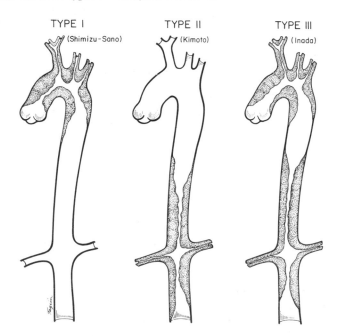

TYPE I (Shimizu-Sano)   TYPE II (Kimoto)   TYPE III (Inada)

Type I involves primarily the aortic arch and brachiocephalic vessels. **Type II** affects the thoracoabdominal aorta and particularly the renal arteries. **Type III** combines features of both Types I and II. Types I and III may be complicated by aortic regurgitation.

From Braunwald E (ed): Heart Disease: A Textbook of Cardiovascular Medicine, 3rd ed. Philadelphia, W.B. Saunders, 1988, p 1563; with permission.

99. Which age group and sex of patients are most typically affected with Takayasu's arteritis? How does this differ from atherosclerosis and giant cell arteritis?

Takayasu's arteritis typically affects young women, with a female:male ratio of 8:1. In about three-fourths of all cases, onset is in the teenage years. This is in sharp contrast to atherosclerotic aortic disease, which usually affects older men, and giant cell arteritis, which usually affects women over age 50 years.

	Takayasu's Arteritis	*Atherosclerosis*	*Giant Cell Arteritis*
Synonyms	Pulseless disease, reversed coarctation	—	Granulomatous arteritis
Age at onset	15–25 yrs	>50 yrs	>50 yrs
F:M ratio	8:1	1:4	2–3:1
Systemic prodrome	Fever, weight loss	None	Headache, fever
Site of involvement	Aortic arch, thoracoabdominal	Large arteries	Temporal arteries
Complications	Pulseless arms, aortic hypertension	Stroke, MI, claudication (leg)	Blindness, jaw or arm claudication, polymyalgia

100. What is the classic clinical prodrome associated with Takayasu's arteritis?

1. Fever and night sweats
2. Anorexia and weight loss
3. Malaise and fatigue
4. Arthralgias
5. Pleuritic pain

101. What is the holiday heart syndrome?

The holiday heart syndrome is characterized by the presence of supraventricular arrhythmias in alcoholic patients following an acute alcoholic binge, sometimes associated with holiday parties or long weekends. These arrhythmias are often transient and do not require long-term antiarrhythmic drug therapy. The most common arrhythmias are AF and atrial flutter. Digitalis and β-blockers produce an effective and rapid therapeutic response. Supportive care is also essential to prevent alcohol withdrawal symptoms in these patients.

102. Which of the cardiac chambers is most frequently involved in an atrial myxoma?

Frequency of Location of Myxomas

1. Left atrium	86%
2. Right atrium	10%
3. Left ventricle	2%
4. Right ventricle	2%
5. Multiple locations	10%

The most common site of origin of atrial myxomas is the fossa ovalis. To prevent recurrence of myxoma, a wide resection of the fossa ovalis area of the interatrial septum is performed during surgical excision.

103. What is the most common cause of chronic mitral regurgitation in the U.S.?

Mitral valve prolapse. This has replaced rheumatic heart disease, which was the most common cause of chronic mitral regurgitation in the 1950s and 1960s.

104. What are the physical examination findings in mitral regurgitation?

Mitral regurgitation is associated with an apical holosystolic murmur. The intensity and radiation of the murmur vary with the cause and severity. Physical examination may also reveal an S_3, peripheral pulses with a quick upstroke and short duration, a widened pulse pressure, and a hyperdynamic precordium.

105. How is mitral regurgitation treated?

Medical management includes afterload reduction (to maximize "forward" cardiac output), salt restriction and diuretics (in the face of CHF), and digitalis (in the face of AF). Surgical mitral valve replacement should be performed in patients refractory to medical management before they enter the severely symptomatic stage.

PACING

106. Describe the three-letter code used to indicate the essential functions of a cardiac pacemaker.

The Three-Letter Pacemaker Code

First letter	Chamber(s) paced	A–atrial V–ventricle D–dual chamber
Second letter	Chamber(s) sensed	A–atrial V–ventricle D–dual chamber
Third letter	Mode of response to sensed event	O–no response I–inhibition T–triggering D–dual response

The letters in the pacing code describe the different pacer functions. The first letter indicates the chamber paced, the second is the chamber in which electrical activity is sensed, and the third represents the response to a sensed event. Thus, for the two most commonly used pacemakers today, the code indicates:

VVI, a pacemaker that can pace and sense the right ventricle (VV), and has an inhibited mode of response (I).

DDD, the so-called dual-chamber AV sequential pacemaker, can pace and sense either right ventricle or right atrium (DD) and has both inhibited and triggered modes of response (D).

107. What do the different modes of response indicate?

I — Inhibited: Pacemakers with an inhibited mode of response do not pace when a spontaneous depolarization (atrial or ventricular) is sensed by the pacemaker. Following a fixed interval, if no spontaneous depolarization is sensed, pacing occurs. The inhibited mode of response is most commonly used.

T — Triggered: These pacemakers pace shortly after a spontaneous depolarization is sensed. After a fixed interval, pacing will occur if no spontaneous depolarization is sensed.

D — Dual-response: The pacemakers have both inhibited and triggered modes of response.

108. Who generally receives dual-chamber pacemakers?

Dual-chamber pacemakers (DDD) are more expensive, are more difficult to implant, and require greater expertise from the clinician in charge of the patient's follow-up as compared to ventricular-demand pacemakers (VVI). Insertion of a dual-chamber pacemaker is therefore reserved for patients who are not good candidates for ventricular-demand pacemakers. These include older patients, patients with CHF or LV hypertrophy, and physically active young adults who would not tolerate fixed-rate ventricular pacing. On the other hand, patients who have a history of recurrent SVT are not good candidates for any pacing modality that involves atrial sensing, such as dual-chamber pacemakers. The latter would be better served by a simpler ventricular-demand pacemaker (VVI).

109. What are the manifestations and pathophysiology of pacemaker syndrome?

Patients suffering from symptomatic bradyarrhythmias who receive ventricular demand pacemakers (VVI) sometimes report dizziness, palpitations, a pounding sensation in the chest or neck, and/or dyspnea associated with ventricular pacing. The underlying mechanism is thought to be related to loss of the normal AV synchrony during ventricular pacing. An improvement in cardiac output has been documented in various studies when the pacing modality was changed from ventricular to dual-chamber or AV sequential pacing. It is likely that patients with LV hypertrophy or LV failure or older patients who have a large atrial contribution to LV filling are most prone to develop pacemaker syndrome, and they may therefore be better candidates for AV sequential pacing using a DDD pacemaker.

AORTA

110. What are the causes of acute, severe aortic regurgitation (AR)?

Infective endocarditis
Dissecting aneurysm
Rupture or prolapse of aortic leaflet(s)
Traumatic rupture
Spontaneous rupture of myxomatous valve
Spontaneous rupture of leaflet fenestrations
Sudden sagging of a "normal" leaflet
Postoperative—faulty incision of a stenotic aortic valve

Morganroth J, et al: Acute severe aortic regurgitation. Ann Intern Med 87:225, 1977.

111. Why is a wide pulse pressure, typically present in chronic severe AR, unlikely to be observed in patients with acute AR?

The absence of a wide pulse pressure, as well as the concurrent absence of the characteristic arterial auscultatory signs of chronic AR, in patients presenting with acute AR is thought to be due to the much higher LV end-diastolic pressure (LVEDP) in the acute form. The acute development of a severe aortic valvular leak causes a much higher LVEDP in the normal-sized LV of patients with acute AR. Patients with chronic AR commonly have a dilated LV with increased compliance capable of accommodating large blood volumes without a significant rise of LVEDP.

Salient Hemodynamic Features of Severe Aortic Regurgitation

	ACUTE	CHRONIC
LV compliance	Not ↑	↑
Regurgitant volume	↑	↑
LV end-diastolic pressure	Markedly ↑	May be normal
LV ejection velocity	Not signif. ↑	Markedly ↑
Aortic systolic pressure	Not ↑	↑
Aortic diastolic pressure	→ to ↑	Markedly ↓
Systemic arterial pulse pressure	Slightly to moderately ↑	Markedly ↑
Ejection fraction	Not ↑	↑
Effective stroke volume	↓	↔
Effective cardiac output	↓	↔
Heart rate	↑	↔
Peripheral vascular resistance	↑	Not ↑

↔ = unchanged, ↑ = increased, ↓ = decreased.
Morganroth J, et al: Acute severe aortic regurgitation. Ann Intern Med 87:225, 1977.

As a result of the rapid elevation of LVEDP in acute AR and its rapid equilibration with aortic pressure, the diastolic rumble of acute AR is much shorter and softer than that of chronic AR. Another auscultatory manifestation of the rapid rise of LVEDP is premature mitral valve closure. This is considered a reliable echocardiographic sign of acute AR.

112. What are the signs of chronic AR? What are their mechanisms?

Chronic AR is characterized by a dilated LV due to longstanding volume overload, with a large stroke volume and a wide pulse pressure. The peripheral arterial auscultatory signs of chronic regurgitation are primarily due to this wide pulse pressure of chronic AR.

Peripheral Arterial Signs of Chronic Aortic Regurgitation

1. **de Musset's sign:** bobbing of the head with each heartbeat
2. **Corrigan's pulse:** abrupt distension and quick collapse of femoral pulses (also called water-hammer pulse)
3. **Traube's sign:** booming, "pistol-shot" systolic and diastolic sounds heard over the femoral pulse
4. **Müller's sign:** systolic pulsations of the uvula
5. **Duroziez's sign:** systolic murmur over femoral artery when compressed proximally and diastolic murmur when compressed distally
6. **Quincke's sign:** capillary pulsations of fingertips
7. **Hill's sign:** popliteal cuff systolic pressure exceeding brachial cuff pressure by >60 mm Hg

113. What are the three types of aortic dissection according to the DeBakey classification? What are their clinical and therapeutic significance?

The DeBakey classification divides aortic dissections into three groups based on their location, with each type requiring a different therapeutic approach. In general, Types I and II are best managed surgically, whereas Type III is best managed medically. These differences are based largely on the disparate natural history of proximal (types I and II) and distal (type III) dissections. Even minimal progression of a proximal dissection can cause potentially fatal complica-

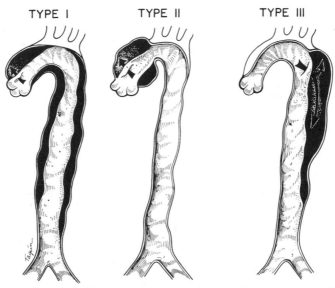

TYPE I   TYPE II   TYPE III

"PROXIMAL" or "ASCENDING"   "DISTAL" or "DESCENDING"

tions, such as cardiac tamponade, acute aortic regurgitaton, or neurologic compromise. On the other hand, patients with distal aortic dissections often have advanced cardiovascular and cardiopulmonary disease and are therefore poor surgical candidates.

(From Braunwald E (ed): Heart Disease: A Textbook of Cardiovascular Medicine, 3rd ed. Philadelphia, W.B. Saunders, 1988, p 1554; with permission.)

114. What are the most common sites of aortic coarctation?
In descending order of frequency:
1. Postductal (adult-type coarctation)
2. Localized juxtaductal coarctation
3. Preductal (infantile-type coarctation)
4. Ascending thoracic aorta
5. Distal descending thoracic aorta
6. Abdominal aorta

115. Which congenital cardiac lesions are associated with coarctation of the aorta?
Aortic coarctation is frequently associated with other congenital cardiac lesions, including:
1. Bicuspid aortic valve
2. Patent ductus arteriosus
3. Ventricular septal defect
4. Berry aneurysms of circle of Willis

DRUG THERAPY

116. Which antiarrhythmic agent is likely to initially worsen the arrhythmia it is used to treat? Why?
Bretylium, used parenterally for the treatment of serious ventricular tachyarrhythmias, causes an initial release of norepinephrine from adrenergic nerves followed by inhibition of norepinephrine release. It is this initial effect that can cause a transient increase in ventricular irritability and hypertension, especially in digitalized patients.

117. Give the mechanisms of action and usual doses of vasodilator drugs.

Effects and Dosages of Major Vasodilators

AGENT	MECHANISM OF ACTION	VENOUS DILATING EFFECT	ARTERIOLAR DILATING EFFECT	USUAL DOSAGE
Nitroglycerin	Direct	+++	+	25–500 μg/min IV
Isosorbide dinitrate	Direct	+++	+	5–20 mg q2h subling. 10–60 mg q4h po
Hydralazine	Direct	—	+++	10–100 mg q6h po
Minoxidil	Direct	—	+++	10–40 mg/day po
Sodium nitroprusside	Direct	+++	+++	5–150 μg/min IV
Epoprostenol (prostacyclin)	Direct	+++	+++	5–15 ng/kg/min IV
Phenoxybenzamine	α-blockade	++	+	10–20 mg q8h po
Phentolamine	α-blockade	++	+	50 mg q4–6h po
Prazosin	α-blockade	+++	++	1–10 mg q8h po
Captopril	Inhibition of ACE	+++	++	6.25–50.0 mg q6–8h po
Enalapril	Inhibition of ACE	+++	+++	5–20 mg bid po
Lisinopril	Inhibition of ACE	+++	++	10–40 mg/day po
Quinapril	Inhibition of ACE	+++	++	10–40 mg/day po

From Rubenstein E, Federman D (eds): Scientific American Medicine. New York, Scientific American, 1988; with permission.

118. What is the mechanism of action of digitalis?

Digitalis and all the cardiac glycosides act by inhibiting Na^+-K^+ ATPase activity (the sodium pump). This blocks the transport of sodium and potassium across cell membranes, leading to an intracellular increase in sodium and decrease in potassium. The increase in intracellular sodium in turn leads to an exchange for calcium. The increased intracellular calcium, the contractile element of muscle, leads to increased contractility (positive inotropic effect).

The antiarrhythmic effects of the cardiac glycosides are probably not due to any direct effect of the drug. Rather, they are mediated by an increase in vagal tone in the atria and AV junction.

119. What factors contribute to digitalis toxicity?

Hypokalemia	Drugs
Hypercalcemia	Quinidine
Hypomagnesemia	Verapamil
Renal insufficiency (digoxin)	Amiodarone
Hepatic insufficiency (digitoxin)	Others

120. What are the elimination half-lives of digoxin and lidocaine? How can you use this information to guide you in the initiation of digoxin or lidocaine therapy?

Lidocaine is metabolized in the liver, and its elimination is prolonged by old age, liver failure, CHF, and cardiogenic shock. Because its elimination half-life is 1–2 hours in healthy individuals, initiation of an IV infusion of lidocaine without a preceding bolus will not result in a steady-state serum level until about 6 hours later. Thus, an IV loading dose of 3 mg/kg is given over the first 15–20 minutes to bring the lidocaine blood level to a therapeutic range as soon as possible.

The **digoxin** elimination half-life is about 36 hours. In the absence of loading, a steady-state level would be reached in 5–6 days. Therefore, a loading dose of 0.75 mg is given over the first 6–24 hours to provide a steady-state serum level more rapidly. The duration of initial digitalization depends on the urgency of digitalis therapy. In patients with acute pulmonary edema, digitalization with a full IV loading dose of 0.75 mg should be completed within the first 4–6 hours, whereas in patients with chronic CHF, digitalization can be performed over 24–48 hours. Digoxin is primarily eliminated by the kidneys, so the oral maintenance dose should be reduced in the presence of renal failure.

121. Patients maintained on digitalis commonly exhibit some changes on ECG referred to as "digitalis effect." What are these changes, and how do they compare with those in myocardial ischemia?

Digitalis is to the ECG what syphilis once was to medicine, a great imitator. Digitalis can cause a variety of ECG abnormalities depending on the serum digoxin level. Administered in therapeutic doses, digoxin causes a characteristic sagging of the ST segment and flattening and inversion of the T waves. These changes typically occur in the inferolateral ECG leads.

These ST and T-wave changes are difficult to distinguish from those of subendocardial myocardial ischemia; however, some subtle differences exist. Typically, horizontal or downsloping ST-segment depression, sharp-angled ST-T junctions, and U-wave inversion are present in patients with subendocardial ischemia (coronary insufficiency). Less commonly, tall T waves may be a subtle ECG sign of myocardial ischemia.

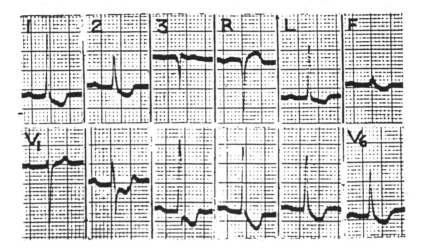

Digitalis effect. Note sagging ST segments in most leads with short QT interval. (From Marriott HJL: Practical Electrocardiography, 8th ed. Baltimore, Williams & Wilkins, 1988, pp 478; with permission.)

122. In primary prevention trials aimed at reducing cardiovascular mortality with cholesterol-lowering drugs, which drugs have been shown to lower the risk of death from cardiac causes?

Coronary Primary Prevention Trials: LRC-CPPT vs. HHS

	LRC-CPPT[1]	HHS[2]
Cholesterol-lowering drug	Cholestyramine	Gemfibrozil
Average daily dose	24 gm	600 mg bid
Duration of follow-up	7.4 yrs	5 yrs
Reduction in cholesterol	8.5%	10%
Reduction in LDL cholesterol	13%	10%
Increase in HDL cholesterol	2%	10%
Reduction in CV mortality	19%	34%

Two primary prevention trials, the Lipid Research Clinic Coronary Primary Prevention Trial (LRC-CPPT) and the Helsinki Heart Study (HHS), were designed to test the hypothesis that a reduction of serum cholesterol decreases cardiovascular mortality. Both clinical trials showed that cholesterol-lowering drugs, such as cholestyramine and gemfibrozil, effectively reduced serum cholesterol and decreased cardiovascular mortality.

A 1% reduction in serum cholesterol in the LRC-CPPT was associated with a 2% reduction in cardiovascular mortality. Overall, about a 10% reduction in serum cholesterol was accompanied by a 20% decrease in cardiovascular mortality. One of the most interesting findings in this trial was that the reduction in cardiovascular mortality was highest in those patients who had the lowest reduction in serum cholesterol levels, supporting the causal relationship between cholesterol and cardiovascular disease.

1. Lipid Research Clinics Program: The Lipid Research Clinics Coronary Primary Prevention Trial results: Reduction in incidence of coronary heart disease. JAMA 251:351, 1984.

2. Frick MH, et al: Helsinki Heart Study: Primary prevention trial with dyslipidemia. N Engl J Med 317:1237–1245, 1987.

123. Most lipid-lowering drugs lower serum cholesterol levels by reducing the LDL fraction, but some are capable of raising the serum HDL-cholesterol level as well. Which lipid-lowering drug is most effective in raising HDL cholesterol levels? Does this affect coronary mortality?

Among all available lipid-lowering drugs, **gemfibrozil** results in the most marked increase in HDL-cholesterol levels. A 600 mg-dose, taken twice a day, resulted in a 10% increase in HDL in the Helsinki Heart Study. In this trial, 4,081 asymptomatic men with hyperlipidemia were randomly assigned to receive gemfibrozil or placebo over 5 years. Unlike patients in the LRC-CPPT, who received cholestyramine and experienced almost no change in the serum HDL level, gemfibrozil-treated patients experienced a 10% increase in HDL and a remarkable 34% reduction in coronary mortality. Cholestyramine-treated patients had only 19% reduction in mortality.

The 10% increase in HDL cholesterol levels induced by gemfibrozil likely accounted for the additional 15% reduction in CHD mortality. This led to the so-called "HDL hypothesis,"—i.e., that an increase in HDL alone can decrease the risk of death from CAD.

124. Does lowering LDL-cholesterol reduce the risk of further mortality in patients with preexisting CAD?

The first published randomized controlled clinical trial of the effect of lipid-lowering therapy on CAD and all-cause mortality is the 4S (Scandinavian Simvastatin Survival Study). In this clinical trial of 4,444 men and women, aged 35–70 years, with a history of angina pectoris or acute MI and serum cholesterol of 5.5–8 mmol/l (220–320 mg/dl), simvastatin lowered total cholesterol and LDL cholesterol by 25% and 35%, respectively, and increased HDL by 8%. This was accompanied by a 30% reduction in overall mortality (from 12% to 8%), a 42% reduction in CAD deaths (from 28% to 19%), and a 37% reduction in the need for myocardial revascularization procedures (coronary bypass or angioplasty).

Unlike the LRC-CPPT, the 4S study showed a 3-fold greater reduction in cardiovascular mortality over a shorter follow-up period (5 vs. 10 years). It is hypothesized that simvastatin lowered CAD events primarily by stabilizing atherosclerotic lesions, accounting for a lower incidence of CAD events as early as 2 years after starting lipid-lowering drug therapy.

Scandinavian Simvastatin Survival Study Group: Randomized tiral of cholesterol lowering in 4444 patients with coronary heart disease: The Scandinavian Simvastatin Survival Study (4S). Lancet 344:1383–1389, 1994.

125. What does cardioselectivity of a β-blocking drug mean? Which β-blockers are cardioselective, and what are the clinical implications of this pharmacologic property?

Cardioselective β-blockers	Noncardioselective β-blockers
Atenolol (Tenormin)	Propranolol (Inderal)
Metoprolol (Lopressor)	Timolol (Blocadren)
Acebutolol (Sectral)	Pindolol (Visken)
	Nadolol (Corgard)

Cardioselectivity refers to the predominant blockade of the β_1- adrenergic receptors, which are mostly present in the heart. Cardioselective β-blockers, in low doses, have minimal blocking effects on β_2-receptors, the predominant β receptors in the lungs. However, cardioselectivity is only relative; when administered in large doses, cardioselectivity is markedly diminished. Despite these limitations, cardioselective β-blockers are much safer than noncardioselective β-blockers in patients with obstructive lung disease.

126. What is the importance of intrinsic sympathomimetic activity (ISA) as it applies to β-blockers? Which β-blockers possess ISA?

ISA refers to the partial β-adrenergic agonist properties of some β-blockers. When sympathetic activity is low (at rest), these β-blockers produce low-grade β-stimulation. However, under conditions of stress (exercise), β-blockers with ISA behave essentially as conventional β-blockers without ISA. The clinical significance of ISA is not clearly established.

Pindolol and acebutolol demonstrate ISA. All other β-blockers presently available do not have any significant ISA.

127. Prior to elective cardioversion of a patient with atrial fibrillation (AF), a 2-week course of anticoagulation decreases the risk of thromboembolic events during and shortly after cardioversion. Is anticoagulation similarly required in a patient with AF with a fast ventricular rate of 230/bpm and systolic BP of 70 mm Hg?

The risks and benefits of cardioversion and anticoagulation must be weighed very carefully prior to elective cardioversion. A 10–14-day period of adequate anticoagulation is desirable before elective cardioversion of a patient with AF. However, in a patient with AF with a fast ventricular response rate, the most important question is how urgent is cardioversion? Whenever there is clinical evidence of hemodynamic compromise (such as CHF, hypotension or systemic hypoperfusion, acute anginal symptoms, or acute MI), urgent cardioversion should be administered *immediately,* regardless of left atrial or LV size, systolic LV function, or prior anticoagulation. In the patient in question with AF with a fast ventricular response rate of 230/bpm and severe hypotension, cardioversion should *absolutely not* be delayed.

128. How is acute pulmonary edema managed with digitalis, diuretics, and vasodilators?

The therapeutic approach to any patient with acute pulmonary edema must be individualized, but some general guidelines for therapy are helpful:

1. IV diuresis with a loop diuretic such as furosemide (20 to 60 mg IV push, to be repeated as necessary): IV furosemide lowers venous tone and thus lowers pulmonary wedge pressure even *before* inducing effective diuresis.

2. IV, cutaneous, or oral preload-reducing drug therapy: Nitrates are effective venodilators. In single oral doses of 40–60 mg (to be repeated 3 or 4 times daily), they are effective in lowering pulmonary capillary wedge pressure and thus improving congestive symptoms of dyspnea, orthopnea, paroxysmal nocturnal dyspnea, and nocturnal cough.

3. IV digitalization is recommended in patients with acute pulmonary edema with or without associated AF.

4. Oxygen therapy, depending on results of arterial blood gas measurements.

5. Bed rest and salt restriction.

6. Afterload-reducing drugs are effective in alleviating the signs and symptoms of CHF. ACE inhibitors, such as captopril, enalapril, or lisinopril, are effective afterload and preload-reducing drugs and can be administered orally in patients with overt CHF.

BIBLIOGRAPHY

1. Braunwald E (ed): Heart Disease; A Textbook of Cardiovascular Medicine, 6th ed. Philadelphia, W.B. Saunders, 1996.
2. Hurst JW (ed): The Heart, 8th ed. New York, McGraw-Hill, 1994.
3. Marriott HJL: Practical Electrocardiography, 9th ed. Baltimore, Williams & Wilkins, 1994.
4. Johnson RA, et al: The Practice of Cardiology. Boston, Little, Brown, 1980.
5. Isselbacher KJ, et al (eds): Harrison's Principles of Internal Medicine, 13th ed. New York, McGraw-Hill, 1994.

4. INFECTIOUS DISEASES

Richard J. Hamill, M.D.

Men take diseases, one of another. Therefore let me take heed of their company.

William Shakespeare
Henry-IV

Throughout nature, infection without disease is the rule rather than the exception.

Rene Dubos
Man Adapting

1. What is Luria's law?

Three antibiotics equals one fungal infection.

Matz RP: Principles of medicine. NY State J Med 77:99–101, 1977.

2. What role does the horseshoe crab, *Limulus polyphemus,* play in infectious diseases?

In 1956, Bang reported that gram-negative bacterial endotoxin caused gelation of a lysate prepared from the blood cells (amebocytes) of the *Limulus* crab. This limulus amebocyte lysate reaction is the basis of an assay now used to detect the presence of endotoxin in various body fluids, pharmacologic products, and medical devices.

Bang FB: A bacterial disease of *Limulus polyphemus*. Bull Johns Hopkins Hosp 98:325–350, 1956.

3. What is Vincent's angina?

This is a necrotizing pharyngitis caused by a mixture of anaerobes and spirochetes. *Streptococcus pyogenes* and *Staphylococcus aureus* may also play a role. Symptoms include an extremely sore throat, fever, and foul breath. Physical examination reveals pharyngeal ulcerations that are covered with a purulent exudate. Treatment with penicillin is curative.

4. Where and when was the last naturally occurring case of smallpox identified?

In Merka Town, Somalia, in October 1977.

5. What are the tick-borne infectious diseases seen in the U.S.?

Tick-borne Infectious Diseases in the U.S.

DISEASE	ORGANISM
Lyme disease	*Borrelia burgdorferi*
Q fever	*Coxiella burnetii*
Human ehrlichiosis	*Ehrlichia chaffeensis, E. equi*-like agent
Rocky Mountain spotted fever	*Rickettsia ricketsii*
Tularemia	*Francisella tularensis*
Babesiosis	*Babesia microti*
Relapsing fever	*Borrelia hermsii*
Tick-borne encephalitis	A flavivirus
Colorado tick fever	An orbivirus

Rathore MH: Human ehrlichiosis: Spotless Rocky Mountain spotted fever. Infect Med 10:21–22, 1993.

6. What is tick paralysis?

Tick paralysis is a complication of prolonged attachment of certain species of ticks (*Dermacentor andersoni* and *D. variabilis* in the U.S.). It is an ascending paralysis that begins in the lower extremities and rapidly progresses to involve the upper extremities and head. It is thought to be caused by a neurotoxin in the tick's saliva, and it usually resolves quickly after the tick is removed.

7. Post-splenectomy sepsis is caused by what organisms?

Splenectomy predisposes patients to sepsis by encapsulated organisms, including:

Streptococcus pneumoniae   *Neisseria meningitidis*
Haemophilus influenzae   *Escherichia coli*

Occasional cases due to *Staphylococcus aureus* and *Capnocytophaga canimorsus* (DF-2) have been described.

8. Infective endocarditis due to *Pseudomonas aeruginosa* occurs almost always in what risk group?

P. aeruginosa causes infective endocarditis on native heart valves in intravenous drug abusers. Rarely, it is a cause of prosthetic valve endocarditis. The occurrence of *P. aeruginosa* endocarditis varies regionally. The source of the organism is thought to be standing water that contaminates drug paraphernalia.

9. What are the causative organisms of prosthetic valve endocarditis and their time of appearance relative to the valve replacement surgery?

Traditionally, prosthetic valve endocarditis has been classified according to the time of onset with respect to the replacement surgery, with 2 months being the division between early- and late-onset endocarditis:

Prosthetic Valve Endocarditis (PVE)

ORGANISM	EARLY PVE (%)	LATE PVE (%)	OVERALL (%)
Staphylococci			
S. epidermidis	35	26	29
S. aureus	17	12	14
Streptococci			
Group D and enterococci	3	9	7
S. pneumoniae	1	< 1	1
Other (incl. viridans streptococci)	4	25	17
Gram-negative bacilli	16	12	13
Diphtheroids	10	4	7
Other bacteria	1	2	2
Candida	8	4	5
Aspergillus	2	1	1
Other fungi	1	< 1	1
Culture-negative	1	4	3

Mayer KH, et al: Evaluation and management of prosthetic valve endocarditis. Prog Cardiovasc Dis 25:43–62, 1982.

10. What are the causes of biologic false-positive RPRs?

The causes of biologic false-positive rapid plasma reagent (RPR) tests for syphilis can be divided into those of acute or chronic duration:

Acute (positive < 6 mos)   **Chronic (> 6 mos' duration)**
Acute febrile illnesses   Chronic infections (lepromatous leprosy)
Recent immunizations   Autoimmune diseases (e.g., lupus)
Pregnancy   IV drug addiction

When false-positive tests occur, the titer is usually low (<1:8).

11. Do the specific treponemal serologic tests for syphilis (i.e., MHA-TP, FTA-ABS) return to undetectable levels after appropriate antimicrobial therapy for syphilis?

No, the treponemal tests remain positive for life after initial infection. These tests should not be used to assess response to therapy.

12. What is the expected rate of fall of nontreponemal serologic tests after appropriate treatment of primary, secondary, and early latent syphilis?

Expect a 4-fold decline in VDRL or RPR titers at 3 months and an 8-fold decline at 6 months.

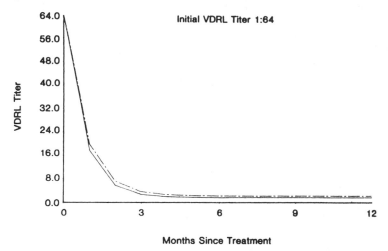

VDRL titer decline after treatment of primary or secondary syphilis with penicillin or tetracycline. (From Brown ST, et al: Serologic response to syphilis treatment. JAMA 253.1296–1299, 1985; with permission.)

13. What are the clinical settings and risk factors associated with *Candida* infections?

Clinical Settings and Risk Factors for Candida Infections

CLINICAL SETTING	RISK FACTORS
Chronic mucocutaneous infections	Defects in T-lymphocyte immunity, congenital (e.g., chronic mucocutaneous candidiasis) or acquired (e.g., AIDS)
	Qualitative defects in neutrophil function (e.g., myeloperoxidase deficiency)
Deeply invasive, disseminated infections	Peripheral neutrophil count < 500/mm³
	Mucosal barrier breakdown (burn, cytotoxic agents, GI surgery, IV catheter sites)
	Candidal overgrowth (broad-spectrum antibiotics)
Colonization of a catheter, with fever	Indwelling catheter

The difference between the first two categories may be difficult to distinguish clinically, and if there is doubt the patient should be treated for disseminated disease.

Crislip MA, et al. Candidiasis. Infect Dis Clin North Am 3:103–133, 1989.

14. Endophthalmitis is present in what percentage of patients with candidemia?

10–37%. Endophthalmitis is an important clue that the infection is disseminated.

15. Which species of *Candida* most commonly colonizes the skin?

C. parapsilosis. Its identification in blood cultures may suggest a contaminated intravascular line.

16. Which occupations are associated with *Erysipelothrix rhusiopathiae* infection?

Fishermen, fish handlers, butchers, meat-processing workers, poultry workers, farmers, veterinarians, and abattoir (slaughterhouse) workers. There are two major clinical syndromes: (1) localized cutaneous and (2) disseminated/endocarditis.

Gorby GL, et al: *Erysipelothrix* endocarditis: Microbiologic, epidemiologic and clinical features of an occupational disease. Rev Infect Dis 10:317–325, 1988.

17. What are the infusion-related syndromes associated with IV vancomycin administration?

1. **Red-man syndrome** is a histamine-mediated phenomenon that occurs with too rapid an infusion of vancomycin. It is characterized by the development of erythema, hives, and pruritus across the upper trunk and face.

2. The **pain and spasm syndrome** is characterized by throbbing chest pain that resolves when the antibiotic infusion is stopped. The pain is not secondary to myocardial ischemia.

3. **Hypotension,** a very rare infusion-related syndrome, can usually be treated with antihistamines, although pressor agents are occasionally needed.

18. How is the "bedside" cold agglutinin test performed? What does a positive result indicate?

Four to five drops of blood are added to a blood collection tube containing sodium citrate. The tube is immersed in an ice bath for 1–2 minutes. Floccular hemagglutination observed on the side of the tube is indicative of a positive reaction. Confirmation is provided if the agglutination disappears when the tube is warmed to 37°C. A positive test correlates with a cold agglutinin titer of >1:64, seen with *Mycoplasma pneumoniae* infections.

19. The commercial Monospot test for detection of heterophile antibodies is reactive in what percentage of patients with acute infectious mononucleosis?

Heterophile antibodies, as detected by the Monospot test, are present in approx. 90% of cases at some point in the illness.

20. What are the causes of a false-positive Monospot test?

Serum sickness, lymphoma, and acute hepatitis. One can distinguish false-positives from true-positives with differential adsorptions using guinea pig kidney and beef red cells as follows:

	UNADSORBED	ADSORPTION WITH GUINEA PIG KIDNEY	ADSORPTION WITH BEEF RBCS
Inf. mononucleosis	4+	3+	0
Lymphoma	3+	0	0
Serum sickness	3+	0	0
Hepatitis	3+	0	0
Normal	1+	0	1+

21. What is the differential diagnosis of exudative pharyngitis?

- Groups A, C, and G streptococci
- *Corynebacterium hemolyticum,*
  C. diphtheriae
- Anaerobic bacteria
- *Yersinia enterocolitica*
- *Mycoplasma pneumoniae*
- Adenovirus, herpes simplex virus, Epstein-Barr virus

22. Patients with multiple myeloma are prone to develop infections due to what types of organisms?

Infections in patients with myeloma demonstrate a biphasic pattern. Infections with *Streptococcus pneumoniae* and *Haemophilus influenzae* occur at the time of initial presentation of myeloma, early in the disease, and during response to chemotherapy. Infections with *Staphylococcus aureus* and gram-negative bacilli (including *Escherichia coli, Pseudomonas aeruginosa, Klebsiella pneumoniae, Enterobacter* sp. and *Serratia marcescens*) cause approx. 80% of infections seen after diagnosis of myeloma and 92% of infectious deaths. These latter infections occur in patients with active and advancing disease and in those responding to chemotherapy in the period in which they are neutropenic.

Savage DG, et al: Biphasic pattern of bacterial infection in multiple myeloma. Ann Intern Med 96:47–50, 1982.

23. When examining a sputum specimen, how can you determine if a specimen originates from the lower respiratory tract and is adequate for culture?

Generally, a sputum is considered adequate when there are <10 epithelial cells and >25 polymorphonuclear leukocytes per low-power (×100) field.

24. What is the differential diagnosis of trismus ("lockjaw")?

While tetanus is the best-known cause of trismus, other disorders must be considered in a patient with tonic spasm of the masticatory muscles:

- Tetanus
- Inflammatory lesions of the floor of the mouth, cheeks, pharynx, or external auditory canal (peritonsillar or dental abscess, Ludwig's angina, trichinosis)
- Malignancies (sarcoma of the jaw, squamous cell carcinoma of the oral cavity)
- Psychiatric disorders (hysteric tetanus)
- Mechanical problems (temporomaxillary ankylosis, dislocation of the jaw)
- Strychnine poisoning (a late manifestation)
- Phenothiazines (part of a dystonic reaction)
- Encephalitis

25. Describe the different clinical presentations of tetanus in the adult.

Tetanus may present in three clinical forms:

1. **Generalized tetanus,** the most common form of the disease, is characterized by trismus, nuchal rigidity, dysphagia, irritability, and rigidity of the abdominal muscles.

2. **Localized tetanus** is manifested by persistent rigidity of a group of muscles close to the site of injury. It occasionally progresses to generalized tetanus.

3. **Cephalic tetanus** is a severe form of localized tetanus that occurs when the injury is on the head or neck. It usually presents with cranial motor nerve dysfunction (most commonly CN VII) and has a poor prognosis.

Bleck TP: Tetanus: dealing with the continuing clinical challenge. J Crit Illness 2:41–52, 1987.

26. If a patient with no prior history of tetanus vaccination recovers from an episode of tetanus, is he or she at risk for a second episode?

Yes. The occurrence of tetanus does not prevent second episodes of clinical disease from occurring, because the amount of toxin needed to produce the clinical syndrome is so small that it is usually not immunogenic. Hence, persons recovering from tetanus should be vaccinated with tetanus toxoid against future episodes of the disease.

27. What are the 3 types of antimicrobial resistance mechanisms displayed by *Staphylococcus aureus* for β-lactam antibiotics?

1. Plasmid-mediated production of extracellular enzymes (β-lactamases) that act on the β-lactam ring.

2. Chromosomally mediated resistance (methicillin-resistance or intrinsic resistance) that results from production of penicillin-binding proteins with altered affinity for β-lactam antibiotics.

3. Tolerance, defined by a minimal bactericidal concentration to minimal inhibitory concentration (MBC/MIC) ratio >32, which results from an inability of β-lactam antibiotics to activate autolytic enzymes.

28. *Staphylococcus saprophyticus* is most commonly associated with what infectious problem?

Urinary tract infections (UTI), usually in young women. There is a high correlation between genitourinary mucosal colonization with this organism and the subsequent development of UTI. Symptoms and urinalysis findings are indistinguishable from those of infections due to enteric organisms. This bacterium accounts for 20% of UTIs in women 16–35 years old.

29. Discuss the etiologic and epidemiologic associations in the toxic shock syndrome (TSS).
Approx. 70% of cases occur in women < 30 years old in association with their menstrual period. Approx. 30% of cases are not associated with menses but occur in association with:

IV drug abuse   Nonsurgical traumatic wounds
Homosexuals   Parturition
Staphylococcal sepsis   Staphylococcal pneumonia
Surgical wound infections

The toxins elaborated by *Staphylococus aureus* are responsible for the clinical manifestations (TSST-1). There is a strong association between TSS and the recovery of *S. aureus* from vaginal cultures.

Broome CV: Epidemiology of toxic shock syndrome in the United States: Overview. Rev Infect Dis 11:S14-S21, 1989.

30. How is the diagnosis of toxic shock syndrome made?
The diagnosis is a clinical diagnosis based on the presence of certain signs and symptoms:
Definite TSS (all criteria must be present)
1. Temperature ≥ 38.9°C (102°F)
2. Rash (diffuse or palmar erythroderma) with desquamation of palms or soles 1–2 weeks after onset of illness.
3. Hypotension—manifested by one of the following:
   a. Systolic BP < 90 mm Hg
   b. Orthostatic decrease in systolic BP ≥ 15 mm Hg
   c. Orthostatic dizziness or syncope
4. Clinical or laboratory abnormalities in three or more organ systems:
   a. Mucous membrane   e. Renal
   b. GI   f. Muscular
   c. Hepatic   g. Cardiovascular
   d. CNS

Probable TSS (at least 3 criteria with desquamation or at least 5 criteria without desquamation)
1. Temperature ≥ 38.9°C (102°F)   6. Mucous membrane inflammation
2. Diffuse or palmar erythroderma (rash)   (conjunctivitis, pharyngitis, or vaginitis)
3. Hypotension, orthostatic dizziness,   7. Clinical or laboratory abnormalities in two
   or syncope   or more organ systems
4. Myalgia   8. Reasonable evidence for the absence of
5. Vomiting, diarrhea, or both   other causes of illness

Tofte RW, et al: Toxic shock syndrome in the United States: Evidence of a broad clinical spectrum. JAMA 246:2163–2167, 1981.

31. What is the significance of bacteremia or endocarditis due to *Streptococcus bovis?*
A strong association exists between lesions of the GI tract, particularly bowel carcinoma, and *S. bovis* bacteremia or endocarditis. Patients in whom this organism is identified should have a thorough evaluation of the GI tract.

32. Infection with *Streptococcus agalactiae* is most commonly seen in what epidemiologic setting?
Infection with group B streptococci is seen in postpartum women and neonates.

33. How often is a current or past history of diarrhea evident in patients with amebic liver abscess?
Approx. one-third of patients with amebic liver abscess have a history of past or present diarrhea. The major presenting manifestations are those referable to the abscess itself or its extension and rupture into adjacent structures. *Entamoeba histolytica* is found in the stool in less than one-third of patients with an abscess.

34. Which part of the liver is most commonly involved with amebic liver abscess?

Amebic liver abscesses are most commonly single lesions involving the right superior or superior-posterior aspect of the liver.

35. Primary amebic meningoencephalitis due to *Naegleria fowleri* occurs predominantly in what epidemiologic setting?

Children or young adults who have been swimming, diving or water-skiing in small fresh-water lakes, usually in the southern United States. The organism is associated with freshwater having heavy growths of algae and bacteria, probably resulting from high concentrations of sewage components in the water.

36. Why should aminoglycoside antibiotics be given with careful monitoring to patients with neuromuscular diseases such as myasthenia gravis?

Aminoglycoside antibiotics demonstrate neuromuscular blockade properties by inhibiting presynaptic release of acetylcholine and blocking postsynaptic receptors for acetylcholine. Patients with myasthenia gravis have shown increased sensitivity to the paralytic effects of these agents, as have patients simultaneously receiving other neuromuscular blockading agents (e.g., succinylcholine, D-tubocurare). The paralytic effects can be overcome with anticholinesterases and calcium.

Snavely SR, et al: The neurotoxicity of antibacterial agents. Ann Intern Med 101:92–104, 1984.

37. How can acute paralytic polio and Guillain-Barré syndrome be differentiated clinically?

	Polio	*Guillain-Barré*
Fever	+	−
Acute illness	+	−
Signs of meningeal infection	+	−
Symmetrical paralysis	−	−
Motor loss	+	+
Sensory loss	Rare	80%
Pattern of progression of paralysis	No pattern	Ascending
Duration of progression of paralysis	3–4 days	Up to 2 wks in stages

38. Name five different disease manifestations in humans secondary to the dimorphic fungus *Histoplasma capsulatum*.

1. Acute pulmonary histoplasmosis
2. Disseminated histoplasmosis
3. Mediastinal granuloma or fibrosis
4. Chronic cavitary pulmonary histoplasmosis
5. Histoplasmoma

39. Why does herpes simplex recur in small areas but varicella-zoster recurs in a dermatomal region?

Both herpes simplex (HSV) and varicella-zoster viruses (VZV) cause latent infections in human sensory nerve ganglia. However, the cells that are latently infected are different. HSV causes a latent infection of individual neuronal cells. With reactivation, infection does not spread well from cell to cell but does spread easily to the skin. Hence, only a small area of skin is involved during reactivation.

VZV, on the other hand, causes a latent infection in the satellite cells, and during reactivation, the infection readily spreads throughout the sensory ganglia. The virus then spreads to all areas of the sensory dermatome.

Croen KD, et al: Patterns of gene expression and sites of latency in human nerve ganglia are different for varicella-zoster and herpes simplex viruses. Proc Natl Acad Sci USA 85:9773–9777, 1988.

40. What sexually transmitted diseases commonly cause genital ulceration with regional adenopathy?

Syphilis	Genital herpes
Chancroid	Lymphogranuloma venereum
Granuloma inguinale (donovanosis)	

Krockta WP, Barnes RC: Genital ulceration with regional adenopathy. Infect Dis Clin North Am 1:217–233, 1987.

41. What is hydrophobia? Why is it significant?

Patients with rabies encephalitis often have violent, jerky contractions of the diaphragm and accessory muscles of inspiration that are triggered by attempts to swallow liquids or other stimuli. Hydrophobia is pathognomonic of rabies.

42. What animal vectors are involved in human rabies?

Dogs account for >90% of reported human cases of rabies in areas of the world where domestic rabies is not well controlled. Other domestic animals contribute 5–10% worldwide; these include cats, cattle, horses, sheep, and pigs. In the U.S., the principal vectors are wild mammals, including the striped skunk, raccoon, foxes, and insectivorous bats. Small rodents, birds, and reptiles are not known to be reservoirs of rabies.

King AA, Turner GS: Rabies: A review. J Comp Pathol 108:1–39, 1993.

43. In which STD does the "groove sign" appear?

The "groove sign" is the occurrence of adenopathy above and below the inguinal ligament. Though it has been said to be pathognomonic of lymphogranuloma venereum, it is seen in only 15% or less of cases and also occurs in other infectious and neoplastic conditions.

Krockta WP, Barnes RC: Genital ulceration with regional adenopathy. Infect Dis Clin North Am 1:217–233, 1987.

44. How often does perinatal transmission of hepatitis B occur in offspring of women who are chronically hepatitis B surface antigen (HBsAg)-positive?

Women who are HBsAg-positive and hepatitis B e antigen (HBeAg)-positive transmit the virus to their offspring 50–70% of the time, whereas those who are HBsAg-positive but HBeAg-negative transmit it approx. 10% of the time. Neonates who acquire hepatitis B in the perinatal period tend to become chronic carriers and are at significantly increased risk for cirrhosis and hepatocellular carcinoma. These complications are potentially preventable with passive and active immunization of the infant.

45. What criteria are suggestive of UTI on the microscopic examination of a clean-catch urine specimen?

Type of Urine	Method of Observation	Finding	Indication
Uncentrifuged	Hemocytometer	$\leq 10^3$ WBC/ml	Normal
		$>10^4$ WBC/mL	Infection
	Low-power magnification (10 × objective)	> 2–3 WBC/field	Correlates with $> 10^4$ WBC/mL
	High-power magnification (45 × objective)	1–2 WBC/ field	$\geq 10^5$ WBC/ml
		Bacteria	$\geq 10^5$ bacteria/mL
		WBC cast	Suggests renal involvement (pyelonephritis)
Uncentrifuged or centrifuged	High-power magnification	WBC cast	(Same as above)
		RBC cast	Indicates glomerunephritis

From Musher DM: Urinary tract infection. In Dupont H, Pickering L (eds): Infectious Diseases Handbook. Menlo Park, CA, Addison-Wesley, 1986, p 450; with permission.

46. Which organisms are likely to cause a chronic UTI with urinary pH ≥ 7.5?

Urinary pH is elevated in chronic UTIs caused by organisms that are urease-producers. *Proteus* sp. are the most common organisms that cause this clinical presentation. Others include *Corynebacterium urealyticum, Staphylococcus saprophyticus, Ureaplasma urealyticum,* and *Providencia* sp. *Klebsiella* and *Serratia* sp. are rare causes.

O'Leary JJ, et al: The importance of urinalysis in infectious diseases. Hosp Physician 27:25–30, 1991.

47. Linear calcifications seen in the wall of the urinary bladder on a roentgenogram are indicative of what chronic infection?

Shistosoma haematobium infection may result in bladder wall calcifications due to the deposition of eggs in the submucosa and mucosa of the bladder. The consequent inflammatory response leads to scarring and calcium deposition.

48. Which antibiotics can be found in cyst fluid in patients with polycystic kidney disease?

Trimethoprim-sulfamethoxazole and chloramphenicol occur in significant concentrations in cyst fluid. Patients with polycystic disease and UTI may fail to improve with other antibiotics. Surgical aspiration or drainage of infected cysts may be necessary.

49. What factors are necessary for methenamine to function effectively as a urinary tract antiseptic?

Methenamine itself is not bactericidal but depends on hydrolysis, at an acid pH, to liberate ammonia and formaldehyde by the following reaction:

$$N_4(CH_2)_6 + 6H_2O \rightarrow 4NH_4^+ + 6HCHO$$

Formaldehyde is the bactericidal agent. For this reaction to work optimally, the urine pH needs to be <7.0 and the hydrolysis needs sufficient time to occur, usually hours. Consequently, the drug is ineffective in patients with indwelling bladder catheters.

50. Which organism appears as delicate, weakly gram-positive, beaded filaments that also are acid-fast if 1% sulfuric acid is used to decolorize instead of acid-alcohol?

Nocardia species (e.g., *No. asteroides*).

McNeil MM: The medically important aerobic actinomycetes: epidemiology and microbiology. Clin Microbiol Rev 7:359–379, 1994.

51. What are the most common etiologic agents in the acute sinusitis syndrome?

Microbial Etiology of Acute Community-Acquired Antral Sinusitis

MICROBIAL AGENT	ADULTS (%)	CHILDREN (%)
Bacteria		
S. pneumoniae	31 (20–35)	36
H. influenzae (unencapsulated)	21 (6–26)	23
Mixed *S. pneumoniae* and *H. influenzae*	5 (1–9)	—
Anaerobic bacteria (*Bacteroides, Peptostreptococcus, Fusobacterium,* etc.)	6 (0–10)	—
S. aureus	4 (0–8)	—
S. pyogenes	2 (1–3)	2
M. catarrhalis	2	19
Gram-negative bacteria	9 (0–24)	2
Viruses		
Rhinovirus	15	—
Influenza virus	5	—
Parainfluenza virus	3	2
Adenovirus	—	2

Hamory BH: Etiology and antimicrobial therapy of acute maxillary sinusitis. J Infect Dis 139:197–202, 1979.

52. What percentage of patients with pneumococcal pneumonia also have bacteremia?
25–30%

53. What are the radiographic changes associated with osteomyelitis?
1. Deep soft tissue swelling and obliteration of muscle planes (usually the earliest radiographic changes seen)
2. Periosteal reaction
3. Cortical irregularity
4. Rarification of bone
5. Sequestrum (devitalized area of bone following loss of vascular supply)
6. Involucrum (periosteal new bone formation in response to infection)

54. Which bacterial species usually causes osteomyelitis in patients with sickle cell disease?
Approx. 80% of cases of osteomyelitis complicating sickle cell disease are due to *Salmonella* species.

55. How reliable are sinus tract cultures for determining the etiologic agent of chronic osteomyelitis?
The likelihood that a sinus-tract isolate corresponds with an operative isolate is high if *Staphylococcus aureus* is the organism isolated from a sinus tract culture (78%); however, only 44% of sinus tract cultures from patients with biopsy-proven *S. aureus* osteomyelitis will yield this organism. The predictive values for the Enterobacteriaceae, *Pseudomonas aeruginosa,* and mixed cultures of *Streptococcus* species isolated from sinus tracts are <50%, and only a small number of cultures from sinus tracts of patients with chronic osteomyelitis caused by these organisms will yield the operative pathogen.

56. In a young, healthy patient who presents with *Pseudomonas aeruginosa* osteomyelitis of the calcaneus bone, what is the most likely cause of this disorder?
A puncture wound to the foot. Almost 90% of cases of osteomyelitis that result from puncture wounds to the feet are due to *P. aeruginosa;* the remaining 10% are due to various other gram-negative organisms, staphylococci, streptococci, and atypical mycobacteria.
Riley HD: Puncture wounds of the foot: their importance and potential for complications. J Okla State Med Assoc 77:3–6, 1984.

57. Bacterial endophthalmitis secondary to penetrating trauma to the eye is associated with which pathogens?

S. epidermidis, S. aureus, streptococci	60%
Bacillus sp.	25%
Gram-negative rods	10%
Fungi	5%

Bacillus cereus causes a particularly fulminant form of the disease, with enucleation not uncommon. Given all the episodes of trauma that occur to the eye, secondary infection is relatively uncommon.
Davey RT Jr., et al: Post-traumatic endophthalmitis: The emerging role of *Bacillus cereus* infection. Rev Infect Dis 9:110–123, 1987.

58. Acute gastric anisakiasis results from what dietary habit?
Eating raw or smoked fish, most commonly mackerel. Symptoms consist of the acute onset of severe epigastric pain, nausea, and vomiting within 12 hours of ingestion. Treatment involves the endoscopic removal of the larvae.
Sugimachi K, et al: Acute gastric anisakiasis: Analysis of 178 cases. Arch Intern Med 253:1012–1013, 1985.

59. What is the most common cause of nonepidemic viral encephalitis in the U.S.?
Herpes simplex type 1, which causes a focal encephalitis.

60. Who should receive prophylaxis after exposure to persons with *Neisseria meningitidis* meningitis?

1. Household contacts

2. Individuals in closed populations, such as military barracks, nursery schools, college dormitories, and chronic care hospitals

3. Hospital personnel who have intimate exposure to infected patients (but not other personnel without such exposure)

61. Define fever of undetermined origin (FUO).

The classic definition of FUO as defined by Petersdorf and Beeson is:

1. Illness of >3 weeks' duration: This eliminates any acute, self-limited illnesses.

2. Documented fever >101°F or 38.3°C on several occasions

3. Uncertain diagnosis after 1 week in the hospital to allow completion of routine laboratory examinations

Petersdorf RG, Beeson PB: Fever of unexplained origin: Report of 100 cases. Medicine 40:1–29, 1961.

62. What are the major causes of FUO?

Causes of Fever of Undetermined Origin

I. Infection	**II. Cancer**
A. Generalized	A. Hematologic
1. Tuberculosis	1. Lymphoma
2. Histoplasmosis	2. Hodgkin's disease
3. Typhoid fever	3. Acute leukemia
4. Cytomegalovirus	B. Tumors with propensity to cause fever
5. Epstein-Barr virus	1. Hepatoma
6. Miscellaneous:	2. Renal cell carcinoma
a. Syphilis	3. Atrial myxoma
b. Brucellosis	
c. Malaria	**III. Rheumatologic disorders**
B. Localized	1. Rheumatoid arthritis
1. Infective endocarditis	2. Systemic lupus erythematosus
2. Empyema	3. Vasculitis
3. Intra-abdominal infection	
a. Peritonitis	**IV. Miscellaneous**
b. Cholangitis	1. Drug-induced
c. Abscess	2. Immune complex (SLE, RA)
4. Urinary tract	3. Vasculitis
a. Pyelonephritis	4. Alcoholic hepatitis
b. Perinephric abscess	5. Granulomatous hepatitis
c. Prostatitis	6. Inflammatory bowel disease, Whipple's disease
5. Decubitus ulcer	7. Recurrent pulmonary emboli
6. Osteomyelitis	8. Factitious fever
7. Thrombophlebitis	9. Undiagnosed

From Larson EB, et al: Fever of undetermined origin: Diagnosis and follow-up of 105 cases, 1970–1980. Medicine 61:269–292, 1982; with permission.

63. What types of reactions to penicillin may be predicted by skin testing prior to antibiotic use?

Skin testing is predictive of IgE-mediated reactions. Such reactions, including accelerated urticaria or anaphylaxis, occur with varying frequency depending on the skin test result. Among patients with a positive skin test, the frequency of these reactions varies from 10% in those without a previous history of penicillin allergy to 50–70% in those with a past history of penicillin allergy. In patients with a negative skin test, accelerated urticaria occurs in only 1% and anaphylaxis does not occur.

Skin test reactivity is not predictive of other types of reactions, such as serum sickness, maculopapular rash, exfoliative dermatitis, hemolytic anemia, or interstitial nephritis.

Sogn DD, et al: Results of the NIAID collaborative clinical trial to test the predictive value of skin testing with major and minor penicillin derivatives in hospitalized adults. Arch Intern Med 152:1025–1032, 1992.

64. What chest roentgenogram findings are very suggestive of thoracic actinomycosis?
  1. Lesions extending through the chest wall
  2. Involvement of adjacent lobes by transgression through an interlobar fissure
  3. Periostitis or destruction of bones such as ribs or sternum adjacent to a pulmonary process
  4. Vertebral destruction, with disc space sparing, due to extension from mediastinal or thoracic involvement.

65. Name a parasitic disease that mimics pulmonary tuberculosis (TB). How is it diagnosed?
  The trematode lung fluke *Paragonimus westermani* can cause a pulmonary syndrome consistent with pulmonary TB. Chronic bronchitis, bronchiectasis, lung abscess, and pleural effusion are other clinical syndromes related to paragonimiasis. Examination of the sputum may show the characteristic operculated eggs.
  Harinasuta T, et al. Trematode infections: Opisthorchiasis, clonorchiasis, fascioliasis, and paragonimiasis. Infect Dis Clin North Am 7:699–716, 1993.

66. What is a Simon focus?
  During primary infection with *Mycobacterium tuberculosis,* apical and subapical pulmonary foci may undergo necrosis when delayed hypersensitivity develops. These foci then develop tiny calcific deposits, within which latent but viable mycobacteria persist. These foci can later reactivate.

67. What is Pott's disease?
  Spinal tuberculosis. Percival Pott, an English surgeon, in 1779 first wrote the classic description of the disease that bears his name.

68. What are the clinical features of genitourinary tuberculosis?

Sterile pyuria	50%
Painless hematuria	40%
Fever	10%
Perinephric abscess	10%
Positive sputum culture	20–40%
Positive urine culture	80%

69. What is Poncet's disease?
  A polyarticular arthritis that occurs during active TB in which no infectious or other cause of the arthritis can be demonstrated. *Mycobacterium tuberculosis* cannot be isolated from the affected joint spaces. The disorder is felt to have an immunologic basis.
  Dall L, et al: Poncet's disease: Tuberculous rheumatism. Rev Infect Dis 11:105–107, 1989.

70. Name the most important prognostic factor in tuberculous meningitis.
  The patient's neurologic exam at clinical presentation appears to indicate the outcome. Patients who are stuporous or hemiplegic have a mortality rate around 80%, while patients with only meningismus and fever have a mortality rate around 5–9%. Patients with a more severe neurologic deficit should probably receive steroids.
  Ogawa SK, et al: Tuberculous meningitis in an urban medical center. Medicine 66:317–326, 1982.

71. What is the differential diagnosis of eosinophilic meningitis?
  • CNS infection caused by parasites (*Toxoplasma gondii, Trypanosoma* sp., *Trichinella spiralis, Toxocara canis, Toxocara cati, Taenia solium, Fasciola hepatica, Paragonimus westermani, Angiostrongylus cantonensis, Gnathostoma spinigerum*)
  • *Mycobacterium tuberculosis*
  • Fungi (*Coccidioides immitis, Histoplasma capsulatum*)
  • Viruses (lymphocytic choriomeningitis virus)
  • Rickettsiae
  • Neoplasia (leukemia, lymphoma, meningeal tumors)
  • Multiple sclerosis
  • Hypereosinophilic syndrome

- Collagen vascular disease
- Allergic reaction to foreign body or direct instillation of drugs or contrast agent into the CSF
- Drug allergy (e.g., ibuprofen, ciprofloxacin)

Asperilla MO, et al: Eosinophilic meningitis associated with ciprofloxacin. Am J Med 87:589–590, 1989.

72. How many patients with tuberculous meningitis will have a positive PPD skin test?

The purified protein derivative PPD skin test is positive in 50–95% of patients with TB meningitis. Stated another way, the PPD is negative in up to 50% of patients with TB meningitis.

Molavi A, LeFrock JL: Tuberculous meningitis. Med Clin North Am 69:315–331, 1985.

73. Most cases of Rocky Mountain spotted fever (RMSF) occur in what region of the U.S.?

The south Atlantic states. Despite its name, few cases of RMSF occur in the Rocky Mountain states.

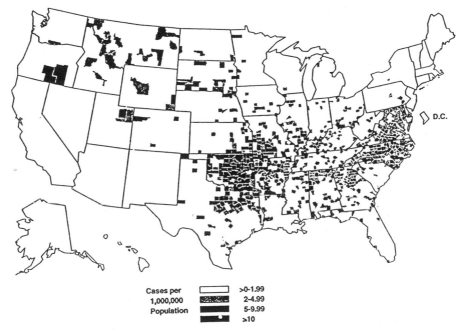

Cases per 1,000,000 Population		>0-1.99
		2-4.99
		5-9.99
		>10

From Dalton MJ, et al: National surveillance for Rocky Mountain spotted fever, 1981–1992: Epidemiologic summary and evaluation of risk factors for fatal outcome. Am J Trop Med Hyg 52:405–413, 1995; with permission.

74. What are the major pulmonary syndromes associated with Aspergillus sp.? How are they treated?

1. **Allergic bronchopulmonary aspergillosis** (ABPA) occurs in patients with asthma who have eosinophilia, transient pulmonary infiltrates thought to be due to bronchial plugging, and elevated total serum IgE and IgG antibody to *Aspergillus*. Corticosteroids have been used to treat this disorder, although anecdotal reports suggest itraconazole may have a role.

2. **Aspergilloma** (fungus ball) results from colonization and growth of *Aspergillus*, usually within a preexisting pulmonary cavity. No specific treatment is usually given unless significant hemoptysis occurs, in which case surgical excision is performed.

3. **Invasive aspergillosis** usually occurs in individuals with profound granulocytopenia and is also being described more frequently in individuals with AIDS. Amphotericin B, with or without surgical excision, is the therapy of choice.

4. **Chronic necrotizing aspergillosis** is a slowly progressive form of invasive aspergillosis

that occurs in patients who have some underlying pulmonary disease (chronic obstructive pulmonary disease, sarcoidosis, penumoconiosis, or inactive TB) or mild systemic immunocompromising illness (low-dose corticosteroids, diabetes mellitus, alcoholism). Patients have a chronic infiltrate that may slowly progress to cavitation or aspergilloma formation.

Levitz SM. Aspergillosis. Infect Dis Clin N Amer 3:1–18, 1989.

75. What is the Fitz-Hugh–Curtis syndrome? What organisms cause it?

The Fitz-Hugh–Curtis syndrome is a perihepatitis caused usually by either *Neisseria gonorrhoeae* or *Chlamydia trachomatis*. It is thought to occur by spread of organisms from the fallopian tubes to the surface of the liver. This should be considered one of the causes of right-upper-quadrant pain in young, sexually active persons. It occasionally has been reported in males, probably as a result of bacteremic spread.

76. Are fever patterns helpful in establishing the cause of fever?

There have been multiple classifications of fever patterns. For the most part, the pattern of fever is not helpful in establishing its cause. Two exceptions are fever secondary to cyclic neutropenia and fever secondary to malaria. Patients with cyclic neutropenia have fevers every 3 weeks, coincident with their neutropenia. Patients with malaria may have paroxysms of fever every 2 or 3 days, depending on the infecting parasite.

77. Which organisms most commonly cause infectious complications after a human bite?

Streptococci (alpha and group A β-hemolytic), *Staphylococcus aureus, Eikenella corrodens, Peptostreptococcus* sp., *Bacteroides* sp., and *Fusobacterium* sp. are the most common organisms cultured from human bite wounds.

Goldstein EJC: Bite wounds and infection. Clin Infect Dis 14:633–640, 1992.

78. Which other organisms should be considered after dog or cat bites?

Pasteurella multocida and *Capnocytophaga canimorsus* (DF–2). Several other pathogens have been transmitted after bites by these animals, including rabies, tularemia (cats), brucellosis (dogs), EF-4 (dogs), and blastomycosis (dogs).

Goldstein EJC: Bite wounds and infection. Clin Infect Dis 14:633–640, 1992.

79. What is the Jarisch-Herxheimer reaction?

It is a self-limited systemic reaction that occurs within 1–2 hours after the initial treatment of syphilis with antimicrobial agents. It is particularly common in patients treated for secondary syphilis but can occur when any stage is treated. The reaction consists of the abrupt onset of chills, fever, myalgias, tachycardia, hyperventilation, vasodilatation with associated flushing, and mild hypotension. It is probably due to the release of pyrogens from the spirochetes.

80. Which agents should be considered in the differential diagnosis of necrotizing pneumonia?

Staphylococcus aureus, aerobic gram-negative bacilli (excluding *Haemophilus influenzae*), and anaerobes. *Aspergillus* sp. and *Mycobacterium tuberculosis* may also cause this clinical picture.

81. What is typhlitis?

Typhlitis, also known as necrotizing enterocolitis or neutropenic enterocolitis, is a fulminate, necrotizing process that occurs in the GI tract of individuals with profound neutropenia. The disease is manifested by fever, abdominal pain, distention, and copious diarrhea. Involvement of the cecum and terminal ileum is characteristic.

82. What is Blackwater fever?

Blackwater fever refers to the dark-colored urine associated with the clinical syndrome of acute and massive hemolysis seen during *Plasmodium falciparum* malaria. It may be etiologically related to the therapeutic use of quinine.

83. Which species of malaria is associated with the occurrence of febrile paroxysms every 72 hours?

Plasmodium malariae. The other species of malaria that infect humans — *P. vivax, P. ovale,* and *P. falciparum* — have 48-hour erythrocyte cycles and, therefore, a 48-hour fever pattern.

Hoffman SL: Diagnosis, treatment and prevention of malaria. Med Clin North Am 76:1327–1355, 1992.

84. Which species of malaria have exoerythrocytic stages from which late relapses may occur if treatment is not adequate?

Plasmodium vivax and *P. ovale* have exoerythrocytic stages in the liver. Relapse may occur months to years later.

Zucker JR, et al. Malaria: Principles of prevention and treatment. Infect Dis Clin North Am 7:546–567, 1993.

85. What causes "swimmer's itch"?

Schistosome cercariae. Migratory birds, particularly ducks, harbor the adult worms and deposit the organism in freshwater, where snails become infected. Cercariae break out of the snails and penetrate the skin of warm-blooded animals. The cercariae are walled off and destroyed in the skin, which evokes an acute inflammatory response that results in the associated pruritus.

86. Where are Osler's nodes found? In what conditions are they seen?

Osler's nodes are small, painful, nodular lesions (2–15 mm in size) that usually appear in the pads of the fingers or toes. They may be seen in association with infective endocarditis (subacute), gonococcal infections, marantic endocarditis, hemolytic anemia, systemic lupus erythematosus, and intra-arterial catheters (distal to the cannulation site).

87. What organism is associated with the consumption of water chestnuts?

The intestinal fluke *Fasciolopsis buski*, which is endemic in the Far East and Southeast Asia. Infection occurs in individuals who ingest water chestnuts on which the metacercariae have encysted.

88. Extrusion of "sulfur granules" from a draining wound is characteristic of which infection?

Infections with *Actinomyces* sp. characteristically form external sinuses which discharge "sulfur granules." These consist of conglomerate masses of branching filaments of the organism cemented together and mineralized by host calcium phosphate stimulated by tissue inflammation. They do not contain sulfur.

89. What is the causative agent of Whipple's disease?

Tropheryma whippelii, a gram-positive actinomycete that is not closely related to any other known bacterial genus. Whipple's disease is a multisystemic disorder characterized by migratory polyarthritis, diarrhea, malabsorption, weight loss, generalized lymphadenopathy, hyperpigmentation, and occasional neurologic abnormalities.

Relman DA, et al. Identification of the uncultured bacillus of Whipple's disease. N Engl J Med 327:293–301, 1992.

90. How often is the Gram stain likely to be positive in patients with bacterial meningitis?

The Gram stain of the CSF in patients with bacterial meningitis demonstrates the etiologic agent in most cases. The following table demonstrates the sensitivity of the Gram stain for each pathogen:

Organism	*Positive (%)*
Neisseria meningitidis	66%
Streptococcus pneumoniae	83%
Haemophilus influenzae	76%
Listeria monocytogenes	42%

91. Rhinocerebral mucormycosis occurs most commonly in what setting?

Rhinocerebral mucormycosis occurs almost exclusively in patients with diabetes mellitus, particularly when poorly controlled or with ketoacidosis. Occasional cases have been described in patients with hematologic neoplasms or renal insufficiency and in infants with severe diarrhea. The disease is characterized by black, necrotic lesions of the palate or nasal mucous membranes that rapidly involve the paranasal sinuses with extension into the brain. The organism has a particular predisposition to invade vascular structures.

Sugar AM: Mucormycosis. Clin Infect Dis 14(suppl):S126-S129, 1992.

92. The intermediate stage of which tapeworm causes the clinical syndrome of cysticercosis?

Cysticercus cellulosae is the intermediate stage of *Taenia solium,* the pork tapeworm, and causes the clinical syndrome of cysticercosis.

93. Why are anti-streptolysin O (ASO) antibodies of little help in the diagnosis of cutaneous infections by *Streptococcus pyogenes*?

The ASO response after skin infections is weak, probably because of inactivation of streptolysin O by skin lipids. Antibody responses to DNase B are brisk, as is the response to hyaluronidase. Antibodies to the latter two substances can be helpful in the serodiagnosis of streptococcal skin infections.

94. What is the most common cause of secondary pneumonia following illness due to influenza?

Streptococcus pneumoniae most commonly causes pneumonia after influenza virus infection. However, the incidence of pneumonia caused by *Staphylococcus aureus* is also increased, and so this agent must also be considered when treating a patient with this clinical syndrome.

95. What are the symptoms of scombroid fish poisoning? What causes it?

Scombroid, or histamine fish poisoning, is characterized by symptoms of a histamine reaction: flushing, headache, nausea, vomiting, abdominal cramps, diarrhea, and dizziness. It is thought to be due to histamine formed in the fish meat, in addition to the presence of substances that inhibit the degradation of histamine.

Marrow JD, et al: Evidence that histamine is the causative toxin of scombroid fish poisoning. N Engl J Med 324:716–720, 1991.

96. What are the symptoms of ciguatera fish poisoning? What causes it?

Ciguatera fish poisoning is characterized by the onset of nausea, vomiting, diarrhea, abdominal cramps, and numbness or paresthesias of the structures of the oropharynx 1–6 hours following the ingestion of "poisoned" fish. Other symptoms may also be present, including shooting pains in the legs and pain in the teeth. It is caused by accumulation of ciguatoxin in the fish from the food chain. The source of the toxin in the food chain is a dinoflagellate (*Gambierdiscus toxicus*). The illness may last for days to months.

Underman AE, et al: Fish and shellfish poisoning. Curr Clin Top Infect Dis 13:203–225, 1993.

97. Which infectious diseases are associated with raw shellfish ingestion?

Raw shellfish may be the source of several pathogens. Viral diseases that may be acquired after raw shellfish ingestion include hepatitis A and Norwalk virus gastroenteritis. Bacterial pathogens include *Vibrio* sp. (cholera and noncholera) and, less commonly, *Campylobacter, Salmonella, Shigella,* and *Escherichia coli.*

Eastaugh J, et al: Infectious and toxic syndromes from fish and shellfish consumption. Arch Intern Med 149:1735–1740, 1989.

98. What is the significance of infection due to *Escherichia coli O157:H7*?

E. coli O157:H7 has emerged as a major cause of both sporadic cases and outbreaks of diarrheal disease in North America. The most outbreaks have been associated with the consumption of beef, most commonly undercooked ground beef. Other outbreaks have been associated with fecally contaminated drinking water supplies. It can cause either bloody or nonbloody diarrhea.

In addition, *E. coli* O57:H7 is responsible for most cases of hemolytic-uremic syndrome, a major cause of acute renal failure in children.

Boyce TG, et al: *Escherichia coli* O157:H7 and the hemolytic-uremic syndrome. N Engl J Med 333:364–368, 1995.

99. Which group of patients develops keratitis due to to *Acanthamoeba*?

Acanthamoeba sp. cause a severe and difficult-to-treat keratitis in individuals who wear soft contact lenses. The incidence is much higher in those individuals who prepare their own saline solutions and also in persons who wear their lenses while swimming in lakes and swimming pools.

100. What causes acute hemorrhagic conjunctivitis?

Enterovirus 70 and coxsackie virus A24. It is characterized by ocular pain, swelling of the eyelids, and subconjunctival hemorrhage. The incubation period is 1 day, and the duration of illness is approx. 1 week. These facts distinguish it from adenovirus infection (epidemic keratoconjunctivitis), which has an incubation of 5–7 days and may have symptoms present for 2–3 weeks.

Syed NA, et al. Infectious conjunctivitis. Infect Dis Clin North Am 6:789–805, 1992.

101. What is the "hyperinfection" syndrome associated with *Strongyloides stercoralis?*

Hyperinfection syndrome due to *S. stercoralis* is the result of systemic dissemination by the filariform larval stage of the organism. This usually occurs in individuals who are immunocompromised, primarily due to defects in cell-mediated immunity. Patients present with abdominal pain, diarrhea, vomiting, shock, fever, cough, and decreased mental status. Bacteremia is a frequent accompanying event, usually with enteric organisms which are thought to accompany the larva as they migrate through the bowel wall.

102. What is hepatitis C? Hepatitis E? Hepatitis G?

Hepatitis C and E are two of the non-A, non-B hepatitis viruses. **Hepatitis C** is due to an RNA virus and is spread in a manner similar to the hepatitis B virus (by the parenteral route). It is probably the major cause of transfusion-associated hepatitis.

Hepatitis E is also due to an RNA virus, but it is spread in a manner more like the hepatitis A virus (by the fecal-oral route). It is a significant cause of epidemic hepatitis in Asia and Africa, and is increased in severity in pregnant women.

Hepatitis G is an RNA virus of global distribution that is transmitted parenterally. It causes a very mild acute hepatitis, rarely resulting in jaundice. Chronic hepatitis does occur.

Martin P, Friedman LS (eds): Viral hepatitis. Gastroenterol Clin North Am 23(3), 1994 (entire issue).

103. When does the window period occur during hepatitis B infection?

The window period occurs during acute infection when the patient no longer has detectable hepatitis B surface antigen (HBsAg). However, the patient will have antibody to the core antigen (anti-HBc) and should develop anti-HBsAg in the following month.

104. What preexisting or concurrent condition is necessary for the delta agent to cause infection in humans?

The delta agent is a defective RNA virus and is the causative agent of hepatitis D. It requires the presence of HBsAG for infection to occur, so it is seen as a coinfection with acute hepatitis B infection or as a superinfection in a chronic carrier of hepatitis B. It is generally spread by the parenteral route in the U.S., but other modes of spread seem to occur in other parts of the world.

Rizzetto M, et al: Delta hepatitis—present status. J Hepatol 1:187–193, 1985.

105. Which infection occurs in nursery workers who handle sphagnum moss?

Outbreaks of lymphocutaneous infection due to *Sporothrix schenkii* have occurred in nursery and forestry workers who handle seedlings packed in sphagnum moss. Disease has also been associated with contaminated hay, timbers, and thorny bushes, such as roses.

106. What are the infectious causes of parotitis?

Acute Viral Parotitis	Acute Suppurative Parotitis
Mumps virus	*Staphylococcus aureus*
Influenza	*Streptococcus pneumoniae*
Parainfluenza types 1 and 3	Enteric gram-negative bacilli
Coxsackievirus A and B	*Haemophilus influenzae*
ECHO virus	*Actinomyces* sp.
Lymphocytic choriomeningitis	*Mycobacterium tuberculosis*
	Anaerobic organisms
	Salmonella typhi

107. What are the most common causes of infection in the first month following solid organ transplantation?

Infections in the first month following solid organ transplantation generally are not secondary to immunosuppression; they are the infections seen in most postoperative patients:

Pneumonia due to gram-negative bacilli, *Staphylococcus aureus,* or aspiration
Bacteremia (catheter-related)
Wound infections
Herpes simplex infections (usually reactivation)
Preexisting infections (e.g., strongyloidiasis, tuberculosis, or systemic mycoses)

108. What are the most common pathogens seen in months 2–6 following solid organ transplantation?

They are more typical of the pathogens seen in immunocompromised hosts:

Viruses	Others
Cytomegalovirus	Aspergillus
Epstein-Barr virus	Nocardia
Varicella-zoster virus	Toxoplasma
Papovavirus (BK and JC)	Cryptococcus
Adenovirus	*Pneumocystis carinii*
Herpes simplex virus	Legionella
Non-A, non-B hepatitis	*Listeria monocytogenes*

109. Which infectious diseases have been reported to be transmitted by blood transfusion?

The most common transmissible pathogens are viruses, but others have been implicated.

• Hepatitis A, hepatitis B, hepatitis D
• Non-A, non-B hepatitis (including hepatitis C and G)
• HIV-1, HIV-2, HTLV-1
• Cytomegalovirus, Epstein-Barr virus
• Syphilis
• Babesiosis
• Toxoplasmosis
• Malaria
• American trypanosomiasis (Chagas' disease)
• *Yersinia enterocolitica*

Berkman SA: Infectious complications of blood transfusion. Blood Rev 2:206–210, 1988.

110. What is a chagoma?

A chagoma (from Chagas) is the lesion caused by replication of *Trypanosoma cruzi* at the site of inoculation, i.e., at the site of the reduviid bug bite.

111. *Vibrio vulnificus* has been described primarily with which two clinical syndromes?

1. A cutaneous localized cellulitis after a localized inoculation
2. A high-mortality sepsis syndrome with bacteremia, usually occurring after raw-oyster ingestion and seen in immunocompromised patients, particularly cirrhotics

112. What organism shares a common epidemiologic niche and the same tick vector as *Borrelia burgdorferi*?

Babesia microti, a protozoan that parasitizes human erythrocytes, shares some of the same geographic distribution as *B. burgdorferi* (Lyme disease). *Ixodes dammini [scapularis]* is the most important tick vector, with *Dermacentor variabilis* being a less frequent vector. Some of this same geographic distribution is also shared by the agent causing human granulocyte ehrlichiosis, for which *I. dammini [scapularis]* is also the vector. Consequently, it is theoretically possible to see infection with all three agents.

113. What infections are seen in individuals with cats?

Toxoplasmosis	Cat scratch disease (*Bartonella* sp.)
Hookworm	Pasteurellosis (usually bite wound)
Rabies	Toxocariasis (visceral larval migrans)
Strongyloidiasis	Tularemia
Dermatomycoses	

Elliot DL, et al: Pet-associated illness. N Engl J Med 313:985–995, 1985.

114. How do corticosteroids interfere with the immune system? What are the infectious consequences?

Corticosteroids predominantly influence cell-mediated immunity by interfering with mononuclear cell migration and bactericidal capacities. The consequences of this are increased numbers of infections with organisms that are normally controlled through cell-mediated immune mechanisms:

Viruses	**Bacteria**
Herpes simplex virus	*Legionella*
Varicella-zoster virus	*Salmonella*
Cytomegalovirus	*Mycobacterium*
JC virus	*Listeria monocytogenes*
Fungi	**Parasites**
Cryptococcus neoformans	*Strongyloides stercoralis*
Histoplasma capsulatum	*Toxoplasma gondii*
Coccidioides immitis	
Pneumocystis carinii	

115. What is the differential diagnosis for fever and pulmonary infiltrates in a patient with Hodgkin's disease?

Patients with Hodgkin's disease can become infected with the normal respiratory flora, such as *Streptococcus pneumoniae,* particularly following courses of chemotherapy. Classically, these patients are infected with organisms that are normally controlled by cell-mediated immunity. In addition, noninfectious entities such as tumor invasion, hemorrhage, radiation pneumonitis, and drug reactions have to be considered.

Rosenow EC III, et al: Pulmonary disease in the immunocompromised host. Mayo Clin Proc 60:473–487, 610–631, 1985.

116. Which infectious diseases are associated with fecal leukocytes?

Fecal polymorphonuclear leukocytes are seen with:

Shigella	Enteroinvasive *Escherichia coli*
Salmonella enteritidis	*Vibrio parahemolyticus*
Clostridium difficile	*Campylobacter jejuni*
Entamoeba histolytica	

Fecal mononuclear leukocytes are seen with:

Salmonella typhi	*Yersinia enterocolitica*
Campylobacter fetus	

Guerrant RL: Principles and syndromes of enteric infection. In Mandell GL, et al (eds): Principles and Practice of Infectious Diseases. New York, Churchill Livingstone, 1995, pp 945–962.

117. Which infectious agents have been implicated in cervical carcinoma?

Cancer of the cervix behaves epidemiologically as if it were a sexually transmitted disease. Strong epidemiologic associations exist between cervical infections with herpes simplex virus and *Chlamydia trachomatis,* but the strongest association exists with infection with *human papillomavirus.* HPV types 16 and 18 have the strongest link with subsequent malignancy.

Paavonen J, et al: Cervical neoplasia and other STD-related genital and anal neoplasia. In Holmes KK, et al (eds): Sexually Transmitted Diseases, 2nd ed. New York, McGraw-Hill, 1990, pp 561–592.

118. What are the infectious causes of an eosinophilic pleural effusion?

1. Bacterial pneumonia (usually *Streptococcus pneumoniae*)
2. Fungi: *Cryptococcus neoformans, Histoplasma capsulatum, Coccidioides immitis*
3. *Mycobacterium tuberculosis*

Some authors feel that pleural fluid eosinophilia offers no help in differential diagnosis. Other common associations with eosinophils in the pleural fluid are spontaneous pneumothorax or repeated thoracenteses.

119. Name two types of bone marrow toxicity associated with the use of chloramphenicol.

1. Reversible bone marrow suppression due to inhibition of mitochondrial protein synthesis. It can be manifested by reticulocytopenia, anemia, leukopenia, or thrombocytopenia. Vacuolization of erythroid and myeloid precursors in the bone marrow occurs. This form of toxicity is dose related and seen most frequently in patients receiving > 4 gm/day.

2. An idiosyncratic response, frequently manifested as an aplastic anemia. It is estimated to occur once in 24,500–40,800 patients who receive chloramphenicol. It may occur weeks to months after cessation of the drug.

120. Which viral illnesses are more severe in pregnancy?

Pregnant patients have been noted to have increased morbidity and/or mortality from varicella, influenza, hepatitis C, polio, and measles. Rubella, while associated with increased fetal defects, has not been noted to be more severe in pregnancy.

121. What is the significance of a methylthiotetrazole (MTT) side chain in certain cephalosporins? Which cephalosporins have one?

MTT side chains are associated with an increased risk of bleeding after antibiotic administration and with the occurrence of disulfiram-like reactions after ethanol ingestion. Cefamandole, cefoperazone, cefotetan, and moxalactam all have MTT side chains.

122. Other than allergy, what is the most important adverse effect of imipenem?

Seizures occur in up to 1% of patients on imipenem. Patients with a history of preexisting seizure disorder, recent head trauma, or chronic alcoholism are at increased risk. Seizures are also seen in patient with renal failure when the dose is not adjusted. Treatment consists of withdrawal of the drug and anticonvulsants.

Eng RHK, et al: Seizure propensity with imipenem. Arch Intern Med 149:1881–1883, 1989.

123. What are the two most important drug–drug interactions associated with ciprofloxacin?

1. Coadministration of ciprofloxacin with theophylline may result in increased theophylline levels and theophylline toxicity.

2. **Magnesium**- and **aluminum-containing antacids** decrease the bioavailability of ciprofloxacin, causing the peak serum levels to be in the subtherapeutic range.

Hendershot EF: Fluoroquinolones. Infect Dis Clin North Am 9:715–730, 1995.

124. Are any important drug-drug interactions associated with erythromycin?

Yes. Erythromycin alters the metabolism of a number of drugs, resulting in increased drug effect and possible toxicity. These drugs include:

Oral anticoagulants
Phenytoin
Cyclosporine
Digoxin

Carbamazepine
Corticosteroids
Theophylline
Ergot alkaloids

125. Describe the mechanisms of resistance to acyclovir.
Acyclovir triphosphate is a potent inhibitor of viral DNA polymerase. It enters the infected cell as acyclovir and is phosphorylated to a monophosphate by viral thymidine kinase (TK). Further phosphorylation is accomplished by cellular enzymes. The major mechanism of resistance is alteration in viral TK. Alterations in the DNA polymerase as a cause of resistance are much less common.

Whitley RJ, et al: Acyclovir: a decade later. N Engl J Med 327:782–789, 1992.

126. How frequently will a single stool smear be diagnostic in a patient with symptomatic giardiasis?
The diagnosis of giardiasis usually can be made by careful examination of the stool for trophozoites or cysts. The diagnosis is confirmed 50–70% of the time after only 1 stool examination and > 90% of the time after examination of 3 stool specimens.

127. An immigrant from Mexico who presents with a seizure disorder and has multiple small ring-like lesions on a head CT scan is likely to have what disorder?
Neurocysticercosis. This is invasion of the CNS by the larval form of the pork tapeworm, *Taenia solium*. CT scans typically show cystic lesions that do not usually enhance with contrast and, in many cases, hydrocephalus. It is the most common cerebral parasitic infection in humans.

128. Name the etiologic agents of the STDs, chancroid, lymphogranuloma venereum, and granuloma inguinale.

Chancroid   *Haemophilus ducreyi*
Lymphogranuloma venereum   *Chlamydia trachomatis,* serovars L1–3
Granuloma inguinale (donovanosis)   *Calymmatobacterium granulomatis*

129. What percentage of older patients with salmonella bacteremia will have an endovascular source of infection?
Approx. 25% of patients over age 50 will have an endovascular source. Salmonella organisms tend to "seed" abnormal tissues (e.g., hematomas, tumors, cysts, stones, and altered endothelium such as aortic aneurysms) during bacteremia.

130. Which organisms may be confused with *Listeria monocytogenes* on Gram stain or blood agar plates?

1. *Corynebacterium* spp.   4. *Streptococcus pneumoniae*
2. β-Hemolytic streptococci   5. *Erysipelothrix rhusiopathiae*
3. *Enterococcus*   6. *Lactobacillus* sp.

One should always make certain these organisms are not overlooked in clinical specimens submitted to the laboratory, especially spinal fluid.

Sen P, et al: Human listeriosis. Infect Med (May/June): 204–215, 1987.

131. How is disease due to *Corynebacterium diphtheriae* produced?
Certain strains of *C. diphtheriae,* when infected by a lysogenic bacteriophage, produce a toxin that enters cells and interrupts protein synthesis, resulting in neuritis and myocarditis.

132. Infection with *Chlamydia psittaci* should be considered an occupational hazard for what group of individuals?
Petshop employees, pigeon fanciers, zoo workers, veterinarians, and poultry processors. It causes an atypical pneumonia.

133. Describe the serologic response to Epstein-Barr virus (EBV) infections.

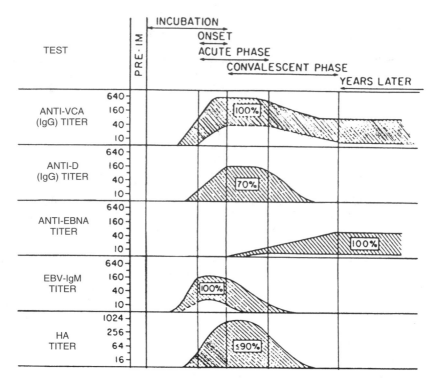

The typical sequence of serologic events following exposure to EBV. The incubation period ranges from 30–50 days. Antibody to viral capsid antigen (anti-VCA, difficult to detect in some labs) can be demonstrated at the time of clinical presentation and is diagnostic of acute infection. The EBV nuclear antigen (anti-EBNA) characteristically appears 3–4 weeks after the onset of clinical illness. Both the anti-VCA and anti-EBNA antibodies are present lifelong following infection. (HA, heterophile antibody; anti-D, antibody to early antigen) (From Schooley RT: Chronic fatigue syndrome: A manifestation of Epstein-Barr virus infection? In Remington JS, Swartz MN (eds): Current Clinical Topics in Infectious Disease, vol 9. New York, McGraw-Hill, 1988, pp 126–146; with permission.)

134. What is the differential diagnosis of infectious causes of monocytosis?

Infectious Causes	Noninfectious Causes
Tuberculosis	Myeloproliferative disorders
Epstein-Barr virus mononucleosis	Lymphomas
Rocky Mountain spotted fever	Solid tumors
Diphtheria	Gaucher's disease
Subacute bacterial endocarditis	Regional enteritis
Histoplasmosis	Ulcerative colitis
Typhus	Sprue
Brucellosis	Rheumatoid arthritis
Kala-azar	Systemic lupus erythematosus
Malaria	Polyarteritis nodosa
Syphilis	Post-splenectomy
Recovery from neutropenia	Sarcoidosis
Recovery from chronic infection	

From Calubiran O, et al: The significance of lymphocytes, monocytes, and platelets in infectious diseases. Hosp Physician 26:10–12, 1990, with permission.

135. What is the differential diagnosis of atypical lymphocytosis?

Disorders Associated with Atypical Lymphocytes

> 20% Atypical Lymphocytes	< 20% Atypical Lymphocytes	
	INFECTIONS	NON-INFECTIOUS CAUSES
Epstein-Barr mononucleosis	Varicella	Drug hypersensitivity
Viral hepatitis	Rubella	reactions
CMV mononucleosis	Herpes simplex	Drug fever
	Varicella-zoster	Dermatitis herpetiformis
	Tuberculosis	Radiation therapy
	Brucellosis	Stress
	Smallpox	Lead intoxication
	Babesiosis	
	Ehrlichiosis	
	Rubeola	
	Roseola infantum	
	(HHV-6)	
	Influenza	
	Syphilis	
	Toxoplasmosis	
	Malaria	
	Rocky Mountain spotted fever	

From Calubiran O, et al: The significance of lymphocytes, monocytes, and platelets in infectious diseases. Hosp Physician 26:10–12, 1990; with permission.

136. Identify the sites and mechanisms of action of the various classes of antibiotics. Which are bactericidal and which are bacteriostatic?

Mechanism of Action of Antimicrobial Agents

CLASS	SITE OF ACTION	EFFECT	BACTERI-CIDAL	BACTERIO-STATIC
Penicillins cephalosporins	Cell wall	Inhibit cross-linking of pepidoglycan, resulting in spheroplast formation	+	Occ.
Vancomycin	Cell wall	Block transfer of pentapeptide from cytoplasm to cell membrane	+	Occ.
Polymyxin B, colistin	Cytoplasmic membrane	Bind phospholipid and disrupt cell membrane	+	—
Aminoglycosides	Ribosome	Bind to 30S subunit, thereby inhibiting attachment of m RNA; also affects tRNA	+	—
Tetracyclines	Ribosome	Bind to 30S subunit and inhibit binding of tRNA	—	+
Chloramphenicol	Ribosome	Bind to 50S subunit and inhibit mRNA translation	Occ.	+
Erythromycin, clindamycin	Ribosome	Inhibit mRNA translation	Occ.	+
Rifampin	Nucleic acid synthesis	Impaired RNA formation by inhibiting DNA-dependent RNA-polymerase	+	Occ.
Metronidazole	Nucleic acid synthesis	Damages nucleic acid structure	+	—
Quinolones	Nucleic acid synthesis	Inhibit DNA gyrase	+	—
Sulfonamides	Nucleic acid synthesis	Competitive inhibition of *para*-amino benzoic acid (PABA), thereby blocking formation of thymidine and purines	—	+

Occ. = occasionally (From Wyngaarden JB, Smith LH (eds): Cecil Textbook of Medicine, 18th ed. Philadelphia, W.B. Saunders, 1988, p 113; with permission.)

137. What is the MIC? MBC?

MIC—minimum inhibitory concentration: minimum concentration of a given antibiotic that will inhibit the growth of a given pathogen but will not kill it (usually expressed in μg/ml).

MBC—minimum bactericidal concentration: minimum concentration of a given antibiotic that will kill a given pathogen

138. What causes hand-foot-mouth disease? Describe the clinical findings of this disease.

Hand-foot-mouth disease may be caused by a number of viruses in the picornavirus family. It has been most often associated with coxsackievirus A16, but outbreaks have also been attributed to coxsackieviruses A4, A5, A9, A10, B2, and B5 and enterovirus 71. It is characterized by an ulcerative exanthem, usually occurring on the buccal mucosa, which is followed by a vesicular exanthem on the hands and feet.

139. Discuss the epidemiologic aspects of *Penicillium marneffei* infection.

P. marneffei is endemic in Southeast Asia, particularly Vietnam, Thailand, Hong Kong, and the adjacent areas of China. Human disease almost always occurs as a disseminated infection in immunocompromised patients, and in recent years, most reported infections have been in patients with AIDS. Clinical manifestations include fever, anemia, weight loss, skin lesions, cough with pulmonary infiltrates, lymphadenopathy, and hepatomegaly.

Hilmarsdottir I, et al: Disseminated *Penicillium marneffei* infection associated with human immunodeficiency virus: A report of two cases and a review of 35 published cases. J AIDS 6:466–471, 1993.

140. What are the diagnostic criteria for the chronic fatigue syndrome (CFS)?

According to the Centers for Disease Control and Prevention's consensus definition, in order to be diagnosed with CFS, a patient must have *both* of the following major criteria, *and* (1) at least 6 of the 11 symptom criteria and at least 2 of the 3 physical criteria or (2) they must have 8 or more of the symptom criteria:

Major criteria:

1. New onset of persistent or relapsing, debilitating fatigue or easy fatigability in a person who has no previous history of similar symptoms, that does not resolve with bedrest, and that is severe enough to reduce or impair average daily activity below 50% of the patient's premorbid activity level for a period of at least 6 months.

2. Other clinical conditions that may produce similar symptoms must be excluded by thorough evaluation based on history, physical exam, and appropriate laboratory findings.

Minor criteria:

A. *Symptom criteria:*

1. Mild fever (oral temperature 37.5–38.6°C, if measured by patient) or chills
2. Sore throat
3. Painful lymph nodes in the anterior or posterior cervical or axillary distribution
4. Unexplained generalized muscle weakness
5. Muscle discomfort or myalgia
6. Prolonged generalized fatigue after levels of exercise that would have been easily tolerated in the patient's premorbid state
7. Generalized headaches
8. Migratory arthralgia without joint swelling or redness
9. Neuropsychologic complaints including:

     a. Photophobia   e. Confusion
     b. Transient visual scotomata   f. Difficulty thinking
     c. Forgetfulness   g. Inability to concentrate
     d. Excessive irritability   h. Depression

10. Sleep disturbance (hypersomnia or insomnia)
11. Description of the initial symptom complex as initially developing over a period of a few hours to a few days

B. *Physical criteria:*

1. Low grade fever (oral temperature 37.6–38.6°C or rectal temperature 37.8–38.8°C)
2. Nonexudative pharyngitis

3. Palpable or tender anterior or posterior cervical or axillary lymph nodes generally < 2 cm in diameter

From Schooley RT: Chronic fatigue syndrome. In Mandell GL, Bennett JE, Dolin R (eds.), Principles and Practice of Infectious Disease, 4th ed. New York, Churchill Livingstone, 1995, p 1306; with permission.

141. What precautions are needed when administering rifampin?

1. Rifampin has a significant first-pass effect after ingestion. Consequently, drug levels are optimal if the total daily dose is taken once instead of divided.

2. Rifampin stains secretions orange-red; individuals who wear soft contact lenses should be warned about staining of the lenses.

3. Rifampin reduces the serum concentration of a number of drugs because of its potent induction of hepatic microsomal enzymes, which may result in clinically important consequences:

- Decreased digoxin levels can result in decompensated heart failure.
- Decreased warfarin levels can result in inadequate anticoagulation.
- Exacerbation of hyperglycemia may result from decreased serum concentrations of oral hypoglycemic agents.
- Decreased efficacy of oral contraceptive agents may occur.
- Ketoconazole and itraconazole levels are substantially reduced.
- Thyroid replacement therapy may be inadequate due to decreased levels of L-thyroxine in patients with hypothyroidism.
- Rejection of solid organ transplants may result from decreased cyclosporine concentrations.
- Asthma or Addison's disease may relapse during glucocorticosteroid therapy.

Baciewicz AM, et al: Rifampin drug interactions. Arch Intern Med 144:1667–1671, 1984.

142. Which individuals are candidates for pneumococcal immunization?

Candidates for the Pneumococcal Vaccine

ADULTS
1. Immunocompetent adults at increased risk for pneumococcal disease or its complications because of chronic illnesses:

Cardiovascular disease	Diabetes mellitus	Cirrhosis
Pulmonary disease	Alcoholism	CSF leaks

2. Individuals ≥ 65 years old
3. Immunocompromised adults at increased risk for pneumococcal disease or its complications:

Splenic dysfunction (e.g., sickle cells anemia) or anatomic asplenia	Lymphoma	Nephrotic syndrome
	Multiple myeloma	Conditions, associated with
Hodgkin's disease	Chronic renal failure	immunosuppression, (e.g., organ transplantaion)

4. Adults with HIV infection, asymptomatic or symptomatic

CHILDREN
1. Children ≥ 2 years old with chronic illnesses specifically associated with increased risk for pneumococcal disease or its complications:

Anatomic or functional asplenia (including sickle cell anemia)	Nephrotic syndrome	Conditions associated with
	CSF leaks	immunosuppression

2. Children ≥ 2 years old with HIV infection, asymptomatic or symptomatic

SPECIAL GROUPS
1. Persons living in special environments or social settings with an identified increased risk of pneumococcal disease or its complications (e.g., certain Native American populations)

CDC. Recommendations of the Immunization Practices Advisory Committee: Pneumococcal polysaccharide vaccine. MMWR 38:64–76, 1989.

143. What is ecthyma gangrenosum?

Ecthyma gangrenosum are skin lesions that occur in association with gram-negative bacteremia, most commonly in neutropenic patients. *Pseudomonas aeruginosa* is the most commonly implicated bacteria, but other species have produced this lesion, including *Aeromonas hydrophila* and *Escherichia coli*. The lesions typically begin as painless erythematous macules which rapidly progress to papules and develop central vesicles or bullae. Eventually, they ulcerate to form gangrenous ulcers. The characteristic histologic appearance demonstrates large numbers of bacteria in and around blood vessels, but an absence of an inflammatory response.

144. Why is the use of astemizole, terfenadine, and cisapride absolutely contraindicated in individuals receiving itraconazole or ketoconazole?

Itraconazole and ketoconazole interfere with the metabolism of these three drugs, causing an elevation in their serum levels. This can lead to prolongation of the QT interval on the ECG, torsades de pointes, and even sudden cardiac death.

145. What animal is the reservoir for the agent causing the hantavirus pulmonary syndrome?

The deer mouse, *Peromyscus maniculatus,* is the reservoir for the Sin Nombre virus that causes the hantavirus pulmonary syndrome.

Childs JE, et al: Serologic and genetic identification of *Peromyscus maniculatus* as the primary rodent reservoir for a new hantavirus in the southwestern United States. J Infect Dis 169:1271–1280, 1994.

146. Which infection causes "owl's eye" of intranuclear inclusions in histopathologic specimens of involved tissues?

Cytomegalovirus infection produces a characteristic cytopathologic effect resulting in the "owl's eye" appearance of infected cells. Cytomegalic cells are large 25–35 μm cells and contain basophilic intranuclear inclusions that are frequently surrounded by a clear halo, producing the "owl's eye" effect.

147. Describe the spectrum of illness caused by Bartonella species.

Originally, *B. bacilliformis* was the only *Bartonella* species associated with human disease. Recently, however, the various organisms classified as *Rochalimaea* have been reclassified as *Bartonella,* and a number of different clinical syndromes are associated with these organisms:

1. *B. bacilliformis* infection manifests as 2 different syndromes:
    * **Oroyo fever,** in which patients experience fever, chills, diaphoresis, myalgias, arthralgias, and headaches. Generalized, nontender lymphadenopathy may occur. The patients develop hemolytic anemia, jaundice, and secondary infections.
    * **Verruga peruana** is a cutaneous, eruptive lesion that may or may not be preceded by Oroyo fever. The nodules appear over exposed parts of the body usually, but may involve mucous membranes and internal organs.

2. *B. quintana* is the causative agent of **trench fever.** Recently, a similar syndrome with endocarditis has been described in homeless men living in Seattle. *B. quintana* may also cause some of the same clinical manifestations as *B. henselae.*

3. *B. henselae* has been associated with several clinical presentations:
    * **Cat-scratch disease,** which most commonly presents as localized lymphadenopathy, but may have systemic findings such as hepatitis, encephalopathy, and neuroretinitis.
    * **Bacillary angiomatosis,** which occurs most commonly in immunocompromised patients (e.g., AIDS and organ transplant recipients). These neovascular, proliferative lesions may involve the skin, liver, spleen, bone, and brain.
    * **Peliosis hepatis** are blood-filled cystic structures that involve visceral organs, such as the liver, spleen, and lymph nodes.
    * A febrile, bacteremic syndrome that occurs most commonly in immunocompromised patients and may be relapsing.

4. *B. elizabethae* has been described in one patient with **endocarditis.**

5. *B. vinsonii* has not yet been associated with human disease.

148. What are the "flesh-eating" bacteria?

"Flesh-eating" bacteria is the term coined by the British press to describe invasive necrotizing infections caused by *Streptococcus pyogenes* (group A streptococci). These infections are characterized by aggressive soft-tissue infection, shock, adult respiratory distress syndrome, and renal failure. The mortality is 30–70%. The pathophysiology of these infections is thought to involve bacterial production of pyrogenic exotoxins, which function as superantigens to stimulate T-cell production of cytokines responsible for many of the clinical manifestations.

Stevens DL: Streptococcal toxic-shock syndrome: spectrum of disease, pathogenesis, and new concepts in treatment. Emerging Infect Dis 1:69–78, 1995.

149. Which upper GI lesions are associated with *Helicobacter pylori*? Which are not?

Lesion	Association with H. pylori
Peptic esophagitis	No association
Barrett's esophagitis	May colonize distal-most gastric epithelium in patients with gastric colonization
Chronic diffuse superficial gastritis	Nearly always associated
Type A (pernicious anemia) gastritis	Negative association
NSAID gastropathy	Negative or no association
Acute erosive gastritis (alcohol, aspirin, etc.)	No association
Gastric ulceration	Nearly universally observed in patients who are not ingesting NSAIDs or aspirin
Duodenal ulceration	Nearly universally associated with "idiopathic" lesions
Gastric adenocarcinoma	Associated with cancers of the body and antrum but not cardia
Gastric lymphoma	Strongly associated with MALT-type B-cell lymphomas

From Blaser MJ. *Helicobacter pylori* and related organisms. In Mandell GL, Bennett JE, Dolin R (eds): The Principles and Practice of Infectious Diseases, 4th ed. New York, Churchill Livingstone, 1995, p 1957; with permission.

150. Which conditions predispose patients to the development of cellulitis due to group A streptococci?

Cellulitis due to the group A streptococci (and sometimes B, C, or G) has been described in a number of clinical settings in which there has been **impairment of venous and lymphatic drainage.** These situations include:

- Extremities from which the saphenous vein has been harvested for CABG
- Following mastectomy with axillary lymph node dissection for breast cancer
- Following vulvectomy and inguinal lymphadenectomy for cancer of the vulva
- After regional lymph node dissection for melanoma
- Following traumatic injuries to extremities
- Following retroperitoneal lymph node dissections for genitourinary tumors

Simon MS, et al: Cellulitis after axillary lymph node dissection for carcinoma of the breast. Am J Med 93:543–548, 1992.

151. How long does it take for resolution of chest x-ray changes in patients who have been treated for pneumococcal pneumonia?

The great majority of patients who have been treated for *Streptococcus pneumoniae* pneumonia should have complete resolution of radiographic consolidation by 8–10 weeks. Findings such as volume loss, stranding, and pleural disease may take longer to resolve. Patients who are < 50 years old and do not have underlying alcoholism or preexisting airway disease will have earlier resolution.

152. In adults presenting with a sore throat, what clinical findings may suggest the possibility of infectious mononucleosis?

The presence of palatine petechiae, posterior auricular adenopathy, marked axillary adenopathy, or inguinal adenopathy substantially increases the possibility that the patient has infectious mononucleosis. If none of these findings is present, the chances are remote.

153. List the infectious causes of adrenal insufficiency.

Mycobacterium tuberculosis

Histoplasma capsulatum

Other fungi (*Cryptococcus neoformans, Coccidioides immitis, Sporothrix schenkii, Blastomyces dermatitidis, Paracoccidioides brasiliensis*)

Neisseria meningitidis (in Waterhouse-Friderichsen syndrome)

In HIV infection, *Mycobacterium avium* complex and cytomegalovirus

Painter BF: Infectious causes of adrenal insufficiency. Infect Med 11:515–520, 1994.

154. What is the significance of *Clostridium septicum* infection?

There is a very strong association between *C. septicum* infection and underlying malignancy. Approx. 40% of cases will have a hematologic malignancy and 34% colorectal carcinoma. These patients frequently present with myonecrosis, often at sites distant from the presumed source of entry.

Kornbluth AA, et al: *Clostridium septicum* infection and associated malignancy: Report of 2 cases and review of the literature. Medicine 68:30–37, 1989.

155. How many blood cultures should be done for patients with suspected bacteremia or endocarditis in order to make a diagnosis?

If 20–30 ml of blood is drawn during each venipuncture (to be divided between 1 aerobic and 1 anaerobic blood culture bottle or between 2 aerobic bottles), one set of blood cultures will identify the offending pathogen approx. 91.5% of the time and two sets will be positive in > 99%. Consequently, two separate sets of blood cultures are normally recommended.

Smith-Elekes S, et al. Blood cultures. Infect Dis Clin North Am 7:221–234, 1993.

156. What is erythema nodosum leprosum?

This complication of therapy is seen in patients with the full lepromatous (LL) form of leprosy and most commonly occurs within the first year of treatment. It is manifested as nodular skin lesions that histopathologically resemble arthus-type reactions, with localized vasculitis in the veins and arteries characterized by PMN and eosinophilic infiltrates. It may also be associated with neuritis, polyarthritis and immune-complex glomerulonephritis.

Jacobson RR, et al: The diagnosis and treatment of leprosy. South Med J. 69:979–985, 1976.

BIBLIOGRAPHY

1. Fields BN, Knipe DM (eds): Field's Virology, 3rd ed. New York, Lippincott-Raven, 1996.
2. Mandell GL, Bennett JE, Dolin R (eds): Principles and Practice of Infectious Diseaes, 4th ed. New York, Churchill Livingstone, 1995.
3. Rubin RH, Young LS (eds): Clinical Approach to Infection in the Compromised Host, 2nd ed. New York, Plenum Publishers, 1988.
4. Sande MA, Volberding PA (eds): The Medical Management of AIDS, 4th ed. Philadelphia, W.B. Saunders, 1995.
5. Warren KS, Mahmoud AAF (eds): Tropical and Geographical Medicine, 2nd ed. New York, McGraw Hill, 1990.

5. GASTROENTEROLOGY

Rhonda A. Cole, M.D.

Indigestion is charged by God for enforcing morality on the stomach.
Victor Hugo
Les Miserables

A good digestion turneth all to health.
George Herbert
The Temple

GASTROINTESTINAL BLEEDING

1. What are the five ways in which GI bleeding presents?

1. **Hematemesis:** Vomiting of blood. The blood may be a fresh, bright red in color or like coffee grounds.
2. **Melena:** Black, tarry, foul-smelling stool.
3. **Hematochezia:** Bright red blood per rectum, blood mixed with stool, bloody diarrhea, or clots.
4. **Occult GI blood loss:** Normal-appearing stool that is hemOccult-positive.
5. **Symptoms only:** Syncope, dyspnea, angina, palpitations, or shock.

2. Describe the initial approach to the patient who presents with acute GI bleeding.

In any patient presenting with acute GI bleeding, the key is **resuscitation!** The initial approach should include a rapid assessment to gauge the urgency of the situation, including whether the patient is hemodynamically stable or unstable. Venous access should be obtained with a large-bore IV cannula, and fluids such as normal saline should be begun immediately. Blood should be obtained for a complete blood count, clotting studies, platelets, routine chemistry, and type and cross-match.

Clearly, the urgency of management depends on the results of this initial assessment. If the patient appears hemodynamically stable with minor bleeding, further management can be undertaken electively. If there are signs of an acute, life-threatening bleed and an unstable condition, aggressive resuscitation and evaluation for the source must be under taken immediately. Placement of a nasogastric (NG) tube to assess rapidity of bleeding and to clear the stomach of blood for endoscopic evaluation should be done at this time. Close monitoring of vital signs and urinary output in an ICU setting is important. The patient must be monitored for signs of concomitant heart, lung, renal, or CNS disease. Blood transfusions should be given as indicated for massive bleeding in the patient who is hemodynamically compromised.

Once the patient has been stabilized, a search can be carried out to localize the source of bleeding and perform any indicated endoscopic therapy.

The presence of a GI bleed should be confirmed by inspecting the stool for melena or hematochezia and the NG tube aspirate for blood. The site of bleeding can frequently be determined from the patient's complaints. Upper GI bleeding often presents with hematemesis combined with melena, hematochezia with a negative NG aspirate suggests a lower GI source.

3. What are the common causes of upper GI bleeding?

1. Duodenal and gastric ulcers
2. Esophageal or gastric varices in the cirrhotic patient

3. Mallory-Weiss tears (most commonly seen in the alcoholic population or patients with forceful vomiting)

4. Erosive gastritis as a result of nonsteroidal anti-inflammatory drugs (NSAIDs) or in intubated ICU patients.

4. What questions addressed in the history and physical examination can help identify the source of an upper GI bleed?

1. Is there a history of prior bleeding episodes?

2. Is there a family history of diseases that cause bleeding?

3. Are there other superimposed illnesses that may lead to bleeding, such as cirrhosis, carcinoma, coagulopathy, a known connective tissue disorder, or amyloidosis?

4. Has the patient had prior surgery of the intestinal tract, such as gastric surgery for peptic ulcer or the placement of an arterial bypass graft?

5. Is the patient an alcoholic or does he or she take ulcerogenic drugs, such as aspirin or NSAIDs?

6. Has the patient recently had a caustic ingestion?

7. Was the bleeding episode preceded by abdominal pain, dyspepsia, or retching?

8. Have there been recent nose bleeds?

5. Is examination of the skin helpful in identifying the source of an upper GI bleed?

The skin examination can be helpful for suggesting a potential source if certain stigmata are present. Lymphadenopathy or abdominal masses may suggest sources for intra-abdominal pathology.

Skin Findings in Conditions Which Cause GI Bleeding

DISEASE	ASSOCIATED SKIN FINDINGS
Peutz-Jeghers	Pigmented macules on lips, palms, soles
Malignant melanoma	Melanoma
Hereditary hemorrhagic telangiectasias	Telangiectasias on lips, mouth, palms, soles (Osler-Weber-Rendu)
Blue rubber bleb nevus	Dark, blue soft nodules
Bullous pemphigoid	Oral and skin bullae
Neurofibromatosis	Café -au-lait spots, axillary freckles, neurofibromas
Cronkhite-Canada	Alopecia; hyperpigmentation of creases, hands, and face
Cirrhosis	Spider angiomata, Dupuytren's contracture
Neoplasm	Acanthosis nigricans
Kaposi's sarcoma	Cutaneous Kaposi's sarcoma
Ehlers-Danlos	Skin fragility, keloids, paper thin scars
Pseudoxanthoma elasticum	Yellow "chicken fat" papules and plaques in flexural areas
Turner's	Webbing of neck, purpura, skin nodules

From Berger T, Silverman S: Oral and cutaneous manifestations of gastrointestinal disease. In Sleisenger MH, Fordtran JS (eds): Gastrointestinal Disease, 5th ed. Philadelphia, W.B. Saunders, 1994, pp 268–285; with permission.

6. When should endoscopy be performed in upper GI bleeding?

Endoscopy is the procedure of choice in an active GI bleed, as it allows clinical decisions to be made regarding further therapy for the bleeding lesion. Endoscopy is usually performed within the first 24 hours following admission. The timing depends in some respects on the stability of the patient and whether or not bleeding continues. Patients who show evidence of ongoing bleeding despite resuscitative efforts should have emergent endoscopy while resuscitation is occurring in order to define the source and institute endoscopic therapy. If the bleeding has stopped, elective endoscopy can be done after full resuscitation has been achieved.

Contraindications to endoscopy include suspected perforation and an uncooperative patient.

7. Which therapeutic modalities for GI bleeding can be performed during endoscopy?

Hemostasis of actively bleeding ulcers can be achieved by two categories of endoscopic therapy: thermal or nonthermal. Multiple trials comparing the various modalities have demonstrated no significant differences in achieving hemostasis, rebleeding rates, or mortality.

THERMAL	NONTHERMAL	
Heater probe	Absolute alcohol	
Bipolar or multipolar electrocoagulation	Epinephrine	
BiCap	Sclerosing agents:	
Gold probe	50% dextrose in water	Ethanolamine
Nd:YAG laser	Normal saline	Pilodocanol
Argon laser	Sodium morrhuate	Sodium tetradecyl

From Cook DJ, et al: Endoscopic therapy of acute non-variceal upper GI hemorrhage: A meta-analysis. Gastroenterology 102:139, 1992; with permission.

8. Which patients are at high risk for continued bleeding and should undergo emergency upper GI endoscopy?

Elderly patients (age >60)

Patients with fresh blood per NG tube or rectum

Patients who remain hemodynamically unstable despite aggressive resuscitative measures

Patients who rebled during the same hospital admission

Patients who have multiple comorbid illnesses, such as cardiac disease, liver disease, diabetes, etc.

Silverstein FE, et al: The national ASGE survey on upper gastrointestinal bleeding: II. Clinical prognostic factors. Gastroint Endosc 27:80, 1981.

9. What are the common causes of lower GI bleeding?

Hemorrhoids are the most common cause but rarely present with massive bleeding requiring hospitalization.

Diverticulosis accounts for approx. 50% of all cases severe enough to warrant angiographic examination. Diverticular bleeding may occur from either the right or left colon.

Angiodysplasia or **vascular ectasias** are increasingly well-recognized causes and tend to occur in older patients. They are commonly found in the cecum and ascending colon.

Neoplasms of the large bowel usually present with chronic occult bleeding but occasionally will bleed acutely.

Other less common causes include Meckel's diverticulum, ischemic or inflammatory bowel disease, solitary ulcers of the cecum and rectum, and aortoenteric fistulas.

10. Describe the diagnostic approach to a patient with lower GI bleeding.

A complete **history** and **physical examination** may yield important information regarding the source of the bleeding. A history of hemorrhoids, inflammatory bowel disease, preceding crampy abdominal pain (suggesting ischemia), and painless faucet-like bleeding (suggesting a diverticular source) may be key findings.

Rigid proctoscopy or **flexible sigmoidoscopy** follow. Low-lying lesions, such as hemorrhoids, anal fissures, rectal ulcers, colitis, or rectal tumors, can be identified easily. If the patient is bleeding from a lower tract source, the next test is **colonoscopy,** unless the bleeding is too massive to allow preparation and examination.

If the bleeding site is localized at colonoscopy, local **endoscopic therapy** may be undertaken to achieve hemostasis of certain lesions. If only diverticulosis is found, it is unlikely the endoscopist will be able to localize the specific diverticulum that bled, but the value of the procedure is in ruling out other lesions as the bleeding site, as well as potentially localizing an area if surgery must be performed.

With bleeding too rapid to perform colonoscopy or with a negative colonoscopy despite continued brisk bleeding, **arteriography** should be the next step. With active bleeding, (0.5–1 ml/min), arteriography may reveal the site and localize it to the right or left colon or small bowel, helping to direct the surgeon to the correct location for resection. Additionally, the radiologist may be able to institute therapy by selective infusion of vasopressin or embolization of the bleeding vessel.

If the bleeding rate is too slow to yield a positive arteriogram, a **radionuclide bleeding scan** using ^{99m}Tc–sulfur colloid may be an effective means of detecting ongoing bleeding (0.1 ml/min). The technetium **"tagged" RBC scan** can detect even slower rates of bleeding, and the scan can be repeated at a later time if the initial scan is negative.

Any patient with a lower GI bleed in whom an obvious source cannot be found should have a diagnostic upper GI endoscopy to rule out an upper tract source. This should be done before any surgical procedure.

Britt LG, et al: Selective management of lower gastrointestinal bleeding. Am Surg 49:121, 1983.

11. Does melena indicate a right-sided colonic source and hematochezia indicate a left-sided source?

Usually. The color of stool depends on colonic transit time. If the stool remains in contact with bacteria that degrade hemoglobin, the resulting stool will be melanic. Although right-sided lesions are usually associated with melena (dark, tarry stools) and left-sided lesions with hematochezia (the passage of bright red blood per rectum), the opposite can also be seen. Therefore, the evaluation of a patient with hematochezia must include examination of the proximal colon.

Cuellar RE, et al: Gastrointestinal trace hemorrhage. Arch Intern Med 150:1381, 1990.

12. What are the possible causes of esophageal varices?

Elevation of pressure in the hepatic portal system leads to the development of varices. This increased pressure may be due to diseases of the hepatic vasculature (e.g., Budd-Chiari syndrome), portal or splenic vein thrombosis, or intrinsic liver disease (e.g., cirrhosis). The most common cause in the Western world is alcohol-related cirrhosis.

13. Which two factors determine whether esophageal varices will develop and whether they will bleed?

Portal pressure and **variceal size.** The portal to hepatic vein pressure gradient must be $\geq$ 12 mm Hg (normal = 3–6 mm Hg) for varices to develop. Beyond this level, there is poor correlation between the portal pressure and the likelihood of bleeding.

The best predictor of impending variceal hemorrhage is size. When varices reach a large size > 5 mm in diameter, they are more likely to rupture and bleed. At any given pressure, the wall of a large varix is under greater tension than that of a small varix and must be thicker to withstand the pressure.

14. What is the mortality rate of bleeding esophageal varices? What is the rebleeding rate during hospitalization?

The mortality rate for bleeding esophageal varices during the initial hospitalization approaches 30%. This rate is in part due to the fact that approx. 50–70% of patients will experience a rebleeding episode during that hospitalization. At least 33% of patients will rebleed within 6 weeks after discharge, and only 33% will survive beyond the first year following the index bleed.

15. What percentage of patients with upper GI bleeding and known esophageal varices have a bleeding source other than varices at endoscopy?

In the patient with upper GI bleeding and a strong suspicion of esophageal varices, endoscopy must be performed to determine the site of bleeding, since 30–50% of these patients will be bleeding from a source other than varices. Other common causes of bleeding in patients with varices include peptic ulcer disease, Mallory-Weiss tears, and portal hypertensive gastropathy.

16. How do you treat a patient with bleeding esophageal varices?

In patients with suspected bleeding varices, the first line of therapy after volume resuscitation and blood transfusion is **upper GI endoscopy.** The objectives of endoscopic therapy are to control acute bleeding, minimize therapy-induced complications, and prevent rebleeding. Upper GI endoscopy should be done as soon as possible to document the site of bleeding and to perform either **endoscopic esophageal sclerotherapy** (EST) or **band ligation** (EVL) if the bleeding site is found to be variceal. In EST, the endoscopist injects a sclerosing solution into and around the bleeding varix; this results in rapid occlusion of the varix by thrombus or perivariceal edema so that active bleeding ceases in 80–90% of patients. In EVL, tiny rubber bands are used to ensnare varices, causing strangulation and eventual sloughing and obliteration.

If sclerotherapy or ligation is unsuccessful, the next step is **balloon tamponade** of the bleeding varices using a Sengstaken-Blakemore tube, with the addition of IV vasopressin or somatostatin (if these medications have not already been previously added). The next step would be performing **transjugular intrahepatic portosystemic shunt** (TIPS) by interventional radiology. **Surgery** (either a portosystemic shunt or esophageal transection) is the last resort since these patients have a >50% mortality when shunts are performed emergently.

Steigmann G, et al: Endoscopic sclerotherapy as compared with endoscopic ligation for bleeding esophageal varices. N Engl J Med 326:1527, 1992.

Zemel G, et al: Percutaneous transjugular portosystemic shunt. JAMA 266:390, 1991.

17. When is medical therapy instituted for a suspected variceal hemorrhage?

Many physicians begin immediate medical therapy of suspected variceal hemorrhage, consisting of vasopressin, somatostatin, or either of their analogues. The addition of nitroglycerin to the vasopressin has decreased the incidence of systemic ischemic complications. These agents may also be administered after the initial endoscopy has been performed.

Burroughs AK. Randomized, double-blind, placebo controlled trial of somatostatin for variceal bleeding: Emergency control and prevention of variceal rebleeding. Gastroenterology 99:1388, 1990.

18. How does the Sengstaken-Blakemore tube work?

This tube is a double-balloon system, one of which inflates in the stomach and the other in the esophagus to tamponade the bleeding site. Between 75–90% of patients stop bleeding with this technique. However, there is a high incidence of complications related to balloon tamponade, including esophageal perforation, pulmonary aspiration, and malfunction of the tube requiring replacement, and 30–60% of patients rebleed after the tube is deflated. This technique should be reserved for the patient who fails to stop bleeding using standard measures.

19. Can any therapeutic procedures prevent rebleeding from varices?

Surgical variceal systemic shunting diverts blood from the esophageal or gastric veins and from the high-pressure portal circulation into the lower-pressure systemic circulation. This can be accomplished by portacaval, splenorenal, or mesocaval shunting.

Endoscopic long-term repeated injection sclerotherapy requires the patient to return for endoscopy every 2–4 weeks to undergo repeated sclerotherapy or ligation until the varices have been obliterated (usually 3–4 sessions).

Esophageal variceal band ligation requires fewer endoscopic sessions to achieve obliteration and has fewer procedure-associated complications (e.g., strictures, pulmonary infections, and ulcers), but the patient still must return for endoscopy every 3–4 weeks.

Transjugular intrahepatic portosystemic shunt (TIPS) is a relative newcomer. This procedure, performed by interventional radiologists, involves placing an expanding metal stent between branches of the portal and hepatic venous systems.

β-Blocker therapy has been given in doses to decrease the heart rate by 25%. The portal pressure is decreased as a result of propranolol's decreasing the splanchnic blood flow.

Hayes PC, et al: TIPS: The immediate problems solved. Am J Gastroenterol 90:533, 1995.

Laine L, et al: Endoscopic ligation compared with sclerotherapy for treatment of esophageal variceal bleeding: A meta-snalysis. Ann Intern Med 123:280, 1995.

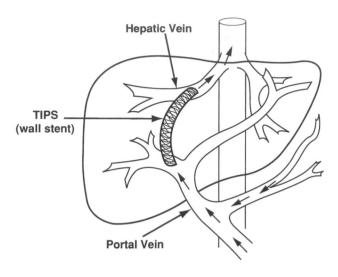

TIPS procedure involving placement of a metallic wire stent between the hepatic and portal viens (From Mc-Nally PR (ed): GI/Liver Secrets. Philadelphia, Hanley & Belfus, 1996; with permission.)

20. What is Dieulafoy's lesion?

Dieulafoy's lesion (exulceratio simplex) is an uncommon cause of massive GI bleeding. In it, a large submucosal artery erodes through the mucosa without any overlying ulceration or other obvious mucosal damage. Dieulafoy's lesion has the potential to bleed profusely but intermittently, and thus it is easily missed at endoscopy unless it is actively bleeding. In most cases, Dieulafoy's lesion is located in the proximal stomach within 6 cm of the gastroesophageal junction, but it may occur in the antrum, duodenum, jejunum, colon, and rectum. Treatment is initially endoscopic thermal coagulation or injection sclerotherapy. Surgical wedge resection remains the definitive management.

Dy NM, et al: Bleeding from the endoscopically identified Dieulafoy lesion of the proximal small intestine and colon. Am J Gastroenterol 90:108, 1994.

HEPATITIS

21. What are the differences between hepatitis A, B, and C?

Hepatitis A, called infectious hepatitis, is easily spread by the fecal/oral route. HAV causes a short-lived, benign, acute hepatitis that is not followed by chronic liver disease. IgG antibodies to HAV remain positive for life. To determine if the hepatitis is acute, one must look for IgM antibodies in the serum.

Hepatitis B, called serum hepatitis, is contracted by contact with blood or other bodily secretions from an infected individual, usually through a break in the skin or use of a contaminated needle. Unlike hepatitis A, hepatitis B may go on to cause chronic disease and cirrhosis. It also predisposes to hepatocellular carcinoma (hepatoma). A carrier state is possible in which patients demonstrate persistent hepatitis B surface antigenemia (HBsAg) without clinically evident disease but are able to transmit the disease.

Hepatitis C had been previously included in the non-A, non-B hepatitis category. It is the form of hepatitis most commonly contracted from blood transfusion. It also is the most common viral cause of chronic liver disease and increases the patient's risk for developing hepatoma. The most widely available marker of disease is anti-HCV, which denotes chronic infection. HCV-RNA can be used to determine the level of disease activity and to measure response to therapy.

22. How is hepatitis A virus (HAV) transmitted?

HAV is typically transmitted through contaminated water supplies and is most common in developing countries with poor hygiene and inadequate sanitation. Transplacental or perinatal transmission of the virus has not been documented. Homosexual men have a higher prevalence of antibodies to HAV, which suggests possible sexual transmission.

23. Describe the symptoms and duration of illness in hepatitis A. How is it diagnosed and treated?

The symptoms of hepatitis A are relatively nonspecific and are similar to those of any cause of hepatitis: anorexia, fatigue, malaise, right-upper-quadrant abdominal discomfort, and jaundice. The duration of illness tends to vary, but most patients recover within 4 weeks of the onset of clinical disease.

Hepatitis A can be diagnosed by the detection of HAV-specific IgM in the blood; this antibody is always present when symptoms from hepatitis A are present. Treatment is purely supportive, and no effective antiviral agent has been identified that will accelerate recovery.

Mijch AM, et al: Clinical, serologic, and epidemiologic aspects of hepatitis A virus infection. Semin Liver Dis 16:42, 1986.

24. A teacher was exposed to a child with hepatitis A at a daycare center on the previous day. How should you treat her?

The patient plus his or her household and sexual contacts, as well as other daycare center exposures, should receive immunoglobulin for prevention of hepatitis A. This should be administered within 2 days after known contact. The adult dose is 0.02 mg/kg given in a single intramuscular (IM) dose. The hepatitis A vaccine is newly released, and recommendations for its appropriate use are being defined.

25. What is the usual serologic response after naturally acquired hepatitis B infection?

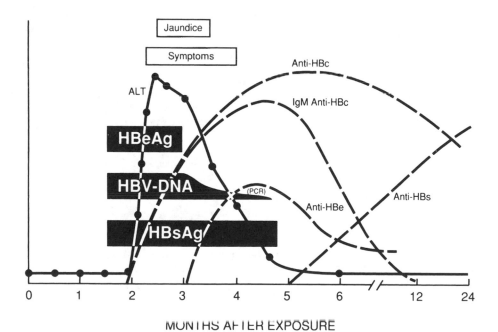

Clinical and serologic course of a typical case of acute hepatitis B. HBsAg, hepatitis B surface antigen; HBeAg, hepatitis B e antigen; DNA-p, DNA polymerase; HBV-DNA, hepatitis B virus DNA; ALT, alanine aminotransferase (SGPT); anti-HBC, antibody to hepatitis B core antigen; anti-HBe, antibody to HBeAg; anti-HBs, antibody to HBsAg. (From Hoofnagle JH: Acute viral hepatitis. In Mandell GL, et al (eds): Principles and Practice of Infectious Diseases, 4th ed. New York, Churchill Livingstone, 1995, p 1143.)

26. Which serologic marker indicates protection in a person who has completed the hepatitis B vaccine protocol?

The currently available hepatitis B vaccine is composed only of HBsAg and induces an antibody response only to HBsAg. The anti-HBsAg response correlates well with protection against HBV infection. Of healthy persons vaccinated by the IM route, 95% develop protection against HBV.

27. How should you treat a health care worker with a recent (<48 hour) needlestick exposure to hepatitis B?

The worker should receive hepatitis immunoglobulin (HBIg), 0.06 ml/kg IM, as soon as possible and within 7 days of exposure. If the worker has not previously received the hepatitis B vaccine, the vaccination program should be initiated with the usual three doses—the first dose within 14 days after exposure and again at 1 and 6 months.

28. How is hepatitis C virus (HCV) transmitted? What are the possible courses of this disease?

HCV is the primary cause of parenterally transmitted non-A, non-B hepatitis, which is classically transmitted by blood transfusion or by contaminated needles among IV drug abusers. Approx. 10% of patients who have had multiple transfusions develop hepatitis, and >90% of these cases are due to HCV. To date, there is little consistent evidence for vertical (mother to baby) or sexual transmission. Because > 30% of patients give no history of parenteral exposure, a second major route of transmission through nonpercutaneous or covert percutaneous exposure may exist.

Significant liver disease develops in 50% of persons infected, and they are at risk for the development of hepatocellular carcinoma. Available serologic markers include anti-HCV, which is present in chronic disease, and HCV-RNA, which is present in both acute and chronic infection.

29. How effective is treatment of hepatitis C?

Antiviral therapy is with alpha-interferon, administered at a dose of 3 MU subcutaneously three times a week for a minimum of 6 months. Data are still evolving on whether longer treatment or maintenance therapy is effective. One-third of patients treated respond to interferon therapy with complete resolution of active disease, one-third respond during therapy but relapse, and one-third do not respond.

Maddrey WC: Chronic hepatitis. DM 39(2):96–108, 1993.

30. How is hepatitis D virus (delta virus) transmitted?

Hepatitis D virus (HDV) is a very small RNA virus that contains a defective genome and requires HBsAg to become pathogenic. Infection may occur under two circumstances:

1. In conjunction with simultaneous infection with hepatitis B in a previously unexposed patient **(coinfection)**

2. In the chronic carrier of HBsAg **(superinfection).**

Hepatitis D is diagnosed by detecting IgM antibody to HDV in acute serum or an increase in IgG antibody to HDV in convalescent serum.

31. What is hepatitis E? What is hepatitis G?

Hepatitis E virus causes enterically transmitted non-A, non-B hepatitis. It is endemic to Southeast and Central Asia, Africa, and Mexico but is rare in the U.S. No serologic test for it is currently available. Hepatitis E is most severe in pregnant women, in whom the mortality is ≥20%.

Hepatitis G is an RNA virus that appears to be similar in transmission to hepatitis C (i.e., blood borne) but to date has not been documented to produce chronic liver disease.

NUTRITION

32. Name the six common vitamins and trace minerals and the clinical manifestations of their respective deficiency states.

Thiamine	Beriberi, muscle weakness, tachycardia, heart failure
Niacin	Pellagra, glossitis
Vitamin A	Xerophthalmia, hyperkeratosis of skin
Vitamin E	Cerebellar ataxia, areflexia
Zinc	Hypogeusia, acrodermatitis
Chromium	Glucose intolerance

33. Name the two most common nutritional deficiencies seen in patients with intestinal disease.

Deficiencies of folate and calcium. When the small bowel is diseased, intestinal loss of calcium is excessive, and the rate of bone resorption is insufficient to maintain serum calcium.

Severe folate deficiency occurs most often in association with chronic alcoholism, celiac sprue, tropical sprue, and blind loop syndrome. Minor deficiencies can be found in Crohn's disease and following partial gastrectomy. Since folate absorption is largely completed in the upper small intestine, malabsorption is worse in disorders that affect the upper gut. However, any intestinal disorder accompanied by a decrease in dietary intake or rapid transport may result in folate deficiency.

34. An elderly white man presents with profound peripheral neuropathy and a markedly low serum B_{12}. Physical examination reveals an abdominal scar consistent with previous laparotomy, but the patient doesn't remember what kind of surgery was done. What two possible operations would result in B_{12} deficiency? Why?

1. **Gastrectomy:** Vitamin B_{12} absorption starts in the stomach, where it binds to intrinsic factor and R-proteins produced there. In the duodenum, the R-proteins are hydrolyzed off the vitamin B_{12} in the presence of an alkaline environment, which then allows for further binding of B_{12} with intrinsic factor. Vitamin B_{12} cannot be absorbed unless it is bound to intrinsic factor. If the patient's stomach was completely or partially removed, he would have insufficient intrinsic factor.

2. **Terminal ileal resection:** This patient may have had Crohn's disease and undergone resection of a large portion (>100 cm) of terminal ileum, the site of absorption of the vitamin B_{12}–intrinsic factor complex.

Both mechanisms of deficiency can be easily treated with supplemental IM vitamin B_{12} injections.

35. What is the most common disorder of carbohydrate digestion in humans?

Lactase deficiency. Lactase-deficient adults retain 10–30% of intestinal lactose activity and develop symptoms (diarrhea, bloating, and gas) only when they ingest sufficient lactose. Symptoms result from the colonic bacteria metabolizing lactose to methane, CO_2, and short-chain fatty acids.

36. After avoiding dairy products, the patient's symptoms have disappeared. Does this confirm the diagnosis of lactose deficiency?

No. The diagnosis cannot be made simply by advising the patient to avoid dairy products for 2 weeks to determine if the altered bowel habits revert to normal, because many patients who respond to these manipulations are actually *not* lactase-deficient. The diagnostic test to be used is the lactose hydrogen breath test.

37. What are medium-chain triglycerides (MCTs)? In which intestinal diseases are they used as therapy?

MCTs are lipids containing only medium-length fatty acid chains (C6–C12) and are absorbed in a different manner from long-chain triglycerides, which are more common in the diet. MCTs can be absorbed intact by enterocytes and pass directly into the portal circulation. Patients with a variety of small intestinal diseases—short bowel syndrome, biliary obstruction, and pancreatic insufficiency—absorb MCTs more efficiently than long-chain triglycerides.

38. Outline the fundamental principles of total parenteral nutrition (TPN).

Fundamental Principles of Total Parenteral Nutrition

1. Patients generally require 25–35 kcal/kg for maintenance.
2. The optimal calorie/nitrogen ratio appears to be ~160 cal/gm N.
3. The average adult requires ~30 ml water/kg body weight/day.
4. IV lipid emulsions are a suitable source of nonprotein calories that contribute to conservation of body protein. A regimen in which calories are supplied by both dextrose solution and lipid emulsions, with fat providing 20–30% of the total calories, appears to be the most effective form of parenteral nutrition.

39. What are the most common complications of TPN? How are they treated?

The most common complications are those related to **catheter placement** and **management.** These include infections, thrombosis, nonthrombotic occlusion, and other mechanical complications during line placement. Catheter-related complications can be minimized by maintaining strict and reproducible technique as well as meticulous line care.

In prolonged TPN, especially when excessive carbohydrate calories are given, patients frequently develop **liver tenderness** and **transaminase elevations.** The increased liver values are thought to reflect hepatic steatosis. AST and ALT abnormalities should return to normal when TPN is discontinued. If TPN is continued, one should decrease the dextrose infusion and increase the amount of fat calories provided.

A complication of long-term (home) TPN is **metabolic bone disease** which is similar to osteomalacia and osteoporosis. The addition of acetate or phosphate may offset the urinary calcium losses and restore positive calcium balance in these patients.

An increased incidence of **cholecystitis** and **cholelithiasis** related to gallbladder stasis is seen in patients on TPN.

40. Which vitamin deficiencies might develop in a patient maintained on long-term TPN (>6 mos) containing only Na^+, K^+, Cl^-, HCO_3^-, glucose, and amino acids?

This TPN solution clearly is lacking in vitamins and trace minerals. In a matter of weeks, this patient would be expected to develop deficiencies in magnesium, zinc, essential fatty acids, and water-soluble vitamins (with the exception of B_{12}). Over several months, vitamin K and copper deficiencies would develop. Over a period of years, deficiencies in the fat-soluble vitamins A and D as well as selenium, chromium, and vitamin B_{12} would result.

CANCER

41. A patient presents with an "apple core" lesion in the sigmoid colon which on biopsy is found to be adenocarcinoma. Which tests should be included in the routine preoperative evaluation for this patient?

If carcinoma is detected either by radiographs or sigmoidoscopy, a full **colonoscopic exam** should be done because of the high incidence of synchronous lesions. Half of patients with a single cancer of the colon have additional polyps, which may require modification of treatment.

Preoperative serum **carcinoembryonic antigen** (CEA), liver **aminotransferases,** and **alkaline phosphatase** tests should be ordered. If the preoperative CEA is elevated, it will usually fall to a normal level postoperatively if all tumor has been removed. Patients with a rising CEA level after total resection should be suspected of having a recurrence. Elevated AST and ALT levels suggest clinically silent liver metastases, and an elevated alkaline phosphatase may point to bone metastases.

An **abdominal CT scan** should be performed with and without contrast to exclude clinically silent liver metastases. The presence of metastases does not prevent palliative surgery, but it will affect postoperative therapy.

42. The primary therapy for colorectal carcinoma is surgical resection, but radiation therapy is useful for tumors arising in part of the colon. Which part and why?

Patients with colorectal cancer who have lesions penetrating the bowel wall or who have regional lymph nodes involved by tumor are at particularly high risk for recurrence following resection. Radiation therapy used preoperatively or postoperatively may decrease the local recurrence rate. It is uncertain whether pre- or postoperative radiation to the rectum prolongs survival.

43. Name the most common malignant neoplasms of the small intestine.

Adenocarcinoma	45%
Carcinoid	34%
Leiomyosarcoma	18%
Lymphoma	3%

Maglinte DDT, et al: The role of the physician in the late diagnosis of primary malignant tumors of the small intestine. Am J Gastroenterol 86:304, 1991.

44. Name the most common benign neoplasms of the small intestine.

Adenoma   >   leiomyoma   >   lipoma

45. What are adenomatous polyps and what is their significance?

Adenomatous polyps are neoplastic polyps found most often in the colon that give rise to symptoms only when they become large. They are frequently detected incidentally on colono-scopic exam or barium enema. Their importance relates to their malignant potential; nearly all colonic carcinomas arise from adenomatous polyps. Approx. 75% of adenomatous polyps are tubular adenomas, 15% are tubulovillous adenomas, and the rest are villous adenomas. Villous tumors are more likely to be malignant than tubular adenomas. Other factors that relate to ma-lignant potential include tumor size >1 cm, degree of cellular atypia, and number of polyps pre-sent.

Patients having adenomatous polyps diagnosed usually have them removed with endoscopic polypectomy. They should undergo colonoscopy at routine intervals so that additional polyps may be removed before they progress to malignancy.

Itzkowitz SH: The adenomatous polyp. Semin Gastrointest Dis 3:3, 1992.

INFLAMMATORY BOWEL DISEASE

46. Explain the differential diagnosis in a young patient with Crohn's disease of the ileum who presents with right-upper-quadrant discomfort and jaundice.

In the patient with inflammatory bowel disease (IBD) who presents with jaundice, the diag-nostic considerations include pericholangitis, sclerosing cholangitis, choledocholithiasis, and pri-mary hepatocellular disease. **Pericholangitis** is a histologic finding representing inflammatory changes of the small bile ductules and may be one end of the spectrum of sclerosing cholangitis. **Sclerosing cholangitis** is focal narrowing and inflammation of the intra- and extrahepatic biliary tree. These diseases have been reported only with IBD affecting the colon and are much more common with ulcerative colitis than with Crohn's colitis.

A more likely consideration is **choledocholithiasis.** Patients with longstanding ileal disease or ileal resection are unable to resorb bile salts and therefore have a diminished bile salt pool. This results in supersaturation of bile with cholesterol with subsequent precipitation of cholesterol crystals and gallstone formation. With these possibilities in mind, this patient should be evaluated for extrahepatic duct obstruction or hepatocellular disease.

47. How do Crohn's disease and ulcerative colitis differ?

Distinguishing Features of Ulcerative Colitis and Crohn's Disease

	CROHN'S DISEASE	ULCERATIVE COLITIS
Symptoms	Pain is more common; bleeding is uncommon	Diarrhea with a bloody-mucosal discharge, cramping
Location	Can affect the GI tract from mouth to anus	Limited to the colon
Pattern of colonic involvement	Skip lesions	Continuous involvment
Histology	Transmural inflammation, granu-lomas, focal ulceration	Mucosal inflammation, crypt ab-scesses, crypt distortion
Radiologic	Terminal ileal involvement, deep ulcerations, normal haustra be-tween involved areas, strictures fistulas	Rectum involved, shortened colon, absence of haustra (lead-pipe sign)
Complications	Obstruction, fistulas, abscesses, kidney stones, gallstones, B_{12} deficiency	Bleeding, toxic megacolon, colon cancer

Podolsky DK: Inflammatory bowel disease. N Engl J Med, 325:928–937, 1008–1016, 1991.

ULCERS

48. What are the two major functions of acid secretion in the stomach?
1. Acid activates the enzyme pepsin by converting pepsinogen to pepsin, initiating the first stages of protein digestion.
2. Acid serves as an antibacterial barrier to protect the stomach from colonization.

49. How does the pathogenesis of duodenal and gastric ulcers differ?
Duodenal ulcer disease, with a peak incidence in young adults, has frequent recurrences over a period of 10–20 years. The precise pathogenesis is not completely understood but has been associated with the following:
- *Helicobacter pylori* infection in >90% of cases. Recurrence rates are dramatically reduced after eradication of the bacteria.
- Increased acid secretion that correlates with an increased number of parietal cells in the gastric mucosa.
- Increased responsiveness of the parietal cells of the stomach to stimulation factors, such as food, gastric acid, or histamine.
- Increased vagal activity.

Gastric ulcer disease, with a peak incidence in the elderly, is not associated with these factors. These patients have normal or even decreased gastric acid secretion. Gastric ulcers probably develop because of a change in the mucosal resistance to the acid. NSAIDs play a prominent role in the etiology of gastric (more than duodenal) ulcer disease.

Walsh JH, Peterson WL: The therapy of *Helicobacter pylori* infection in the management of peptic ulcer disease. N Engl J Med 333:984, 1995.

50. What are the five major indications for peptic ulcer surgery?
1. **Intractability:** This relates to the symptoms and not to delayed healing. The diagnosis of intractability requires clinical confirmation that an ulcer is responsible for the patient's symptoms.

2. **Hemorrhage:** Surgery to control bleeding is occasionally necessary but carries a high mortality rate. It should be considered in patients who require a large-volume blood transfusion (6–8 units/24 hrs) to correct losses, who have one or more rebleeding episodes occurring in the hospital, or who have persistent bleeding requiring transfusion over 48–72 hours in the hospital.

3. **Perforation:** This requires immediate surgery.

4. **Penetration:** This represents erosion of an ulcer through the entire thickness of the wall of the stomach or intestine without leakage of digestive contents into the peritoneal cavity. The diagnosis is usually suggested by a change in symptoms experienced by the patient, and treatment is surgical if complicated penetration exists.

5. **Obstruction:** Gastric outlet obstruction as a result of ulcer disease occurs in 2% of all ulcer patients. Standard therapy has been surgical, but endoscopic balloon dilatation of the stenotic pylorus may be another possibility.

51. What are the reasons for recurrent ulcer in patients who have undergone previous ulcer surgery?
- Untreated *Helicobacter pylori* infection
- NSAIDs use
- Incomplete vagotomy
- Adjacent nonabsorbable suture that acts as an irritant
- "Retained antrum" syndrome, in which antral tissue left behind at surgery produces a continued source of gastric production
- Antral G-cell hyperplasia (uncommon)
- Zollinger-Ellison syndrome (gastrinoma)
- Gastric cancer

Other factors that may contribute to recurrent ulcers but have not necessarily been implicated as primary causes include smoking, enterogastric reflex (bile acid reflex), primary hyperparathyroidism, and gastric bezoar.

52. Discuss the relationship between *Helicobacter pylori* infection and duodenal ulcer disease.

H. pylori is a microaerophilic bacterium found primarily in the gastric antrum of humans. It appears to be the most common infection worldwide. *H. pylori* is the primary cause of chronic active gastritis, which is a crucial predictive factor for peptic ulcer disease. *H. pylori* infection alone does not invariably cause duodenal ulcer disease, because most patients with *H. pylori* gastritis do not have peptic ulcer disease. Other factors contributing to ulcer formation may include NSAIDs, cigarette smoking, hereditary tendency, and acid hypersecretion.

53. Review the current recommended therapies for *Helicobacter pylori* infection.

No available therapy results in 100% cure rates, but it is recommended that all patients who have either a duodenal or gastric ulcer and documented *H. pylori* infection should be treated with antimicrobial therapy. Patients with nonulcer dyspepsia who are *H. pylori*-positive do not require treatment. Suggested regimens include:

    1. Triple therapy: >90% successful, given with meals × 7–14 days
      Tetracycline HC1, 500 mg qid
      Metronidazole, 250 mg tid
      Bismuth subsalicylate (PeptoBismol), 2 tablets qid
      And H_2 receptor antagonist
    2. MOC therapy: >90% successful, × 7–14 days
      Metronidazole, 500 mg bid
      Omeprazole, 20 mg bid; or lansoprazole, 15 mg bid
      Clarithromycin, 250 mg bid
    3. Dual therapies: (FDA approved): 70–80% successful, given with meals × 14 days
      Clarithromycin, 500 mg tid
      Omeprazole, 40 mg q AM; or lansoprazole, 30 mg q AM
        or
      Ranitidine bismuth (Tritec), 400 mg bid
      Clarithromycin, 500 mg tid

Yousfi MM, Cole RA, Graham DY: Metronidazole, omeprazole and clarithromycin: An effective combination therapy of *Helicobacter pylori* infection. Aliment Pharmacol Ther 9:209, 1995.

54. Which diseases are strongly associated with *Helicobacter pylori* infection?

    Peptic ulcer disease (duodenal >> gastric)
    Chronic active gastritis
    MALToma (mucosa-associated lymphoid tissue)
    Gastric carcinoma

NIH Consensus Development Panel: *Helicobacter pylori* in peptic ulcer disease. JAMA 272:65, 1994.

55. What is the most common presenting symptom of peptic ulcer disease in the elderly?

Melena. Epigastric pain occurs in <50% of elderly patients, and many are asymptomatic. A fatal hemorrhagic event may be the first sign of an ulcer in the elderly.

Shamburek K, et at: Disorders of the digestive system in the elderly. N Engl J Med 322:438, 1990.

56. What is the clinical triad of the Zollinger-Ellison syndrome (ZES)?

Gastric acid hypersecretion, severe ulcer disease of the upper GI tract as a direct result of acid hypersecretion, and a non-β cell tumor of the pancreas that secretes the hormone gastrin (gastrinoma). The other common feature of ZES is diarrhea, which may precede the diagnosis of ZES by many years. The diagnosis should be suspected in patients with a compatible clinical history and gastric acid hypersecretion.

PANCREATITIS

57. What are the most common causes of acute pancreatitis in the U.S.?

Acute pancreatitis is due to choledocholithiasis, ethanol abuse, or idiopathic causes in 90% of cases in the U.S. Most patients who previously were felt to have an idiopathic etiology actually have been found to have diminutive gallstones (microlithiasis) as the etiology. In the private hospital setting, 50% of patients with acute pancreatitis have gallstones (gallstone pancreatitis). In public hospitals, up to 66% of first episodes are caused by excessive alcohol consumption.

Marshall JB: Acute pancreatitis: A review with emphasis on new developments. Arch Intern Med 153:1185, 1993.

58. Which drugs can cause acute pancreatitis?

Drugs Causing Acute Pancreatitis

Ethanol, methanol	6-Mercaptopurine
Didanosine (ddI)	Pentamidine
Azathioprine	Sulfasalazine
Hydrochlorothiazide	Furosemide
Sulfonamides	Tetracyclines
Estrogens	Valproic acid
L-Asparaginase	?Cyclosporine

59. List Ranson's criteria for the prognosis in acute pancreatitis.

Ranson initially published criteria that could be used to prognosticate in cases of acute pancreatitis in 1974. These are still used in practice today. When there are fewer than 3 positive signs, the patient has mild disease and an excellent prognosis. The mortality rate is 10–20% with 3–5 signs and >50% with 6 or more signs.

Prognostic Criteria in Acute Pancreatitis

ON ADMISSION	IN INITIAL 48 HOURS
Age > 55 yrs	Hematocrit decrease of > 10%
WBC > 16,000/mm^3	BUN rise of > 5 mg/dl
Serum LDH > 350 IU/l	Serum calcium < 8 mg/dl
Blood glucose > 200 mg/dl	Arterial PO$_2$ < 60 mm Hg
SGOT/AST > 250 IU/l	Base deficit > 4 meq/l
	Estimated fluid sequestration > 6 liters

Ranson JH: Etiologic and prognostic factors in human acute pancreatitis: A review. Am J Gastroenterol 77:633, 1982.

60. What are the causes of an increase in serum amylase?

Several conditions other than acute pancreatitis can cause an increase in serum amylase, including:

Macroamylasemia	Perforated peptic ulcer disease
Renal failure	Ruptured ectopic pregnancy
Mesenteric infarction	Diabetic ketoacidosis
Parotitis	Peritonitis
Burns	Tumors of pancreas, salivary glands, ovary, lung, prostate
Cholecystitis	Pancreatitis complications (pseudocyst, abscess, ascites)
Post-ERCP	

61. What are Cullen's and Grey Turner's signs?

These signs are associated with acute hemorrhagic pancreatitis:
Cullen's sign: ecchymotic discoloration in the umbilicus
Grey Turner's sign: ecchymotic discoloration around the flanks

62. Why is meperidine indicated for analgesia in acute pancreatitis?

Meperidine is indicated over other narcotic analgesic agents in acute pancreatitis because it has minimal effects on the ampulla of Vater. Other narcotic analgesics can cause increased ampullary pressure and theoretically may worsen pancreatitis.

63. How is gallstone pancreatitis treated?

Gallstone or biliary pancreatitis refers to acute pancreatitis resulting from choledocholithiasis. Most commonly, these patients are elderly, appear seriously ill, and have a bilirubin > 3.0 mg/dl and amylase > 500 IU. Imaging studies such as ultrasound will document dilated biliary ducts or the presence of cholelithiasis in most patients.

The initial management is conservative therapy with IV antibiotics, nothing per mouth (NPO), and close monitoring. Patients who do not respond within 48 hours are deemed to have severe pancreatitis and endoscopic retrograde cholangiopancreatography (ERCP) is performed. ERCP can document the offending stone and provide definitive therapy, such as sphincterotomy with stone removal. Following resolution of the acute symptoms, the patient should undergo a cholecystectomy, as the recurrence rate is > 35% within 6–8 weeks following the index attack.

Fan ST, et al: Early therapy of acute biliary pancreatitis by endoscopic papillotomy. N Engl J Med 328:228, 1993.

VASCULAR DISEASE

64. What is intestinal angina?

When occlusive vascular disease, usually atherosclerosis, affects two of the three major arteries supplying the gut, it may be associated with a syndrome of intermittent, cramping, midabdominal pain commonly called intestinal angina. Symptoms worsen during eating, often causing patients to lose weight simply by avoiding meals or eating small meals. The diagnosis is facilitated by angiography, which documents significant stenosis of vessels. Treatment for patients with a significant gradient across the stenosis is surgical bypass, endarterectomy, or percutaneous transluminal angioplasty.

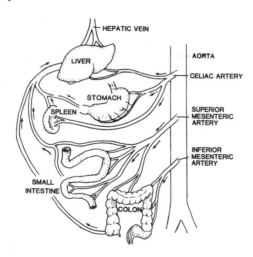

Major splanchnic organs and blood vessels. (From McNally PR (ed): GI/Liver Secrets. Philadelphia, Hanley & Belfus, 1996; with permission.)

65. Which two colonic segments are most commonly involved in ischemic colitis? Why?

Ischemic colitis most commonly occurs in the regions lying in the "watershed" areas between two adjacent arterial supplies. These are the **splenic flexure,** which lies between the inferior and superior mesenteric arteries, and the **rectosigmoid junction,** which lies between the inferior mesenteric and interior iliac arteries.

Brandt LJ, et al: Colonic ischemia. Surg Clin North Am 72:203, 1992.

66. What are the classic signs and symptoms of ischemic colitis?
1. Sudden onset of mild, crampy, left-sided abdominal pain
2. Painless hematochezia within 24 hours of onset of pain

DIARRHEA

67. What differentiates osmotic from secretory diarrhea? Give examples of each.

Osmotic diarrhea is caused by ingestion of excessive amounts of a poorly absorbable but osmotically active solute. Commonly implicated substances include mannitol or sorbitol (seen in patients chewing large quantities of sugar-free gum), magnesium sulfate (Epsom salt), and some magnesium-containing antacids. Carbohydrate malabsorption also may cause osmotic diarrhea through the action of unabsorbed sugars (lactulose). Clinically, osmotic diarrhea stops when the patient fasts (or stops ingesting the poorly absorbable solute).

Secretory diarrhea involves a disruption of normal bowel function. Small intestinal epithelial cells normally secrete less than they absorb, ultimately leading to a net absorption of fluid and electrolytes. If this process is interrupted by a pathologic process that stimulates increased secretion or inhibits absorption, secretory diarrhea may occur. Causes of secretory diarrhea include enterotoxin-mediated secretion, such as with *Vibrio cholerae* and enterotoxigenic *Escherichia coli* infection, hormone production by tumors such as VIPomas, and use of laxatives containing phenolphthalein. Unabsorbed bile acids and fatty acids also may induce colonic secretion and diarrhea.

Fedorak RN, et al: Basic investigation of a patient with diarrhea. In Field M (ed): Textbook of Diarrheal Diseases. New York, Elsevier, 1991, pp. 191–218.

68. Which three diagnostic features can distinguish secretory from osmotic diarrhea?
1. The stool osmolar gap is <50 mOsm/kg in secretory diarrhea but is >50 mOsm/kg in osmotic diarrhea. Normal stool osmolality is ~290 mOsm/kg.
2. Secretory diarrhea is typically unrelated to ingested foods or solutes and persists during a 24–72-hour fast, whereas osmotic diarreha stops when ingestion of the offending solute ends.
3. Patients with a pure secretory diarrhea do not have WBCs, RBCs, or fat in their stool.

69. What are the two basic mechanisms by which bacteria cause infectious diarrhea? Give examples of each type.
1. **Enterotoxigenic**: Bacteria adhere to the mucosa and then secrete an enterotoxin that stimulates epithelial cell secretion. Examples include enterotoxigenic *Escherichia coli* (ETEC) and *Vibrio cholerae*.
2. **Enteroinvasive:** Organisms adhere to epithelial cells in preparation for invasion of the mucosa. Many of the invasive organisms also release toxins that stimulate secretion by the intestinal cell, but by a mechanism that does not involve activation of adenylate cyclase. Organisms that invade the mucosa and result in diarrhea include *Salmonella, Shigella,* enteroinvasive *E. coli* (EIEc), *Campylobacter,* and *Yersinia.*

The toxigenic bacteria do not induce visible changes in the intestinal mucosa during infection. In contrast, mucosal damage, inflammatory infiltrate, and ulceration are commonly seen with the invasive organisms. For this reason, fecal leukocytes are typically present in infections with enteroinvasive organisms, whereas few or no WBCs are seen in the stool of patients infected with enterotoxigenic organisms.

70. What organisms are responsible for bacillary dysentery?

The term *dysentery* refers to a diarrheal stool that contains inflammatory exudate (pus) and blood. Bacillary dysentery refers to infectious diarrhea caused by invasive pathogens, most commonly, *Shigella, Salmonella, Campylobacter,* and enteroinvasive or enterohemorrhagic *Escherichia coli.*

71. A 50-year-old woman complains of 6–8 loose stools per day for 1 month. The etiology is not immediately evident after a careful history and physical. What diagnostic tests should be performed at this stage?

If performed early in the disease course, a compltete blood count, serum chemistry profile, and urinalysis may help pinpoint the likely causes of diarrhea. For example, the patient who has an anemia with a very high MCV may be suspected of having malabsorption and diarrhea based on the presence of ileal disease and inability to absorb vitamin B_{12}.

Basic stool studies, including bacterial culture and sensitivity, Sudan stain for fat, Wright's stain for WBCs, test for occult blood, and a phenolphthalein test for the presence of laxative ingestion, are simple and quickly obtainable tests that may give valuable results.

Proctosigmoidoscopy is a very important part of the examination in most patients with chronic and recurrent diarrhea. Examination of the rectal mucosa may reveal pseudomembranes seen with antibiotic-associated diarrhea, discrete ulceration typical of amebiasis, or a diffusely inflamed granular mucosa seen in ulcerative colitis. Biopsy specimens can be obtained through the scope for histologic examination, and fresh stool samples can be collected for cultures.

72. A 28-year-old man returns from a camping trip in the Colorado mountains complaining of cramping abdominal pain and diarrhea. His stool contains no RBCs or WBCs. What could account for his symptoms?

Giardia lamblia is a protozoan parasite found in water systems that fail to filter out the cysts (which resist chlorination). Although giardiasis can be contracted in any part of the country, it is most commonly associated with camping and backpacking in the mountainous west. Routine physical and laboratory findings are normal. Examination of the stools may reveal *Giardia* cysts or trophozoites. Duodenal aspiration and small bowel biopsy often show trophozoites. Most patients may be successfully treated with quinacrine or metronidazole.

73. What are the possible causes of diarrhea seen in a homosexual man who is HIV-negative? One who has AIDS?

The evaluation of diarrhea in the homosexual population is complicated by the various enteric organisms to which they are frequently exposed. Many organisms potentially carried by homosexual men may not be involved in clinical illness (such as *Neisseria gonorrhoeae, Entamoeba histolytica,* and *Giardia lamblia*). Organisms that must be considered in the differential diagnosis of homosexual men include:

HIV negative men

Amebiasis	Giardiasis
Shigellosis	*Campylobacter*
Rectal syphilis	Rectal spirochetes other than syphilis
Rectal gonorrhea	*Chlamydia trachomatis* (lymphogranuloma venereum)
Herpes simplex	

With AIDS

All the above organisms *plus:*

Cryptosporidium	*Candida albicans*
Cryptococcus neoformans	*Salmonella typhimurium*
Microsporidia	*Mycobacterium avium complex*
Cytomegalovirus	*Isospora belli*
Clostridium difficile	

74. What is diabetic diarrhea?

"Diabetic diarrhea" is a chronic diarrhea that affects approx. 5% of non-insulin-dependent diabetics (NIDDM). It is characterized by frequent (usually 10–30/day) passage of watery brown stool that occurs during the daytime or at night and is frequently associated with fecal incontinence.

Because diabetics are subject to all of the other causes of diarrhea, diabetic diarrhea is a diagnosis of exclusion. The cause of the diarrhea is not clear in most patients. Bacterial overgrowth may be the etiology in some patients, and treatment with broad-spectrum antibiotics often brings relief. However, diabetic diarrhea is often refractory to antidiarrheal therapy. Chronic pancreatitis with exocrine pancreatic insufficiency is more common in patients with longstanding diabetes. Steatorrhea due to exocrine pancreatic insufficiency may be relieved with pancreatic enzyme replacement therapy. Adult celiac disease is also more common in diabetics than in the general population. Diabetic diarrhea is often refractory to antidiarrheal therapy.

Ogbonnaya KI, Arem R: Diabetic diarrhea: Pathophysiology, diagnosis and management. Arch Intern Med 150:262, 1990.

75. How does the time of onset of illness relate to the possible causes of food poisoning?

Onset	Symptoms and Signs	Agents
≤ 1 hr	Nausea, vomiting, abdominal cramps	Heavy metal poisoning (copper, zinc, tin, cadmium)
≤ 1 hr	Paresthesias	Scrombroid poisoning, shellfish poisoning, Chinese restaurant syndrome (MSG), niacin poisoning
1–6 hrs	Nausea and vomiting	Preformed toxins of *Staphylococcus aureus* and *Bacillus cereus*
2 hrs	Delirium, parasympathetic hyperactivity, hallucinations, disulfiram reaction, or gastroenteritis	Toxic mushroom ingestion
8–16 hrs	Abdominal cramps, diarrhea	In vivo production of enterotoxins by *Clostridium perfringes* and *B. cereus*
6–24 hrs	Abdominal cramps, diarrhea, followed by hepatorenal failure	Toxic mushroom ingestion (*Amanita* sp.)
16–48 hrs	Fever, abdominal cramps, diarrhea	*Salmonella, Shigella, Clostridium jejuni,* invasive *Escherichia coli, Yersinia enterocolitica, Vibrio parahemolyticus*
16–72 hrs	Abdominal cramps, diarrhea	Norwalk agent and related viruses, enterotoxins produced by *Vibrio* sp., *E. coli,* and occasionally *Salmonella, Shigella,* and *C. jejuni*
18–36 hrs	Nausea, vomiting, diarrhea, paralysis	Food-borne botulism
72–100 hrs	Bloody diarrhea without fever	Enterotoxigenic *E. coli,* most frequently serotype O157:H7
1–3 wks	Chronic diarrhea	Raw milk ingestion

Mandell GL, et al (eds): Principles and Practice of Infectious Diseases, 4th ed. New York, Churchill Livingstone, 1995.

NONHEPATITIS LIVER DISEASE

76. List the common causes of jaundice in the pregnant patient.
Viral hepatitis A, B, C, and E (accounts for 50%)
Acute fatty liver of pregnancy
HELLP (hemolysis, elevates liver enzymes, low platelets)
Toxemia (preeclampsia or eclampsia)
Cholestasis of pregnancy
Cholelithiasis/choledocholithiasis
Drug-induced liver disease

77. Describe the two predominant forms of alcoholic liver injury. Which one may progress to cirrhosis?
Mild alcoholism impairs the excretion of triglyceride from hepatocytes, resulting in the typical **fatty liver** with fat globules in parenchymal cells. The fatty liver of alcoholism generally causes hepatomegaly and minimal elevations in aminotransferases. Jaundice is rarely seen unless the disease progresses to severe hepatocellular failure.

The more severe form of alcoholic liver injury is **alcoholic hepatitis,** characterized by focal necrosis of liver cells. Clusters of neutrophils and Mallory bodies (clumps of hyaline) can be seen on liver biopsy. The lesions of alcoholic hepatitis characteristically occur in the center of the lobule and are accompanied by fibrosis. In its severe form, manifestations include marked jaundice and transaminase elevations (up to $10 \times$ normal), which may be accompanied by impaired synthesis of coagulation proteins leading to a prolonged prothrombin time. Typically, in alcoholic hepatitis, unlike viral hepatitis, the AST (SGOT) is greater than the ALT (SGPT) and the AST:ALT ratio is $\geq 2:1$. Alcoholic hepatitis may progress to cirrhosis. Alcohol abuse is the most frequent cause of cirrhosis in the U.S.

78. What are the clinical manifestations of liver disease and their pathogenetic basis?

Clinical Manifestations of Liver Disease

SIGN/SYMPTOM	PATHOGENESIS	LIVER DISEASE
Constitutional		
Fatigue, anorexia, malaise, weight loss	Liver failure	Severe acute or chronic hepatitis Cirrhosis
Fever	Hepatic inflammation or infection	Liver abscess Alcoholic hepatitis Viral hepatitis
Fetor hepaticus	Abnormal methionine metabolism	Acute or chronic liver failure
Cutaneous		
Spider telangiectasias, palmar erythema	Altered estrogen and androgen metabolism	Cirrhosis
Jaundice	Diminished bilirubin excretion	Biliary obstruction Severe liver disease
Pruritus		Biliary obstruction
Xanthomas and xanthelasma	Increased serum lipids	Biliary obstruction/cholestasis
Endocrine		
Gynecomastia, testicular atrophy, diminished libido	Altered estrogen and androgen metabolism	Cirrhosis
Hypoglycemia	Decreased glycogen stores and gluconeogenesis	Liver failure
Gastrointestinal		
RUQ abdominal pain	Liver swelling, infection	Acute hepatitis Hepatocellular carcinoma Liver congestion (heart failure) Acute cholecystitis Liver abscess
Abdominal swelling	Ascites	Cirrhosis, portal hypertension
GI bleeding	Esophageal varices	Portal hypertension
Hematologic		
Decreased RBCs, WBCs, and/or platelets	Hypersplenism	Cirrhosis, portal hypertension
Ecchymoses	Decreased synthesis of clotting factors	Liver failure
Neurologic		
Altered sleep pattern, subtle behavioral changes, somnolence, confusion, ataxia, asterixis, obtundation	Hepatic encephalopathy	Liver failure, portosystemic shunting of blood

From Andreoli TE, et al: Cecil Essentials of Medicine, 2nd ed. Philadelphia, W.B. Saunders, 1990, p 312; with permission.

79. Which drugs have been associated with the development of liver tumors?
Adenoma: oral contraceptives
Angiosarcoma: vinyl chloride, arsenic, Thorotrast, anabolic steroids
Hepatocellular carcinoma: anabolic steroids, estrogens, Thorotrast

80. A patient with known cirrhosis of the liver presents with massive swelling of his abdomen. A fluid wave can be elicited on examination of the abdomen by striking one flank and feeling the transmitted wave on the opposite flank. What is the appropriate diagnostic procedure at this point?

Following the diagnosis of new-onset ascites made on physical examination, all patients should undergo abdominal paracentesis and ascitic fluid analysis. A small amount of fluid is aspirated from the midline of the abdomen between the umbilicus and pubis with a small-gauge needle. The most important tests to order are the albumin and cell count.

The serum albumin value should be measured within a few hours of the paracentesis so as to ensure accuracy. Ascitic fluid with a serum: ascitic fluid albumin gradient (S-A AG) > 1.1 gm/dl is designated as **high-gradient ascites.** Those with values < 1.1 gm/dl are designated as **low-gradient ascites.** Diseases usually associated with high-gradient ascites include portal hypertension (i.e., cirrhosis), congestive heart failure, constrictive pericarditis, inferior vena cava obstruction, hypoalbuminemia, Meigs' syndrome, myxedema, fulminant hepatic failure, nephrotic syndrome (occasionally), and mixed ascites. Low-albumin gradient ascites is commonly seen with peritoneal neoplasms, pancreatic ascites, tuberculosis, nephrotic syndrome, ascites due to bowel obstruction or infarction, and ascites in connective tissue diseases. The terms high-albumin gradient and low-albumin gradient should replace the terms transudative and exudative in the description of ascites.

A large number of RBCs in the fluid or grossly bloody ascites suggests neoplasm. An ascitic fluid and WBC count of >500/ml is strongly suggestive of a peritoneal infection or an inflammatory process. Other tests to be ordered in the appropriate clinical settings include cytologic examination, lactic dehydrogenase, specific tumor markers, glucose, and cultures for bacteria, mycobacteria, and fungi.

Friedman LS, et al: Work-up of the patient with ascites. Hosp Med 31:11, 1995.

81. What are the pathogenetic mechanisms responsible for ascites formation in patients with cirrhosis?

Ascites forms when there is a disturbance in the normal balance between the formation and reabsorption of peritoneal fluid in the direction of net formation. Factors that lead to this in cirrhotic patients are as follows:

1. Increased hydrostatic pressure in the portal circulation due to increased resistance to flow through the cirrhotic liver favors net leakage of fluid into the extravascular space.

2. Increased renal sodium and water retention due to:
   a. Secondary hyperaldosteronism
   b. Increased antidiuretic hormone (ADH) release

3. Impaired hepatic and splanchnic removal of lymphatic fluid due to elevated hepatic sinusoidal pressure.

4. Decreased intravascular oncotic pressure due to decreased hepatic protein (albumin and others) synthesis.

5. Increased plasma vasopressin and epinephrine levels with resultant vasomotor changes.

82. List the treatments available for ascites.

1. Sodium restriction to 22 meq/day (0.5 gms NaCl)
2. Removal by paracentesis
3. Fluid restriction, if dilutional hyponatremia occurs
4. Diuretic agents, used if dietary restriction does not suffice
   a. *Potassium-sparing agents:* spironolactone, triamterene
   b. *Loop diuretics:* furosemide, ethacrynic acid, bumetanide
5. TIPS
6. Peritoneovenous (LeVeen) shunts
7. Extracorporeal ultrafiltration
8. Liver transplantation

Runyon BA: Care of patients with ascites. N Engl J Med 330:337, 1995.

83. How common is drug-induced liver disease?

More than 600 medicines have been reported to cause liver injury. Drug-induced liver disease accounts for 2–5% of hospital admissions for jaundice in the U.S. and 10–20% of cases of fulminant liver failure. Acetaminophen and alcohol are the two most common offending agents.

84. How is acetaminophen toxic to the liver? At what dose?

Acetaminophen is only toxic to the liver when taken in excessive doses or when the protective detoxifying pathway in the liver is overwhelmed. Accumulation of the toxic metabolic, *N*-acetyl-*p*-benzoquinone, is responsible for death of hepatocytes.

Hepatotoxicity of acetaminophen occurs in nonalcoholic patients at doses >7.5 gm. A potentially lethal effect is seen with ingestion of >140 mg/kg (10 gm in a 70-kg man). Chronic alcoholics are at greater risk of acetaminophen injury due to alcohol induction of the cytochrome P450 system and attendant malnutrition and low levels of glutathione. Glutathione is an intracellular protectant naturally found in the hepatocyte. Acetaminophen is the second most common cause of death from poisoning in the United States.

85. What are the indications for liver transplantation?

Advanced cirrhosis	Fulminant hepatic failure
Metabolic liver disease	Cholestatic disorders
Alcoholic liver disease	Hepatic malignancies

86. What are contraindications to liver transplantation?

Systemic septicemia	Extrahepatic malignancy
AIDS	Severe and irreversible extrahepatic organ failure
Ongoing alcoholism	

ESOPHAGEAL DISEASE

87. Describe the approach to treatment of gastroesophageal reflex disease.

Treatment of Gastroesophageal Reflux Disease

1. Dietary and lifestyle changes (Phase I)
   a. Postural therapy
   Elevate head of bed 6–8 inches
   Avoid lying down after eating; remain upright >2 hrs.
   b. Limit intake of foods and drink that reduce lower esophageal sphincter (LES) pressure:

Fatty foods	Peppermint
Acidic foods	Caffeine
Onions	Alcohol
Chocolate	

   c. Avoid medications that reduce LES pressure:

Theophylline	Calcium channel blockers
Nitrates	Anticholinergic agents
Tranquilizers	β-Adrenergic agonists
Progesterone	

   d. Stop smoking
   e. Decrease the size of meals
   f. Weight reduction if obese
   g. Avoid tight-fitting garments around abdomen
2. Medications (Phase II)
   a. Antacids and coating agents: Postprandial antacids and sucralfate increase the pH of gastric contents and promote healing.
   b. Antisecretory agents (H_2 antagonists)
   c. Promotility agents: Increase LES pressure and promote esophageal and gastric emptying. (Cisapride is the drug of choice and has nearly replaced the use of metoclopramide and bethanechol.)
   d. Proton pump inhibitors: The most potent single agent for treating severe reflux esophagitis; these agents (omeprazole or lansoprazole) act to increase the pH of gastric contents and heal esophagitis.
3. Surgery (Phase III)
   a. Procedures aimed to restore LES competence or prevent reflux

Richter J: Severe reflux esophagitis. Gastrointest Endosc Clin North Am 4:677, 1994.

88. Name the three types of esophageal dysphagia. How can a patient's history be used to distinguish between them?

True esophageal dysphagia may be classified into one of three categories:

1. **Transfer**—pathologic alteration in the neuromotor mechanism of the oropharyngeal phase. Patients give a history of difficulty swallowing liquids, while solids pass normally. These are patients having stroke, myasthenia gravis, amyotrophic lateral sclerosis, and botulism.

2. **Transit**—abnormal peristalsis and LES function. Transit dysphagia is due to **motor disorders** in which the primary peristaltic pump of the esophagus fails. Motor disorders often begin with dysphagia to both solids and liquids. This is commonly seen in such entities as achalasia and scleroderma. Dysphagia that worsens upon ingesting cold liquids and improves with warm liquids suggests a motor disorder.

3. **Obstructive**—mechanical narrowing of the esophagus. Obstructive dysphagia may be due to intrinsic lesions blocking the esophagus (e.g., peptic strictures, esophageal webs, carcinoma) or to extrinsic lesions (e.g., mediastinal tumors) compressing the esophagus. This typically presents as dysphagia to solid food that may progress to include liquids. Patients usually give a history of eating only soft foods, chewing foods longer, and avoiding steak, apples, and fresh bread. Solid-food dysphagia associated with a long history of heartburn and regurgitation suggests a peptic stricture. If the bolus can be dislodged by repeated swallowing or drinking water, a motor disorder is usually the cause.

After a thorough history and physical examination, the initial diagnostic step is a barium swallow.

Boyce HW: Clinical update: Dysphagia. ASGE 1:1, 1993.

89. What is achalasia?

Achalasia is the best-known motor disorder of the esophagus. Its usual onset is in patients aged 25–60 years, with an equal frequency between the sexes. Its symptoms include dysphagia (solids and liquids), regurgitation of undigested foods, heartburn, and chest pain. The diagnosis can be made by esophageal manometry, which yields the following characteristic findings:

• Loss of peristalsis (*absolute* requirement)
• Failure of the LES to relax
• Increased LES pressure

90. What is the most frequent form of infectious esophagitis? How does it present?

The most frequent form of infectious esophagitis is **candidal esophagitis.** Most fungal infections occur in immunocompromised patients, especially those with AIDS, but they are also seen in patients with less obvious immune defects (e.g., diabetics, malnourished elderly, alcoholics, patients on antibiotics or steroids). The symptoms include painful swallowing (odynophagia), retrosternal pain, dysphagia, fever, and bleeding. Physical examination may reveal oral thrush.

Sutton FM, et al: Infectious esophagitis. Gastrointest Endosc Clin North Am 4:713, 1994.

91. Which drugs are commonly implicated as causes of pill-induced esophagitis?

Doxycycline	Tetracycline	Slow-release KCl
Ascorbic acid	Quinidine	Aspirin
NSAIDs	Emepronium bromide	Ferrous sulfate

92. How are 24-hour pH monitoring, esophageal manometry, endoscopy, and an acid perfusion test used to assess patients with suspected esophageal disease?

24-Hour ambulatory pH monitoring of the esophagus provides a temporal profile of acid reflux events and acid clearance and correlates these events with symptoms. Specific variables measured include the number of reflux episodes in 24 hours, acid clearance times from the esophagus, and esophageal exposure to acid. These values can be determined while the patient is in the upright or recumbent position.

Esophageal manometry is useful in evaluating patients with noncardiac chest pain and a history suggestive of esophageal motor disorder, achalasia, or esophageal reflux disease.

Endoscopy provides a direct view of the esophageal mucosa and allows directed biopsy when necessary. Endoscopy and biopsy are necessary to make a definitive diagnosis of many esophageal diseases.

The **acid-perfusion** or **Bernstein test** is useful for determining if chest pain is of esophageal origin. In this test, 0.1 N HCl is infused into the distal esophagus at a rate of about 1 ml/min using saline infusion as a control. There appears to be a good correlation between esophagitis symptoms and provocation of heartburn by the esophageal acid infusion test.

Chobanian SJ, et al: Systematic esophageal evaluation of patients with noncardiac chest pain. Arch Intern Med 146:1505, 1986.

93. What is Barrett's esophagus? How should patients with this entity be managed?

Barrett's esophagus is a complication that develops in patients with longstanding reflux peptic esophagitis. It represents a unique reparative process in which the original squamous epithelial cell lining of the esophagus is replaced by a metaplastic columnar-type epithelium. In most adults, this epithelium resembles intestinal mucosa, complete with goblet cells. When the lower esophagus is lined by this columnar-type epithelium, it is termed Barrett's esophagus.

Its clinical significance lies primarily in its malignant potential. There is an increased risk (30–125× above the general population) of esophageal adenocarcinoma arising in the Barrett's epithelium. The actual incidence is unknown, but the average is about 10%.

The management of Barrett's esophagus is the same as the treatment of gastroesophageal reflux disease. Acid suppression with H_2-receptor antagonists or proton pump inhibitors in high doses controls symptoms and heals esophageal damage. Although the inflammatory changes associated with Barrett's epithelium can be healed, once Barrett's epithelium has developed, the process cannot be reversed by any form of antireflux therapy. Early studies appear to indicate that laser ablation of the Barrett's mucosa may result in complete regression of the abnormal mucosa with restoration of squamous epithelium, but more trials need to be performed.

94. Is routine surveillance for esophageal cancer necessary in patients with Barrett's esophagus?

The benefits of periodic endoscopic screening for dysplasia have not been shown. Yearly endoscopic surveillance and four-quadrant biopsies of each 2-cm segment of the esophagus are advocated by many. Only those patients who would be surgical candidates if dysplasia or carcinoma was detected should undergo surveillance.

Castell DO, et al: Barrett's esophagus: A continuing dilemma. Pract Gastroenterol 11:22B, 1995.

MALABSORPTION

95. What is the cause of Whipple's disease?

Whipple's disease is a systemic disease that may affect almost any organ system of the body, but in most cases, it involves the small intestine. The causative agent is the bacterium *Tropheryma whippelii*. Patients present with intestinal malabsorption, weight loss, diarrhea, abdominal pain, fever, anemia, lymphadenopathy, and arthralgias. Nervous system symptoms, pericarditis, or endocarditis may also be present.

The pathologic feature is infiltration of involved tissues with large glycoprotein-containing macrophages that stain strongly positive with a periodic acid–Schiff stain. This diagnosis is most often made by biopsy of the small intestine. One can also see characteristic rod-shaped, gram-positive bacilli that are not acid-fast.

96. How is Whipple's disease treated?

Effective treatment includes prolonged antibiotic therapy, usually with double-strength trimethoprim/sulfamethoxazole given for a minimum of 1 year. Repeat intestinal biopsy should document the disappearance of the Whipple bacillus before therapy is discontinued. Relapses are not uncommon and are treated for a minimum of 6–12 months. Patients allergic to sulfonamides should receive parenteral penicillin.

97. In a small-bowel biopsy, the mucosa shows flat villa with markedly hyperplastic crypts. What is this disease?

Celiac sprue, also called gluten enteropathy, is an allergic disease characterized by malabsorption of nutrients secondary to the damaged small intestinal mucosa. The responsible antigen is gluten, a water-insoluble protein found in cereal grains such as wheat, barley, oats, and rye. Withdrawal of gluten from the diet results in complete remission of both the clinical symptoms and mucosal lesions. Although this disease is present worldwide, the distribution varies; the highest prevalence is in western Ireland.

98. What is dermatitis herpetiformis? How does this disease relate to celiac sprue?

Dermatitis herpetiformis is a pruritic skin condition that also may be reversed with dietary therapy (gluten restriction). It is characterized by papulovesicular lesions in a symmetrical distribution on the elbows, knees, buttocks, face, scalp, neck, and trunk. Although most patients with celiac sprue do not develop skin lesions of dermatitis herpetiformis, patients with dermatitis herpetiformis usually have the sprue-like mucosal lesion in the small bowel. The two diseases appear to be distinct entities that respond to the same dietary restrictions. Unlike the intestinal disease, the skin lesions can be treated with the antibiotic dapsone, with a clinical response within 1–2 weeks.

99. What is the blind-loop syndrome?

The blind-loop syndrome is a constellation of symptoms and laboratory abnormalities that include malabsorption of B_{12}, steatorrhea, hypoproteinemia, weight loss, and diarrhea. These symptoms are attributed to overgrowth of bacteria within the small intestine and have been associated with a number of diseases and surgical abnormalities. The common link between these conditions is abnormal motility of a segment of small intestine, resulting in stasis. The aim of therapy is to reduce the bacterial overgrowth and consists of antibiotics and, when feasible, correction of the small intestinal abnormality that led to the condition.

100. Describe the pathophysiologic mechanisms that can lead to fat malabsorption.

Normal fat absorption requires all phases of digestion to be intact. The process begins with secretion of pancreatic lipase and colipase. These enzymes are activated intraluminally and require an optimal pH of 6–8. Both enzymes are necessary for triglyceride hydrolysis in the duodenum. Any disorder that causes deficiencies of pancreatic enzyme secretion or leads to an acidic intraluminal environment could lead to fat malabsorption.

The products of triglyceride hydrolysis, i.e., fatty acids and monoglycerides, then must be solubilized by bile salts to form micelles, which are subsequently absorbed by the small intestinal epithelium. Any disorder that interrupts the enterohepatic circulation or secretion of bile salts may impair micelle formation and therefore result in fat malabsorption.

If the intestinal epithelial cell is in some way diseased, monoglyceride absorption and processing into chylomicrons for transport out of the small intestine may be impaired, leading to fat malabsorption. Disease of the intestinal lymphatics with impaired chylomicron transport has also been reported to result in fat malabsorption.

101. Which diseases can affect fat absorption?
- Chronic pancreatitis
- Cystic fibrosis
- Pancreatic carcinoma
- Postgastrectomy syndrome
- Biliary tract obstruction
- Terminal ileal resection or disease
- Cholestatic liver disease
- Intestinal epithelial disease, such as Whipple's disease, sprue, eosinophilic gastroenteritis
- Lymphatic disease, such as abetalipoproteinemia, intestinal lymphangiectasia, lymphoma, and tuberculous adenitis

- Small bowel bacterial overgrowth (bile salts are deconjugated and inactivated by bacteria)
- Zollinger-Ellison syndrome (low intraluminal pH)

Weber SA: Malabsorption: An overview. In Lindner AE (ed): Mediguide to Gastrointestinal Disease. Philadelphia, American Society of GI Endoscopy 6:1, 1995.

102. Which conditions are associated with or may result in small bowel bacteria overgrowth?

Any abnormality of the small intestine that results in local stasis or recirculation of intestinal contents is likely to be associated with marked proliferation of intraluminal bacteria. The gold standard for diagnosing bacterial overgrowth is culture of the upper small bowel of $>100,000$ cfu/ml. Associated disorders include:

1. Gastric proliferation of bacteria as seen in hypochlorhydric or achlorhydric states, particularly when these are combined with motor or anatomic disturbances.

2. Small intestinal stagnation associated with anatomic alterations following surgery, such as afferent loop syndrome after a Billroth II procedure.

3. Duodenal and jejunal diverticulosis, particularly as seen in scleroderma.

4. Surgically created blind loops, such as end-to-side anastomoses.

5. Chronic low-grade obstruction secondary to small intestinal strictures, adhesions, inflammation, or carcinoma.

6. Motor disturbances of the small intestine, such as scleroderma, idiopathic pseudo-obstruction, or diabetic neuropathy.

7. Abnormal communication between the proximal small intestine and the distal intestinal tract, as seen in gastrocolic or jejunocolic fistulas or resection of the ileocecal valve.

8. Immunodeficiency syndromes such as AIDS, primary immunodeficiency states, and malnutrition.

103. How does bacterial overgrowth of the small bowel result in fat malabsorption?

The bacterial enzymes deconjugate intraluminal bile salts to free bile acids, which are unable to solubilize monoglycerides and free fatty acids into micelles for absorption by the epithelial cells. The result is impaired absorption of fat and fat-soluble vitamins.

104. What constitutes a normal fecal fat concentration? What is steatorrhea and how is it detected?

The typical U.S. diet consists of 100–150 gm of fat per day. Fat absorption is extremely efficient, and most of the ingested fat is absorbed with very little excretion into the stool. The average fecal fat concentration for the normal individual is 4–6 gm/day, ranging to an upper limit of normal of approx. 7 gm. Patients with steatorrhea, or increased excretion of fecal fat, may have up to 10 times this amount in the stool.

In order to detect steatorrhea, a 72-hour stool sample is collected while the patient is on a defined dietary fat intake of ≥ 100 gm/day. Chemical analysis of the stool collection measures the amount of fat present. This test is highly reliable but neither specific nor sensitive in determining the etiology of steatorrhea.

Weber SA: Malabsorption: an overview. In Lindner AE (ed): Mediguide to Gastrointestinal Disease. 6:1, 1995.

105. Describe the four stages of a Schilling test. What mechanisms of absorption does each stage test for?

The standard Schilling test measures vitamin B_{12} absorption and is used to detect intrinsic factor deficiency in patients with pernicious anemia. The test results are often abnormal in patients with genetic defects in vitamin B_{12} absorption; in bacterial overgrowth of the small bowel; following extensive destruction, resection, or bypass of the terminal ileum; and in pancreatic insufficiency.

Stage 1: An oral dose of radiolabeled vitamin B_{12} is given simultaneously with an IM injection of 1 mg of nonradiolabeled B_{12}. The urine is collected for 24 hours, and the amount of radioactivity is measured. Patients with normal absorption of B_{12} and normal renal function will excrete >7% of the radiolabeled B_{12} in 24 hours.

Stage 2: If the results of stage 1 are abnormal, the test is repeated following oral administration of 60 mg of intrinsic factor. If the level of urinary radiolabeled B_{12} normalizes, it indicates pernicious anemia.

Stage 3: Small intestinal bacterial overgrowth may cause B_{12} malabsorption and an abnormal result in stage 1 of the Schilling test, which is not corrected with intrinsic factor in stage 2. A Broad-spectrum antibiotic is administered for 1 week to eliminate the intestinal bacteria, after which stage 1 of the Schilling test should normalize.

Stage 4: If pancreatic insufficiency exists, B_{12} malabsorption may occur. Normalization of B_{12} absorption after administration of pancreatic enzyme therapy suggests a pancreatic origin of B_{12} malabsorption.

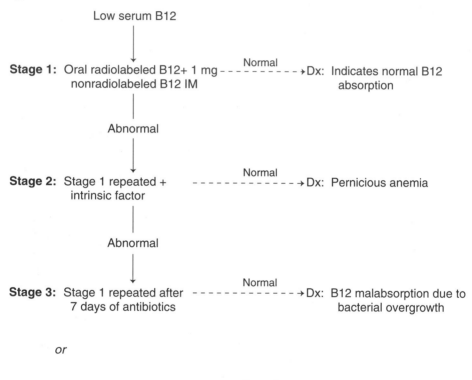

Schilling test for determining the etiology of vitamin B_{12} deficiency. Stage 3 and 4 is done based on clinical suspicion of the etiology.

OBSTRUCTION

106. Name the four most common causes of mechanical small bowel obstruction (SBO) in adults.
1. Adhesions (approx. 74%)
2. Hernias (8%)
3. Malignancies of the small bowel (8%)
4. Inflammatory bowel disease with stricture formation

107. What historical and physical clues may help to determine the location of the obstruction in SBO?

The patient with mechanical SBO typically presents with crampy, intermittent abdominal pain occurring in paroxysms, 4–5 minutes apart. **Proximal obstruction** presents in a more acute fashion, with vomiting as a prominent complaint. The vomiting is typically bilious and nonfeculent, and pain occurs at short-spaced intervals. Abdominal distention may be minimal or absent if the location is high in the small bowel.

Distal obstruction may have a more insidious onset of symptoms. Vomiting is often present but is a less prominent complaint. When present, the vomiting is often feculent. Pain occurs at longer-spaced intervals compared with that seen in proximal SBO. The lower the blockage, the more likely there is to be abdominal distention resulting from accumulation of fluid and gas in the intestine.

108. What findings on the plain film x-ray suggest an SBO?

Plain abdominal x-rays in SBO usually reveal abnormally large quantities of gas in the bowel. This gas can be identified as small intestinal gas by the presence of the valvulae conniventes, which usually occupy the entire transverse diameter of the small bowel. This feature can be distinguished from colonic haustral markings, which occupy only a portion of the diameter of the bowel. Additionally, loops of small bowel are most commonly located in the more central portion of the abdomen, whereas colonic gas is usually seen in the periphery of the x-ray film. In the patient with classic mechanical SBO, there is minimal or no colonic gas. The upright or decubitus abdominal film will reveal multiple air-fluid levels with distended loops of small bowel resembling inverted U's.

109. Is surgery always necessary in a patient with SBO?

In most circumstances, the best therapy for mechanical SBO is surgical correction of the obstruction. The timing of the operation depends on the following three factors: (1) the duration of obstruction and the severity of fluid, electrolyte, and acid-base abnormalities; (2) the improvement of vital organ function (i.e., management of concomitant cardiac and pulmonary disorders); and (3) the risk of strangulation. Because the mortality rate of SBO associated with strangulation is high, operative intervention should be performed early in the course.

However, in certain patients, a short trial of conservative, nonoperative management can be tried. These patients include those in the immediate postoperative period, who may respond to simple nasogastric (NG) suction. Similarly, patients with obstruction caused by disseminated intra-abdominal carcinomatosis, Crohn's disease, radiation strictures, or adhesions following previous surgery may improve with simple management and NG suction. If conservative medical therapy is used, the patient should show continuous improvement during the first 12–24 hours of therapy. If not, surgical relief of the obstruction should be performed.

110. What seven entities may cause small bowel ileus?

Paralytic ileus is a relatively common disorder and occurs when neural, humoral, and metabolic factors combine to stimulate reflexes that inhibit intestinal motility. The result is small bowel and/or colonic distention due to intestinal muscle paralysis. The seven common causes of paralytic ileus are:

1. Abdominal surgery
2. Peritonitis
3. Generalized sepsis
4. Electrolyte imbalance (esp. hypokalemia)
5. Retroperitoneal hemorrhage
6. Spinal fractures
7. Pelvic fractures.

Drugs such as phenothiazines and narcotics inhibit small bowel motility and also may contribute to paralysis. Treatment consists of NG suction to relieve distention and IV fluids to replace losses, followed by correction of the underlying disorder.

111. What conditions may aggravate or be associated with colonic pseudo-obstruction?

Conditions Associated with Colonic Pseudo-obstruction

1. Trauma (nonoperative) and surgery (gynecologic, orthopedic, urologic)
2. Inflammatory processes (pancreatitis, cholecystitis)
3. Infections
4. Malignancy
5. Radiation therapy
6. Drugs (narcotics, antidepressants, clonidine, anticholinergics)
7. Cardiovascular disease
8. Neurologic disease
9. Respiratory failure
10. Metabolic disease (diabetes, hypothyroidism, electrolyte imbalance, uremia)
11. Alcoholism

112. Name the most common cause of gastric outlet obstruction.
Peptic ulcer disease.

113. In what clinical setting are bezoars likely to be seen?
Bezoars are clusters of food or foreign matter that have undergone partial digestion in the stomach, failed to pass through the pylorus into the small bowel, and formed a mass in the stomach. Substances typically comprising bezoars include hair (trichobezoars) and, more commonly, plant matter (phytobezoars). Bezoars may become quite large and can present with abdominal mass, gastric outlet obstruction, attacks of nausea and vomiting, and peptic ulceration. Factors important in the formation of bezoars include the amount of indigestible materials in the diet (pulpy, fibrous fruit or vegetables such as oranges), the quality of the chewing mechanism, and loss of pyloric function, which limits the size of food particles that may enter the duodenum.

Saeed ZA, et al: A method for the endoscopic retrieval of trichobezoars. Gastrointest Endosc 39:698, 1993.

BILIARY TRACT DISEASE

114. How prevalent is asymptomatic cholelithiasis in adult Americans over age 40? How many will ultimately develop symptoms?
40% of Americans over age 40 have gallstones, and 10–30% of these will become symptomatic at some point.

115. Is surgery indicated for asymptomatic cholelithiasis?
Elective surgery is generally not indicated. It has been previously recommended that elective cholecystectomy be performed in diabetic patients with asymptomatic cholelithiasis, but there is evidence that they have a higher complication rate from elective cholecystectomy.

116. Which U.S. ethnic groups have the highest prevalence of cholesterol gallstone formation?
American Indians and Mexican-Americans.

117. What percentage of gallstones are radiopaque?
Pigment gallstones, which account for 20–30% of gallstones in the U.S., are often radiopaque and can be seen on plain radiographs of the abdomen. Cholesterol gallstones, which account for 70–80%, are radiolucent.

118. Describe the therapeutic approach to the patient with cholangitis who has previously undergone cholecystectomy.
Bacterial cholangitis is a life-threatening illness that requires urgent intervention with immediate drainage of the common bile duct and relief of the obstruction. Treatment can be performed via endoscopic retrograde cholangiopancreatography (ERCP) or by percutaneous transhepatic cholangiogram (PTC). The advantages of ERCP include the ability to treat the primary disease process utilizing sphincterotomy, with removal of common bile duct stones or placement

of an internal drain, and avoiding the morbidity associated with percutaneous external drainage. Nonoperative therapy utilizing ERCP and endoscopic drainage in the patient with cholangitis has a mortality rate of only 1–2%, in contrast to emergency surgery in this setting which has a mortality rate as high as 40%. Elective surgery can be done later, if needed, and is associated with a lower mortality than in the acute situation.

119. What is Charcot's triad?

Right-upper-quadrant pain, jaundice, and fever. This triad is present in 70% of patients with bacterial cholangitis.

120. In the initial diagnostic evaluation of a patient with suspected obstructive jaundice, which diagnostic tests are available and how do they compare?

The cause of jaundice can be determined in many cases from clinical data and routine laboratory tests. The only special study that is routinely useful in the early evaluation of obstructive jaundice is an **ultrasound scan** of the gallbladder, bile ducts, and liver. Ultrasound is fairly specific for detecting gallstones and ductal dilatation (the latter signifying ductal obstruction). However, a negative scan does not prove the absence of stones or obstruction, since the sensitivity of ultrasound in detecting obstruction is only about 90%.

Abdominal CT is fairly sensitive for detecting ductal dilatation and can be useful in localizing the site of ductal obstruction. A CT scan is less able to detect stones of the gallbladder and common bile duct than ultrasound, but it is better able to image mass lesions and to evaluate the pancreas.

Liver biopsy in the patient with extrahepatic ductal obstruction is not routinely useful. It may reveal evidence of cholestasis and cholangitis but will not help to determine the cause. A **liver scan** using technetium sulfur colloid is of very little value in the jaundiced patient.

Magnetic resonance imaging (MRI) and **magnetic retrograde cholangiopancreatiography** (MRCP) are two new techniques which are fast becoming more useful as diagnostic tools in the evaluation of these patients.

Richter JM, et al. Suspected obstructive jaundice: A decision analysis of diagnostic strategies. Ann Intern Med 99:46, 1983.

121. If the bile ducts are dilated on the ultrasound or CT scan, what is the next step?

The next step should include an evaluation to determine the cause of the obstruction and an attempt to relieve the obstruction and provide drainage. The two modalities that can achieve these ends are endoscopic retrograde cholangiopancreatography (ERCP) and percutaneous transhepatic cholangiogram (PTC).

ERCP is a relatively simple procedure if a trained endoscopist is available. The common bile duct is cannulated endoscopically and dye is injected, yielding a cholangiogram. If bile duct stones, biliary stricture, or an obstructive lesion is seen, a variety of therapeutic maneuvers can be performed during ERCP, including sphincterotomy with stone removal, dilatation of the stricture, or placement of a biliary stent or nasobiliary catheter.

PTC offers similar advantages, but it adds the additional morbidity and discomfort of percutaneous needlestick and the possibility of external biliary drainage following a procedure. The overall risk of both procedures is fairly low and they compare favorably in their effectiveness.

BIBLIOGRAPHY

1. Barkin JS, O'Phelan CA (eds): Advanced Therapeutic Endoscopy, 2nd ed. New York, Raven Press, 1994.
2. Fenoglio-Preiser CM, et al: Gastrointestinal Pathology: An Atlas and Text. New York, Raven Press, 1989.
3. McNally PR (ed): GI/Liver Secrets. Philadelphia, Hanley & Belfus, 1996.
4. Schiff L, Schiff ER (eds): Diseases of the Liver, 7th ed. Philadelphia, J.B. Lippincott, 1993.
5. Sleisenger MH, Fordtran JS (eds): Gastrointestinal Disease: Pathophysiology, Diagnosis, and Management, 5th ed. Philadelphia, W.B. Saunders, 1993.
6. Spiro HM (ed): Clinical Gastroenterology, 4th ed. New York, McGraw-Hill, 1993.
7. Yamada T (ed): Textbook of Gastroenterology, 2nd ed. Philadelphia, J.B. Lippincott, 1995.
8. Zakim D, Boyer TD (eds): Hepatology: A Textbook of Liver Disease, 3rd ed. Philadelphia, W.B. Saunders, 1996.

6. ONCOLOGY

Mary Anne Doherty, M.D., and Teresa G. Hayes, M.D., Ph.D.

A story circulated at a medical meeting about a man who had decided
gradually to give up everything that scientists have linked to cancer.
The first week he cut out smoked fish and charcoal steaks.
The second week, he cut out smoking.
The third week, he cut out having relations with women.
The fourth week, he cut out drinking.
The fifth week, he cut out paper dolls.

Anonymous
Quoted in the Boston Herald, 9/4/65

GENERAL ISSUES

1. How is carcinogenesis defined?

Carcinogenesis is the alteration of normal cells into malignant cells. It is almost always a multistage evolution of genetic and epigenetic alterations that eventuates in cells that escape the normal growth constraints of the host.

2. What are the known genetically related mechanisms of neoplasia?

Four broad categories of genes can influence the origin and progression of neoplasia:

1. **Oncogenes:** These are genes in humans and other animals that have the capacity to transform normal cells into malignant ones. These genes, acquired at conception or mutated during life, make the patient susceptible to cancer by altering or impairing several processes:

    a. Production of nuclear transcription factors that control cell growth (e.g., *myc*).

    b. Signal transduction within cells (e.g., *ras*).

    c. Interaction of growth factors and their receptors (e.g., *her/neu*).

Almost 100 different oncogenes have been identified, but only some have been associated with human cancers exclusively. Mutations convert proto-oncogenes to oncogenes by amplification, translocation, and point mutation.

2. **Tumor-suppressor genes:** Mutations of these genes must occur in both alleles to cause loss of function and so effect tumor growth. Eight to 10 tumor-suppressor genes have been identified (e.g., *p53* and *RB*), and these are found in many types of cancers. These mutations are the basis of the inherited predispositions to cancers and are inherited in the heterozygous state.

3. **Regulators of cell death:** The cell death genes are involved in the programmed death (**apoptosis**) of cells no longer needed by the body. Mutation in one of these genes (e.g., *bcl*-2) allows cells to live that should have died, causing excess accumulation of cells. Activation of the **telomerase** gene, which controls cell senescence, is thought to cause cells to become immortal by turning off the normal aging process.

4. **Mutator genes:** These are responsible for ensuring the fidelity of the DNA duplication process. When the gene products subsequently fail to function, the mutation rate increases and inherited predispositions to cancers are observed. The tumor suppressor genes and oncogenes are thought to be the target of the faulty DNA editing process.

3. Besides genetic factors, what are some environmental "causes" of cancer?

155

Examples of Carcinogens

Inherited genetic defects—Retinoblastoma, numerous "familial" cancer syndromes
Social agents—Tobacco, alcohol
Occupational exposures—Arsenic, benzenes, CCl_4, chromium, combustion byproducts (engine exhaust), polycyclic hydrocarbons (coal byproducts)
Ionizing radiation—UV-B (sunlight), mining, others
Dietary factors—Aflatoxin B, high-fat diet, nitrates/nitrites (converted endogenously to nitrosamines), smoked foods
Foreign body reactants—Asbestos fiber
Chronic inflammation—Ulcerative colitis
Infectious agents—Epstein-Barr virus, hepatitis B virus, human papillomavirus, human T-lymphotrophic virus
Iatrogenic agents—Cancer chemotherapeutic drugs, DES, estrogens, Thorotrast

4. Are there "protective" factors?

- Some dietary factors, such as a high-fiber diet, are theorized to reduce the risk for large bowel cancer. This may occur by increasing the bulk of the stool, thereby diluting the contents of the colon and promoting rapid emptying.
- Diets high in antioxidants, including many fruits and vegetables (such as broccoli), are felt to protect against cancer development by scavenging for free radicals.
- Some vitamins may modify the effect of chemical carcinogenesis: vitamin A (which promotes the differentiation of epithelial tissues), vitamin C (which blocks the formation of *n*-nitrosocarcinogens from nitrite and secondary amines), and vitamin E (which is a free-radical scavenger).

5. Which cancers tend to cluster in families?

The common cancers—breast, endometrial, colon, prostate, lung, melanoma, and stomach—have a 2–3 times increased risk of development in first-degree relatives. This may be due to hereditary factors, shared exposures to environmental carcinogens, chance associations, or a combination of all three.

- The familial clustering of **breast cancer** may be due, in about 5% of cases, to a genetic locus (17q, BRCA1) that is predictive of familial breast and ovarian cancer.
- In the **Lynch syndrome,** cancer family adenocarcinomatosis, there is an autosomal dominant pattern of predisposition to non-polyposis colorectal cancer as well as an increased incidence of other cancers, including endometrial, ovarian, breast, stomach, small intestine, pancreatic, urinary tract, and biliary tract.
- The **Li-Fraumeni syndrome** is a familial cancer syndrome with an autosomal dominant pattern of inheritance in which there is a variety of mesenchymal and epithelial tumors and multiple primary neoplasms in children and young adults. The gene for this cancer is located on the short arm of chromosome 17.
- Multiple endocrine neoplasia **(MEN) type 1,** associated with a gene on chromosome 11, causes parathyroid, pituitary, and islet cell tumors.
- **MEN type 2** has two phenotypes: medullary thyroid carcinoma, pheochromocytoma, and parathyroid hyperplasia are seen in the A type, and medullary thyroid carcinoma, pheochromocytoma, marfanoid habitus, and mucosal neuromas occur in type B. The gene for MEN2A is on chromosome 10.

6. How are tumor markers used in diagnosing and monitoring cancer?

Tumor markers include enzymes, hormones, gene loci, and oncofetal antigens that are associated with particular tumors. The markers reflect the presence of the tumor or the quantity of the tumor (tumor burden). Many cancers do not produce markers, and those tumors known to produce markers may sometimes fail to do so, particularly if they are very poorly differentiated. Some markers, such as prostate-specific antigen (PSA) and alpha-fetoprotein (AFP), are highly sensitive, highly specific, and of high predictive value. Others, such as lactic dehydrogenase (LDH) or carcinoembryonic antigen (CEA), are nonspecific and elevated in many conditions besides malignancies; the most important use of these markers is in following the effects of therapy on tumor burden and in detecting recurrence of disease after initial therapy.

Tumor Markers Specific for Individual Cancers

TUMOR MARKER	TYPE OF MALIGNANCY
AFP	Hepatocellular carcinoma, nonseminomatous germ cell tumors, GI tumors
HCG	Gestational trophoblastic tumors, germ cell tumors, pancreatic islet cell tumors, lung cancer
CA 19-9	Pancreatic adenocarcinoma, colorectal carcinoma, gastric adenocarcinoma, mucinous ovarian carcinoma
CA-125	Ovarian carcinoma, endometrial carcinoma, hepatocellular carcinoma, lung and pancreatic cancer
CEA	Breast cancer, colorectal carcinoma, gastric adenocarcinoma, lung cancer, medullary thyroid carcinoma, pancreatic adenocarcinoma
PSA	Prostate adenocarcinoma
Thyroglobulin	Papillary/follicular thyroid carcinoma

From Zollo AJ Jr: The Portable Internist. Philadelphia, Hanley & Belfus, 1995, p 106; with permission.

7. Which are the four most common tumor markers? How are they used?

1. **Carcinoembryonic antigen (CEA).** CEA is a glycoprotein of 200,000 daltons that is found in GI mucosal cells and pancreatobiliary secretions. Elevations occur with breaks in the mucosal basement membrane by a tumor but can also occur in smokers and with cirrhosis, pancreatitis, inflammatory bowel disease, and rectal polyps. CEA is most useful in monitoring disease activity in recurrent colorectal cancer.

2. **Prostate-specific antigen (PSA).** PSA is a serine protease found only in the prostate, whose normal function is liquefaction of seminal gel. The serum level of PSA may be elevated in any type of prostate disease, including benign prostatic hypertrophy, prostatitis, and prostate cancer. However, high levels of PSA, especially in patients with small-volume prostates, are a strong indicator of probable prostate cancer.

3. **Alpha-fetoprotein (AFP).** AFP is an α-globulin of 70,000 daltons that is made by the yolk sac and liver of the human fetus. It is elevated in hepatomas and certain germ cell neoplasms and has been found to be a very sensitive marker for disease activity. Although AFP is rather nonspecific and can be elevated in acute viral and chronic hepatitis, very high levels correlate with the presence of these malignancies.

4. **Human chorionic gonadotropin (HCG).** HCG is a glycoprotein normally secreted by the trophoblastic epithelium of the placenta. It is used as a sensitive and specific marker for germ cell tumors of the testes and ovary and extragonadal presentations of these tumors.

8. List the principles used in formulating combination chemotherapy regimens.

Principles of Combination Chemotherapy

1. Drugs used should have activity against the tumor.
2. Drugs should be selected with dissimilar toxicities.
3. Drugs with different mechanisms of action should be used.
4. Several cycles of therapy, with adequate biological effect, should be used before determining efficacy.
5. Recovery time of normal tissues should be allowed before starting the next cycle.

9. What are the mechanisms of drug resistance to chemotherapeutic agents?

Mechanisms of Drug Resistance in Chemotherapy

1. Intrinsic cytokinetic or biochemical resistance
2. Impaired transport of the drug into the cell or active extrusion from the cell
3. Altered drug affinity for the target enzyme
4. Amplification of genes
5. Membrane alterations from overproduction of high-weight glycoproteins

10. What are the toxic effects of chemotherapy?

The most common immediate effects are nausea and vomiting, which vary in presence and degree with the type of drug. Some, such as cisplatin, are very emetogenic, whereas others, like methotrexate, are unlikely to cause emesis.

The most dangerous adverse effect is myelosuppression. Leukopenia predisposes to acute and serious infections; thrombocytopenia predisposes to bleeding; and anemia may worsen other problems, such as chronic obstructive pulmonary disease and atherosclerotic cardiovascular disease.

Toxicities of Chemotherapeutic Agents

DRUG	ACUTE TOXICITY	DELAYED TOXICITY
Bleomycin (Blenoxane)	Nausea/vomiting, fever, hypersensitivity reactions	**Pneumonitis/pulmonary fibrosis,**[*] rash and hyperpigmentation, stomatitis, alopecia, Raynaud's, cavitating granulomas
Carboplatin (Paraplatin)	Nausea/vomiting	**Myelosuppression,**[*] peripheral neuropathy (uncommon), hearing loss, hemolytic anemia, transient cortical blindness
Chlorambucil (Leukeran)	Seizures, nausea/vomiting	**Myelosuppression,**[*] pulmonary infilgrates and fibrosis, leukemia, hepatic toxicity, sterility
Cisplatin (Platinol)	Nausea/vomiting, anaphylactic reaction	**Renal damage,**[*] ototoxicity, myelosuppression, hemolysis, $\downarrow$Mg$^+$/Ca^{2+}/K$^+$, peripheral neuropathy, Raynaud's, sterility
Cyclophosphamide (Cytoxan)	Nausea/vomiting, anaphylaxis, facial burning with IV administration, visual blurring	**Myelosuppression,**[*] alopecia, hemorrhagic cystitis, sterility, lung infiltrates/fibrosis, $\downarrow$Na$^+$, leukemia, bladder cancer, SIADH
Cytarabine (ara-C)	Nausea/vomiting, diarrhea, anaphylaxis	**Myelosuppression,**[*] oral ulceration, conjunctivitis, hepatic damage, fever, pulmonary edema, neurotoxicity (high dose), rhabdomyolysis, pancreatitis with asparaginase
Dacarbazine (DTIC)	Nausea/vomiting, diarrhea, anaphylaxis, pain or administration	**Myelosuppression,**[*] cardiotoxicity,[*] alopecia, flulike syndrome, renal impairment, hepatic necrosis, facial flushing, paresthesias, photosensitivity, urticarial rash
Daunorubicin (Cerubidine)	Nausea/vomiting, diarrhea, red urine, severe local tissue necrosis on extravasation, transient ECG changes, anaphylactoid reaction	**Myelosuppression,**[*] cardiotoxicity,[*] alopecia, stomatitis, anorexia, diarrhea, fever and chills, dermatitis in previously irradiated areas, skin and nail pigmentation
Doxorubicin (Adriamycin)	Nausea/vomiting, red urine, severe local tissue necrosis on extravasation, diarrhea, fever, transient ECG changes, ventricular arrhythmia, anaphylactoid reaction	**Myelosuppression,**[*] cardiotoxicity,[*] alopecia, stomatitis, anorexia, conjunctivitis, acral pigmentation, dermatitis in previously irradiated areas, acral erythrodysesthesia, mucositis
Etoposide (VP16)	Nausea/vomiting, diarrhea, fever, hypotension, allergic reaction	**Myelosuppression,**[*] alopecia, peripheral neuropathy, mucositis and hepatic damage with high doses, leukemia
Floxuridine (FUDR)	Nausea/vomiting, diarrhea	**Oral and GI ulceration,**[*] **myelosuppression,**[*] alopecia, dermatitis, hepatic dysfunction with infusion
Fluorouracil (5-FU)	Nausea/vomiting, diarrhea, hypersensitivity, photosensitivity	**Oral and GI ulcers, myelosuppression,**[*] diarrhea, ataxia, arrhythmias, angina, hyperpigmentation, hand-foot syndrome, conjunctivitis CHF

Toxicities of Chemotherapeutic Agents (cont.)

DRUG	ACUTE TOXICITY	DELAYED TOXICITY
Ifosfamide (lfex)	Nausea/vomiting, confusion, nephrotoxicity, metabolic acidosis, **cardiac toxicity with higher dose**[*]	**Myelosuppression,**[*] **hemorrhagic cystitis,**[*] alopecia, SIADH, neurotoxicity
Mechlorethamine (nitrogen mustard)	Nausea/vomiting, local reaction and phlebitis	**Myelosuppression,**[*] alopecia, diarrhea, oral ulcers, leukemia, amenorrhea, sterility
Methotrexate	Nausea/vomiting, diarrhea, fever, anaphylaxis, hepatic necrosis	**Oral/GI ulceration,**[*] **myelosuppression,**[*] hepatic toxicity, renal toxicity, **pulmonary infiltrates and fibrosis,**[*] osteoporosis, conjunctivitis, alopecia, depigmentation
Mitoxantrone (Novantrone)	Blue-green sclera and pigment in urine, nausea/vomiting, stomatitis	**Myelosuppression,**[*] cardiotoxicity, alopecia, white hair, skin lesions, hepatic damage, renal failure
Paclitaxel (Taxol), docetaxel (Taxotere)	Hypersensitivity, hypotension, nausea, pain on extravasation	**Myelosuppression,**[*] alopecia, peripheral neuropathy, rash and edema (docetaxel)
Vinblastine (Velban)	Nausea/vomiting, local reaction and phlebitis with extravasation	**Myelosuppression,**[*] alopecia, stomatitis, loss of DTRs, jaw pain, muscle pain, paralytic ileus
Vincristine (Oncovin)	Local reaction with extravasation	**Peripheral neuropathy,**[*] alopecia, mild myelosuppression, constipation, paralytic ileus, jaw pain, SIADH

[*]Dose-limiting effects.

Drugs of choice for cancer chemotherapy. Med Lett 37:25–32, 1995.

11. Which chemotherapeutic drugs are associated with cardiotoxicity?

Cardiac toxicity is most frequently associated with **doxorubicin** (Adriamycin), which causes a progressive loss of cardiac muscle cells. In previously normal hearts, this toxicity is dose-related and does not become clinically important until a total dose of approx. 450 mg/m[2] is administered. Of course, in patients with already compromised cardiac function, this toxicity may occur at lower dosages. Cardiac radionuclide gated wall motion studies (multiple-gated acquisition [MUGA] scans) measuring ejection fraction are used to monitor changes in cardiac function.

12. Define the term neoadjuvant therapy.

Neoadjuvant therapy means treatment with chemotherapy is given prior to definitive surgery or radiotherapy. This differs from adjuvant therapy, in which the tumor has been grossly removed by surgery and chemotherapy is administered afterward to prevent recurrence. Patients given neoadjuvant therapy often have large tumors, and the idea is to shrink these tumors to make subsequent surgical removal or radiotherapy easier and more effective.

13. What are radiosensitizers?

Radiosensitizers are chemical agents that increase the sensitivity of cells in vitro to radiation and are usually classified as nonhypoxic cell sensitizers. This class of compounds includes drugs such as halogenated pyrimidine nucleoside analogs, 3-amino-benzamide, diamide, and various platinum compounds, among others. Radiosensitization by these compounds may be mediated by a variety of mechanisms, none of which is precisely known. However, it is often assumed that effects on the induction and/or repair of radiation-induced damage may be involved.

14. Define the term tumor doubling time.

Tumor doubling time refers to the time required for the tumor to double in size. The doubling time varies greatly among cancers.

Tumor Doubling Times for Common Cancers

TUMOR TYPE	DOUBLING TIME
Primary lung cancer	
Adenocarcinoma	21 wks
Squamous cell carcinoma	12
Anaplastic carcinoma (oat cell)	11
Breast cancer	
Primary	14
Lung metastases	11
Soft-tissue metastases	3
Colorectal cancer	
Primary	90
Lung metastases	14

From Tannock IF, Hill RP (eds): The Basic Science of Oncology, 2nd ed. New York, McGraw Hill, 1992, p 155; with permission.

15. How is the doubling time of tumors calculated from chest x-rays?

The doubling time of tumors can be roughly calculated from chest x-rays by measuring the diameter of the lesion (assuming it is approximately spherical) and calculating its volume with the formula: volume = Πr^3, where Π is *pi* and *r* is the radius of the lesion. After the volume is calculated on two separate occasions, doubling time can be extracted from a plot of volume versus time.

This calculation assumes very simple growth kinetics and the absence of other factors affecting the growth, which is rarely, if ever, the case. However, tumor cell populations exhibit a reduction in net fractional growth rate with increasing population size. The Gompertz equation describes this slowing of growth with size and takes into account various other factors, such as decreasing blood supply, with increasing size of tumor.

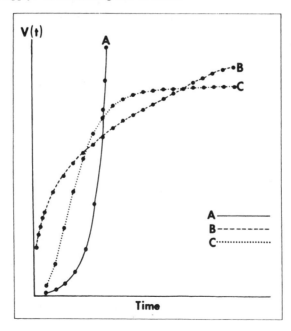

A, Exponential tumor growth curve; *B*, cube-root function growth curve; *C*, tumor growth curve from the Gompertz equation. (From Silver RT, et al: Some new aspects of modern cancer chemotherapy. Am J Med 63:772–787, 1977; with permission.)

16. What phenotype is most highly associated with the development of melanoma? Describe the characteristic lesions of melanoma in the small bowel.

Typical physical characteristics of patients with melanoma are fair skin, reddish hair, and freckles. Familial melanoma families have been described in which > 25% of the kindred are affected with a vertical distribution of disease. There is an early age of onset, from the third to fourth decades. The incidence of multiple primary melanomas is increased, as is the presence of atypical nevi (B-K moles or familial atypical multiple melanoma [FAMM] with melanocyte dysplasia). However, there is a superior overall survival, possibly related to earlier detection. Ocular melanoma is also seen in this group of patients. The gene for the dysplastic nevus syndrome/familial melanoma is located on chromosome 1.

Melanoma often metastasizes to the bowel, where it causes obstruction and bleeding. Lesions seen on barium studies are ulcerated with a central crater and a surrounding heaped-up border, causing the barium to pool in a "target" configuration.

COMPLICATIONS OF CANCER

17. What are the causes of anemia in cancer patients?

The anemia may be secondary to blood loss due to bleeding from tumors or from gastritis caused by the use of nonsteroidal anti-inflammatory drugs (NSAIDs) such as aspirin. It may also be caused by hemolysis (which may be secondary to antibodies associated with the tumor), disseminated intravascular coagulation (DIC), sepsis, or a paraneoplastic syndrome in cases of cancer of the pancreas or prostate.

Anemia can also be caused by bone marrow suppression by chemotherapy or marrow involvement by the tumor. Anemia of chronic disease is common in cancer patients, and the diagnosis is made when no other cause of anemia can be found and plasma iron is < 60 mg/dl, total iron-binding capacity (TIBC) is 100–250 mg/dl, and ferritin is > 60 ng/ml. The hematocrit is generally ~25%, although values as low as 16% are not uncommon. An inadequate erythropoietin response to the anemia has been demonstrated in these patients. An inadequate response to treatment with recombinant human erythropoietin has also been demonstrated in some studies.

Miller CB, et al. Decreased erythropoietin response in patients with the anemia of cancer. N Engl J Med 322:1689–1692, 1990.

18. What are the predisposing factors, organisms, and sources for infection in cancer patients?

Predisposing factors for infection in cancer patients include defects in cellular and humoral immunity, organ compromise due to tumor-related obstruction, chemotherapy-related granulocytopenia, disruption of mucosal (e.g., respiratory and alimentary tract) and integumental surfaces, iatrogenic procedures or placement of prosthetic devices, CNS dysfunction, and hyposplenic or postsplenectomy states.

Organisms currently accounting for the majority of infections in cancer patients are the gram-positive organisms, especially the coagulase-negative staphylococci, *Staphylococcus aureus,* and streptococci. Infections with gram-negative Enterobacteriaceae (*Klebsiella, Enterobactober, Escherichia coli,* and *Pseudomonas* sp.) have declined since the early 1980s. Fungal organisms found in infected cancer patients include *Aspergillus, Candida* sp., and *Cryptococcus.* The most common viral infections are herpes simplex and varicella-zoster.

The vast majority of infections originate from the patients' own endogenous flora. **Sources** of infection in neutropenic cancer patients include the lungs, urinary tract, skin, upper aerodigestive tract (mouth, skin, teeth), CNS, rectum, perirectum, biopsy sites, and GI tract (appendicitis, cholecystitis, perforations). Cultures should include blood, urine, sputum, and, if appropriate, stool, pleural fluid, and peritoneal fluid.

19. Which tumors spread to bone most commonly? Are these lesions osteoblastic or osteolytic?

Cancer of the lung, breast, kidney, prostate, and thyroid, as well as multiple myeloma and malignant melanoma spread to bone most commonly. Renal cell carcinoma and multiple myeloma tend to be purely lytic, prostatic carcinoma tends to be mainly blastic, and the others are mixed. The most frequently involved bones are the spine, ribs, pelvis, and long bones. Tumors that are lytic are most often associated with hypercalcemia, whereas blastic metastases are rarely associated with this complication. The pain of these metastases is characterized by a dull, aching discomfort that is worse at night and improves with physical activity.

20. Which tumors metastasize to the lungs?

All tumors can metastasize to the lungs. Therefore, the more common the tumor, the more commonly it is found to have spread to the lung (e.g., breast cancers). Although they also can spread to the lungs, GI cancers tend to metastasize to the liver and locally before pulmonary involvement is seen. Those tumors that spread via the blood stream, such as sarcomas, renal cell carcinoma, and colon cancer, tend to produce nodular lung lesions. Those that spread via lymphatic routes, such as cancers of the breast, pancreas, stomach, and liver, manifest a pattern of lymphangitic spread.

21. What are the symptoms of intracranial metastases?

Headache occurs in up to 50% of these patients. It is classically described as occurring early in the morning, disappearing or decreasing after arising, and often being associated with nausea and/or projectile vomiting. Other symptoms include focal signs, such as unilateral weakness, numbness, seizures, or cranial nerve abnormaltiies. Nonfocal complaints, such as mental status changes or ataxia, may be seen. The diagnosis is made by CT or MRI of the brain. Treatment consists of decreasing intracranial pressure with steroids, followed by radiotherapy. Surgery is sometimes used in patients with single intracranial lesions, no other sites of metastases, and a long time interval between the primary tumor and the intracranial metastasis.

22. What are the signs and symptoms of malignant pericardial effusion?

The presentation of malignant pericardial effusion can resemble that of heart failure, with dyspnea, peripheral edema, and an enlarged heart on chest x-ray. However, the dyspnea is often out of proportion to the degree of pulmonary congestion seen on the x-ray. Kussmaul's sign, or jugulovenous distention with inspiration, and pulsus paradoxus of > 10 mm Hg with distant heart sounds are clues to the presence of a pericardial effusion. Confirmation of the clinical diagnosis is made by echocardiogram or CT scan. Malignant effusions are usually exudates and are often hemorrhagic. Cytology is helpful if positive but does not exclude cancer if negative.

Treatment is dependent on the patient's condition but should include drainage of the fluid for diagnostic as well as therapeutic reasons. A nonsurgical approach is preferred, with catheter drainage followed by sclerosis of the pericardium, most often with a sclerosing agent such as doxycycline. Other approaches include subxiphoid pericardiectomy, transthoracic catheters, pericardial windows, and pericardial stripping for patients with prolonged life expectancy.

23. Which tumors are associated with nonbacterial thrombotic endocarditis?

This paraneoplastic syndrome is associated with **mucinous adenocarcinomas,** most commonly of the lung, stomach, or ovary, but has been described in other types of cancers as well. It is revealed by the appearance of embolic peripheral or cerebral vascular events causing arterial insufficiency, encephalopathy, or focal neurologic defects. Heart murmurs are often not present. Echocardiograms may often be negative, and the diagnosis is usually made post mortem. Treatment with anticoagulants or antiplatelet drugs has been tried with little success.

24. What are the tumor-related causes of hypercalcemia?

1. **Lytic bone metastases,** which release calcium into the bloodstream. This is the most common cause in solid tumors with bony metastases.

2. **Humoral mediators** of hypercalcemia have been demonstrated in patients without bony metastases. Ectopic parathyroid hormone (PTH) and elevated prostaglandin activity have been described in the past, but the term mediator of **humoral hypercalcemia of malignancy** is now used. This is a non-PTH substance with some PTH-like activity and is associated with squamous cell cancers of many origins, renal cell cancer, transitional cell carcinoma, and ovarian carcinoma.

3. Formerly known as **osteoclast activating factor,** osteolytic substances such as interleukin

1 (IL-1), IL-6, and tumor necrosis factor-α (lymphotoxin) have been shown to cause hypercalcemia in plasma cell dyscrasias.

4. **Vitamin D metabolites** are seen in some lymphomas. These promote intestinal calcium absorption.

25. What is the tumor lysis syndrome?

When rapidly growing tumors are effectively treated with chemotherapy, breakdown products of tumor lysis are released into the vascular system in large amounts. This may cause hyperkalemia, hyperuricemia, hyperphosphatemia, and hypocalcemia. Renal failure may result from the hyperuricemia. This complication is usually seen within a few hours to days following the treatment of tumors such as acute leukemia, Burkitt's lymphoma, and occasionally other rapidly dividing lymphomas. It is rarely, if ever, seen with solid tumors but has been described in small cell carcinoma of the lung.

Treatment is the same as for renal failure, with vigorous hydration, dialysis if necessary, and appropriate treatment of electrolyte disorders. Preventive treatment with allopurinol given before the chemotherapy is the best course.

26. Which medications are commonly used for severe cancer pain?

Oral Nonnarcotic and Narcotic Analgesics for Severe Cancer Pain

	ROUTE	EQUIANAL-GESIC DOSE (MG)	DURA-TION (HR)	PLASMA HALF-LIFE (HR)	COMMENTS
Narcotic agonists					
Morphine	IM	10	4–6	2–3.5	Standard for comparison
	PO, SL, PR	60	4–7	2–3.5	Also available in slow-release tablets and rectal suppositories
Codeine	IM	130	4–6	3	Biotransformed to morphine; useful as initial narcotic analgesic
	PO	200	4–6	3	Same as IM
Oxycodone	IM	15	—		Short-acting; available alone or as 5-mg dose in combination with aspirin and acetaminophen
	PO	30	3–5	—	Same as IM
Levorphanol	IM	2	4–6	12–16	—
	PO	4	4–7	12–16	Good oral potency; requires careful titration in initial dosing because of drug accumulation
Hydromorphone	IM	1.5	4–5	2–3	Available in high-potency injectable form (10 mg/ml) for cachectic patients and as a rectal suppositories; more soluble than morphine
	PO	7.5	4–6	2–3	Same as IM
Meperidine	IM	75	4–5	3–4 (12–16 for nor-meper-idine)	Contraindicated in patients with renal disease; accumulation of active toxic metabolite normeperidine produces CNS excitation
	PO	300	4–6	See IM	Same as IM
Methadone	IM	10	—	15–30	May be limited to narcotic rehab programs; requires careful titration of the initial dose to avoid drug accumulation
	PO	20		15–30	Good oral potency
Fentanyl patch	Skin	—	25–72	17	Long-acting; for patients who cannot take oral or parenteral meds
Mixed agonist-antagonist drug					*May precipitate withdrawal in physically dependent patients.*
Butorphanol	IM	2	4–6	2.5–3.5	Not available orally, but available as an intranasal preparation; Less severe psychotomimetic effects than pentazocine.

IM, intramuscular; PO, oral; SL, sublingual; PR, rectal.

27. What medications are commonly used for mild to moderate cancer pain?

Oral Nonnarcotic and Narcotic Analgesics for Mild to Moderate Cancer Pain

	EQUIANAL-GESIC DOSE (MG)*	DURATION (HR)	PLASMA HALF-LIFE (HR)	COMMENTS
Aspirin	650	4–6	3–5	Standard for nonnarcotic comparisons; GI and hematolgic effects limit use in cancer patients
Acetaminophen	650	4–6	1–4	Weak anti-inflammatory effects; safer than aspirin
Codeine	30–60	4–6	3	Biotransformed to morphine; available in combination with nonnarcotic analgesics
Ibuprofen	400	4–6	2–4	Monitor for renal effects; GI side effects can limit use in cancer patients
Meperidine	50	4–6	3–4	Biotransformed to active toxic metabolite normeperidine; associated with myoclonus and seizures
Pentazocine	30	4–6	2–3	Psychotomimetic effects with escalation of dose; only available in combination with naloxone, aspirin, or acetaminophen (U.S.)

*Relative potency of drugs, as compared with aspirin, for mild to moderate pain.

28. What are the neuromuscular complications of cancer?

Neuromuscular Complications of Malignant Disease

Neuromuscular disorder (common)
Myopathy
    Myositis and dermatomyositis
    Myasthenic syndrome (Eaton-Lambert syndrome)
    Carcinomatous myopathy
Neuropathy
    Distal sensorimotor polyneuropathy (common)
    Carcinomatous sensory neuropathy (rare)
Myelopathy
    Necrotizing myelopathy
    Subacute myelitis
Subacute cerebellar degeneration
Encephalopathy
    Limbic encephalopathy (very rare, ? viral)
    Progressive multifocal leukoencephalopathy (rare)

From Rubenstein E, Federman DD (eds): Scientific American Medicine. New York, Scientific American, 1986; with permission.

GASTROINTESTINAL AND LIVER CANCERS

29. What genetic abnormalities are assŕ ɟiated with esophageal cancer?

Extensive loss of heterozygosity for *p53* (55% cases), *Rb* (48%), *APC* (66%), and *DCC* (24%) have been demonstrated in esophageal cancers. The disturbances of the *p53* and *rb* genes in this disease suggest that dysregulation of normal cell-cycle control plays an important role in its development. In addition, two ligands of epidermal growth factor receptor (EGFR), EGF and transforming growth factor-α (TGF-α), have been demonstrated to be present in esophageal carcinoma cells. Proto-oncogene cyclin D1 has been shown to be amplified 2–5-fold in esophageal carcinomas with the 11q13 amplification.

Rosen, N: Molecular basis of esophageal carcinoma. Semin Oncol 21(4):416–424, 1994.

30. Summarize the risk factors for esophageal cancer.

Squamous cell cancer of the esophagus occurs in the 40–60-year age group, mainly in men. It is more common in blacks and in Far Eastern countries. Risk factors include:

- Geography: Africa, China, Russia, Japan, Scotland, and the Caspian region of Iran have an increased incidence
- Nonwhite male population
- Excessive alcohol use
- Excessive tobacco use
- Native Bantu beer (southern Africa)
- Chronic hot beverage ingestion
- Lye ingestion: > 30% of cases develop esophageal cancer
- Tylosis: > 40% of cases develop esophageal cancer
- Achalasia
- Plummer-Vinson syndrome
- Nontropical sprue
- Oral and pharyngeal cancer
- Occupational exposure to asbestos, combustion products, ionizing radiation. (Seen in waiters, bartenders, metal workers, and construction workers.)
- Decreased dietary intake of fruits and vegetables throughout adulthood

Adenocarcinoma of the esophagus in a younger population without the traditional risk factors has been associated with chronic esophagitis and the development of Barrett's esophagus.

Blot WJ: Esophageal cancer trends and risk factors. Semin Oncol 21:403–410, 1994.

31. How does esophageal cancer present?

Presenting Symptoms of Esophageal Carcinoma

Dysphagia: first with solids, then with liquids	Occult GI bleeding	Choking
	Aspiration pneumonia	Hoarseness
Weight loss	Cough	Chest pain on swallowing
Regurgitation	Fever	GERD

32. How should esophageal cancer be treated?

Treatment depends largely on the patient and his or her physical condition at the time of presentation. The only curative procedure is surgery, but fewer than half of the patients are operable at the time of presentation, and of these, only one-half to two-thirds have tumors that are resectable. Radical radiation therapy has been tried in selected patients, but the 5-year survival rates are < 15%. Local recurrence is reported in about 50% of these patients, and toxicity is high, with complications of radiation pneumonitis, aspiration, tracheoesophageal fistulas, mediastinal perforations, radiation myelitis, hemorrhage, and constrictive pericarditis reported.

Chemotherapy has yet to play a major role in the treatment of this disease, but several studies are investigating the use of chemotherapy in combination with radiotherapy or prior to surgery. To date, encouraging responses have been noted, but no increase has been seen in long-term survival.

33. List the risk factors for gastric cancer.

Precursor Conditions	**Genetic and Environmental Factors**
Chronic atrophic gastritis and intestinal metaplasia	Family history of gastric cancer
	Blood type A
Pernicious anemia	Hereditary nonpolyposis colon cancer syndrome
Partial gastrectomy for benign disease	Low socioeconomic status
Helicobacter pylori infection	Low consumption of fruits and vegetables
Ménétrier's disease	Consumption of salted, smoked, or poorly
Gastric adenomatous polyps	preserved foods
Barrett's esophagus	Cigarette smoking

Fuchs CS, et al: Gastric carcinoma. N Engl J Med. 333:32–41, 1995.

In addition, the role of oncogenes and tumor-suppressor genes is being elucidated. Allelic deletions of the *MCC, APC,* and *p53* tumor-suppressor genes have been reported in 33, 34, and

64% of gastric cancers, respectively, but gastric cancer rarely involves mutations in the *ras* oncogene. Disparities between mutations associated with the intestinal and diffuse types of gastric cancers may account for their different natural histories.

34. What are the symptoms at the time of diagnosis in patients with gastric cancer?

Symptoms at Initial Diagnosis Among 18,365 Patients with Gastric Cancer

SYMPTOMS	FREQUENCY
Weight loss	61.6%
Abdominal pain	51.6
Nausea	34.3
Anorexia	32.0
Dysphagia	26.1
Melena	20.2
Early satiety	17.5
Ulcer-type pain	17.1
Lower-extremity edema	5.9

Fuchs CS, et al: Gastric carcinoma. N Eng J Med. 333:32–41, 1995.

35. What are the risk factors, signs, and symptoms of pancreatic cancer?

Risk Factors for Pancreatic Cancer

- Heredity
- Males > females
- Blacks > whites
- Diabetes mellitus
- Smoking (2–3 times increased risk)
- Surgery for peptic ulcer disease
- High-calorie, high-fat, and high-protein diet (?)
- Occupational exposure to 2-naphthylamine and petroleum products (>10 yrs. increases risk to 5:1)
- Elderly, heavy-smoking, alcoholic men exposed to occupational carcinogens have especially high risk

Three or more risk factors in men increases the risk by 6-fold. A history of alcohol abuse or pancreatitis is *not* a proven risk factor for pancreatic cancer.

Signs and Symptoms of Pancreatic Cancer Based on Tumor Location

	HEAD	BODY/TAIL
Symptoms		
Weight loss	92%	100%
Jaundice	82	7
Pain	72	87
Anorexia	64	33
Nausea	45	43
Vomiting	37	37
Weakness	35	43
Signs		
Jaundice	87	13
Palpable liver	83	—
Palpable gallbladder	29	—
Tenderness	26	27
Ascites	19	20

Adapted from Moossa AR, et al: Tumors of the pancreas. In Moossa AR, et al (eds): Comprehensive Textbook of Oncology, 2nd ed. Baltimore, Williams & Wilkins, 1991, p 964.

36. Which tests are most useful in diagnosing pancreatic cancer?

Test	Diagnostic Yield (Various Series)
CA19–9 >200U/ml	97%*
CT scan of abdomen	83–94%
ERCP	94%
Angiography	90%
Ultrasound of abdomen	75–90%
MRI of abdomen	NA

*Forsmark CE, et al: Diagnosis of pancreatic cancer and prediction of unresectability using the tumor-associated antigen CA19–9. Pancreas 9:731–734, 1994. (ERCP, endoscopic retrograde cholangiopancreatography.)

After a radiographic diagnosis of a mass is made, percutaneous or open biopsy may be done. In various series, a positive cytologic diagnosis has been obtained in 87–100% of cases.

37. Describe the diagnostic and staging evaluation for patients suspected of having pancreatic cancer.

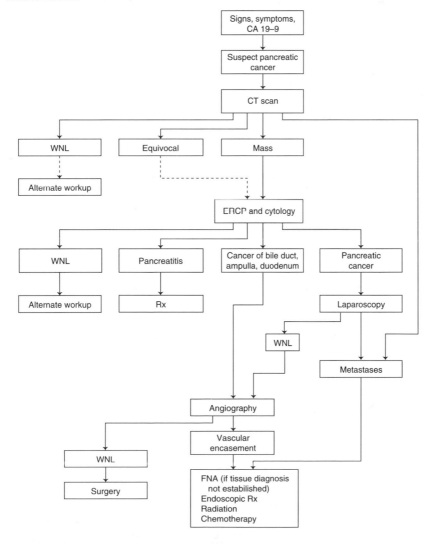

Poutch PG: A diagnostic approach to pancreatic cancer. Dig Dis. 12(3):129–38, 1994.

38. What are the risk factors for hepatocellular carcinoma?

Underlying **cirrhosis** from any cause appears to be the most important risk factor for the development of hepatocellular carcinoma. The evidence available indicates that chronic infection with **hepatitis B or C viruses** is the major etiology for human hepatocellular carcinoma, since it causes development of cirrhosis. Macronodular cirrhosis is found in 85% of patients with hepatocellular carcinoma, and it is theorized that this is a result of the chronic infection with the virus, which may occur as early as the perinatal stage.

There are extensive studies of **aflatoxins** in human foods in Africa that suggest a quantitative relationship between increased human aflatoxin consumption and the incidence of hepatocellular carcinoma around the world. In a small proportion of hepatocellular carcinomas, the cause appears to be related to other factors, including other hepatotropic viruses, tobacco, alcohol, chemicals, mycotoxins, and hepatic parasites. The relative importance of these factors seems to vary among populations.

39. List the common presenting features of primary tumors of the liver.

Common Presenting Features of Primary Liver Tumors

Asthenia	85–90%
Hepatomegaly	50–100%
Abdominal pain	50–70%
Jaundice	45–80%
Fever	9.5%

Hepatomas can present in many unusual ways, as well, including:
* Hemoptysis, secondary to pulmonary metastases
* Rib mass, secondary to bony metastasis
* Encephalitis-like picture, secondary to brain metastasis
* Heart failure, secondary to cardiac metastasis and thrombosis of inferior vena cava
* Priapism, secondary to soft-tissue metastasis
* Bone pain and pathologic fractures, secondary to bony metastases

40. What are the systemic manifestations of hepatocellular carcinoma?

Hepatoma

Endocrine

Erythrocytosis	Hypercalcemia

Nonendocrine

Hypoglycemia	Hyperlipidemia
Porphyria cutanea tarda	Dysfibrinogenemia
Cryofibrinogenemia	Alpha-fetoglobulin synthesis
Osteoporosis	

Hepatoblastoma

Precocious puberty	Hemihypertrophy
Cystinuria	

Margolis S. et al: Systemic manifestations of hepatoma. Medicine 51:381–390, 1972.

41. Which environmental factors are thought to be related to the development of colon cancer?

There are abundant epidemiologic data to support the link between environmental factors and colorectal cancer:

1. The disease is more frequent among upper socioeconomic classes living in urban areas.

2. There is a direct correlation with calorie consumption and with dietary fat, oil, and meat protein.

3. A direct correlation is seen between mortality from coronary artery disease and mortality from colorectal cancer.

4. Migrant groups tend to assume the incidence rates of their new environments.

5. Burkitt noted years ago that in South Africa, the low incidence of large bowel cancer was correlated with a diet high in roughage. Others have correlated a diet high in cruciferous vegetables with a lower incidence of this cancer.

6. Regular use of nonsteroidal anti-inflammatory drugs (NSAIDS), especially aspirin, significantly decreases the risk of developing colorectal cancer.

Nevertheless, as with all epidemiologic data, confounding factors may be significant.

42. Besides environmental factors, are there other risk factors associated with the development of colon cancer?

Up to 25% of patients with colorectal cancer have a **family history** of the disease, suggesting the involvement of a genetic factor or factors. Genes so far identified for their involvement in colorectal carcinogenesis are *K-ras, APC, DCC, hMSH2, hMLH1, hPMS1, hPMS1,* and *p53.*

Two clinical types of cancer are seen. **Familial adenomatous polyposis, Gardner's syndrome,** and **hereditary nonpolyposis colorectal cancer** are autosomal dominant syndromes: the first two account for < 1% of all colorectal cancers, and the last for 6–15%. Hereditary nonpolyposis colorectal cancer is a familial cancer syndrome that differs in natural history and genetic characteristics from sporadic colorectal cancer.

Familial polyposis coli is characterized by thousands of adenomatous polyps throughout the large bowel. If left untreated, cancer will develop in all patients with this syndrome. The cancer will usually manifest under age 40. The more common nonpolyposis syndrome also involves the proximal large bowel. The median age at presentation is <50 years, and patients with a strong family history should be intensively screened.

Toribara NW, et al: Screening for colorectal cancer. N Engl J Med 332:861–867, 1995.

Nonenvironmental Risk Factors in Colorectal Cancer

Age	>40 in symptomatic patients
Associated disease	Ulcerative colitis
	Granulomatous colitis
	Peutz-Jeghers syndrome
	Familial polyposis syndrome
Past history	Colon cancer or polyps
	Female genital or breast cancer
Family history	Juvenile polyps
	Colon cancer or polyps
	Familial polyposis syndrome

Winawer S: Early diagnosis of colorectal cancer. Curr Concepts Oncol (Mar/Apr):8, 1981.

43. Compare the TNM and Dukes classification systems for colon cancer. Give the 5-year survivals.

Colon Cancer Classification and Five-Year Survivals

	TNM				5-YR
STAGE	T	N	M	DUKES	SURVIVAL
Stage 0	T0	N0	M0	—	
Stage I	T1: invades submucosa	N0	M0	A	>90%
Stage I	T2: invades muscularis	N0	M0	B_1	85%
Stage II	T3: through wall	N0	M0	B_2	70–75%
Stage II	T4: perforates visceral peritoneum, or invades other structures	N0	M0	C_1: invades muscularis, positive nodes	30–65%
Stage III	Any T	N1: 1–3 pericolic or perirectal nodes positive	M0	C_2: through wall, positive nodes	30–65%
Stage III	Any T	N2: ≥ 4 pericolic or perirectal nodes positive N3: any node along vascular trunk positive	M0	C_2: through wall, positive nodes	30–65%
Stage IV	Any T	Any N	M1	D	<5%

44. What are the presenting symptoms of colon cancer?

The presenting symptoms depend on the location of the lesion. Lesions in the **ascending colon,** where the stool is still quite liquid, do not present with mass effects. However, these tumors frequently ulcerate, leading to chronic blood loss, and patients present with guaiac-positive stools on screening tests or with symptoms of anemia. In the **transverse bowel,** the stool is more concentrated and formed, so that symptoms of obstruction such as abdominal cramping, abdominal pain, or perforation may occur. Cancers in the **rectosigmoid** present with tenesmus, narrowing of the stool, and hematochezia. Anemia is unusual.

45. What are the uses and limitations for carcinoembryonic antigen (CEA) level testing?

CEA is an antigen produced by many colon cancers. It cannot be used for screening because it usually (in 85% of cases) is normal in patients with stage A disease (those who are most amenable to curative surgery). It has also been found to be elevated in cancers of the stomach, pancreas, breast, and lung and with various nonmalignant conditions such as alcoholic liver disease, inflammatory bowel disease, heavy cigarette smoking, chronic bronchitis, and pancreatitis.

Testing should be done preoperatively in patients undergoing resection for colon cancer, so that the data can be used to follow the course of the disease and treatment. CEA returns to normal in 30–45 days after complete resection of tumors producing it. Thus, postoperative measurement should not be made prior to this time. If a preoperative elevated level, which returns to normal after surgery, subsequently becomes elevated, it is a very reliable indicator of tumor recurrence. CEA can also be used as a marker for response to chemotherapy.

46. How is chemotherapy used in the treatment of colon cancer?

Chemotherapy has two roles in its treatment. The first, and broader, role is in the treatment of **metastatic disease,** where the agent most commonly used is 5-fluorouracil (5-FU). Response rates to this drug in metastatic disease are only 15–20%. Many different schedules and combinations with other drugs, such as methyl CCNU, levamisole, and leucovorin, are used to improve response rates.

The second use of chemotherapy is in an **adjuvant setting.** In patients who had curative-intent resections of Stage III colon cancer, treatment with 5-FU and levamisole reduced the recurrence rate by 40% and the death rate by 33% over non-chemotherapy-treated controls, and this regimen is now considered standard postoperative therapy for stage III patients. In patients with stage II disease, treatment can be given to high-risk patients, as judged by DNA flow studies. Several large cooperative groups have used 5-FU with leucovorin in early-stage disease, but this indication is still in need of further testing.

Tumor vaccines and other immunotherapy are still under investigation.

Moertel CG, et al: Fluorouracil plus levamisole as effective adjuvant therapy after resection of Stage II colon carcinoma: A final report. Ann Intern Med 122:321–326, 1995.

47. What is the mechanism of action of 5-fluorouracil ? What are its side effects?

5-FU is a potent inhibitor of thymidylate synthetase. Thymidylate synthetase binds strongly to 5-fluorodeoxyuridylate, one of the metabolites of 5-FU. Without thymidylate synthesis, tumor cells cannot form dTMP, a precursor of DNA synthesis.

Side effects of 5-FU include myelosuppression, cerebellar ataxia, dacryocystitis, angina, mucositis, and hyperpigmentation.

PROSTATE CANCER

48. What tests are available for the diagnosis and staging of prostate cancer? How do their results correlate with the stage?

Diagnostic Evaluation and Staging of Prostate Cancer

STAGE	HISTOLOGY OF PROSTATE BIOPSY SPECIMEN	URINARY SYMPTOMS	NONINVASIVE ASSESSMENT OF METASTIC DISEASE*					SURGICAL LN SAMPLING
			SAP	PSA	CXR	BONE SCAN	PELVIC CT SCAN	
A1	Well-differentiated cancer present in <5% of specimens	Compatible with BPH	N	Sometimes ↑	−	−	−	Usually not performed
A2	Well-differentiated cancer present in ≥ 4 chips or cancer not well-differentiated	Compatible with BPH	N	Often ↑	−	−	−	+ in 25% (indicating stage D1 disease)
B	Well-differentiated nodule	Absent	N	May be ↑*	−	−	−	+ in 8% (indicating stage D1 disease)
	Nodule not well differentiated	Absent	N	May be ↑*	−	−	−	+ in 25% (indicating stage D1 disease)
C	Local, contiguously extended lesion that is not poorly differentiated	Present	N	Always ↑*	−	−	−	+ in 40–50% (indicating stage D1 disease)
	Local, contiguously extended lesion that is poorly differentiated	Present	Possibly ↑	Always ↑*	−	−	−	+ in 95% of patients who have elevated sAP
D0	Cancer present	Variable	Always ↑	Often ↑	−	−	−	Usually +; high risk of relapse in 2–4 yr
D1	Cancer present	Usually present	Often ↑	Always ↑*	−	−	−/+	+ below aortic bifurcation
D2	Cancer present	Usually present	↑ in 80%	Always ↑*	−/+	Usually +	−/+	Usually not performed

sAP, serum alkaline phosphatase; PSA, prostate specific antigen; CXR, chest x-ray; LN, lymph node; BPH, benign prostatic hypertrophy; ↑, elevated; −, negative; +, positive.
*PSA levels increased proportionate to tumor volume.
From Rubenstein E, Federman DD (eds): Scientific American Medicine. New York, Scientific American, 1993, p 12(IXA):5; with permission.

49. What is the long-term survival of patients with prostate cancer?

Survival in Prostate Cancer by Stage

AUA STAGE	SURVIVAL
A	Lower than general population
B	5-yr, 75–55%; 10-yr, 57–61%, 15-yr, 28–40%
C	5-yr, 64%; 10-yr, 35%; 15-yr, 20%
D	Median survival 2.5 yr

AUA, American Urological Association.

50. How are the prostatic acid phosphatase and prostatic-specific antigen (PSA) used in the treatment of prostate cancer?

PSA is a glycoprotein found in the ductular epithelium of normal and malignant prostate tissue. Serum levels reflect the volume of the prostate and therefore may be elevated in large benign prostates as well as tumors. PSA can be a useful immunohistochemical marker when the primary site of tumor is occult. It is currently used as a screening method. The America Cancer Society and the American Urological Association recommend yearly rectal exam and PSA in men age > 50 or age > 40 for high-risk groups (blacks, strong family history).

Acid phosphatases are enzymes that hydrolyze esters of orthophosphoric acid in an acidic milieu. One of these, the prostatic acid phosphatase, is elevated in most patients with advanced or stage D prostatic cancer, and its level correlates with the disease activity. It thus may be used as a marker for treatment response. It is not useful as a screening test in early-stage disease and is a much less sensitive marker than PSA.

51. How do the TNM and AUA staging systems relate?

TNM		AUA	
T0	No evidence of primary tumor	A	No palpable lesion
T1a	Incidental histologic finding in <5% of resected tissue	A1	Focal
T1b	Incidental histologic finding in >5% of resected tissue	A2	Diffuse
T1c	Identified by needle biopsy (e.g., because of elevated PSA values) but not palpable or visible by imaging		
T2	Tumor present clinically or grossly, limited to gland	B	Confined to prostate
T2a	Involves ½ lobe or less	B1	Small, discrete nodule
T2b	Involves >½ lobe but not both lobes	B2	Large or multiple nodules or areas
T2c	Involves both lobes		
T3	Extends through prostatic capsule	C	Localized to periprostatic area
T3a	Extends unilaterally	C1	No involvement of seminal vesicles, <70 gm
T3b	Extends bilaterally		
T3c	Invades seminal vesicle (or vesicles)	C2	Involvement of seminal vesicles, >70 gm
T4	Fixed or invades adjacent structures other than seminal vesicles	D	Metastatic disease
T4a	Invades bladder neck, external sphincter, or rectum	D1	Pelvic lymph node metastases or urethral obstruction causing hydronephrosis
T4b	Invades levator muscles or is fixed to pelvic wall (or both)		
N1	Metastasis in a single regional lymph node (largest dimension, ≤2 cm)		
N2	Metastasis in a single regional lymph node (largest dimension, >2 cm but <5 cm) or multiple nodes (largest dimension in all nodes, <5 cm)		
N3	Metastasis in a regional lymph node (largest dimension, >5 cm)		
M1	Distant metastasis	D2	Bone or distant lymph node or organ or soft-tissue metastases
M1a	Nonregional lymph node (or nodes)		
M1b	Bone (or bones)		
M1c	One or more other sites		

52. What are the effects and mechanisms of the various androgen-deprivation therapies for prostate cancer?

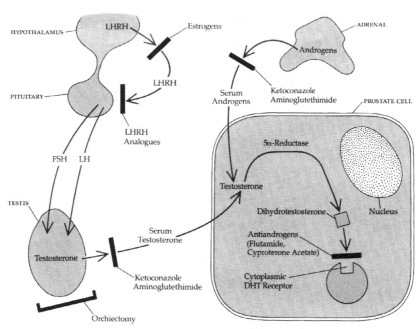

Androgen deprivation, which prevents the trophic influence of testosterone on the prostate in advanced prostate carcinoma, can be effected in a variety of ways. Estrogens such as diethylstilbestrol (DES) inhibit the release of luteinizing hormone-releasing hormone (LHRH) from the hypothalamus, thus diminishing the release of follicle-stimulating hormone (FSH) and luteinizing hormone (LH) from the anterior pituitary and reducing the signal that stimulates testosterone production by the testes. LHRH analogues such as leuprolide initially stimulate but ultimately inhibit the release of FSH and LH from the anterior pituitary and thus have an estrogenlike effect. The testes, which produce most of the testosterone, can be removed by orchiectomy. Ketoconazole and aminoglutethimide inhibit a variety of steroid synthetic pathways, including those that produce androgens in the testes and adrenal glands. In the prostate cells, testosterone is converted into dihydrotestosterone (DHT) by the enzyme 5α-reductase. Antiandrogens such as flutamide, cyproterone acetate, and certain progestational agents block the binding of DHT to its cytoplasmic receptor. (From Rubenstein E, Federman DD (eds): Scientific American Medicine. New York, Scientific American, 1993, p 12(IXA):8; with permission.)

53. What is the appropriate therapy for prostate cancer at each stage?

Therapy for Prostate Cancer by Stage

STAGE	THERAPY
A1	Transurethral resection followed by close observation
A2	Radiation therapy or radical prostatectomy
B	Radical prostatectomy or radiation therapy
C	Radiation therapy
D1	For urinary obstruction, transurethral prostatectomy (TURP) or radiation therapy
	For asymptomatic patients, endocrine manipulation or close observation
D2	Close observation for asymptomatic disease
	Hormonal therapy for symptomatic disease
	Chemotherapy for disease refractory to hormonal therapy
	Palliative radiation therapy for symptomatic areas

GENITOURINARY CANCERS

54. List the risk factors for the development of bladder cancer.

Environmental factors

Occupational hazards
   Workers in dye industry
   Hairdressers
   Painters
   Leather workers
   Geographic
   Endemic schistosomiasis

Self-ingested toxins
   Tobacco
   Phenacetin
   Artificial sweeteners (possibly)
Miscellaneous
   Alkylating agent (cyclophosphamide)

Cytogenetic abnormalities

Presence of the Ha-*ras* oncogene
Alterations in *p53* suppressor gene

Methylation of *myc* oncogene
Abnormalities on chromosomes 1,5,7,9,11,17

Previous cancers

Especially those of uroepithelial tract

55. What are the most common causes of isolated hematuria?

Major Causes of Isolated Hematuria

TYPE OF BLEEDING	CAUSES
Glomerular bleeding	Mild forms of glomerulonephritis: IgA nephropathy, hereditary nephritis, thin basement membrane disease, postinfectious glomerulonephritis
	Long-distance running
Extraglomerular renal bleeding	Pelvic calculi
	Hypercalciuria
	Carcinoma: renal cell, transitional cell (esp. with analgesic abuse)
	Sickle cell trait or disease
	Cystic diseases: polycystic kidney disease, medullary sponge kidney
	Coagulation disorders: hemophilia, anticoagulation therapy
	Trauma
	Vascular malformation
	Venereal diseases: emboli, vasculitis
Extrarenal bleeding	Ureters: calculi
	Bladder: catheterization, carcinoma, infection by common bacteria or *Mycobacterium tuberculosis,* cyclophosphamide
	Prostate: hypertrophy, carcinoma
	Urethra: trauma, urethritis

Rubenstein E, Federman DD (eds): Scientific American Medicine. New York, Scientific American, 1993, 10:III:10.

56. How does renal cell cancer present?

Presenting Signs and Symptoms of Renal Cell Cancer

Classic triad	9%	Anemia	21%
Gross hematuria		Tumor calcification on x-ray	13%
Abdominal mass		Symptoms from metastases	10%
Pain		Fever	7%
Hematuria	59%	Asymptomatic	7%
Abdominal mass	45%	Erythrocytosis	3%
Pain	41%	Hypercalcemia	3%
Weight loss	28%	Acute varicocele	2%

Skinner DG, et al: Diagnosis and management of renal cell carcinoma: A clinical and pathologic study of 309 cases. Cancer 28:1165, 1971.

Despite the classic triad of presenting features, renal cell cancer has been called the 'internist's tumor" due to its various unusual presentations. These include amyloidosis, hypercalcemia, hypertension, hepatopathy without liver metastases, enteropathy, heart failure, and immune complex glomerulonephritis, among others.

57. What is the prognosis for renal cell cancer?

Survival depends on the stage as well as grade of the tumor:

Stage	Description	5-year Survival
I	Confined to the renal parenchyma	76%
II	Confined to Gerota's fascia	65%
III	Involves the renal vein, inferior vena cava regional lymph nodes	35%
IV	Spread to adjacent organs or distant metastases	5%

Grade	Description	5-year survival
I	Highly differentiated tumors, sharply demarcated from surrounding tissue	100%
IIA	Moderately differentiated tumors, locally well-circumscribed but not necessarily provided with capsule	59%
IIB	Moderately differentiated tumors, poorly circumscribed but not diffusely infiltrating or markedly polymorphous and mitotic	36%
III	Poorly differentiated, markedly polymorphous tumors that are diffusely infiltrating; tumors with abundant growth in capillary vessels	0%

Bottiger LE: Prognosis in renal cell carcinoma. Cancer 26:780–787, 1970.

58. What treatments are available for advanced stage renal cell cancer? How effective are they?

There are few effective therapies for advanced stage renal cell cancer. Some data suggest a hormonal influence in these tumors, theorized to be related to the embryonic origins of the tissue. **Megestrol acetate** has been used with variable success, resulting in responses of 10–15%. A few **chemotherapeutic agents** (e.g., vinblastine) have been slightly active, with response rates in the same range as the hormonal treatments. Currently, **biological-response modifiers** such as interferon, interleukins, tumor necrosis factor, and activated lymphocytes are being used; under strict selection criteria, overall response rates of 15–30% have been achieved. The most effective therapy is early diagnosis and **surgery.**

59. How common is testicular cancer in the U.S.?

Testicular cancer is responsible for approx. 1.14% of all cancers in U.S. males. Most of these are in patients aged 29–35 years, with 7,100 new cases annually. The incidence is higher in patients with cryptorchidism, Klinefelter's syndrome, and testicular feminization syndrome.

The etiology of this cancer is unknown, but age, genetic influences, repeated infection, radiation, and possible endocrine abnormalities have been suggested. Cytogenetic markers associated with germ cell cancer of the testes include the presence of isochromosome 12p. When this marker is present in multiple copies, a poorer prognosis is indicated.

Wingo PA, et al: Cancer statistics, 1995. CA 45(1):8–30, 1995.

60. What are the presenting features of testicular cancer?

Tumors that present locally are detected as a mass in the scrotum. The mass is often painless, although pain is noted in about 25% of reported cases. When the tumor has already spread (5–15%), symptoms of metastases to the lungs and liver are seen. Other diagnostic possibilities of a scrotal mass include epididymitis, hydrocele, inguinal hernia, hematocele, hematoma, testicular torsion, spermatocele, varicocele, and gumma.

61. Which pathologic types are most commonly seen among testicular cancers?

Current Pathologic Classification of Germinal Tumors of the Testes

HISTOLOGY	FREQUENCY
Tumors of one histologic type	
Seminoma (germinoma)	
Typical	35%
Anaplastic	4
Spermatocytic	1
Embryonal carcinoma	20
Teratoma	10
Choriocarcinoma	1
Tumors of mixed histologic types	
Embryonal carcinoma and teratoma (teratocarcinoma)	24
Other combinations	5

62. Outline the stages of testicular cancer.

IA: Tumor confined to the testes

IB: Microscopic involvement of retroperitoneal lymph nodes

II: Macroscopic involvement of retroperitoneal lymph nodes

III: Extension beyond retroperitoneal lymph nodes

Survival cannot be determined on the basis of stage but is much more dependent on the response to therapy. In patients who respond, the survival curves plateau at about 90%.

63. How should testicular cancer be treated?

Transinguinal orchiectomy is performed in all patients with testicular carcinoma. This serves to make the pathologic diagnosis and is the treatment for stage I cancer.

For **pure seminoma,** limited cases are treated with radiation to the retroperitoneal nodes. Disseminated disease is treated with combination chemotherapy.

For **nonseminomatous tumors,** retroperitoneal lymphadenectomy is most commonly done. If nodes are positive, the patients may be treated with two courses of adjuvant chemotherapy.

For patients with **stage III disease** or earlier-stage disease with bulky mediastinal or retroperitoneal masses, three to four courses of chemotherapy are given, followed by resection of any residual disease.

Tumor markers—AFP and HCG— are followed for evidence of recurrent disease. These are quite sensitive for the presence of disease, although normal values do not rule out disease.

64. List the possible long-term effects of therapy for testicular cancer.

1. Impotence
2. Infertility
3. Renal dysfunction
4. Raynaud's phenomenon
5. Pulmonary fibrosis
6. Generalized vascular disorders (acute myocardial infarction, deep venous thrombosis, stroke)
7. Leukemia

65. Describe the extragonadal germ cell syndrome.

The extragonadal germ cell syndrome is characterized by germ cell tumors found in the mediastinum, retroperitoneum, or pineal gland in relatively young males, with elevated HCG or AFP, and marked elevation of lactic dehydrogenase (LDH). These patients often respond to treatment with chemotherapy developed for testicular cancer. It is very important that a careful search for an occult testicular primary be carried out, since the testes is thought to be a relative sanctuary from the effects of chemotherapy. Ultrasound evaluation is useful in this setting.

LUNG CANCER

66. What is the most common cancer in the U.S. today, excluding skin cancer?

Lung cancer. See cancer incidence percentages in the figure on the next page.

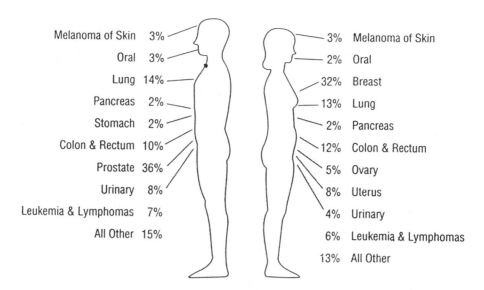

1995 estimated new cancer cases, United States—percent distribution of sites by sex (excluding basal and squamous cell cancers and in situ carcinomas except bladder). (From CA 45(1):1, 1995; with permission.)

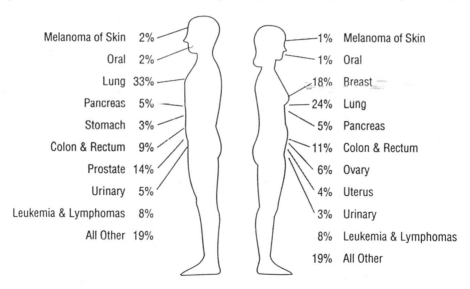

1995 estimated cancer deaths, United States—percent distribution of sites by sex.

67. What are the common presenting signs and symptoms of lung cancer?

1. Symptoms secondary to central or endobronchial growth of the primary tumor:

Cough

Wheeze and stridor

Hemoptysis

Dyspnea from obstruction

Pneumonitis from obstruction (fever, productive cough)

2. Symptoms secondary to peripheral growth of the primary tumor:

Pain from pleural or chest wall involvement

Cough

Dyspnea on a restrictive basis

Lung abscess syndrome from tumor cavitation

3. Symptoms related to regional spread of tumor in the thorax by contiguity or by metastasis to regional lymph nodes:

Tracheal obstruction	Esophageal compression with dysphagia
Recurrent laryngeal nerve paralysis with hoarseness	Phrenic nerve paralysis with elevation of the hemidiaphragm and dyspnea
Sympathetic nerve paralysis with Horner's syndrome	C8 and T1 nerve compression with ulnar pain and Pancoast's syndrome
Superior vena cava syndrome from vascular obstruction	Pericardial and cardiac extension with resultant tamponade, arrhythmia, or cardiac failure
Lymphatic obstruction with pleural effusion	Lymphangitic spread through the lungs with with hypoxemia and dyspnea

4. Symptoms due to distant metastases or systemic effects:

Bone pain	Hemiparesis
Painful lymphadenopathy	Weight loss
Hypercalcemia	

Cohen MH: Signs and symptoms of bronchogenic carcinoma. In Straus MJ (ed): Lung Cancer: Clinical Diagnosis and Treatment, 2nd ed. New York, Grune & Stratton, 1983, pp 97–111.

68. What are the accepted and proposed risk factors for lung cancer?

- **Cigarette smoking** causes 85% of lung cancers in men. In women, its incidence is increasing steadily, and it now has surpassed breast cancer as the leading cause of cancer deaths. Passive smoking (side-stream smoke) also increases the risk of lung cancer, causing 25% of the lung cancers seen in nonsmokers.
- **Radon exposure** increases the risk of lung cancer, especially in smokers, who have a 10-fold higher risk. An estimated 25% of lung cancers in nonsmokers and 5% in smokers is attributed to radon daughter exposure in the home.
- **Marijuana smoking** increases the risk of lung cancer in smokers.
- **Emphysema,** which develops in smokers, is associated with an increased risk.
- **Other agents**

Bis-chloromethyl ether	Arsenic	Nickel
Ionizing radiation	Asbestos	Chromates

69. Which chromosomal defects are associated with lung cancer?

Deletion of 3p (usually 3p14–23) is found in virtually all cases (93%) of small cell lung cancer (SCLC, both classic and variant), in 100% of bronchial carcinoids, and 25% of non-SCLC. Also seen are absent or reduced expression of the *rb* gene at 13q14, increased production of the c-*jun* oncogene product, and constitutive expression of c-*raf*-1 gene on 3p25. More than 50% of all lung cancers contain a mutation of the *p53* tumor-suppressor gene. A *ras* family oncogene is mutated in about 20% of non-SCLC cases, but not in SCLC.

Various tumor markers can be used to assess prognosis. Elevated levels of CA-125, expression of blood group antigen A in tumor cells, expression on tumor cells of the carbohydrate antigen H/Le^y/Le^b, activation of the K-*ras* oncogene, and increased expression of p186*neu* have all been associated with poorer prognosis of patients with lung cancer.

70. Which tests are used for the evaluation of lung cancer?

The primary evaluation should include a chest x-ray and sputum cytology. If the expectorated sputum cytology is negative, bronchoscopy with biopsy or percutaneous biopsy may be done. Preoperative evaluation includes CT scanning of the chest and upper abdomen to evaluate for mediastinal and hilar nodes and for liver and/or adrenal metastases. Routine hematology and biochemical tests suggest the presence of bone marrow or liver metastases, and screening for the presence of brain metastases can be done using CT or MRI. Elevated alkaline phosphatase suggests bony metastases if the liver CT is normal, and a bone scan should be done. Pulmonary function tests and mediastinoscopy should be done if surgical resection is considered.

71. What are the 5-year survival rates for the different pathologic types of lung cancer?

Survival in Lung Cancer

HISTOLOGICAL TYPE	5-YEAR SURVIVAL	
	ALL CASES	RESECTABLE
Epidermoid carcinoma	11%	30%
Adenocarcinoma	5	17
Large cell carcinoma	4	15
Small cell carcinoma (oat cell)	1	5

72. Which paraneoplastic syndromes are associated with lung cancer?

Paraneoplastic Syndromes in Lung Cancer

1. Systemic symptoms
   Anorexia-cachexia (31%)
   Fever (21%)
   Suppressed immunity
2. Endocrine (12%)
   Ectopic PTH: hypercalcemia (epidermoid)
   SIADH (SCLC)
   Ectopic secretion of ACTH: Cushing's syndrome (SCLC)
3. Skeletal
   Clubbing (29%)
   Hypertrophic pulmonary osteoarthropathy: periostitis (1–10%) (adenocarcinima)
4. Coagulation-thrombotic
   Migratory thrombophlebitis, Trousseau's syndrome: venous thrombosis
   Nonbacterial thrombotic endocarditis: arterial emboli; DIC: hemorrhage
5. Neurologic-myopathic
   Lambert-Eaton syndrome (SCLC)
   Peripheral neuropathy
   Subacute cerebellar degeneration
   Cortical degeneration
   Polymyositis
   Retinal blindness
6. Cutaneous
   Dermatomyositis
   Acanthosis nigricans
7. Hematologic (8%)
   Anemia
   Granulocytosis
   Leukoerythroblastosis
8. Renal (<1%)
   Nephrotic syndrome
   Glomerulonephritis

Cohen MH: Signs and symptoms of bronchogenic carcinoma. In Straus, MJ (ed): Lung Cancer Clinical diagnosis and treatment. Grune & Stratton, New York, 1977, pp 85–94.

73. Describe the TNM staging system for lung cancer.

TNM Classification for Lung Cancer

Tumor
T1	≤3 cm
T2	>3 cm; visceral pleura invasion
T3	Direct extension to chest wall, mediastinal pleura, or pericardium
T4	Malignant pleural effusion, superior vena cava syndrome, or involvement of the heart, great vessels, trachea, esophagus, or vertebral bodies

Nodes
N0	Negative regional lymph nodes
N1	Peribronchial or ipsilateral hilar nodes
N2	Ipsilateral mediastinal nodes
N3	Contralateral hilar or mediastinal nodes; any supraclavicular nodes

Metastasis (M)
M0	No distant metastases
M1	Distant metastases

Comparison of Lung Cancer Staging Systems

PREVIOUS AJC SYSTEM		NEW INTERNATIONAL SYSTEM			
STAGE	TNM	STAGE	TNM	MEDIAN SURVIVAL (MOS)	FIVE-YEAR SURVIVAL (%)
I	T1 N0 M0	I	T1 N0 M0	48	48
	T2 N0 M0		T2 N0 M0		
	T1 N1 M0				
II	T2N1M0	II	T1 N1 M0	20	28
			T2 N1 M0		
III-M0	T3 (any N)	IIIA	T1–3 N2 M0	12	12
			T3 N0 M0		
			T3 N1 M0		
	N2 (any T)	IIIB	N3 (any T) M0	9	3
	M0		T4 (any N) M0		
III-M1	Any T or N M1	IV	M1 (any T or N)	5	2

From: Rubenstein E, Federman DD (eds): Scientific American Medicine. New York, Scientific American, 1994, p 12:VI:13; with permission.

An international TNM system is used in the clinical evaluation of lung cancer. Staging is significant in determining prognosis and treatment. The new four-stage system attempts to unify the various systems in use throughout the world and to correct deficiencies in the older American Joint Commission (AJC) system.

Note that in SCLC, a simpler staging system is sometimes used:

Limited: Disease confined to one hemithorax with or without ipsilateral supraclavicular, hilar, and mediastinal lymphadenopathy.

Extensive: Anything beyond limited disease. Includes recurrent disease, wherever the location.

74. Which drugs and other treatment modalities are used to manage SCLC?

Because of early hematogenous spread and because 40% of patients present with limited unresectable Stage III disease, **chemotherapy** (CAVVP—cyclophosphamide, doxorubicin [Adriamycin], vincristine, etoposide [VP-16], and cisplatin) and **radiotherapy** are used. These combinations have resulted in complete remission rates of 40–60%, median survival of 14–18 months, and 2-year survivals of 10–20%. Radiotherapy to the brain remains somewhat controversial, and timing, dose, and long-term complications continue to be argued. **Hematopoietic growth factors,** such as G-CSF, GM-CSF, and IL-3, have been added to some regimens in an effort to give higher doses and prevent the development of resistance.

75. How effective is the treatment of advanced Stage IV SCLC?

Approx. 15–20% of patients with limited disease survive 3 years, but few patients with extensive disease reach this point. The median survival for patients with extensive disease who respond to treatment is 7 months. For patients with limited disease, the median survival is 14 months.

76. What is the superior vena cava (SVC) syndrome? What is its significance in lung cancer?

SVC syndrome results when flow of blood in the SVC is obstructed due to thrombosis within the vessel or compression of the vein externally. Seventy-five to 85% of cases are due to compression by a tumor, with lung cancer, especially SCLC, accounting for up to 80% of these. Lymphoma and other mediastinal malignancies account for the remaining cases.

Although obstruction of the vena cava has been considered a life-threatening **oncologic emergency,** only rarely does it progress to cause laryngeal edema, seizures, coma, and death. Usually, patients present with dyspnea, facial edema and a sense of fullness in the head, and cough. Collateral circulation often develops, leading to the finding of prominent veins over the neck and chest and limiting the severity of symptoms.

Abner A: Approach to the patient who presents with SVC obstruction. Chest 103:39-45, 1993.

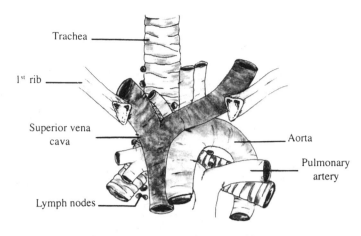

Trachea

1ˢᵗ rib

Superior vena
cava

Aorta

Pulmonary
artery

Lymph nodes

Anatomy of the superior vena cava

From Wood ME, Bunn PA Jr: Hematology/Oncology Secrets. Philadelphia, Hanley & Belfus, 1994, p 240; with permission.

77. How is non-small cell lung cancer treated?

The first decision to be made is whether the patient is a candidate for resection. If the patient is medically able to undergo resection, then it should be performed only if the following are *not* present:

1. Distant metastases
2. Pleural effusion
3. Superior vena cava obstruction
4. Involvement of supraclavicular, cervical, or contralateral mediastinal nodes
5. Recurrent laryngeal nerve paralysis
6. Involvement of the tracheal wall or mainstem bronchus < 2 cm from carina
7. Small cell carcinoma histology

Recent evidence suggests that in Stage IIIA disease (large tumor or involvement of mediastinal nodes), preoperative chemotherapy significantly improves survival. If patients are not able to undergo surgery and they do not have small cell cancer, then radiotherapy is indicated. The only contraindication is the presence of such bulky disease that treatment would compromise remaining lung tissue.

78. What are the acute and long-term complications of chemotherapy and radiotherapy used in the treatment of lung cancer?

Acute	Long term
Tumor lysis syndrome	Neurologic damage with resultant:
Myelosuppression predisposing to:	Confusion
Infection	Episodic hemiparesis
Bleeding	Ataxia
Hemorrhagic cystitis (cyclophosphamide)	Progressive organic brain syndrome
Cardiotoxicity (doxorubicin)	Leukemia
Renal toxicity (cisplatin)	Second primary carcinomas and sarcomas
Peripheral neuropathy (cisplatin,	Pulmonary fibrosis
vincristine)	Constrictive pericarditis
Radiation pneumonitis	

HEAD AND NECK CANCERS

79. What are the presenting symptoms of head and neck cancer?

Presenting Signs and Symptoms of Head and Neck Cancer by Site

SITE	SYMPTOMS/SIGNS
Oral cavity: lips, buccal mucosa, alveolar ridge, retromolar trigone, floor of mouth, hard palate, anterior 2/3 of tongue	Mass, ulcer, leukoplakia, bleeding, pain, loose teeth, earache, trismus, halitosis
Larynx: supraglottic (false cords, arytenoid), glottic (true vocal cords), subglottic	Hoarseness, bleeding, sore throat, thyroid cartilage pain
Pharynx: nasopharynx, oropharynx, soft palate, uvula, tonsil, base of tongue, hypopharynx, pyriform sinus	Sore throat, earache, epistaxis, nasal voice, dysphagia, masses, hearing loss, blood-streaked saliva
Maxillary sinus	Sinusitis, epistaxis, headache
All sites	Bleeding (oral or nasal), neck nodes, pain at site of tumor or referred pain

80. What are the risk factors for squamous cell cancer of the head and neck area?

Tobacco use is the most significant contributing factor to the development of head and neck cancers. Nine of 10 patients with cancer in this area are smokers. Snuff dipping and tobacco chewing are also causally related to the development of oral cancer. Smokers have an increased mortality related to head and neck cancer once it has been diagnosed, showing a 2-fold increase in mortality over nonsmokers.

Alcohol is also strongly correlated with the development of head and neck cancer. About half of the patients with these cancers have cirrhosis, and three-quarters drink alcohol excessively.

Another factor is poor dental hygiene. Woodworkers have an increased incidence of nasopharyngeal cancer. Syphilitic glossitis predisposes to tongue cancer, and nickel compounds to nasal sinus cancer. The Epstein-Barr and Herpes simplex type I viruses have been implicated in up to 15% of new cases.

81. Describe the evaluation and initial staging of patients with head and neck cancer.

Initial staging of head and neck cancer includes a thorough **triple endoscopy** of upper and lower airway and upper aerodigestive tract, with biopsy of any suspicious lesions. Measurement and biopsy, if indicated, of any cervical or supraclavicular nodes should be performed. A **CT scan** of the area contributes to the determination of the extent of disease. If elements of the routine blood counts and biochemical profile are abnormal, a **bone scan** and/or **liver scan** may be done. If there is a history of alcohol abuse, liver scans in the face of abnormal liver function tests are usually only useful if there is hepatomegaly.

The most common sites of metastases of these tumors are local lymphatics, followed by lung metastases. Bone metastases occur in about 15% of the patients. Brain metastases are rare and are seen mainly in those patients with nasopharyngeal cancer. It is also important to remember that second primaries in the lung are not uncommon. Depending on the tobacco and alcohol history, another cancer, usually of the esophagus or lung, may be seen in up to 20% of patients at some time in the course of their disease.

82. Currently, what is the most appropriate treatment of head and neck cancer?

Traditionally, head and neck cancers have been treated primarily with surgery, usually involving extensive and radical dissection and often accompanied by postoperative radiotherapy. Radiotherapy also was used for recurrences that were no longer amenable to surgery. However, the current trend is to treat with **multimodality therapy,** using chemotherapy, either in combination with radiotherapy or prior to surgery or radiotherapy. The optimum combination of these agents and modalities has not yet been determined, and trials are ongoing. One problem is that the natural history of these tumors is quite divergent, meaning that results will vary depending on the patient mix. Stopping smoking and alcohol consumption, combined with the use of retinoic acid derivatives, may help prevent occurrences of second primary cancers in the head and neck region.

83. Which chemotherapeutic agents are used in the treatment of squamous cell cancers of the head and neck? How effective are they?

Several agents are effective, and include methotrexate, bleomycin, cisplatin, carboplatin, paclitaxel, mitomycin C, and 5-fluorouracil. Response rates for these agents vary from 25–80%, depending on the agent, schedule, tumor type, previous treatment, and performance status. Combination chemotherapy regimens usually show higher initial response rates but have yet to show an increase in survival rates.

BREAST CANCER

84. What are the current recommendations for screening for breast cancer?

Currently, several sets of recommendations are available from the various specialty organizations whose members are engaged in breast cancer screening. These are as follows:

Recommended Frequency of Screening for Breast Cancer

ORGANIZATION	AGE >50		AGE <50	
	MAMMOGRAM	BREAST EXAM	MAMMOGRAM	BREAST EXAM
American Cancer Society	Annual	Annual	Age 35–40, baseline Age 40–50, every 1–2 yrs	Age 40–50, annual Age 20–40, every 3 yrs
National Cancer Institute	Annual	With every periodic physical exam	Starting at age 40, every 1–2 yrs*	With every periodic exam
American Coll. of Obstetricians and Gynecologists	As determined by woman's doctor		Age 35–50, baseline*	Age 35–50, exams recommended
American College of Radiology	Annual	Annual	<40 yrs, baseline Then every 1–2 yrs as determined by doctor	—
American College of Physicians	Age 50–59, on "routine" basis Age ≥ 60, as determined by doctor and patient	—	Not recommended	—
U.S. Preventive Services Task Force	Annual	Annual	Not recommended	Age 40–50, annual

*Mammography recommended more frequently for women with high risk factors.

In addition, it is important for the physician to identify high-risk patients who may have a mutation in a dominant breast cancer susceptibility gene. Such families have a history of breast or ovarian cancer in as many as half of all female relatives, with early age of onset and/or bilateral or multifocal disease. These patients have been shown to have a high incidence of the *BRCA*1 and *BRCA*2 genes on chromosome 17 and 13, respectively. Their cumulative lifetime risk of breast cancer ranges up to 87%.

85. How is the diagnosis of breast cancer established?

By tissue examination. Tissue may be obtained by percutaneous fine-needle aspiration, with or without x-ray direction, or by incisional or excisional biopsy. While mammograms are essential in screening and localizing tumors, up to 15% of breast cancers may not be seen on mammograms, and the diagnosis cannot be made definitively without tissue confirmation. Any clinically suspicious mass must be biopsied.

86. At what age does the incidence of breast cancer peak?

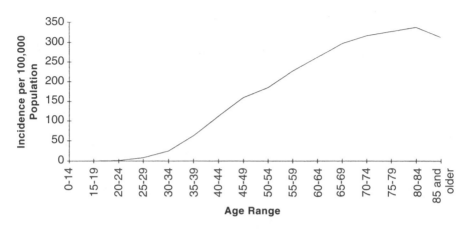

Annual age-specific incidence of breast cancer, 1983–1985. (Modified from Eddy DM: Screening for breast cancer. Ann Intern Med 111:389–399, 1989.)

87. What are the risk factors for breast cancer?

High risk factors (associated with a 3x or more increase)
- a. Age (> 40 years old)
- b. Previous cancer in one breast
- c. Breast cancer in a first- or second-degree family member
- d. Gross cystic disease, multiple papillomatosis, and atypical hyperplasia, probably only if associated with family history
- e. Parity: Nulliparous or first pregnancy after age 31 years
- f. Lobular carcinoma in situ

Intermediate risk (1.2 to 1.5x risk)
- a. Early menarche and/or late menopause
- b. Oral estrogens
- c. History of cancer of ovary, uterus, or colon
- d. Alcoholic beverages (?)

88. Which factors confer a poor prognosis in primary breast cancer?

1. Estrogen receptor-negative tumor
2. Positive HER-2/*neu* oncogene
3. Premenopausal patient
4. Large tumor size
5. Positive lymph nodes
6. Local skin involvement
7. Fixed axillary nodes
8. Distant metastasis
9. *BRCA*1 or *BRCA*2 markers
10. Aneuploidy and high cathepsin D
11. Nuclear grade 3 (poor)
12. High S-phase fraction

89. Describe the appropriate treatment of local-regional breast cancer.

Although there is no single "right" way to treat localized breast cancer, and a great deal of controversy exists, the following guidelines are available:

Stage I—Lumpectomy with axillary dissection and radiation, or modified radical mastectomy. **Modified radical mastectomy** is used if cosmesis is not important, lesion size is large relative to breast size, or radiotherapy is not technically possible. **Lumpectomy/radiotherapy** is used if cosmesis is important, complete excision is possible, and >6000 rads can be delivered to the tumor bed.

Stage II—Modified radical mastectomy with postoperative chemotherapy for patients with positive nodes. The benefit of chemotherapy in node-negative patients is not clear at present. The value of postoperative hormonal therapy in postmenopausal patients is also being explored.

Stage III—Preoperative radiation, possibly with chemotherapy or hormonal therapy, followed by modified radical mastectomy and then chemotherapy. Or simple mastectomy with postoperative radiotherapy and/or chemotherapy or hormonal therapy

Stage IV—Systemic chemotherapy or hormone therapy, reserving surgery and radiotherapy for local control.

90. How is adjuvant therapy used in the management of breast cancer?

Current Recommendations for the Use of Adjuvant Systemic Therapy in Breast Cancer[*]

	PREMENOPAUSAL	POSTMENOPAUSAL
Node-positive:		
ER-negative	CMF × 6 mos	CMF × 6 mos
ER-positive	CMF × 6 mos	Tamoxifen × 2–5 yrs
Node-negative:		
ER-negative	None, or CMF × 6 mos[*]	None, or CMF × 6 mos[*]
ER-positive	None, or CMF × 6 mos[*]	None, or CMF × 6 mos + tamoxifen

[*]Adjuvant treatment recommended for poor-prognosis tumors (large tumor size, poor nuclear grade, high S phase fraction). ER = estrogen receptor; CMF = cyclophosphamide, methotrexate, 5-fluorouracil.

The National Cancer Institute study that was conducted between 1979 and 1987 now has a median follow-up of 10 years and shows that in the management of stage I and II breast cancer, breast conservation with lumpectomy and radiation offers results at 10 years that are equivalent to those with mastectomy.

The Bonadonna study, begun in 1973, now has an almost 20-year median follow-up of women who received adjuvant combination chemotherapy with CMF following radical mastectomy for breast cancer with histologically positive axillary nodes. Long-term results show that those who received therapy had an adjusted relative risk of relapse-free survival of 0.65 and a total survival of 0.76 as compared with controls. Benefit from adjuvant therapy was evident in all subgroups of patients except postmenopausal women.

Jacobson JA, et al: Ten-year results of a comparison of conservation with mastectomy in the treatment of stage I and II breast cancer. N Engl J Med 332:907–911, 1995.

Bonadonna G, et al: Adjuvant cyclophosphamide, methotrexate, fluorouracil in node-positive breast cancer. N Engl J Med 332:901–906, 1995.

91. Which agents are used in the treatment of metastatic breast cancer? How effective are they?

The most commonly used agents with clinical activity in breast cancer are doxorubicin, epirubicin, cyclophosphamide, methotrexate, fluorouracil, vinorelbine, paclitaxel (Taxol), and prednisone. Various combinations of these agents are used in the treatment of advanced or metastatic breast cancer.

Overall induction response rates range from 55–65%. Median survival times are 14–18 months. The survival rates, however, depend more on the site of the metastatic disease than on the treatment, with visceral disease faring more poorly than bony or soft-tissue metastases. Most patients receive more than one treatment regimen, since the median time to failure of most programs is about 6 months.

GYNECOLOGIC CANCERS

92. What are the current recommendations for screening for carcinoma of the cervix?

Recommendations concerning periodic screening of women in the U.S. using Pap smears have been developed for the various risk groups. **Low-risk** groups are those women who have never had sexual activity, have had a hysterectomy for nonmalignant reasons, or have reached the age of 60 and have never had a positive Pap smear. **High-risk** patients are those who are sexually active early, have had many partners, or are in low socioeconomic groups.

The American Cancer Society recommends that asymptomatic women over age 18 years and those under age 18 years who are sexually active have annual screening for at least 3 years. Following this, some suggest at least one screening every 3 years until age 65, while others suggest yearly screening as long as the patient is sexually active. High-risk patients should be screened yearly.

93. What is the appropriate management of a patient with an abnormal Pap smear?

An abnormal Pap smear should lead to colposcopy and/or biopsy. If **carcinoma in situ** or **dysplasia** is found, cryotherapy, laser therapy, cone biopsy, or hysterectomy should be performed, depending on the size and extent of the lesion.

If **invasive cancer** is found on biopsy, a metastatic workup is indicated. Stage I disease is treated with radical hysterectomy or radiation therapy, whereas all other stages are further evaluated with a CT scan. If the para-aortic nodes are enlarged, a needle biopsy should be done. Those with a positive biopsy are treated with pelvic radiation therapy and chemotherapy and/or radiation therapy to para-aortic nodes. If nodes are normal on the CT scan or if the needle biopsy is negative, then laparotomy with para-aortic node biopsies should be considered to determine the actual state of the nodes. If the biopsy is positive, then treatment should proceed as for other positive-node biopsies. If the biopsy is negative, treatment is radiotherapy with two intracavitary radium implants.

94. Which studies are used in the staging of carcinoma of the cervix?

Pelvic exam	Barium enema, for advanced stage, or age
Biochemical profile	> 40 years
Chest x-ray	CT scan, to evaluate retroperitoneal nodes, or
Cystoscopy	for planning radiotherapy of bulky lesions
Proctosigmoidoscopy	Lymphangiograms in selected cases
Intravenous pyelogram (IVP)	MRI in selected cases

95. What are the 5-year survival rates, relative to stage, for carcinoma of the cervix?

Stage	Description	5-Year Survival
I	Tumor confined to the cervix	80%
II	Tumor extends beyond cervix but has not extended onto pelvic wall. Tumor involves vagina but not lower third	55–60%
III	Tumor extends to pelvic wall Tumor involves lower third of vagina All cases with hydronephrosis or nonfunctioning kidney (unless known to be due to another cause)	32–32%
IV	Tumor extends beyond true pelvis or has involved bladder or rectal mucosa	8–10%

96. How is carcinoma of the cervix treated?

Stage	Treatment
IA	Simple hysterectomy or intracavitary radiation
IB, IIA	Radical abdominal hysterectomy with pelvic lymphadenectomy or radiation therapy
IIB, III	Radiation therapy
IVA	Pelvic exenteration plus radiation
IVB	Chemotherapy

97. Name the risk factors for carcinoma of the endometrium.

1. Infertility
2. Obesity
3. Failure of ovulation
4. Dysfunctional bleeding
5. Prolonged estrogen use
6. Diabetes mellitus
7. Hypertension
8. Polycystic ovaries
9. Familial cancer syndrome (Lynch)

98. What are the 5-year survival rates for the various grades and stages of endometrial cancer?

Grades and Stages of Endometrial Cancer

	DESCRIPTION	5-YEAR SURVIVAL
Grade		
I	Differentiated	81%
II	Intermediate	74%
III	Undifferentiated	50%
Stage		
I	Tumor confined to corpus	70%
II	Tumor involves corpus and cervix	47%
III	Tumor extends outside corpus, but not outside true pelvis (may involve vaginal wall or parametrium but not bladder or rectum)	28%
IV	Tumor involves bladder or rectum or extends outside pelvis	5%

99. Name the risk factors for ovarian cancer.
- Nulliparity or low parity
- Presence of basal cell nevus syndrome
- Family history of ovarian cancer or ovarian cancer syndromes
- Gonadal dysgenesis (46XY type)
- History of breast, endometrial, or colon cancer
- Asbestos exposure
- Presence of Peutz-Jeghers syndrome
- Use of fertility drugs (?)

NIH Consensus Development Panel on Ovarian Cancer: Ovarian cancer: Screening, treatment and follow-up. JAMA 273:491–497, 1995.

100. What is the appropriate use of the CA-125 antigen?
CA-125 serum tumor marker is an antigenic determinant detected by radioimmunoassay and is elevated in 80% of epithelial ovarian cancers. Because it is elevated in only half of patients with stage I cancers and is elevated in a significant proportion of healthy women and women with benign disease, it is not a sensitive or specific screening test. In high-risk patients or patients suspected of having an ovarian cancer, it should be used in conjunction with bimanual rectovaginal pelvic examination and transvaginal ultrasonography. It is also useful as a marker of disease recurrence after surgical resection of ovarian cancer.

101. List the paraneoplastic syndromes associated with ovarian cancer.

1. Neurologic
   Peripheral neuropathy
   Organic brain syndrome
   AML-like syndrome
   Cerebellar ataxia
2. Cross-matching of blood antigens
3. Cushing's syndrome
4. Hypercalcemia
5. Thrombophlebitis

102. What are the 5-year survival rates for the various stages of carcinoma of the ovary?

Stage	Description	5-Year Survial
I	Growth limited to ovaries	50–70%
II	Growth involving 1 or 2 ovaries with pelvic extension	40–50%
III	Tumor involving ovaries with peritoneal implants outside pelvis and/or positive retroperitoneal or inguinal nodes	10–15%
	Patients with superficial liver metastases	
	Tumors limited to true pelvis but with histologically verified malignant extension to small bowel or omentum	
IV	Tumor involving ovaries with distant metastases	3–5%

103. What is the treatment for advanced stage ovarian cancer?

Patients with stage III and IV epithelial ovarian cancers are treated with regimens including cyclophosphamide combined with cisplatin or carboplatin, or cisplatin combined with paclitaxel (Taxol). Clinical response rates are approx. 60–70%, with 5-year survivals of 10–20%.

104. What is a molar pregnancy?

Molar pregnancies refer to a group of benign and malignant gestational trophoblastic neoplasms. The most malignant of these is choriocarcinoma, which was fatal within 1–2 years prior to the advent of chemotherapy. The most common variant, hydatidiform mole, occurs in only 1 in 2000 pregnancies in the U.S.

LYMPHOMAS

105. What are some unusual epidemiologic features of Hodgkin's disease?

The epidemiology of Hodgkin's disease is scientifically intriguing, suggesting an infective agent. It occurs more frequently in individuals from small families and in children raised in hygienic, isolated environments. Reports of epidemics of Hodgkin's disease in neighborhoods and among school classes are not completely convincing. Genetic predisposition, as well as infective agents, could explain the increased incidence in some families. Hodgkin's disease is more common in some tropical countries and in the Middle East in children < 10 years old.

106. Which are the "favorable" lymphomas?

The low-grade (or "favorable") lymphomas of the Rappaport classification are:
Diffuse, well-differentiated lymphocytic
Nodular, poorly differentiated lymphocytic
Nodular, mixed lymphocytic-histiocytic
They are described as favorable because their natural history is characterized by a relatively long survival, indolent course, and easy response to minimal therapy.

107. Which are the "unfavorable" lymphomas? What is their prognosis?

The unfavorable, or high-grade, non-Hodgkin's lymphomas are:
Large cell immunoblastic
Lymphoblastic
Burkitt's
All the other types (nodular histiocytic, diffuse poorly differentiated lymphocytic, diffuse mixed lymphocytic and histiocytic, and diffuse large cell) are called intermediate grade, as their aggressiveness and responsiveness to treatment are intermediate between the other two groups. CNS lymphomas and lymphomas associated with HIV infection are particularly difficult to treat, the latter due to the immunocompromised status of the host.

108. Which three cytogenetic abnormalities are associated with lymphomas?

Three recurrent chromosomal aberrations have been found to correlate with certain histologic types of lymphoma:

1. A translocation between chromosome 18 and 14 is found in 85% of patients with follicular lymphoma (small cleaved cell, mixed cell, and large cell). If, in addition, a deletion 13q32 is found, these patients have an accelerated course and a leukemic phase.

2. A translocation between chromosomes 8 and 14 is found in 85% of patients with small non-cleaved cell (Burkitt's or non-Burkitt's) lymphoma. The remaining 15% of patients have 2:8 or 8:22 translocations. These three translocations place the c-*myc* oncogene on chromosome 8, next to the immunoglobulin heavy-chain (chromosome 14) or light-chain (chromosomes 2 and 22) genes.

3. A trisomy 12 in patients with small-cell lymphocytic lymphoma, more commonly seen in chronic lymphocytic leukemia.

109. How are lymphomas staged?

Stage I—Single node region or single extranodal site
Stage II—Two or more node regions, same side of diaphragm

Stage III—Nodal disease above and below diaphragm
Stage IV—Disseminated extranodal disease
Additional designations:
S   Splenic involvement
E   Localized extranodal involvement
A   Absence of constitutional symptoms
B   Presence of ≥ 10% weight loss in preceding 6 months, fever, and/or night sweats
CS   Clinical stage
PS   Pathologic stage

110. How does the natural history of Hodgkin's disease compare with that of the non-Hodgkin's lymphomas?

	Hodgkin's Disease	*Non-Hodgkin's Lymphomas*
Age	Bimodal: 5–34 and >50 yrs	Median age 50 yrs
Symptoms	B symptoms are more common in older age and higher state; in mixed cellularity and lymphocyte depleted, may have severe symptoms with minimal nodes	< 0% have B symptoms
Signs		
Nodes	Seen in > 90% at presentation	Least common in histiocytic type
Waldeyer's	Uncommon	30% in some series
Cervical	65%	10–20%
Mediastinal	10%	2–3%
Abdominal	Retroperitoneal	Mesenteric
Extranodal	3%	Up to 60% in histiocytic
GI	4%	20–40%
CNS	Uncommon except in immunocompromised	Common, esp. lymphocytic
Pleural effusion	From obstruction due to mediastinal nodes	Chylous

111. What are the 5-year survival rates relative to grade of the non-Hodgkin's lymphomas?

Grade	*5-Year Survival*
Small lymphocytic	59%
Follicular, small cleaved	70%
Follicular mixed	50%
Follicular, large cell	45%
Diffuse, mixed small and large cell	38%
Diffuse, large cell	35%
Immunoblastic	32%
Lymphoblastic	26%
Small, noncleaved cell	23%

BIBLIOGRAPHY

1. Beahrs O, Hensen DE, Hutter RVP, Myers MH (eds): Manual for Staging of Cancer, 4th ed. Philadelphia, J.B. Lippincott, 1992.
2. Calabresi P, Schein PS, Rosenberg SA (eds): Basic Principles and Clinical Management of Cancer, 2nd ed. New York, McGraw-Hill, 1993.
3. Casciato DA, Lowitz BB (eds): Manual of Clinical Oncology, 3rd ed. Boston, Little, Brown, 1995.
4. DeVita T Jr, Hellman S, Rosenberg SA (eds): Cancer: Principles and Practice of Oncology, 4th ed. Philadelphia, J.B. Lippincott, 1993.
5. Haskell CM: Cancer Treatment, 4th ed. Philadelphia, W.B. Saunders Co., 1995.
6. Moossa AR, Schimpff SC, Robson MC (eds): Comprehensive Textbook of Oncology, 2nd ed. Baltimore, Williams & Wilkins, 1991.
7. Tannock IF, Hill RP (eds): The Basic Science of Oncology, 2nd ed. New York, McGraw-Hill, 1992.
8. Wood ME, Bunn PA Jr (eds): Hematology/Oncology Secrets. Philadelphia, Hanley & Belfus, 1994.

7. NEPHROLOGY

Sharma Prabhakar, M.D.

Bones can break, muscles can atrophy, glands can loaf, even the brain can go to sleep without immediately endangering our survival; but should the kidneys fail . . . neither bone, muscle, gland nor brain could carry on.

Homer W. Smith (1895–1962)
From Fish to Philosopher, Ch. 1

Too much attention has been paid to the excretory offices of the kidney to the neglect of its conservative services.

John P. Peters
Yale Journal of Biology & Medicine, 1953

ASSESSMENT OF RENAL FUNCTION

1. What is the glomerular filtration rate?

Glomerular filtrate is the ultrafiltrate of plasma that exits the glomerular capillary tuft and enters the Bowman's capsule to begin the journey along the tubule of the nephron. It is the initial step in the formation of urine. The volume of this filtrate formed per unit time is called the **glomerular filtration rate** (GFR) and is usually expressed in ml/min.

2. How is the GFR measured clinically? Describe the rationale.

The GFR is measured indirectly with a marker substance contained in glomerular filtrate, which is then excreted in the urine. The amount of this substance leaving the kidney (urinary mass excretion) must equal the amount of marker substance entering the kidney as glomerular filtrate; it must not be reabsorbed, secreted, or metabolized after entering the kidney tubule. Then, the volume of glomerular filtrate, represented by the urinary mass excretion of the marker substance, can be calculated by dividing the urinary mass excretion of the marker substance by the concentration of the substance in the glomerular filtrate.

The marker substance is chosen so that its concentration in the glomerular filtrate is equal to its concentration in the plasma, i.e., the substance is freely filterable across the glomerular capillary. Therefore, the amount of substance X entering the kidney equals the GFR multiplied by the plasma concentration of the substance (P_X). Likewise, the amount of the substance leaving the kidney in the urine equals the urinary concentration of the substance (U_X) multiplied by the urine flow in ml/min (V). Therefore, the formula for calculating GFR using our marker substance X becomes:

$$GFR \times P_X = U_X \times V$$

or

$$GFR = \frac{U_X \times V}{P_X}$$

A stable plasma concentration of the substance (steady-state situation) is required to make the above equation useful.

3. Name two marker substances used to measure GFR.

The polysaccharide **inulin** is often used in laboratory determinations of GFR. However, it requires constant intravenous infusion, making it somewhat impractical for routine clinical use in patients. **Creatinine** is used as a marker substance in clinical settings.

4. Why is creatinine used as a marker substance for GFR determinations in clinical settings?

Creatinine is an endogenous substance, derived from the metabolism of creatine in skeletal muscle, that fulfills almost all of the requirements for a marker substance: it is freely filterable, not metabolized, and not reabsorbed once filtered. There is a small amount of tubular secretion that makes the creatinine clearance a slight overestimate of the GFR, but this overestimate becomes quantitatively important only at low levels of GFR.

Creatinine is released from muscle at a constant rate, resulting in a stable plasma concentration. The creatinine clearance is commonly determined from a 24-hour collection of urine. This time period is used to average out the sometimes variable creatinine excretion that may occur hour to hour. Creatinine is easily measured, making it a nearly ideal marker for GFR determination.

5. Can the completeness of a 24-hour urine collection be judged?

Since total creatinine excretion in the steady state is dependent on muscle mass, day-to-day creatinine excretion remains fairly constant for an individual and is related to lean body weight. In general, men excrete 20–25 mg creatinine/kg body weight/day, whereas women excrete 15–20 mg/kg/day. Therefore, a 70–kg man excretes ~1400 mg creatinine/day. Creatinine excretion levels measured on a 24-hour urine collection that are substantially less than the estimated value suggest an incomplete collection.

6. What is the relationship between the plasma creatinine concentration and GFR?

Because creatinine production and excretion remain constant and equal, the amount of creatinine entering and leaving the kidney remains constant. Thus:

$$GFR \times P_{Cr} = U_{Cr} \times V = constant$$

or

$$GFR = \frac{1}{P_{Cr}} \times constant$$

Creatinine excretion remains constant as GFR declines until the GFR reaches very low levels. Therefore, the GFR is a function of the reciprocal of the plasma creatinine concentration.

7. Does a given plasma creatinine concentration reflect the same level of renal function in different patients?

Not necessarily. Remember that creatinine production is directly proportional to muscle mass, and that the plasma creatinine concentration (P_{Cr}) is determined in part by creatinine production. Examination of the creatinine clearance (CrCl) for an 80-kg man compared to that of a 40-kg woman, assuming both individuals have P_{Cr} of 1.0 mg/dl (0.01 mg/m) shows the following:

For the 80-kg man, creatinine excretion should be:

$$80 \text{ kg} \times 20 \text{ mg/kg/day} = 1600 \text{ mg/day} = 1.11 \text{ mg/min}$$

$$GFR = \frac{1.11 \text{ mg/min}}{0.01 \text{ mg/ml}} = 1.11 \text{ ml/min}$$

For the 40-kg woman, creatinine excretion should be:

$$40 \text{ kg} \times 15 \text{ mg/kg/day} = 600 \text{ mg/day} = 0.42 \text{ mg/min}$$

$$GFR = \frac{0.42 \text{ mg/min}}{0.01 \text{ mg/ml}} = 42 \text{ ml/min}$$

This demonstrates that the same P_{Cr} can represent markedly different GFRs in different individuals. The difference in creatinine excretion is related to differences in muscle mass, which are related to lean body weight and age. The following formula was devised to provide a rough estimate of the GFR in situations where a measured CrCl is not immediately available:

$$CrCl = \frac{140 - Age \times Lean\ body\ wt\ (in\ kg)}{P_c \times 72}$$

If we use this formula to estimate the GFR of the above individuals and assume an age of 50 years for each, we get a GFR of 100 for the man and 50 for the woman. These estimates are in the range of those determined previously and serve to illustrate the relative differences in the GFR calculated for two individuals with the same P_{Cr}. Recognizing this fact and using this formula to estimate GFR could prevent a serious error when selecting the dose of a drug that is excreted by the kidneys.

8. How does the blood urea nitrogen (BUN) relate to the GFR?

BUN is excreted primarily by glomerular filtration. Its level in the plasma tends to vary inversely with GFR. BUN, however, is a much less ideal marker of GFR than is creatinine. Its production may not be constant, in that it varies with protein intake, liver function, and catabolic rate. In addition, urea can be reabsorbed once filtered into the kidney, and this reabsorption increases in conditions with low urine flow, such as volume depletion. This latter circumstance is one cause of a high ($> 15:1$) BUN: creatinine ratio in plasma. Thus, creatinine is the better marker for GFR. But the plasma level of BUN can be used along with the CrCl to indicate the presence of certain states, such as volume depletion.

9. What is the difference between clearance and excretion?

Urinary **excretion** of a substance is simply the total amount of a substance excreted per unit time. It is usually expressed in mg/min. **Clearance** expresses the efficiency with which the kidney removes a substance from the plasma. It is the volume of plasma that would have to be completely cleared of a substance per unit time to account for the amount of that substance appearing in the urine per unit time. It is expressed in volume per unit time, usually ml/min.

For example, substance (X) having plasma concentration (P_x) of 1.0 mg/ml, urine concentration (U_x) of = 10 mg/ml, and urine flow (V) of 1.0 ml/min has the following clearance:

$$Cl_x = \frac{U_X}{P_X} \times V = \frac{10\ mg/ml \times 1\ ml/min}{1.0\ mg/min} = 10\ ml/min$$

The calculated clearance of 10 ml/min indicates that the amount of substance X appearing in the urine is the same as if 10 ml of plasma were completely cleared of the substance and excreted in the urine each minute. The urinary excretion of X is 10 mg/min, but this measurement does not indicate the efficiency with which the substance is removed from the plasma.

10. How does measurement of urinary protein excretion help in the evaluation of renal disease?

Normal urinary protein excretion is < 150 mg/day, with albumin constituting $< 50\%$ of this protein. Failure of the tubules to reabsorb the normally filtered small-MW proteins leads to **tubular proteinuria.** This occurs in diseases that affect tubular function, and the proteins are almost entirely of smaller MW rather than albumin.

Glomerular proteinuria occurs when the normal glomerular barrier to the passage of plasma proteins is disrupted. This results in variable quantities of albumin and sometimes larger MW proteins spilling into the urine.

Quantitatively, tubular proteinuria is usually < 1 g/24 hr, and glomerular proteinuria is usually > 1 g/24 hr. When the proteinuria is > 3.5 g/1.73 m^2 body surface area, it is said to be in the **nephrotic range.** Significant degrees of proteinuria (> 150 mg/day) usually indicate intrinsic renal disease. Quantification and characterization of the proteinuria is useful in detecting not only the presence of renal disease but also in determining involvement of the tubule, glomerulus, or both.

11. What information can be gained from examining urine sediment?

Urine sediment is normally almost cell-free, is usually crystal-free, and contains a very low concentration of protein ($< 1+$ by dipstick). Examination of this sediment is a very important part of the workup of any patient with renal disease. The examination should be performed by the physician prior to diagnostic or therapeutic decisions. The information obtained must be correlated with all other aspects of the patient's history, physical, and laboratory database. The examination can provide evidence of many conditions, including renal inflammation (cells, protein), infection (WBCs, bacteria), stone disease (crystals), and systemic diseases (bilirubin, myoglobin, hemoglobin, etc.).

ACUTE RENAL FAILURE

12. What is acute renal failure (ARF)?

ARF is a syndrome of many etiologies characterized by a sudden decrease in renal function leading to a compromise in the kidney's ability to regulate normal homeostasis. This inability is multifactorial. The kidney is unable to maintain the content and volume of the extracellular fluid or perform its routine endocrine functions. In most cases, ARF is a potentially reversible process.

13. Why is it important to distinguish acute from chronic renal failure (CRF)?

- The clinical manifestations of ARF are generally more severe than those associated with CRF.
- Unlike CRF, a cause for ARF can usually be identified and must be addressed to prevent further kidney or other organ damage.
- ARF is a potentially reversible disorder if the causative factor or factors are identified and corrected, and appropriate supportive care must be given to optimize the chances for recovery of renal function.

14. What is meant by oliguria?

Oliguria refers to a urine volume that is inadequate for the normal excretion of the body's metabolic waste products. Since the daily load of metabolic products amounts to approx. 600 mOsm and the maximal urine concentrating ability of the human kidney is about 1200 mOsm/kg H_2O, there is a minimal obligate urine volume of 500 ml/day for most individuals. Therefore, a 24-hour urine volume of < **500 ml/day** is said to represent oliguria. When associated with ARF, oliguria portends a poorer prognosis than does nonoliguric ARF.

15. What is anuria? Why is it important to distinguish it from oliguria?

Anuria refers to a 24-hour urine volume of < 100 ml. It denotes a severe reduction in urine volume that is commonly associated with obstruction, renal cortical necrosis, or severe acute tubular necrosis (ATN). It is important to make the distinction between oliguria and anuria so that these diagnostic entities will be considered and appropriate therapy planned.

16. Describe the diagnostic work-up for a patient with ARF.

From an etiological standpoint, ARF can be divided into three categories: prerenal, renal, and postrenal failure. This approach is important because pre- and postrenal causes of ARF can often be corrected rather quickly, and if corrected, further renal injury can frequently be avoided. Placement into the renal category should lead to a search for the agents, factors, or processes that may have resulted in acute renal injury, such as acute tubular necrosis. This approach not only aids in diagnosis but also leads to the appropriate therapy.

17. What are some common causes of ARF in the U.S.?

A. Prerenal
1. True volume depletion
   a. GI losses (vomiting, diarrhea, bleeding)
   b. Renal losses (diuretics, osmotic diuresis [glucose], hypoaldosteronism, salt-wasting nephropathy, diabetes insipidus)
   c. Skin or respiratory losses (insensible losses, sweat, burns)
   d. Third-space sequestration (intestinal obstruction, crush injury or skeletal fracture, acute pancreatitis)

2. Hypotension (shock)
3. Edematous states (heart failure, hepatic cirrhosis, nephrosis)
4. Selective renal ischemia (hepatorenal syndrome, NSAIDs, bilateral renal artery stenosis, calcium channel blockers)

B. Renal causes
1. Postischemic (all causes of severe prerenal disease, esp. particularly hypotension)
2. Nephrotoxins
   a. Drugs and exogenous toxins
      Common: Aminoglycoside antibiotics, radiocontrast media, cisplatin, NSAIDs
      Rare: Cephalosporins, rifampin, amphotericin B, polymyxin B, methoxyflurane, acetaminophen overdose, heavy metals (mercury, arsenic, uranium), carbon tetrachloride, EDTA, tetracyclines
   b. Heme pigments
      Rhabdomyolysis (myoglobinuria)
      Intravascular hemolysis (hemoglobinuria)

C. Postrenal causes
1. Obstruction due to strictures, stones, malignancies, prostatic enlargement

18. What is meant by prerenal failure?

This syndrome refers to a decrease in renal function resulting from a decrease in renal perfusion. The decrease in renal perfusion leads to functional changes within the kidney, which in turn compromise the kidney's ability to perform its homeostatic functions. This disorder is potentially correctable by addressing the factors leading to renal hypoperfusion. In severe cases, renal hypoperfusion can be severe enough and prolonged enough to result in structural damage, and hence lead to the "renal" category of ARF. Therefore, it is important that the prerenal syndrome be identified and corrected promptly.

19. What is acute tubular necrosis (ATN)?

ATN is a syndrome with multiple etiologies that is characterized by structural and functional damage of the renal tubules and a functional decrease of glomerular function. If the patient survives, ATN is self-limited, with most patients recovering renal function within 8 weeks. It is most commonly caused by ischemia, but there is a multitude of other causes.

20. How can the use of urinary indices help to distinguish prerenal failure from ATN?

Patients with prerenal azotemia have intact tubular function. The kidney, in this setting, is attempting to minimize solute and water excretion in an effort to preserve extracellular fluid volume. By contrast, the tubules of patients with ATN do not properly recover solutes and water that have been filtered into the kidney. Thus, the urine of patients with prerenal azotemia typically reveals:

1. Low urinary sodium concentration (< 20 meq/l)
2. Low fractional excretion of sodium ($< 1.0\%$)
3. Low free-water excretion (high urine osmolality > 500 and high urine specific gravity > 1.015).

By contrast, the urinary indices of patients with ATN reveal the kidney's relative inability to reabsorb sodium (urinary Na > 40 meq/l and fractional Na excretion of $> 3.0\%$) and to reabsorb water (urine osmolality < 350 mOsm/l and urine specific gravity < 1.010). Remember that there is considerable crossover between renal and prerenal failure with regard to these indices, and hence no value absolutely indicates one or the other diagnosis. The indices should be used along with other data (i.e., history, physical exam) to arrive at a clinical impression.

21. What is meant by the fractional excretion of sodium (FE_{Na+})? What is its relevance to the diagnosis of ARF?

FE_{Na}^+ is calculated by using the following equation:

$$FE_{Na}^+ = \frac{U_{Na}^+ \times P_{Cr} \times 100}{P_{Na}^+ \times U_{Cr}}$$

where U_{Na}^+ and P_{Na}^+ = urinary and plasma sodium concentrations (in meq/L) and U_{Cr} and P_{Cr} = urinary and plasma creatinine in mg/dl.

An FE_{Na}^+ value $< 1\%$ favors prerenal states, whereas a value $> 1\%$ indicates intrarenal states or ATN. The test is more accurate than urinary Na measurement in this differentiation. However, it should be noted that an $FE_{Na}^+ < 1\%$ is occasionally reported for various causes of ARF other than prerenal states.

It is also to be noted that an intact sodium reabsorptive capacity is necessary for the use of this test. Thus, in conditions such as underlying chronic renal disease, hypoaldosteronism, diuretic therapy, or metabolic alkalosis with bicarbonaturia, the FE_{Na}^+ will be inappropriately high despite the presence of volume depletion.

22. List the four classic phases of ARF.

- The **initial stage** is usually not recognized clinically and represents the period of exposure to the insult.
- The classic **oliguric phase** is characterized by oliguria, but patients in this phase are commonly nonoliguric. During this phase, the deterioration in renal function becomes evident.
- The **diuretic phase** is characterized by a gradual increase in urine volume, often to very high levels. It is thought to represent movement of filtrate through tubules which have yet to completely recover their absorptive function.
- The **recovery phase** is characterized by the gradual return of glomerular function.

23. What are the indications for dialysis in ARF?

Definite Indications for Dialysis in ARF

1. Uncontrollable hyperkalemia
2. Fluid overload with pulmonary edema
3. Uremic pericarditis
4. Uremia encephalopathy (seizures, coma)
5. Bleeding diathesis due to uremia
6. Refractory metabolic acidosis ($HCO_3^- < 10$ meq/l)
7. Severe azotemia (BUN > 100 mg/dl, serum Cr > 10 mg/dl).

Grantham JJ: Acute renal failure. In: Wyngaarden JB et al (eds): Cecil Textbook of Medicine, 19th ed, Philadelphia, W.B. Saunders, 1992.

24. Is the mortality in ARF significant?

The overall mortality in ARF is very high (40–60%) despite the availability of dialysis. The mortality is worse in the subcategory of patients with a history of surgery or trauma. The prognosis is better in the absence of respiratory failure, bleeding, or infection and also in patients with nonoliguric ATN. ARF occurring in the obstetric setting also has a better prognosis, with only a 10–20% mortality.

25. In which clinical situations does the use of ACE inhibitors lead to ARF?

In bilateral renal artery stenosis and renal artery stenosis of the single kidney or transplant kidney. It is believed that ARF under these conditions is mediated by angiotensin-converting enzyme (ACE) inhibitor-induced poststenotic dilatation of efferent arterioles and consequent reduction of glomerular hydrostatic pressure. In normal persons, this affect is offset by dilatation of afferent sites and maintenance of GFR. In the recent past, there have been reports of reversible renal failure in patients with chronic essential hypertension treated with ACE inhibitors. In these patients with severe nephrosclerosis, GFR depends on angiotensin-induced efferent arteriolar constriction. In patients with decreased effective renal blood flow, as in congestive heart failure, cirrhosis, or nephrosis, systemic hypotension and effective arteriolar dilatation caused by ACE inhibitors result in ARF.

Toto RD, et al: Reversible renal insufficiency due to angiotensin converting enzyme inhibitors in hypertensive nephrosclerosis. Ann Intern Med 115:513–519, 1991.

26. How frequently does nephrotoxicity due to exposure to radiocontrast agents occur?

The incidence of contrast-induced renal failure is variable. Most retrospective studies report an incidence of < 1%, whereas most prospective studies reported an incidence of 4–70%. In one of the more recent prospective studies, the frequency was 12%.

Hou SH, et al: Hospital acquired renal insufficiency: A prospective study. Am J Med 74:243–248, 1983.

27. What are the important risk factors for radiocontrast-associated ARF?

Risk Factors and Prevalence in Contrast-induced ARF

1. Azotemia (Cr > 1.5 mg/dl)	6. Uric acid > 8.0 mg/dl
2. Albuminuria > 2+	7. Multiple studies
3. Hypertension	8. Solitary kidney
4. Age > 60 yrs	9. Contrast medium > 2 ml/kg
5. Dehydration	10. Multiple myeloma with renal insufficiency

Berns AS et al: Nephrotoxicity of contrast media. Kidney Int 36:730–40, 1989.

28. What are the pathogenetic factors responsible for ARF with contrast dyes?

1. Hemodynamic changes
2. Osmolality
3. Proteinuria
4. Tubular obstruction
5. Allergic and immunologic reactions
6. Enzymuria
7. Direct toxicity
8. Altered glomerular permeability

Cronin RE: Southwestern Internal Medicine Conference: Renal failure following radiologic procedures. Am J Med Sci 298:342–356, 1989.

29. Do patients with myeloma have an increased risk of ARF with use of radiocontrast agents?

For several years, multiple myeloma was believed to be an important risk factor for radiocontrast-agent-induced ARF. However, several large studies have noted a prevalence of < 5%. In the absence of preexisting renal failure or proteinuria, multiple myeloma by itself is unlikely to predispose to ARF following exposure to radiocontrast media. Considering the high prevalence of renal disease in patients with myeloma, avoidance of radiocontrast agents is still recommended.

CHRONIC RENAL FAILURE

30. List the stages of progressive renal failure.

1. Reduced renal reserve
2. Renal insufficiency
3. Renal failure
4. Uremic syndrome
5. End-stage renal disease (ESRD)

Patients with normal renal function have nephron mass in excess of that necessary to maintain a normal GFR. Thus, with progressive loss of renal mass, that lost initially is the **renal reserve**, which is not reflected by a rise of BUN and creatinine or in a disturbance of homeostasis.

If the progression continues, this stage is followed by **renal insufficiency**, which is associated with mild elevation of BUN and creatinine and very mild symptoms, including nocturia and easy fatigability.

With further progression, **renal failure** ensues. This stage is characterized by apparent abnormalities of renal excretory function, including disturbances in water, electrolyte, and acid-base metabolism.

Continued worsening of renal function is followed by the **uremic syndrome,** which includes multiple dysfunction of major organ systems in addition to the abnormalities of excretory function described.

Finally, **ESRD** appears, at which time the remaining renal function is unable to sustain normal body function. Renal replacement therapy (dialysis or transplantation) is required.

31. How do the remaining intact nephrons adapt in the diseased kidney?

When nephron mass is lost, the remaining intact (functioning) nephrons compensate to maintain the same excretory function performed by the normal kidney. The individual nephrons accomplish this task by increasing the GFR and excretion of salt and water compared to levels when there was a full contingent of functioning nephrons. The increased excretory function is accomplished by reducing reabsorption of filtered salt and water, often resulting in polyuria and nocturia.

32. The compensatory mechanisms can help to maintain near-normal excretion for the diseased kidney with a reduced GFR. What is the major disadvantage these patients suffer with respect to excretory function when compared to patients with normal renal function?

Patients with chronic renal insufficiency have a reduced ability to respond to changes in intake with appropriate changes in excretory function. For example, if a person with normal renal function suddenly increases salt intake, the kidney quickly adjusts its function, allowing for increased excretion of salt which returns total body salt to or toward normal. The remaining functioning nephrons of persons with decreased GFR are chronically excreting a higher salt load and are thus much closer to their maximum salt-excreting ability. Hence, these patients are less able to adjust to an increased salt intake by increasing salt excretion.

At the opposite extreme, the remaining nephrons of the patient with a decreased GFR are less able to reduce their high salt excretion to compensate for a reduction in salt intake. These patients are more at risk of becoming salt-depleted in response to salt restriction than are patients with normal renal function.

33. Explain the "trade-off" concept of progressive renal disease.

This concept refers to compensatory mechanisms intended to alleviate the renal abnormalities resulting from compromised renal function, leading to adverse consequences in other organ systems. For example, the hyperphosphatemia and hypocalcemia occurring with progressive renal insufficiency result in increased parathyroid hormone secretion in an attempt to increase phosphate excretion and increase serum calcium levels. This secondary hyperparathyroidism has the desired effect on calcium and phosphate but leads to increased bone resorption and the bone disease called osteitis fibrosa cystica.

34. Why is the renal potassium excretory ability usually well-maintained down to very low (10–15 ml/min) levels of GFR in patients with progressive CRF?

As is the case for salt excretion, the remaining intact nephrons significantly increase potassium excretion such that the level of excretion per nephron is much higher than when there was a full contingent of nephrons. This allows for a total renal K excretion that is nearly normal. In addition, there is evidence that the extrarenal K excretion, especially by the colon, is increased in patients with CRF. By these mechanisms, patients with a significant decrease in GFR are unlikely to be hyperkalemic purely as a result of chronic renal insufficiency. In this clinical situation, if hyperkalemia is seen, consideration should be given to acute rather than chronic renal insufficiency, hormonal disorders (i.e., hyporenin hypoaldosteronism), or tubular disorders (i.e., obstructive uropathy).

35. Name the common causes of CRF.

The major causes of CRF found in patients entering the end-stage renal disease (ESRD) program in the U.S. are listed below. Note that diabetes and hypertension together account for about two-thirds of ESRD cases.

Common Causes of Chronic Renal Failure

Diabetes mellitus	31%
Hypertension	27%
Glomerulonephritis	14%
Polycystic kidney disease and other interstitial diseases	4%
Obstructive uropathy	5%
Others	19%

Alfrey AC, et al: Chronic renal failure. In: Schrier RW (ed): Renal and Electrolyte Disorders, 4th ed. Boston, Little, Brown and Co., 1992, p 541.

36. How does protein restriction affect the progression of CRF?

Many studies in animals and humans have shown that dietary protein restriction slows the progression of CRF. In diabetics, several studies show that protein restriction retards the progression of CRF. Nutritional status should be monitored regularly, regardless of the protein intake prescribed, to ensure that patients do not become malnourished.

For patients with a moderate loss of renal function (GFR 25–55 ml/min), there is no conclusive data that low-protein diet is beneficial. In such patients, it is recommended to prescribe a standard protein diet (>0.8 g/kg/day), unless there is evidence of progression of renal insufficiency, at which time a protein intake of 0.8 g/kg/day is indicated. For patients with more severe CRF (GFR 13–25 ml/min), dietary protein restriction to 0.6 g/kg/day delays progression in compliant patients. In a recent multicenter prospective study involving nondiabetic patients, dietary further protein restriction to < 0.6 gm/kg/day did not confer additional benefit.

Klahr S, et al: Modification of diet in renal disease study group. N Engl J Med 330:877–884, 1994.

37. What are the postulated mechanisms of the hypertension commonly observed in patients with renal disease?

Most patients with renal disease have an expanded extracellular fluid volume that is felt to contribute to hypertension. Other contributing mechanisms that have been postulated include stimulation of the renin-angiotensin system and increased catecholamines.

38. Do ACE inhibitors have renal protective effects in diabetics?

Yes. Sufficient data now exist supporting the use of ACE inhibitors, especially in diabetic patients with clinical or subclinical renal involvement, to retard the progression of diabetic nephropathy (both in terms of proteinuria as well as renal failure). A recent, large-scale, multicenter, prospective study concluded that captopril treatment was associated with a 50% reduction in the risk of death, dialysis, or transplantation in diabetics, an effect independent of blood pressure control. It is therefore recommended to initiate therapy with ACE inhibitors in patients with IDDM who have either microalbuminuria (30 300 mg/day in at least 2 of 3 measurements) or overt albuminuria (>300 mg/day). ACE inhibitor therapy should be instituted in these circumstances regardless of the presence of hypertension or renal failure.

Lewis EJ, et al: The effect of angiotensin converting enzyme inhibition on diabetic nephropathy. N Engl J Med. 329:1456–1462, 1993.

39. What is meant by uremia?

Uremia refers to a symptom complex that results from severe renal insufficiency. It is characterized by some degree of dysfunction of most organ systems of the body.

DIALYSIS

40. What are the indications for dialysis in a patient with CRF?

Dialytic therapy should be started when conservative management fails to maintain the patient in reasonable comfort. Usually, dialysis is required when the GFR drops to 5–10 ml/min. It is both unnecessary and risky to adhere to strict biochemical indications. Broadly speaking, the development of uremic encephalopathy, neuropathy, pericarditis, and bleeding diathesis are indications to start dialysis immediately. Fluid overload, congestive heart failure, hyperkalemia, metabolic acidosis, and hypertension uncontrolled by conservative measures are also indications for starting patients on dialysis therapy.

41. What is dialysis disequilibrium syndrome? How do you prevent it?

Dialysis disequilibrium syndrome is a neurologic complication that tends to occur during initiation of dialysis. It occurs in the first few dialyses and is characterized by nausea, vomiting, confusion, psychosis, and seizures. These symptoms occur toward the end of dialysis or afterward, when the dialysis has been particularly rapid. The syndrome is attributed to increased hydrogen ion concentration in the brain due to differential diffusion of CO_2 and HCO_3^- across the blood-brain barrier, leading to the generation of idiogenic osmoles and the development of cerebral edema. This complication is prevented by a gradual increase of dialysis time and blood flow rate, the use of slower dialyzers, and use of high dialysate sodium.

42. Which clinical manifestations of uremia (CRF) can be improved with dialysis? Which ones worsen?

Improve	Persist	Develop or worsen
Uremic encephalopathy	Renal osteodystrophy	Dialysis dementia
Seizures	Hypertriglyceridemia	Nephrogenic ascites
Pericarditis	Amenorrhea and infertility	Dialysis pericarditis
Fluid overload	Peripheral neuropathy	Dialysis bone disease
Electrolyte imbalances	Pruritus	Accelerated atherosclerosis
GI symptoms	Anemia	Carpal tunnel syndrome
Metabolic acidosis		(amyloid-related)
		Risk of hepatitis

43. Is there a relationship between dialysis dementia and aluminum?

Dialysis dementia is a rare progressive neurologic disorder seen in patients on chronic dialysis. The syndrome usually consists of disturbances of speech (apraxia, dysarthria) and memory, depression, myoclonus, and seizures. The disorder is progressive, and death occurs in 6–15 months. One of its pathologic hallmarks is a high level of aluminum in brain tissue, derived mostly from ingestion of aluminum-containing phosphate binders. Use of reverse osmosis for dialysate treatment, careful monitoring of aluminum levels in dialysate water, and avoiding aluminum-containing antacids whenever possible reduce the incidence of this disorder.

44. Which poisons and toxins are dialyzable?

The toxins that can be removed by hemodialysis include alcohols (ethanol, methanol, ethylene glycol), salicylates, heavy metals, (Hg, As, Pb), and halides. In addition, hemoperfusion successfully removes barbiturates, sedatives (meprobamate, methaqualone, glutethimide), acetaminophen, digoxin, procainamide, quinidine, and theophylline.

45. What is the principal contraindication for starting chronic dialysis?

The presence of potentially reversible abnormalities. These include volume depletion, urinary tract infection, urinary obstruction, hypercatabolic state, uncontrolled hypertension, hypercalcemia, nephrotoxic drugs, and low cardiac output state.

46. What is chronic ambulatory peritoneal dialysis (CAPD)? What are its indications?

CAPD is a manual form of peritoneal dialysis, usually performed by the patient, in which 1–2 liters of dialysate fluid are infused into the peritoneal space through a Tenckhoff catheter and then drained after a dwell time of 4–6 hours. The exchanges are repeated 4–5 times a day. CAPD is indicated in any patient with ESRD. It is the treatment of choice for diabetics with severe peripheral vascular disease, since they are at increased risk in hemodialysis. This method provides for more independence and motility, and it should be offered to all young patients leading active lives. The contraindications include blindness, severe disabling arthritis, colostomy, poor motivation, and quadriplegia.

47. What are the common complications of CAPD?

Mechanical: Pain, bleeding, leakage, inadequate drainage, intraperitoneal catheter loss, abdominal wall edema, scrotal edema, incisional hernia, other hernia, intestinal hematoma, intestinal perforation

Infections, inflammation: Bacterial or fungal peritonitis, tunnel infection, exit-site infection, diverticulitis, sterile peritonitis, eosinophilic peritonitis, sclerosing peritonitis, pancreatitis

Cardiovascular: Acute pulmonary edema, fluid overload, hypotension, arrhythmia, cardiac arrest, hypertension

Pulmonary: Basal atelectasis, aspiration pneumonia, hydrothorax, respiratory arrest, decreased FVC

Neurologic: Convulsion, ? dialysis disequilibrium syndrome

Metabolic: Hyperglycemia, hyperosmolar nonketotic coma, postdialysis hypoglycemia, hyperkalemia, hypokalemia, hypernatremia, hyponatremia, metabolic alkalosis, protein depletion, hyperlipidemia, obesity

48. Name the common causes of death in dialysis patients.

Despite important technical developments, the mortality in dialysis patients remains significant—about 15% in the first year. The commonest cause of death is cardiovascular failure, with hypotension and diabetes as important predisposing factors. Sepsis is the next leading cause of death, followed by bleeding complications, cerebrovascular accidents, pericardial effusion with tamponade, trauma (accidents), suicides, and others.

49. What are the causes of peritonitis in a patient on peritoneal dialysis?

Peritonitis is an important complication of CAPD. The frequency of infection has decreased considerably since this dialysis method was introduced, to about 1 episode every 18–24 patient months. This decrease is mainly due to the addition of a Luer-Lok adapter between the catheter and tubing and institution of monthly tubing changes. Causative organisms include *Staphylococcus epidermidis* and *S. aureus* (70%), gram-negative organisms (20%), and fungi and tuberculosis (5%).

50. How do you treat peritonitis in a patient on peritoneal dialysis?

The empiric treatment of acute peritonitis involves short lavage (2–3 exchanges drained rapidly), followed by 4 exchanges of 2 liters/day containing antibiotic coverage for both the common gram-positive and gram-negative organisms. 1000 units of heparin is added to each 2 liters if the fluid is fibrinous. If the chosen antibiotic(s) is removed by peritoneal dialysis (i.e., aminoglycosides), the antibiotic must be added to the dialysate at a concentration comparable to the desired trough level in the serum to minimize removal of the drug(s). Appropriate changes in antibiotics can be made after sensitivity patterns are available. Treatment is stopped 1 week after the first negative culture.

51. Discuss developments in the treatment of anemia of CRF.

The most important development is the use of recombinant human erythropoietin (EPO). Studies since 1987 have documented the efficacy of this agent in improving the anemia and minimizing the need for blood transfusion.

Eschbach JW, et al: Recombinant human erythropoietin in anemic patients with end stage renal disease: Results of a phase III multicenter clinical trial. Ann Intern Med 111:992–1000, 1989.

52. What is dialysis bone disease?

The bone disease in uremic patients does not necessarily improve after initiation of chronic dialytic therapy. In fact, additional factors are added that promote and complicate osteodystrophy. For instance, exposure to aluminum (as phosphate binders or, less commonly, in dialysate) superimposes a form of osteomalacia on secondary hyperparathyroidism.

Sherrard DJ, et al: The spectrum of bone disease in end stage renal failure—an evolving disorder. Kidney Int 48:436–442, 1993.

53. What is dialysis-associated amyloidosis?

Long-term dialytic therapy is associated with accumulation and deposition of amyloid fibrils containing β_2-microglobulins. It usually manifests after 5–7 years of chronic dialytic therapy and is seen in most of patients after 10 years of dialysis. Clinically, it manifests as asymptomatic lytic bone lesions, carpal tunnel syndrome (often bilateral), tenosynovitis, scapulohumeral periarthritis, and destructive arthropathy. No satisfactory preventive measures are available.

Koch KM: Dialysis related amyloidosis. Kidney Int 41: 1416–1429, 1992.

54. How does dialysis-induced hypoxemia develop?

A fall in P_aO_2 of 5–35 mm Hg is a frequent and important complication of hemodialysis. It occurs in up to 90% of patients on dialysis and resolves within 1–2 hours after discontinuation of dialysis. This fall is clinically insignificant in the routine dialysis patient but important in people with preexisting respiratory compromise.

The pathogenesis is multifactorial and depends in part on the type of hemodialysis (acetate versus bicarbonate). It is important to remember the CNS-controlled ventilation is normally inhibited by hypocarbia (decreased PaCO2) and alkalemia. Acetate dialysis removes CO_2 gas from the plasma, causing hypocarbia and depressed ventilation. Bicarbonate dialysis causes alkalemia (especially if the dialysate bicarbonate is >35 meq/l) due to diffusion of the bicarbonate into the patient and subsequent depressed ventilation. In addition, the cuprophane membrane of the artificial kidney can activate complement, leading to leukoagglutination in the pulmonary capillaries. This causes diffusion abnormalities, widening of the alveolar–arterial O_2 gradient, and hypoxemia. It is less common now with the advent of dialyzers using newer synthetic membranes.

Bregman H, et al: Complications during hemodialysis. In Daugirdas JT, Ing TS (eds): Handbook of Dialysis. Boston, Little, Brown & Co., 1994.

PROTEINURIA/NEPHROTIC SYNDROME

55. What factors normally inhibit entry of plasma proteins into the glomerular ultra-filtrate?

The glomerular barrier is functionally a filter whose pores are of a given size and lined by negatively charged particles. Consequently, the features of a given plasma protein that limit its entry into the glomerular ultrafiltrate include large size (MW), negative charge, and noncompact configuration.

56. Describe the four general mechanisms by which abnormally increased urinary protein excretion (>150 mg/day) occurs.

The four general mechanisms are glomerular, tubular, overflow, and secretory.

1. **Glomerular proteinuria** occurs as a result of damage to the glomerular filtration barrier (in glomerulonephritis), leading to excessive leakage of plasma proteins into the glomerular ultrafiltrate.

2. **Tubular proteinuria** occurs when there is suboptimal reabsorption of the normally filtered protein as a result of renal tubular disease. It is this recovery of the small amount of normally filtered protein (usually ~2 g/day) that allows for the normal urinary excretion of < 150 mg/day of protein.

3. **Over-flow proteinuria** results from disease states that lead to excessive levels of plasma proteins (such as in multiple myeloma). The proteins are filtered and overload the reabsorptive capacity of the renal tubules.

4. **Secretory proteinuria** describes the proteinuria that occurs because of the addition of protein to the urine after glomerular filtration. The protein may come from the renal tubules (as with Tamm-Horsfall protein from the ascending limb of the loop of Henle) or from the lower GU tract.

57. Which is the most common mechanism for proteinuria in patients with renal disease?

Glomerular proteinuria.

58. What conditions are associated with heavy proteinuria despite severe reduction in GFR?

Heavy proteinuria is generally indicative of glomerular disease. In most glomerular diseases, proteinuria tends to decrease with diminishing GFR as the filtration of proteins also tends to decrease. However, in certain conditions, such as diabetic nephropathy, amyloidosis, focal glomerulosclerosis, and probably reflex nephropathy, proteinuria (often in the nephrotic range) persists despite severely diminished GFR.

59. A 23-year-old white man has 1.2 gm of proteinuria in 24 hours. His urinalysis and other laboratory studies are otherwise normal. What is the differential diagnosis?

Significant ($>$ 0.5 g/24 hr) but nonnephrotic ($<$ 3.5 g/24 hr) proteinuria can be seen in the following conditions:

1. Benign orthostatic proteinuria
2. Idiopathic glomerular disease (esp. in early stages)

Focal glomerulosclerosis	Membranous nephropathy
IgA nephropathy	Amyloidosis

3. Systemic diseases

Diabetic nephropathy	Congestive heart failure
Essential hypertension	Febrile states

60. The commonly available urinary dipstick is most sensitive to which urinary protein?

Albumin. Excretion of even large amounts of some nonalbumin proteins (such as Bence-Jones proteins) will not be evident on this screening test. A more sensitive quantitative test, such as sulfosalicylic acid, must be used to recognize the presence of nonalbumin urinary proteins. Electrophoresis can then be used to identify the specific protein(s).

61. At what age does orthostatic proteinuria most commonly occur? What is its prognosis?

This term refers to excessive urinary protein excretion that occurs only when standing and normalizes when recumbent. It occurs most commonly in **adolescents** and carries an excellent long-term prognosis. It usually resolves spontaneously.

62. Define nephrotic syndrome.

This syndrome is a symptom complex resulting from various etiologies and characterized by heavy proteinuria (usually $>$ 3.5 g/day), generalized edema, and lipiduria with hyperlipidemia. Because all the other features are a consequence of marked proteinuria, some authorities restrict the definition of "nephrosis" to heavy proteinuria alone.

63. What is the nephritic syndrome?

The nephritic syndrome is a renal disorder that results from diffuse glomerular inflammation. It is characterized by the sudden onset of gross or microscopic hematuria, decreased GFR, low urine output (oliguria), hypertension, and edema. It can result from many different etiologies but is traditionally represented by postinfectious glomerulonephritis following infections with certain strains of group A β-hemolytic streptococci.

64. What are the various causes of an acute nephritic syndrome?

Postinfectious glomerulonephritis
    Poststreptococcal glomerulonephritis
        Postinfectious (nonstreptococcal) glomerulonephritis
            Bacterial: Pneumococci, *Klebsiella,* staphylococci, gram-negative rods, meningococci, secondary syphilis, brucellosis, *Leptospira, Mycoplasma, Salmonella*
            Viral: Varicella, infectious mononucleosis, mumps, measles, hepatitis B, coxsackievirus
            Rickettsial: Rocky Mountain spotted fever, typhus
            Parasitic: *Falciparum* malaria, toxoplasmosis, trichinosis
Idiopathic glomerular diseases
    Membranoproliferative glomerulonephritis
    Mesangial proliferative glomerulonephritis
    IgA nephropathy
Multisystem diseases
    Systemic lupus erythematosus (SLE)
    Henoch-Schönlein purpura

Essential mixed cryoglobulinemia
Infective endocarditis
Miscellaneous
Guillain-Barré syndrome
Postirradiation of renal tumors

65. Which four catogories of diseases cause the idiopathic nephrotic syndrome?
Minimal change disease
Focal and segmental glomerulosclerosis
Membranous nephropathy
Proliferative glomerulonephritides.

66. What is the most common cause of nephrotic syndrome in children? In adults?
Children: minimal change disease (also called lipoid nephrosis or nil lesion)

Adults: diabetes mellitus and idiopathic membranous nephropathy among primary glomerular diseases

67. In evaluating patients with nephrotic syndrome, which disease must you rule out before considering the syndrome to be due to a primary renal disease? Why?
The general disease categories to be ruled out include:
• Drugs that may result in excessive urinary protein excretion (gold, penicillamine)
• Systemic infections: e.g., hepatitis B and C, HIV, malaria
• Neoplasia (lymphomas)
• Multisystem collagen vascular diseases (SLE)
• Diabetes (nephropathy is classically associated with nephrotic syndrome)
• Heredofamilial diseases, such as Alport's syndrome.

The distinction between the above causes and primary renal disease is important for a number of reasons. Diagnostically, identification of some of these processes may help to identify the renal lesion without the need for a renal biopsy (as in diabetes). Therapeutically, treatment of such disorders may involve simple discontinuation of the offending agent (such as a drug). And management may need to be directed at a systemic disease (infection) rather than at the renal lesion itself.

68. Name the common complications of the nephrotic syndrome.
1. **Edema and anasarca**

2. **Hypovolemia** with acute prerenal and/or parenchymal renal disease. In the nephrotic syndrome, decreased effective arterial blood volume can lead to various degrees of renal underperfusion, resulting in renal failure in severe cases.

3. **Protein malnutrition,** due to massive protein losses in excess of dietary replacement.

4. **Hyperlipidemia,** which raises the risk of atherosclerotic cardiovascular disease.

5. **Increased susceptibility to bacterial infection,** which often involves the lungs, meninges (meningitis), and peritoneum. Common organisms include *Streptococcus* (including *S. pneumoniae*), *Haemophilus influenzae,* and *Klebsiella* sp.

6. **Proximal tubular dysfunction,** which may lead to Fanconi syndrome with urinary wasting of glucose, phosphate, amino acids, uric acid, potassium, and bicarbonate.

7. **Hypercoagulable state** manifested by an increased incidence of venous thrombosis, particularly in the renal vein. The mechanism may in part involve urinary loss of factors that normally inhibit clotting.

69. Are the syndromes of nephritis and nephrosis mutually exclusive?
No. Some forms of glomerular diseases are characteristically nephrotic in their presentation (e.g., nil lesion). On the other hand, some aggressive forms of proliferative glomerulopathies present as nephritic syndrome. Some others manifest mixed features.

Interrelationship of Morphologic and Clinical Manifestations of Glomerular Injury

	Nephrosis	
Minimal change glomerulopathy	++++	
Membranous glomerulopathy	+++	
Focal glomerulosclerosis	++	+
Mesangioproliferative glomerulopathy	++	++
Membranoproliferative glomerulopathy	++	+++
Proliferative glomerulonephritis	+	+++
Acute diffuse proliferature glomerulonephritis	+	++++
Crescentic glomerulonephritis		++++
		Nephritis

Adapted from Mandal AK, et al: Diagnosis and Management of Renal Disease and Hypertension. Philadelphia, Lea & Febiger, 1988, p. 248.

70. A 62-year-old man with nephrotic syndrome is found to have no systemic etiology. What is the differential diagnosis?

As opposed to that seen in children, minimal lesion on renal biopsy in an elderly patient warrants an extensive search to rule out underlying malignancy, especially lymphomas (both Hodgkin's and non-Hodgkin's) and other solid tumors, (such as renal cell carcinoma). One-third of elderly patients with membranous nephropathy have underlying malignancy (colon, stomach, or breast).

NEPHROLITHIASIS

71. What three mechanisms are believed important in determining the development of nephrolithiasis?

Urinary tract stones occur in a wide variety of diseases and as a consequence of a variety of physiologic and pathologic processes. The three mechanisms currently thought to contribute to urinary stones formation are:
1. Precipitation-crystallization from supersaturated solutions
2. Absence of inhibitors of stone formation normally present in urine
3. Presence of a macromolecular matrix

Precipitation of a substance to form stones depends on many factors, including solubility, concentration, and urine characteristics (i.e., pH). Normal constituents of urine that inhibit stone formation include citrate, pyrophosphate, and magnesium. Reduced concentrations of these substances are felt to contribute to stone formation. Protein matrix contributes to the formation, growth, and/or aggregation of stones. This matrix derives in part from renal tubular epithelial cells and from the uroepithelium.

72. What are the common constituents of urinary stones in the U.S.?

Calcium oxalate	35%
Calcium apatite	35%
Magnesium ammonium phosphate (struvite)	18%
Uric acid	6%
Cystine	3%

73. How does urine pH affect urinary stone formation?

In general, an alkaline urine pH favors precipitation of inorganic stones—calcium phosphate (which undergoes rearrangement into hydroxyapatite) and magnesium ammonium phosphate (struvite). An acid pH favors precipitation of organic stones—uric acid and cystine. Urine pH has little effect on calcium oxalate solubility and therefore little influence on formation of these stones.

74. Which factors predispose to the formation of magnesium ammonium phosphate (struvite) stones?

Alkaline urine pH and high concentrations of urinary ammonia lead to supersaturation of this substance. This environment is created by the presence of urea-splitting bacteria (commonly *Pro-*

teus, Pseudomonas, Klebsiella, and *Staphylococcus),* which contain the enzyme urease and convert urea to ammonia and CO_2.

75. Which common metabolic conditions predispose to the formation of urinary stones?

- **Idiopathic hypercalciuria** is present in approx. 50% of stone-forming patients in the U.S. It is divided into absorptive (due to excessive GI absorption of calcium) and renal (due to renal leak of calcium) types.
- **Hyperuricosuria** (with and without gout) is present in approx. 30% of stone-formers. Increased uric acid excretion can also contribute to the formation of calcium-containing stones.
- **Hyperoxaluria** of various causes is present in about 15%.
- **Low urinary citrate excretion** is present in about 50% and can contribute to stone formation in most states.

Less common causes include chronic UTI, primary hyperparathyroidism, cystinuria, and distal renal tubular acidosis. Typically more than one of the above conditions is present in a stone-forming patient.

76. Name the three common sites in the genitourinary tract where urinary stones are retained and obstruct urine flow.

The ureteropelvic junction, the mid-ureter as it crosses the iliac artery, and the ureterovesical junction.

77. What are the consequences of urinary obstruction by a stone?

A stone acutely lodged in the GU tract can cause severe, colicky pain that radiates toward the lower abdomen and genital area. In women who have children, the pain is often described as more severe than the pain of labor. The increased pressure inside the collecting system decreases the net pressure for glomerular filtration, resulting in a decreased GFR. The resulting urinary stasis predisposes to infection.

All of these problems correct toward normal if the stone passes or is removed from the urinary tract within a few days. If the obstruction becomes chronic, permanent renal injury can ensue, with an irreversible reduction in GFR and chronic dilatation of the collection system. This dilated collecting system is less efficient in delivering urine to the bladder (because of compromised peristalsis), predisposing to urinary stasis and infection.

78. How should you manage the patient with acute urinary tract obstruction due to a stone?

Most stones pass spontaneously in a few hours to days. Supportive management with analgesics and oral fluids will usually suffice. Such patients should have serum chemistries done to document the degree of renal dysfunction (if any) and an imaging procedure (intravenous, pyelography, renal ultrasound, etc.) to locate the stone and estimate its size in order to help determine the possible need for surgical intervention. Once the acute phase ends with exit of the stone, evaluation should be aimed at identifying the condition that led to the formation of the stone, which will lead to a protocol for long-term management.

79. Are patients often successful in recovering stones that are passed at home?

A reasonable percentage will recover stone material from their urine. However, laboratory analysis is usually not readily available, and the approach to management is more often empirical than based on analysis of recovered stones.

80. What conservative, nonmedical management is recommended for patients with a propensity to form renal stones?

In general, such patients should maintain a dilute urine, which can be accomplished by a high intake of hypotonic fluids. Recovery and characterization of stones, if possible, help to diagnose the predisposing condition and guide management.

Except for the oxalate stones, whose formation is not much influenced by urine pH, maintenance of an acid urine inhibits the formation of inorganic stones (calcium apatite, struvite) and maintenance of an alkaline urine inhibits formation of organic stones (uric acid, cysteine). Increasing the urinary concentration of natural inhibitors (citrate, pyrophosphate, magnesium) can limit aggregation and growth of crystals.

81. What drugs are useful in managing these patients?
More specific management depends on the predisposing condition:
- Absorptive hypercalciuria can be managed by reducing dietary calcium (type 2 only) or by using cellulose sodium phosphate, which binds intestinal calcium and prevents its absorption (type 1), or the diuretic thiazide, which promotes renal calcium absorption.
- Renal hypercalciuria can also be treated with thiazides.
- Primary hyperparathyroidism should be treated with parathyroidectomy.
- Uricosuric states resulting from the overproduction of uric acid should be treated with allopurinol, or with potassium citrate if patients have hyperuricosuria associated with calcium oxalate stones.
- Conditions associated with excessive intestinal oxalate absorption can be treated with a low oxalate diet and use of magnesium or calcium salts, which bind oxalate and inhibit its reabsorption.
- Cystinuria can be managed conservatively (i.e., dilute or alkaline urine) or with penicillamine (increases the solubility of cystine) if the conservative measures are ineffective.
- Patients with struvite stones must have their UTIs treated with antibiotics and may also be given the urease inhibitor acetohydroxamic acid.

82. What are the three forms of lithotripsy?
Litho-(stone or calculus) *tripsy* (crushing) is a way of breaking up stones by use of shockwaves or ultrasound and may serve as an alternative to operation or cystoscopy for the removal of stones in the kidney and urinary tract. The three forms now available clinically are:
1. Extracorporeal shock-wave lithotripsy
2. Percutaneous ultrasonic lithotripsy
3. Endoscopic ultrasonic lithotripsy

URINARY TRACT OBSTRUCTION

83. List the common causes of ureteric obstruction in adults.

Renal stones	Blood clot
Prostatic, bladder, or pelvic malignancy	Pregnancy
Retroperitoneal lymphoma, metastasis, or fibrosis	Stricture
Accidental surgical ligation	

84. How do unilateral and bilateral obstruction differ in their effects on the GFR?
Unilateral obstruction does not necessarily lead to a clinically measurable decrease in GFR, but bilateral obstruction quite often does. In patients with normal renal function, unilateral obstruction with complete obliteration of ipsilateral function will force recruitment of the nephron reserve of the unaffected, contralateral kidney, resulting in no changes or only small changes in total GFR. Relatively large reductions in functioning nephron mass (about 40%) are necessary to elicit an appreciable rise in the plasma creatinine (P_{Cr}) concentrations when baseline renal function is normal (P_{Cr} 0.8–1.2 mg/dl). The relatively small change in GFR, in patients with normal baseline renal function who are subjected to unilateral obstruction, likely will not be reflected by a rise in P_{Cr}.

The response is different for patients with baseline renal insufficiency. Such patients have already lost their reserve nephron mass and are likely using compensatory mechanisms to maintain their GFR. Unilateral obstruction in such patients may result in a significant fall in GFR and is more likely to be associated with a rise in P_{Cr}.

Bilateral obstruction leads to a decreased GFR in patients with both normal and abnormal renal function.

85. Describe the differences in clinical presentation between acute and chronic obstruction of the urinary tract.

Partial or complete obstruction of the urinary tract compromises urine passage whether it is acute or chronic. Nevertheless, the urinary findings and clinical consequences differ depending on the duration of the obstruction. After release of an **acute (<24 hrs) obstruction,** there is commonly a decrease in excretion of sodium, potassium, and water. This results in excretion of a urine low in sodium and with increased osmolarity, a situation also seen with volume depletion. In contrast, release of **chronic obstruction** commonly results in *increased* excretion of sodium and water and decreased excretion of acid (with urinary loss of bicarbonate) and potassium. These abnormalities can lead to volume depletion, free-water deficit (reflected by hypernatremia), and hyperkalemic non-anion-gap metabolic acidosis.

86. What abnormalities of tubular function can occur with chronic obstruction?

Chronic obstruction affects primarily distal rather than proximal nephron functions, including reabsorption of sodium and water and secretion of acid and potassium. The decreased **water** reabsorptic results from decreased responsiveness of the collecting tubule to antidiuretic hormone (ADH), yielding a form of nephrogenic diabetes insipidus. The **acid** secretory defect results in incomplete bicarbonate recovery from the urine and a non-anion-gap metabolic acidosis. The **potassium** secretory defect results in potassium retention and hyperkalemia. Therefore, obstructive nephropathy is a common cause of hyperkalemic, hyperchloremic, non-anion-gap metabolic acidosis. These abnormalities usually resolve after correction of the obstruction but may require weeks or months to do so.

87. Which components of the polyuria (postobstructive diuresis) are seen immediately after correction of chronic obstruction?

The patient with obstruction and compromised renal function accumulates solute and water that are ordinarily excreted by the normally functioning kidney. Correction of the obstruction results in appropriate excretion of the accumulated urea, NaCl, and water in an effort to return the volume and content of the extracellular fluid to normal. This polyuria is physiologic. However, a minority of such patients will have a pathologic polyuria, resulting from poor salt and/or water reabsorption. These abnormalities commonly resolve within a few hours but may last for days.

88. How do you tell if the postobstructive polyuria is physiologic or pathologic?

Usually the polyuria is physiologic, but the patient must be observed. The pathologic polyuria may occur because of either salt or water loss (or both). Pathologic salt loss will be reflected by continued excretion of a large amount of urinary sodium in the setting of volume depletion. Pathologic water loss will be reflected by excretion of large volumes of dilute urine in the face of rising serum osmolality. In pathologic polyuria, appropriate fluid replacement therapy should be instituted. If replacement is instituted during the physiologic polyuria, one will "chase" the patient's volume status such that the polyuria will continue as a result of the fluids being administered.

89. What are some complications of urinary tract obstruction?

In addition to the decrease in GFR and the potential tubular abnormalities, the resulting urinary stasis can predispose to infection, renal stones, and papillary necrosis. The salt and water retention can lead to hypertension.

90. What is "functional" obstruction of the urinary tract?

This refers to abnormalities that compromise the exit of urine from the kidney in the absence of anatomic obstruction of the outflow tract. Two examples are an atonic bladder and vesicoureteral reflux.

An **atonic bladder** is unable to empty itself completely and hence contains urine, continuously yielding a higher than normal hydrostatic pressure. This high bladder pressure is transmitted via the ureters and may cause the abnormalities described above.

Patients with **vesicoureteral reflex** have retrograde flow of urine into the ureter and/or kidney during voiding. This occurs because of an incompetent vesicoureteral valve. The transmitted pressure is felt to contribute to the renal abnormalities. Both of these conditions also predispose to infection.

91. How is the diagnosis of lower urinary tract obstruction (LTO) made?

The history, clinical setting, and the laboratory findings provide important clues:

- A palpable urinary bladder on examination is strong evidence for LTO or an atonic bladder.
- The distended bladder as well as hypertrophied kidneys can sometimes be demonstrated on plain abdominal x-rays.
- A post-void residual urine of > 100 ml obtained upon Foley catheter insertion is supportive of LTO.
- Renal ultrasound is a relatively sensitive, noninvasive procedure that is commonly used to investigate the possibility of LTO.
- Retrograde pyelography (selective catheterization and insertion of contrast dye into both ureters via cystoscopy) is occasionally necessary when the above studies do not yield a diagnosis and clinical suspicion remains strong for obstruction. Intravenous pyelograms (IVPs) should be avoided due to the risk of additional renal injury from the contrast dye.
- Abdominal CT scan is helpful but is more expensive than ultrasound.
- Radionuclide renal scans suggest LTO when there is prompt uptake of the dye with prolonged excretion.

PRIMARY GLOMERULAR DISORDERS

92. What is a primary glomerulopathy?

Primary glomerular disease (or primary glomerulopathy) denotes a heterogeneous group of kidney diseases in which the glomeruli are the predominantly involved elements. Extrarenal involvement, if present, is usually secondary to consequences of the glomerular insult. Most of these disorders are idiopathic. The cardinal manifestations of the primary glomerular disorders are proteinuria, hematuria, alterations in GFR, and salt retention leading to edema, hypertension, and pulmonary congestion.

93. Which clinical syndromes are manifested by the primary glomerulopathies?

The clinical features of the primary glomerulopathies appear in various combinations in any given glomerular disorder and present as one of the following clinical syndromes:

1. **Acute glomerulonephritis** (AGN): An acute illness of abrupt onset characterized by variable degrees of hematuria, proteinuria, decreased GFR, and fluid and salt retention. It is usually associated with an infectious agent and tends to resolve spontaneously.

2. **Nephrotic syndrome:** An illness of insidious onset characterized primarily by heavy proteinuria of usually > 3.5 g/day in an adult and usually associated with hypoalbuminemia, lipidemia, and anasarca.

3. **Chronic glomerulonephritis:** A vague illness of insidious onset characterized primarily by progressive renal insufficiency, with a protracted downhill course of 5–10 years' duration. Varying degrees of proteinuria, hematuria, and hypertension.

4. **Rapidly progressive glomerulonephritis** (RPGN): A clinical disorder of rather subacute onset but with rapid progression to renal failure and no tendency toward spontaneous recovery. Patients are usually hypertensive, hematuric, and oliguric.

5. **Asymptomatic urinary abnormalities:** Patients have microscopic hematuria and/or proteinuria (usually < 3 g/day) but with no clinical symptoms.

94. Which strains of streptococci cause poststreptococcal glomerulonephritis (PSGN)? What factors determine the nephritogenicity?

Only certain serotypes of group A (β-hemolytic) streptococci are nephritogenic. Type 12 is the most common type, but types 1, 2, 3, 18, 25, 49, 55, 57, and 60 are also nephritogenic. In contrast, all strains of streptococci can cause acute rheumatic fever, which is why the incidence of nephritis differs from that of rheumatic fever in outbreaks of streptococcal infection.

The M-protein in streptococci is poorly linked to nephritogenicity. Recent evidence indicates that nephritogenicity is more closely related to endostreptosin, a cell membrane antigen. Other streptococcal cytoplasmic antigens and autologous antigens also have been implicated.

95. Describe the typical urine sediment from a patient with PSGN. Does a normal urinalysis rule out this diagnosis?

The urinalysis in PSGN is characterized by a nephritic sediment (see Question 98), high specific gravity, and nonselective proteinuria. The proteinuria is <3 g/day in > 75% of patients, although proteinuria in the nephrotic range is occasionally seen. Pyuria is often noted, indicating glomerulitis. Hematuria is almost always present in either gross (smoky urine) or microscopic form. Red cell casts, if present, are very diagnostic. Dysmorphic erythrocytes are found in abundance. However, a benign urinary sediment does not rule out acute PSGN if clinical features are suggestive. In some cases, biopsy studies have confirmed PSGN.

96. What is the prognosis in acute PSGN? What are the poor prognostic signs?

In children, the immediate and late prognosis is quite favorable in both epidemic and sporadic cases. A diuresis occurs in 1 week, and serum creatinine returns to normal in 3–4 weeks. The mortality in acute cases is < 1%, and chronic sequelae are uncommon. Microscopic hematuria may last 6 months, and proteinuria may persist for as long as 3 years in 15% of patients. The factors indicating a poor prognosis include persistent heavy proteinuria, extensive crescents or atypical humps in initial biopsy, and severe disease in the acute phase requiring hospitalization.

In adults, the prognosis is good in epidemic forms but less predictable in sporadic cases. Severe impairment of renal function at the onset, persistent proteinuria, elderly age, and crescent formation on biopsy are poor prognostic factors.

97. How do you treat hypertension associated with acute PSGN?

Fluid and salt retention are the basis for hypertension in PSGN. Therefore, loop diuretics, such as furosemide, are very useful. Potassium-sparing diuretics are to be avoided. Other antihypertensives are rarely indicated. When needed, vasodilators such as hydralazine, diazoxide, and nitroprusside are most useful. Plasma renin activity levels are often decreased, and hence β-blockers and ACE inhibitors are less useful alone but may be used in conjunction with vasodilators. Clonidine, methyldopa, or nifedepine can also be used.

98. What is rapidly progressive glomerulonephritis (RPGN)? Is it synonymous with crescentic nephritis?

The term RPGN is used to denote the clinical syndrome associated with rapid and progressive deterioration of renal function, often terminating, if untreated, in ESRD within a period of weeks to months. Histologically, it is characterized by extensive glomerular crescent formation, in most cases involving over 75% of glomeruli. The cells of the crescents are thought to be derived from blood-borne monocytes.

RPGN is strictly a clinical expression, whereas crescentic nephritis denotes the histologic picture in such patients. Several primary glomerulopathies demonstrate variable degrees of crescent formation, but they do not progress rapidly as in RPGN.

99. How does routine urinalysis help in the evaluation of a primary glomerular disease?

In glomerular disease, the urinary sediment usually conforms to one of three different forms:

Nephrotic	Nephritic	Chronic
Heavy proteinuria	Red cells	Less proteinuria and hematuria
Free fat droplets	Red cell casts	Broad, waxy casts
Oval fat bodies	Variable proteinuria	Pigmented granular casts
Fatty casts	Frequent white cell and	
Variable hematuria	granular cells	

Schreiner GE: The identification and clinical significance of casts. Arch Intern Med 99:356–369, 1957.

100. How is a patient with recurrent hematuria evaluated?

The first step is to exclude urinary stones and other structural lesions such as tumors of upper and lower urinary tract. This may involve renal imaging and urinary instrumentation. The presence of dysmorphic erythrocytes or red cell casts help to distinguish glomerular bleeding from lower tract bleeding. Glomerular bleeding accounts for recurrent hematuria in over a quarter of patients below age 40 years. The main causes of recurrent isolated glomerular hematuria include IgA nephropathy or Berger's disease (the most common primary glomerulopathy worldwide), thin basement membrane nephropathy, and idiopathic hypercalciuria. Demonstration of the first two entities may require renal biopsy.

RENAL BONE DISEASE

101. What is Bricker's "trade-off" hypothesis?

Early in the course of renal failure, the kidney fails to excrete phosphorus, leading to a transient and often undetectable rise in serum phosphorus. This tends to lower the serum ionized calcium temporarily, leading to stimulation of parathyroid hormone (PTH) secretion. The increased levels of PTH reduce tubular reabsorption of phosphate, leading to phosphate excretion and thereby tending to normalize the serum calcium and phosphorus levels. However, this is occurring at the expense of an elevated PTH level. With further declines in renal function, the serum phosphorus tends to rise, and the whole cycle is repeated.

With advancing renal failure, these changes tend to keep serum calcium and phosphorus levels below normal at the expense of increasing serum PTH levels. The serum level of PTH is increased in an attempt to normalize serum phosphate and calcium levels, but the "trade-off" is the bone disease caused by the elevated PTH levels (osteitis fibrosa cystica). This is the so-called "trade-off" hypothesis propounded by Neil Bricker and is the basis for the secondary hyperparathyroidism seen in renal failure.

102. List the three major bone histologic subtypes found in renal osteodystrophy.

Osteitis fibrosa cystica, which is a result of high bone turnover (bone changes due to secondary hyperparathyroidism), osteomalacia, and occasionally, osteosclerosis. With better management of patients with ESRD, the long-term course of renal bone disease and its clinical features have changed, and newer entities have emerged. Adynamic or aplastic bone disease or low bone turnover has become a fairly common bone disease. Aluminum accumulation causes osteomalacia, which is one cause of adynamic bone disease. Decreased vitamin D, diabetes, and iron accumulation are other factors associated with adynamic bone disease.

103. What is the role of aluminum in renal bone disease?

Recent evidence has shown that aluminum accumulation in the bone is a major factor in causing osteomalacia and anemia in patients with CRF and in those on dialysis. After the dialysate concentration of aluminum was lowered to insignificant amounts, it became obvious that oral ingestion of aluminum in the form of aluminum-containing phosphate binders was an important cause of aluminum-related bone disease. Orally ingested aluminum can accumulate over time to levels significant enough to cause aluminum bone disease. The mechanism of the aluminum effect on bone is believed to be due to deposition of the metal along the mineralization front, leading to interference with mineralization. In addition, aluminum may impair the function of osteoblasts.

104. Why will a patient with CRF and marked hypocalcemia often fail to manifest tetany?

Tetany is a clinical manifestation of severe hypocalcemia in adults. Ionized calcium is decreased in the presence of alkalemia, so that tetany usually manifests only in the presence of an alkalemic pH. The degree of ionization is favorably increased by the acidemia seen in CRF, the result being that the ionic calcium is usually not reduced enough to cause tetany. However, if the acidosis is excessively treated with alkalizing agents, tetany may become manifest.

105. Does bone disease improve with dialysis or renal transplantation?

Renal osteodystrophy is not always improved with dialytic therapy. Indeed, the symptoms may worsen or progress because a number of additional factors are introduced that either directly or indirectly influence the severity of renal bone disease, including the aluminum content of dialysate, heparin administration, and administration of large amounts of acetate.

In patients who undergo renal transplantation, the uremic bone disease improves to a great extent. Increased osteoclastic and osteoblastic activity are noted within a few weeks after transplantation. However, in some patients, osteoporosis and the effects of secondary hyperparathyroidism may persist for as long as 1–2 years. In addition, steroid therapy may be responsible for osteoporosis and osteonecrosis that complicate the later phases of the post-transplant period. Another abnormality that may develop in the post-transplant phase is a renal phosphate leak, which if severe may contribute to osseous abnormalities.

RENAL TRANSPLANTATION

106. When should renal transplantation be considered?
Renal transplantation is indicated in all patients with ESRD who need some form of renal replacement therapy.

107. What are some important contraindications?
Absolute contraindications

Reversible renal disease	Active infection
Recent malignant disease	Active glomerulonephritis
Presensitization to donor Class I	AIDS
major transplantation antigens	

Relative contraindications

Fabry's disease	Oxalosis
Advanced age	Psychiatric problems
Presence of anatomic urologic abnormality	Iliofemoral occlusion
	Chronic active hepatitis

108. What are the donor-selection criteria in living-related transplantation?
Donors for should have a normal physical examination, be under age 65, and have the same ABO blood group as the recipient (or be type O). An angiogram is necessary to exclude the presence of multiple or abnormal renal arteries, because such abnormalities make the surgery prolonged and difficult. In general, the left kidney is preferred because of the longer renal vein. Some relative contraindications for kidney donation include severe hypertension, diabetes mellitus, HIV positivity, active medical illness, urologic abnormalities, persistently abnormal urinalyses, and family history of nephritis, polycystic kidney disease, or other renal disease.

109. What factors are considered important in evaluating suitability of a cadaver kidney?
The donor should have been free of neoplastic or infectious disease, preferably under 60 years of age, and have had good urine output and a normal serum creatinine before death. Urinalyses should be normal, and urine cultures should be negative. The kidney should be transplanted as early after harvesting as possible. The graft function tends to be worse after 24 hours following harvesting. Of course, the donor should be free of infection with hepatitis B virus and HIV.

110. Give the current survival figures for renal transplant recipients in the U.S.
The 1-year patient survival rate for living-related renal transplantation is now around 95–100%, and for cadaveric transplantation, about 90%. With cyclosporine therapy, graft survivals are 90% and 80%, respectively, for living and cadaveric kidney transplants.

DIABETIC RENAL DISEASE

111. What is the incidence of renal involvement in diabetes mellitus?
CRF is an important cause of morbidity and mortality in all diabetics. Diabetes contributes to up to 50% of all cases of ESRD in the U.S. Of type I diabetics, 40–60% develop CRF between

10–30 years after onset of diabetes. Although about one-third of type II diabetics develop protein-uria, only 4% develop nephrotic syndrome and 6% develop ESRD. However, due to the large number of type II diabetics, they constitute the majority of diabetics on dialysis. The difference between the behavior of type I and II diabetes is probably dependent on the age of onset of the disease.

112. What is the earliest evidence of renal involvement in diabetes mellitus?

The earliest renal changes in diabetes consist of an increase in GFR of 25–50% and a slight en-largement of the kidney that persists for 5–10 years. At this stage, there may be a slight increase in al-bumin excretion rate (microalbuminuria), but the total protein excretion remains in the normal range.

113. Why is diabetic nephropathy associated with large kidneys?

Diabetic nephropathy is one of the causes of CRF associated with normal-sized or large kid-neys. Renal size is increased early in the course of diabetic renal disease and involves hypertrophy and hyperplasia. Elevated levels of growth hormone, often seen with uncontrolled hyperglycemia, are incriminated in this renal hypertrophy. However, the exact etiology remains unknown.

114. Do patients with microalbuminuria develop overt renal disease more often than others?

The course of diabetic nephropathy is characterized by a preclinical phase, followed by a clin-ical phase. The clinical phases start with the appearance of proteinuria on urine dipstick. Even in the preclinical phase, there is an increased amount of albumin excretion over the normal (20–40 μg/min), measurable by sensitive radioimmunoassays. Studies indicate that patients with this "microalbuminuria" are more likely to develop overt diabetic nephropathy than those who do not exhibit microalbuminuria.

115. What is the most important factor influencing the course of diabetic nephropathy?

Hypertension. In the proteinuria phase, 50–75% of all diabetics develop hypertension, and by the time they reach ESRD, almost all diabetics have hypertension. In the proteinuric phase, if hyperten-sion is controlled, the rate of decline of GFR can be decreased from 1 ml/min/mo to 0.39 ml/min/mo.

Parving et al: Early aggressive anti-hypertensive treatment in diabetic nephropathy. Lancet i:1175, 1983.

116. How do you treat hypertension in diabetes mellitus?

Many studies have shown that calcium channel blockers and ACE inhibitors are very well-tolerated and effective in diabetes. **ACE inhibitors** should be the first-line agents in therapy for hypertension in DM. Shortly after ACE inhibitors are started, serum creatinine and potassium should be monitored to detect patients who develop hyperkalemia or an abrupt reduction in GFR. If no adverse effects are seen for at least 2 weeks, ACE inhibitors can be safely continued.

ACE inhibitors have been shown in recent large-scale clinical trials to reduce proteinuria and slow the progression of CRF in diabetes. It is unclear whether **calcium channel blockers** are as ef-fective as ACE inhibitors in achieving these objectives, but they are effective in controlling the blood pressure in renal failure. β-blockers may be effective, but their effects on the lipid profile and need for dose modification in renal failure and dialysis make them less desirable. Other agents, while be-ing effective, may not offer any advantages over ACE inhibitors or calcium channel blockers.

117. Do diabetics with renal failure tolerate dialysis as well as nondiabetics?

Several years ago, it was thought that diabetics were not good candidates for dialytic ther-apy, because about 80% of diabetics with ESRD who were placed on hemodialysis died in the first year. Over the last 15 years, results have improved significantly. One recent report indicates a 1-year survival of 85% and a 3-year survival of 60% in diabetics on hemodialysis. However, even today, diabetics tend to do poorly compared to nondiabetics. Their 3-year survival is 20–30% less, and their mortality is 2.25 times higher than that of nondiabetics. Atherosclerotic cardiac dis-ease is the commonest cause of death, with infections a close second.

118. Does diabetic nephropathy recur following renal transplantation?

Histologic lesions typical of diabetic renal disease appear in kidneys transplanted into dia-betics in as early as 1–3 years. However, clinical deterioration of kidney function attributable to these lesions is uncommon.

119. What is pseudodiabetes of uremia?

In nondiabetics with CRF, there is a peripheral resistance to the action of endogenous insulin, resulting in hyperglycemia. If a glucose tolerance test is performed, the resulting curve resembles that of diabetes. This phenomenon is called pseudodiabetes of uremia. The absence of fasting hyperglycemia and the typical changes of diabetic retinopathy distinguish this pseudodiabetes from diabetic uremia.

120. Can meticulous control of blood sugar levels prevent diabetic renal disease?

The hyperfiltration and hypertrophy seen early in the course of diabetic nephropathy can be corrected with insulin treatment. Strict glycemic control can reverse the elevated GFR and renal hypertrophy and also can decrease the spontaneous or exercise-induced microalbuminuria seen in the preclinical phase. Intensive control of blood sugar is recommended in all type I diabetics. The goal is to maintain a blood glucose level within or close to the normal range while avoiding hypoglycemic attacks. These goals frequently require 2–3 insulin injections per day or use of an insulin pump with close monitoring of blood glucose levels. However, once overt nephropathy begins and progressive renal insufficiency ensues, the benefit of tight glycemic control is still observed, although less pronounced than in the preclinical phase.

Diabetes Control and Complications Trial (DCCT) research group: The effects of intensive treatment of diabetes on the development and progression of long-term complications in insulin dependent diabetes mellitus. N Engl J Med 329:977–986, 1993.

MISCELLANEOUS RENAL DISORDERS

121. What are the risk factors associated with aminoglycoside nephrotoxicity?

1. Dose and duration of drug therapy
2. Recent aminoglycoside therapy
3. Preexistent renal or liver failure
4. Elderly age
5. Volume depletion
6. Concurrent nephrotoxin administration
7. Potassium and/or magnesium depletion

Fumes D: Aminoglycoside nephrotoxicity. Kidney Int 33: 900–911, 1988.

122. Which antibacterial agents should be avoided completely in renal failure?

Tetracyclines, nitrofurantoin, nalidixic acid, and bacitracin.

123. How should antibiotic doses be adjusted in patients with renal failure?

Several antibiotics need dosage modification in the presence of renal failure, notably aminoglycosides, most cephalosporins, many penicillins, and vancomycin. The adjustments can be made by maintaining the usual dose and varying the dosing interval, maintaining the dosing interval and varying the dose, or a combination of the two. The objective is to obtain a therapeutic drug concentration–time profile that is therapeutic and not toxic. For most commonly used antibiotics, dosing guidelines have been established and are readily accessible. No adjustment is needed for erythromycin, doxycycline, rifampin, and oral vancomycin.

Benett WM: Drug Prescribing in Renal Failure. Philadelphia, American College of Physicians, 1993, pp 15–35.

124. What are some of the commonly encountered drug–drug interactions seen in renal failure?

Drug interactions are fairly common in patients with renal failure.

- Concomitant use of **metoclopramide** with **digoxin** decreases the absorption of the digoxin due to decreased gastric motility. The digoxin dose may have to be increased. On the other hand, **quinidine** impairs renal excretion of digoxin, and hence the digoxin dose may have to be decreased.

- **Antacids** impair the gastric absorption of β-blockers and **ferrous sulfate.** It is recommended to allow 1–2 hours between the two agents.
- An important interaction occurs between **Scholl's solution,** an alkali that contains sodium citrate, and **aluminum hydroxide.** Citrate increases aluminum absorption so that aluminum toxicity may result. The combination has to be avoided.
- **Azathioprine** levels in the blood are elevated when used in conjunction with **allopurinol** due to decreased xanthine oxidase metabolism of azathioprine. The azathioprine dose therefore has to be decreased and leukocyte counts followed.
- Finally, many drugs alter the **cyclosporine** many drugs alter the cyclosporin levels in the plasma. **Phenytoin, phenobarbitol,** and **rifampin** increase cyclosporine clearance by the liver, and higher dose may be needed. On the other hand, **erythromycin, amphotericin B,** and **ketoconazole** decrease cyclosporine clearance by the liver, and hence the dose may have to be decreased.

125. What is a simple renal cyst? How is it distinguished from a malignant cyst?

Simple cysts represent 60–70% of renal masses. They are common after age 50, most often asymptomatic, and usually detected as incidental findings in radiologic procedures done for other reasons. On sonography, a simple cyst has smooth, sharply delineated margins, no echoes within the mass, and a strong posterior wall echo indicating good transmission through the cyst. These features generally exclude the possibility of malignancy. However, if there is any further suspicion, a CT scan should be done. CT findings consistent with a simple cyst include fluid that is homogeneous with a density of 0–20 Hounsfield units and no enhancement of the cyst fluid following the administration of radiocontrast media.

Characteristics of Renal Cystic Disorders

FEATURE	SIMPLE CYSTS	ADPKD	ARPKD	ACKD	MCD	MSK
Inheritance pattern	None	Autosomal dominant	Autosomal recessive	None	Often present, variable pattern	None
Incidence or prevalence	Common, increasing with age	1/200 to 1/1000	Rare	40% in dialysis patients'	Rare	Common
Age of onset	Adult	Usually adults	Neonates, children	Older adults	Adolescents, young adults	Adults
Presenting symptom	Incidental finding, hematuria	Pain, hematuria, infection, family screening	Abdominal mass, renal failure, failure to thrive	Hematuria	Polyuria, polydipsia, enuresis, renal failure, failure to thrive	Incidental, UTIs, hematuria, renal calculi
Hematuria	Occurs	Common	Occurs	Occurs	Rare	Common
Recurrent infections	Rare	Common	Occurs	No	Rare	Common
Renal calculi	No	Common	No	No	No	Common
Hypertension	Rare	Common	Common	Present from underlying disease	Rare	No
Diagnosis	Ultrasound	Ultrasound, gene linkage analysis	Ultrasound	CT scan	None reliable	Excretory urogram
Renal size	Normal	Normal to very large	Large initially	Small to normal, occ. large	Small	Normal

ADPKD = autosomal dominant polycystic kidney disease; ARPKD = autosomal recessive polycystic kidney disease; ACKD = acquired cystic kidney disease; MCD = medullary cystic disease; MSK = medullary sponge kidney.
Adapted from Gabow PA: Cystic diseases of kidney. In Wyngaarden JB, et al (eds): Cecil Textbook of Medicine, 19th ed. Philadelphia, W.B. Saunders, 1992, pg 609.

126. List the renal manifestations of sickle cell disease.
1. Hematuria
2. Renal infarction and papillary necrosis, which may predispose to UTI
3. Abnormal tubular function:
   a. Reduced concentrating ability
   b. Reduced acid and potassium secretion
   c. Increased uric acid and creatinine secretion
   d. Increased phosphate reabsorption
4. Nephrotic syndrome, which may progress to renal failure

127. What are the causes of papillary necrosis?
Renal papillary necrosis is one of the most common renal complications of sickle cell anemia. The other common conditions in which this renal complication is observed include analgesic nephropathy and diabetes mellitus.

128. What are the renal manifestations of infective endocarditis? What is the pathogenesis of these lesions?
Renal manifestations in infective endocarditis include incidental microscopic or gross hematuria and proteinuria. Renal failure is usually mild or absent. The histologic exam in these cases reveals focal proliferative glomerulonephritis. Rarely, a rapidly progressive renal failure with extensive crescent formation is reported. Nephrotic syndrome is rare. Serum IgG and C3 levels are often decreased, and immunofluorescence often demonstrates IgG, IgM, and in subendothelial and subepithelial deposits, suggesting an immune-complex etiology.

129. What is the "internist's tumor"?
Renal cell carcinoma, because the condition is often diagnosed by its systemic, rather than urologic, manifestations. These systemic effects include fever, anemia, hypercalcemia, galactorrhea, feminization or masculinization, and Cushing's syndrome (see also Chapter 6).

130. Describe the major differences between fibromuscular dysplasia and atherosclerotic renal artery stenosis.

	Fibromuscular Dysplasia	*Atherosclerosis*
Age at onset	<40 yr	>45 yr
Gender	80% female	Primarily males
Distribution of lesion	Distal main renal artery and intrarenal branches	Aortic orifice and proximal main renal artery
Progression	Uncommon	Common, may progress to complete occlusion

131. What history or physical findings suggest renovascular hypertension (HTN)?
Renovascular HTN comprises about 0.2–5% of all cases of HTN. Clues to the presence of renal artery stenosis may be derived from the history and physical exam. Onset of HTN before age 20 or after age 50 should suggest the possibility of renovascular HTN. Similarly, the development of a refractory phase in a previously stable hypertensive, the presence of spontaneous hypokalemia, and the presence of an abdominal bruit makes renovascular HTN very probable. Fibromuscular disease is common in young white females, while atheromatous disease is more likely in middle-aged men, especially when there is evidence of atheromatous vascular disease elsewhere. Family history is not helpful in suspecting renovascular HTN.

132. How do you confirm renovascular HTN? What laboratory tests or imaging techniques are useful in screening for renovascular HTN?
A high **plasma renin** profile is seen in approx. 80% of patients with renovascular HTN, as opposed to 15% in essential HTN. Another screening test often used is the **captopril test.** The

administration of oral captopril causes a reactive rise of renin which is greater in patients with renovascular as opposed to essential HTN. The overall sensitivity is 74% and specificity 89%.

Ultrasound determination of renal size (a difference of >1.5 cm between the two kidneys) is very important in suggesting renal artery stenosis. **Captopril renography** has now replaced **isotope renograph** as the screening procedure of choice, since the sensitivity is 92% and specificity 93%. The rationale for this test is that the GFR and renal blood flow of an ischemic kidney are dependent on the effects of angiotensin on the efferent glomerular arterioles and hence fall markedly with ACE inhibition. Thus, captopril causes decreased isotope uptake by the ischemic kidney.

Mann SJ, Pickering TG: Detection of renovascular hypertension. Ann Intern Med 117:845–853, 1992.

133. And how is the diagnosis confirmed?

The confirmation of renal artery stenosis is by renal angiography.

134. How do you diagnose ARF secondary to rhabdomyolysis? Are there clues to this form of ARF?

Rhabdomyolysis can cause ARF due to acute tubular necrosis (ATN). It occurs in various clinical conditions, including trauma, ischemic tissue damage following a drug overdose, alcoholism, seizures, and heat stroke (especially in untrained subjects or those with sickle cell trait). Hypokalemia and severe hypophosphatemia can also precipitate rhabdomyolysis. It is the most common cause of ARF in patients abusing illicit IV drugs.

Typically, these patients have pigmented granular casts in urine sediment, a positive ortho-tolidine test in the urine supernatant (indicating the presence of heme), and markedly elevated plasma creatine kinase and other muscle enzymes, owing to their release from damaged muscle tissue. Other characteristics of ARF due to rhabdomyolysis include hyperphosphatemia, hyperkalemia, and a disproportionate increase in plasma creatinine (all of these being due to release of cellular constituents). A high anion-gap metabolic acidosis and severe hyperuricemia are also characteristic, and oliguria or anuria is common.

The mechanism of renal failure is not completely understood. Although myoglobin is not directly nephrotoxic, concurrent vasoconstriction or volume depletion decreases the renal perfusion and rate of urine flow in tubules, thereby promoting the precipitation of these pigment casts.

BIBLIOGRAPHY

1. Brenner EM, Rector FC (eds): The Kidney, 5th ed. Philadelphia, W.B. Saunders, 1996.
2. Greenberg A (ed) Primer on Kidney Diseases—National Kidney Foundation. San Diego, Academic Press, 1994.
3. Rose BF: Pathophysiology of Renal Disease, 2nd ed. New York, McGraw-Hill, 1987.
4. Schrier RW (ed): Diseases of the Kidney, 5th ed. Boston, Little, Brown & Co., 1993.
5. Schrier RW (ed): Renal and Electrolyte Disorders, 4th ed. Boston, Little, Brown & Co., 1992.
6. Bennett JC et al (eds): Cecil Textbook of Medicine, 20th ed. Philadelphia, W.B. Saunders, 1996.

8. ACID/BASE AND ELECTROLYTES

Sharma S. Prabhakar, M.D.

In all things you shall find everywhere the Acid and the Alcaly.
Otto Tachenius (1670)
Hyppocrates Chymacus, Ch. 21.

Hence if too much salt is used in food, the pulse hardens.
Huang Ti (The Yellow Emperor) (2697–2597 B.C.)
Nei Chung Su Wen, Bk. 3, Sect. 10, tr. by Ilza Veith,
in The Yellow Emperor's Classic of Internal Medicine.

REGULATION OF SODIUM, WATER, AND VOLUME STATUS

1. List the osmolality and electrolyte concentrations of serum and commonly used intravenous (IV) solutions.

Osmolality and Electrolyte Concentrations of Commonly Used IV Solutions

SERUM AND SOLUTIONS*	OSMOLALITY (MOSM/KG)	GLUCOSE (G/L)	SODIUM (MEQ/L)	CHLORIDE (MEQ/L)
Serum	285–295	65–110	135–145	97–110
5% D/W	252	50	0	0
10% D/W	505	100	0	0
50% D/W	2520	500	0	0
1/2 NS (0.45% NaCl)	154	0	77	77
NS (0.9% NaCl)	308	0	154	154
3% NS	1026	0	513	513
Ringer's lactate	272	0	130	109

*D/W = dextrose in water; NS = normal saline. Ringer's lactate also contains 28 meq/l lactate, 4 meq/l K^+, and 4.5 meq/l Ca^{2+}.

2. How do you estimate a patient's serum osmolality?

A close estimate can be derived from measurements of the serum sodium (Na^+), glucose, and blood urea nitrogen (BUN), using the following equation:

$$\text{Osmolality} = 1.86 \times [Na^+] + \frac{\text{Glucose}}{18} + \frac{\text{BUN}}{2.8} + 9$$

3. What percentage of the adult human body consists of water? What percentage of the water content is intracellular versus extracellular?

Approx. 60% of the adult man and 50% of the adult woman are water. About two-thirds of this volume is intracellular, and one-third is extracellular. About 20% of the extracellular fluid volume is plasma water.

4. What are the sources and daily amounts of water gain and loss?

The average adult male gains and loses 2600 ml of water each day. The **gains** occur from direct fluid ingestion (1400 ml/day), from the fluid content of ingested food (850 ml/day), and as a product of water produced by oxidation reactions (350 ml/day). Water **losses** occur through urine (1500 ml/day), perspiration (500 ml/day), respiration (400 ml/day), and feces (200 ml/day.)

5. Discuss the necessary factors that allow the kidney to adequately excrete free water.

The required factors are:

1. There must be a filtrate formed to allow for renal excretion of free water. The lower the glomerular filtration rate (GFR), the lower the kidney's ability to respond rapidly to a free-water challenge with excretion of free water.

2. Glomerular filtrate must escape reabsorption in the proximal tubule to get to the diluting segment (ascending loop of Henle), where free water is created. Pathologic states involving vigorous fluid reabsorption in the proximal tubule are associated with a compromised ability to excrete free water. Examples include true volume depletion and states of decreased effective arterial blood volume, such as congestive heart failure, cirrhosis, and nephrotic syndrome.

3. An adequately functioning diluting segment must be present. Intrinsic disorders of function of this segment are unusual. Endogenous prostaglandin E_2 and loop diuretics inhibit NaCl transport in this segment and can thereby limit formation of free water.

4. The free water formed by the diluting segment must leave the nephron without being reabsorbed by the collecting tubule. This nephron segment is intrinsically impermeable to water but is made permeable by antidiuretic hormone (ADH).

6. Explain the meaning of serum sodium concentration with respect to sodium balance and water balance.

Serum Na^+ concentration [Na^+], (in meq/l) reflects the concentration of this cation in extracellular fluid (ECF). Because its units are measured as mass per unit volume, [Na^+] indicates the relative relationship between Na^+ and water in the body. It is not indicative of total body Na^+ content but is more an indication of the water status (hydration) of the body. [Na^+] may be low, normal, or increased with any given perturbation of total body Na^+ content.

Alterations of the [Na^+] reflect alterations in free-water balance. Therefore, a true low [Na^+] indicates a free-water excess compared to Na^+ content, and a high [Na^+] indicates a relative free-water deficit.

7. What happens to the serum Na^+ concentration in response to loss of isotonic fluid, as in hemorrhage?

Isotonic fluid losses in and of themselves cause a decrease in ECF volume with no change in [Na^+]. If, however, these losses are replaced with hypotonic fluids, dilutional hyponatremia results.

8. What is meant by a state of "decreased effective arterial blood volume"?

The extracellular space is dynamic, with an ongoing balance between its capacity and its actual volume. Both of these parameters are biologically monitored and normally coordinated to maintain optimal tissue perfusion. A state of decreased effective arterial blood volume occurs when there is a large capacity combined with a smaller volume. This is seen most commonly with congestive heart failure, cirrhosis, and nephrotic syndrome.

9. Why does Na^+ have an effective distribution in total body water despite being confined largely to the extracellular space?

Na^+ is the major determinant of serum osmolality, and changes in its concentration lead to water shifts between the extracellular and intracellular compartments. This osmotic shift of water gives Na^+ an effective distribution greater than its chemical distribution and equivalent to that for total body water.

10. What is the diluting segment of the nephron?

The diluting segment is the thick ascending limb of the loop of Henle. This segment actively reabsorbs NaCl without water. This process leads to urine that is hyposmotic compared to plasma, creating free water for excretion.

11. What is the initial step in evaluating a patient with hyponatremia?

Determining the serum osmolality (either measured or calculated).

- **Hyperosmolar** hyponatremia (serum osmolarity >295 mOsm/kg H_2O) usually results from administration of hypertonic solutions of dextrose or mannitol.

- **Isotonic** hyponatremia (serum osmolality 280–295 mOsm/kg H_2O) is seen with administration of isotonic solutions of dextrose and mannitol.
- **Hyposmolar** hyponatremia (serum osmolality <280 mOsm/kg H_2O) can be associated with low, normal, or increased volume status and is seen with diuretic administration, salt-losing renal conditions, SIADH, chronic renal failure, and a wide range of other causes.
- **Pseudohyponatremia** is artifactual depression of serum Na^+ that results from excessive amounts of lipids and proteins leading to reduction of the plasma fraction of water.

12. How can patients with hyposomolar hyponatremia be categorized according to their history and physical findings?

Patients with hyposmolar hyponatremia can be categorized according to their volume status as estimated from the physical exam and history.

1. **Low volume status:** Supported by a history of volume loss or decreased intake and orthostatic blood pressure changes on examination. These patients need to have the lost volume replaced to turn off the factors that limit the kidney's ability to excrete free water.

2. **Expanded volume:** Supported by a history of a condition with decreased effective arterial blood volume and an examination showing edema. Patients must have therapeutic attention directed to their underlying disorder. If the hyponatremia is mild and symptomatic, free-water restriction, in addition to specific treatment of the underlying disorder, would be the suggested ini-

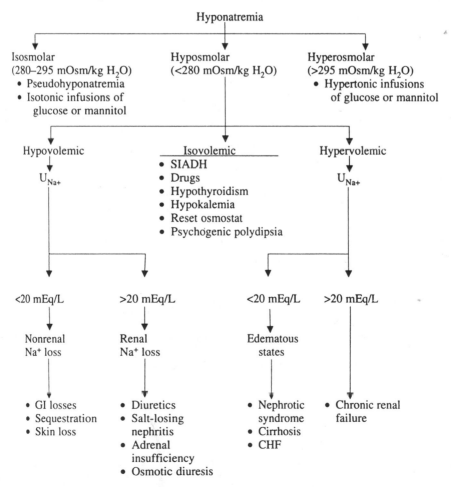

tial therapeutic approach. If the hyponatremia is severe and symptomatic, more aggressive treatment with hypertonic saline and furosemide may be required.

3. **Apparently normal volume status (euvolemia):** A wide variety of pathologic processes must be considered in the diagnostic evaluation, including SIADH and drugs that can limit free-water excretion (e.g., chlorpropamide).

13. How do pseudohyponatremia and spurious hyponatremia differ?

Pseudo-hyponatremia occurs when a quantitative serum Na^+ measurement is performed on a given volume of plasma that contains a greater-than-normal amount of water-excluding particles, such as lipid or protein. In this setting, plasma water (which contains the Na^+) comprises a smaller fraction of the plasma volume, leading to a factitiously low serum Na^+ concentration (when expressed in meq/l). The Na^+ concentration in plasma water is normal, and therefore patients are asymptomatic. Attention should be directed to hyperlipidemia or hyperproteinemia.

Spurious hyponatremia results from hyperosmolality of the serum (i.e., from hyperglycemia), resulting in movement of intracellular water to the extracellular space and subsequent dilution of the Na^+ in the ECF. These patients are not symptomatic from hyposmolality (as are patients with true hyponatremia). If they are symptomatic at all, it is due to their hyperosmolar state. Attention should be directed to correcting the hyperosmolar state.

It is important to distinguish these two categories of hyponatremia from true hyponatremia associated with hyposmolality because the diagnostic workup and therapeutic management are different.

14. How do you correct the serum Na^+ for a given level of hyperglycemia?

Hyperglycemia, one of the causes of spurious hyponatremia, causes a decrease in the measured serum Na^+ concentration. For each increase in serum glucose of 100 mg/dl up to 600 mg/dl (an increase of 500, or 5×100 mg/dl), the serum Na^+ decreases by 8.0 meq/l (5×1.6 meq/l).

15. What is essential hyponatremia?

Essential hyponatremia, or "sick cell syndrome," denotes hyponatremia in the absence of a water diuresis defect. One hypothesis is that the osmoreceptor cells in the hypothalamus are reset so that they maintain a lower plasma osmolality. This is seen in several conditions, such as congestive heart failure cirrhosis, and pulmonary tuberculosis, and is diagnosed by demonstrating normal urinary Na^+ concentration and dilution in the face of hyponatremia. Generally, this entity does not require treatment.

16. What are the signs and symptoms of hyponatremia?

The manifestations are mainly attributable to CNS edema, which is usually not seen until the serum Na^+ falls to 120 meq/l or less. Symptoms range from mild lethargy to seizure, coma, and death.

17. Why would two patients with the same degree of hyponatremia have dramatically different signs and symptoms?

The signs and symptoms of hyponatremia are more a function of the rapidity of the drop in serum Na^+ than the absolute level. In patients with chronic hyponatremia, there has been time for solute equilibration, resulting in less CNS edema and less severe manifestations. In acute hyponatremia, there is no time for equilibration, and so smaller changes in serum Na^+ are accompanied by larger degrees of CNS edema and more severe manifestations.

18. How do you manage hyponatremia in edematous states?

Treatment depends on the underlying etiology, any symptoms, and the rapidity of the drop in serum Na^+. In general, patients with edematous states such as the nephrotic syndrome, who have ECF expansion, have some degree of hyponatremia if they are water-restricted. Generally this condition is asymptomatic and requires no treatment. Treatment is required only if the hyponatremia is severe (<125 meq/ l), and especially if there are symptoms such as lethargy, confusion, stupor, and coma.

19. A 41-year-old black man is hospitalized with acute bacterial meningitis. His chemistry profile shows a BUN and creatinine of 11 and 1.2 mg/dl, respectively, but his serum Na^+ is 127 meq/l. How do you evaluate his hyponatremia and correct it?

Hyponatremia in the setting of bacterial meningitis (or any pathologic CNS process) requires evaluation to rule out the syndrome of inappropriate ADH secretion (**SIADH**). SIADH is a form of hyponatremia involving sustained or spiking levels of ADH that are inappropriate for the osmotic or volume stimuli that normally affect ADH secretion. The essential points in the diagnosis of SIADH are:

1. Presence of hypotonic hyponatremia
2. Inappropriate antidiuresis (urine osmolality higher than expected for the degree of hyponatremia)
3. Significant Na^+ excretion when the patient is normovolemic
4. Normal renal, thyroid, and adrenal function
5. Absence of other causes of hyponatremia, volume depletion, or edema

Thus, the workup includes measurement of serum and urine Na^+ concentration and osmolality. In most cases, urinary osmolality exceeds plasma osmolality, often by > 100 mOsm/l. Urinary Na^+ excretion exceeds 20 meq/l unless the patient is wasting, and it improves with fluid restriction. In the most cases, restriction of fluids to 1000–1200 ml/day is all that is needed. Occasionally, patients with symptomatic and marked hyponatremia may require demeclocycline therapy and/or hypertonic saline.

20. Which conditions are associated with SIADH?

Differential Diagnosis of SIADH

Malignant neoplasia	**Pulmonary disorders**
Carcinoma (bronchogenic, duodenum, pancreatic, urethral, prostatic, bladder)	Tuberculosis
	Pneumonia
Lymphoma, leukemia	Mechanical ventilators with positive pressure
Thymoma, mesothelioma, Ewing's sarcoma	Pneumonia (bacterial, viral, mycobacterial, fungal)
	Asthma, cystic fibrosis
CNS disorders	Pneumothorax
Trauma, subarachnoid hemorrhage, subdural hematoma, Rocky Mountain spotted fever	Lung abscess
Infection (encephalitis, meningitis, brain abscess)	**Drugs**
Tumors	Chlorpropamide
Porphyria	Thiazide diuretics
Guillain-Barré syndrome	Oxytocin
Psychosis, delirium tremens	Vincristine
Stroke	Haloperidol
Multiple sclerosis	Nicotine
	Phenothiazines
	Tricyclic antidepressants
	Others
	Other Conditions
	"Idiopathic" SIADH
	Hypothyroidism

21. What is cerebral salt-wasting?

Due to impaired renal water excretion, this condition is associated with hyposmolar hyponatremia in patients with cerebral trauma or disease. It mimics SIADH in all aspects including hypouricemia, except that in this syndrome patients are volume-deleted while in SIADH patients are euvolemic. The high urinary Na^+ despite hypovolemia reflects renal salt-wasting. The etiology of this salt-wasting is unknown, although increased secretion of cerebral natriuretic factors is one likely explanation. A circulating factor that impairs renal tubular Na^+ reabsorption is another likely possibility.

Al-Mufti H, Arieff AI: Cerebral salt wasting syndrome: Combined cerebral and distal tubular lesion. Am J Med 77:740, 1984.

22. How do you estimate the free-water deficit in a patient with hypernatremia?

It can be assumed that the patient has lost free water without salt, and thus the patient has reduced total body water (TBW) but maintains the same total body Na^+ content. This change results in an increase in the serum Na^+ concentration that is proportional to the decrease in TBW — i.e., the ratio of the initial serum Na^+ (which is assumed to be normal) to the current serum Na^+ (which is higher than normal) is equal to the ratio of the present TBW (which is less than normal) to the initial TBW (which is assumed to have been normal):

$$\frac{\text{Current TBW}}{\text{Initial TBW}} = \frac{\text{Initial } [Na^+]}{\text{Current } [Na^+]}$$

This relationship can be used to calculate the current TBW. Subtracting this value from the intial (normal) TBW yields the estimated free-water deficit. This calculated free-water deficit must be replaced with fluids.

23. What are the manifestations of hypernatremia?

The manifestations of hypernatremia are basically those of hyperosmolality and are similar to the symptoms manifested by other causes of hyperosmolality, such as hyperglycemia. These are produced mainly by fluid shifts from the CNS and increased CNS osmolality, resulting in "shrinking" of the brain. The symptoms range from lethargy to seizures, coma, and death. The severity of the symptoms depends on the severity of the hyperosmolality and the speed with which it develops.

24. What are some common causes of hypernatremia?

Diabetes insipidus

Severe dehydration due to extrarenal fluid losses (e.g., burns, excessive sweating, etc.)

Hypothalamic disorders (e.g., tumors, granulomas cerebrovascular accidents) leading to defective thirst and vasopressin regulation

25. How do you correct hypernatremia?

Once the free-water deficit is calculated, hypernatremia is usually corrected by replacement of the water. In mild cases, this can be accomplished by simply having the patient drink or, if IV fluids are used, dextrose in water can be given. If salt-containing fluids are deemed necessary, the equivalent free-water volume must be given. For example, if half-normal saline is used (1 liter of which contains 500 ml of NS and 500 ml of free water), then twice the amount of the estimated free-water deficit is needed to correct the free-water deficit.

This volume deficit should be replaced slowly. The first half is given over 24 hours. If the patient is hemodynamically unstable, with signs of severe ECF volume depletion, therapy with 0.9% normal saline is warranted before dextrose infusion is started.

POTASSIUM BALANCE

26. How is potassium distributed between the intracellular fluid (ICF) and extracellular fluid (ECF) compartments?

A 70-kg man contains approx. 3500 meq of K^+ ($\sim$ 50 meq/kg body weight). The vast majority of this (98%) is in the ICF space. Therefore, the amount in the ECF compartment (the portion that we routinely measure) represents only a small percentage of the total body K^+.

27. How is the large chemical gradient between intracellular and extracellular K⁺ concentration maintained?

The Na^+, K^+–ATPase pump actively extrudes Na^+ from the cell and pumps K^+ into the cell. This pump is present in all cells of the body. In addition, the cell is electrically negative compared to the exterior, which serves to keep K^+ inside the cell.

28. Given the relatively small extracellular compared to intracellular concentration of K⁺, why are some electrical processes (cardiac conduction, skeletal and smooth muscle contraction) sensitive to changes in the ECF K⁺ concentration?

It is the ratio of the ECF to ICF K^+ concentration more than the absolute level of either that determines the sensitivity of these electrical processes. Because the ECF concentration of K^+ is small compared to the ICF concentration, a small absolute change in ECF K^+ concentration results in a large change in the ECF:ICF K^+ ratio.

29. What are some common factors that influence the movement of K⁺ between the intracellular and extracellular compartments?

1. **Acid-base changes:** Acidemia (increased concentration of H^+ in serum) leads to intracellular buffering of H^+, with subsequent extrusion of K^+ into the ECF, increasing the concentration of K^+ in this compartment.

2. **Hormones:** Insulin, epinephrine (β_2- mediated), growth hormone, and androgens all promote net movement of K^+ into cells.

3. **Cellular metabolism:** Synthesis of protein and glycogen is associated with intracellular K^+ binding.

4. **Extracellular concentration:** All other things being equal, K^+ tends to enter the cell when its extracellular concentration is high and vice versa.

30. How is K⁺ handled by the kidney?

Most of the filtered K^+ is reabsorbed in the proximal tubule, and there is net secretion or net resorption in the distal nephron, depending on the body's K^+ needs. Under most conditions, we are in K^+ excess, and the kidney must excrete K^+ to maintain whole-body K^+ balance. K^+ restriction leads to renal K^+ conservation, but this process is neither as rapid nor efficient as the process for Na^+.

31. How does aldosterone influence K⁺ metabolism?

Aldosterone is the main regulatory hormone for K^+ metabolism. It promotes Na^+ resorption and K^+ secretion in the distal nephron, gut, and sweat glands. Quantitatively, its greatest effect is in the kidney. Its secretion is increased by an increasing K^+ concentration in the ECF and is decreased by low K^+ concentrations.

32. What is meant by transtubular K⁺ gradient (TTKG)? How does it help in evaluating a patient with hyperkalemia?

Asymptomatic hyperkalemia is a common presentation of patients with mineralocorticoid deficiency. Na^+ deficiency and volume depletion are not seen unless there is concomitant glucocorticoid deficiency. Na^+ balance is maintained by other factors, such as angiotensin II and catecholamines, although the ability to conserve Na^+ maximally is generally lost. Thus, urine Na^+ < 10 meq/l is unusual in primary hypoaldosteronism.

To diagnose hypoaldosteronism, the first step is to exclude drug-induced hyperkalemia (such as ACE inhibitors, β-blockers, NSAIDs, heparin, or K^+-sparing diuretics). The next step is to obtain morning samples of plasma for renin, aldosterone, and cortisol measurements. Administration of furosemide (20–40 mg) at 6 PM and 6 AM before samples are drawn enhances the utility of the test by stimulating plasma renin activity in normal persons but not in those with hypoaldosteronism.

TTKG is an indirect method of evaluating the effect of aldosterone on the kidney. The principle is to measure K^+ at the end of the cortical collecting tube, after all the distal K^+ secretion has taken place:

$$\text{TTKG} = \frac{U_{K^+} / (\, U_{osm}/P_{osm}\,)}{P_{K^+}}$$

It is assumed that urine osmolality (U_{osm}) at the end of the cortical collecting tube is the same as that of plasma (P_{osm}) because the interstitium here is iso-osmotic, and that there is no further K^+ secretion or resorption. But, since ADH-mediated water permeability continues in the medullary collecting tubule, the K^+ concentration in this duct rises.

The above formula is applicable as long as the urine Na^+ concentration is >25 meq/l, since Na^+ delivery should not be a limiting factor. The TTKG in normal subjects is 8–10 on a normal diet. On a high K^+ diet, TTKG is > 11 because of increased K^+ secretion. Thus, in a hyperkalemic subject, a TTKG < 5 meq/l indicates impaired tubular K^+ secretion and is highly suggestive of hypoaldosteronism.

Ethier JH, et al: The trans-tubular potassium gradient in patients with hypokalemia and hyperkalemia. Am J Kidney Dis 15:309, 1990.

33. Name seven factors that can lead to increased renal K^+ excretion.

1. Increased dietary K^+ intake
2. Increased aldosterone secretion (as in volume depletion)
3. Alkalosis
4. Increased flow rate in the distal tubule
5. Increased Na^+ delivery to the distal nephron. This promotes Na^+ resorption in exchange for K^+ secretion in the distal nephron. The process is accelerated in the presence of aldosterone.
6. Decreased chloride concentration in tubular fluid in the distal nephron. This allows for Na^+ to be resorbed with a less-permeable ion (e.g., bicarbonate or sulfate) that increases the negativity of the tubular lumen in the distal nephron. The increased negativity of the tubular lumen promotes K^+ secretion.
7. Natriuretic agents. Drugs, such as the loop diuretics, thiazides, and acetazolamide, lead to increased Na^+ delivery to the distal nephron, volume depletion with increased aldosterone secretion, and subsequent increased renal K^+ excretion.

34. How do the potassium-sparing diuretics work?

Some natriuretic agents are K^+-sparing in that they inhibit K^+ secretion in the distal nephron. These agents include spironolactone, triamterene, and amiloride.

35. In addition to the kidney, what is the other major route of K^+ loss?

The GI tract. Fluids in the lower GI tract, particularly those of the small bowel, are high in K^+. Therefore, diarrhea can result in significant losses of K^+. However, upper GI losses, such as vomiting or nasogastric suction, cause *renal* K^+ loss. This renal K^+ loss is multifactorial and includes the following:

- Alkalosis
- Volume depletion, which leads to increased aldosterone secretion.
- Chloride depletion from the loss of HCl in gastric fluid. This leads to a high tubular concentration of HCO_3^-, which is a relatively nonresorbable anion.

36. What can cause a spuriously elevated serum K^+ determination?

1. **Hemolysis,** with the release of intraerythrocytic K^+.
2. **Pseudohyperkalemia,** seen in marked thrombocytosis or leukocytosis. It is due to the disproportionately increased amounts of the normally released K^+ that occurs with clotting. This can be corrected by inhibiting clotting and measuring the plasma K^+ concentration.

37. List the common causes of hyperkalemia.

Causes of Hyperkalemia

1. Inadequate excretion	**3. Shift of K+ from tissues**
Renal disorders	Tissue damage (muscle crush, hemolysis, internal
Acute renal failure	bleeding)
Severe chronic renal failure	Drugs (succinylcholine, arginine, digitalis
Tubular disorders	poisoning, β-blockers)
Hypoaldosteronism	Acidosis
Adrenal disorders	Hyperosmolality
Hyporeninemic (as in tubulointerstitial diseases,	Insulin deficiency
drugs such as NSAIDs, ACE inhibitors,	Hyperkalemic periodic paralysis
β-blockers)	
Diuretics that inhibit K+ secretion	**4. Pseudohyperkalemia**
(spironolactone, triamterene, amiloride)	Thrombocytosis
	Leukocytosis
2. Excessive intake	Poor venipuncture technique
	In vitro hemolysis

Levinksy N: Fluids and electrolytes. In Isselbacher KJ, et al (eds): Harrison's Principles of Internal Medicine, 13th ed. New York, McGraw-Hill, 1994, p 252.

38. Describe the general diagnostic approach to patients who have disturbances in serum K+ concentration.

In the initial approach, it is important to determine whether the disturbance results from:
(1) Abnormal K+ intake or metabolism (excessive catabolism or anabolism)
(2) Intra- and extracellular compartmental shifts
(3) Disturbances in renal excretion or extrarenal loss.

After the patient is placed in one of these three categories, it is possible to narrow the differential diagnosis, order appropriate diagnostic tests, and decide on the appropriate management. Disturbances of intake can be investigated by history and physical examination. The possibility of cellular shifts can be investigated by looking for any of the disturbances that result in compartmental movement of this cation. Determination of the urinary K+ concentration can help in distinguishing renal from nonrenal causes. High urinary K+ excretion in the setting of hypokalemia is compatible with a renal cause for K+ deficiency. In contrast, an appropriately low urinary K+ excretion in the setting of hypokalemia suggests extrarenal (possibly GI) losses.

39. How does hypokalemia present clinically?

The major manifestations are seen in the neuromuscular system. When K+ falls to 2.0–2.5 meq/l, muscular weakness and lethargy are seen. With further decreases, the patient manifests paralysis with eventual respiratory muscle involvement and death. Hypokalemia can also cause rhabdomyolysis, myoglobinuria, and paralytic ileus. Prolonged hypokalemia can lead to renal tubular damage (called hypokalemic nephropathy).

40. How do you manage a patient with hypokalemia?

Management must be directed at the disturbance causing the abnormal K+ concentration. If hypokalemia is associated with alkalosis, then the alkalosis should be corrected in addition to providing K+ supplements.

In general, patients with K+ depletion should be given supplements slowly to replace the deficit. The oral route is preferred because of its safety as well as efficacy. Some instances require more rapid repletion with IV supplements, but this should not exceed 20 meq/hr. Cardiac monitoring should accompany infusions of > 10 meq/hr.

41. What are the manifestations of hyperkalemia besides ECG changes?

The most important manifestation is the increased excitability of cardiac muscle. With severe elevations in K+, a patient can suffer diastolic cardiac arrest. Skeletal muscle paralysis can also be seen. Again, the symptoms produced by hyperkalemia are dependent on the rapidity of the change. Patients with chronically elevated serum K+ levels can tolerate higher levels with fewer symptoms than patients with acute hyperkalemia.

42. How is hyperkalemia managed?

Treatment depends on the extent of the hyperkalemia and the clinical setting. Mild levels of hyperkalemia (5.0–5.5 meq/l) associated with the hyporenin-hypoaldosterone syndrome are tolerated well and usually require no treatment. Higher levels not associated with ECG changes may require treatment with a synthetic mineralocorticoid.

Hyperkalemia occasionally presents as a medical emergency with very high levels (>7.0 meq/l) and cardiac conduction system abnormalities as determined by the ECG changes (see Chapter 3). In this emergent setting, management includes:

1. IV calcium must be administered to immediately counteract the effect of hyperkalemia on the conduction system.

2. This must be followed by maneuvers to shift K+ into cells, thereby decreasing the ratio of extra- to intracellular K+. This can be accomplished by administering glucose with insulin and/or bicarbonate to increase serum pH.

3. Finally, a maneuver to remove K+ from the body must be instituted, such as a cation-exchange resin (Kayexalate) and/or hemodialysis or peritoneal dialysis.

43. A 61-year-old woman with end-stage renal disease (ESRD) missed her dialysis twice and presents to the emergency department with a serum K+ of 6.4 meq/l. How would you manage this patient?

The severity of hyperkalemia is assessed by both the serum K+ level and ECG changes. If the ECG shows only tall T waves and the serum K+ is < 6.5 meq/l, the hyperkalemia is mild, whereas K+ levels of 6.5–8.0 meq/l are associated with more severe ECG changes, including absent P waves and wide QRS complexes. At higher K+ levels, ventricular arrhythmias tend to appear, and the prognosis is grave unless proper treatment is given.

The first step is to obtain an ECG or observe the cardiac monitor. If it shows only tall T waves (as is likely in this situation), the patient can be treated with:

1. **Hypertonic glucose infusion,** along with 10 units of insulin (e.g., 10 units of insulin with 200–500 ml of 10% glucose in 30 min followed by 1 l in the next 4–6 hours).

2. **Sodium bicarbonate,** 50–150 meq given by IV (if the patient is not in fluid overload).

Both of these maneuvers shift K+ into cells and start acting within an hour. Total body K+ can be decreased by using cation-exchange resins, such as sodium polysterone sulfonate; usually, 20 gm with 20 ml of 70% sorbitol solution is started every 4–6 hours.

If the ECG shows the more severe changes, the patient should first receive 10% calcium gluconate (10–30 ml IV) while being monitored. Arrangements must be made to dialyze the patient as soon as possible to correct the hyperkalemia.

44. A 71-year-old diabetic with a nonhealing foot ulcer is on tobramycin and piperacillin. This patient has a resistant hypokalemia. How do you approach this problem?

Aminoglycosides and penicillins are both known to deplete serum K+. The former do this by defective proximal tubular K+ resorption, and the latter by increased renal K+ excretion induced by the poorly resorbable anion (penicillin). With aminoglycosides, magnesium-wasting is another complication. Hence, in addition to K+ repletion, correction of hypomagnesemia is important, since hypokalemia is often resistant to correction unless the magnesium deficit is also corrected.

45. A 67-year-old white man with congestive heart failure treated with furosemide has a serum K+ of 2.4 meq/l. How would you correct his K+ deficit?

Hypokalemia is an important complication of diuretic therapy (except with K+-sparing diuretics). It is important to monitor serum K+ periodically in these patients, especially those with cardiac illness who are likely to be on digoxin because hypokalemia can exacerbate digitalis toxicity. The K+ deficit requires replacement (except in patients who are on minimal doses of diuretics), particularly if serum K^+ is < 3 meq/l. The serum K^+ level is not an exact indicator of the total body deficit, but severe hypokalemia with serum K^+ of <3 meq/l is usually associated with a deficit of approx. 300 meq. KCl elixir or tablets are the treatment of choice. Enteric-coated K^+ supplements are known to cause gastric ulceration.

46. What is Bartter's syndrome?

Bartter's syndrome is a rare disorder characterized by hyperreninemic hyperaldosteronism, hyperplasia of juxtaglomerular apparatus, and hypokalemic alkalosis. There is also hypersecretion of vasodilatory prostaglandins, which help to maintain normal blood pressure despite hyperreninemia. The primary defect seems to be impaired NaCl reabsorption in the thick ascending loop of Henle or distal tubule. The diagnosis is often made by exclusion. Surreptitious use of diuretics and vomiting (urine Cl- is often low!) can mimic most of the findings of this syndrome. Treatment consists of a K^+-sparing diuretic (such as amiloride in higher doses of 10–40 mg) and NSAIDs to raise the plasma K^+ by reversing the physiologic abnormalities.

Stein JH: The pathogenetic spectrum of Bartter's syndrome. Kidney Int 28:85, 1985.

ACID-BASE REGULATION

47. What is the Henderson-Hasselbalch equation? What is its significance?

An acid-base disorder is suspected on clinical grounds and confirmed by arterial blood gas (ABG) analysis of the pH, $PaCO_2$, or bicarbonate concentration. The Henderson-Hasselbalch equation is used to confirm that a given set of these parameters are mutually compatible:

$$pH = pK_a + \log \frac{[HCO_3^-]}{\alpha CO_2 \times PaCO_2} = 61 + \log \frac{[HCO_3^-]}{0.03 \times PaCO_2}$$

The value of pK_a, the negative log of the equilibrium constant K, and the CO_2 solubility coefficient (αCO_2) are constant at any given set of temperature and osmolality. In plasma, at 37°C, the pKa=6.1 and $\alpha CO_2 = 0.03$.

The Henderson-Hasselbalch equation shows that pH is dependent on the ratio of $[HCO_3^-]$ to $PaCO_2$ and not on the absolute individual values alone. A primary change in one of the values usually leads to a compensatory change in the other value. This serves to limit the degree of the resulting acidosis or alkalosis.

48. The integrated action of which three organs is involved in acid-base homeostasis?

The **liver, lungs,** and **kidneys** cooperate to maintain acid-base balance. The liver metabolizes proteins contained in the standard American diet such that net acid (protons) is produced. Hepatic metabolism of organic acids (lactate) can consume acid, which is the equivalent of producing bicarbonate. Acid released into the ECF titrates HCO_3^- to H_2O and CO_2. This CO_2 and the CO_2 produced from cellular metabolism are excreted by the lungs. The kidney reclaims the filtered HCO_3^- and excretes the accumulated net acid.

49. What is the fate of a load of nonvolatile acid administered to the body?

The acid load is initially buffered by extracellular (40%) and intracellular (60%) buffers. These buffers minimize the decrease in pH that otherwise would occur. The major ECF buffer is the HCO_3^- system, and most intracellular buffering is provided by histidine-containing proteins. The administered acid reduces ECF HCO_3^-, and new HCO_3^- is then regenerated by the kidney during the process of proton (acid) secretion. Therefore, the administered acid is initially buffered and eventually excreted by the kidney.

50. Name the two major roles of the kidney in monitoring acid-base balance.

The kidney must **reclaim** the filtered HCO_3^- and **regenerate** the HCO_3^- lost by acid titration. This latter process is equivalent to acid excretion. Reclamation of HCO_3^- is quantitatively a more important process than regeneration (4500 meq/day versus 70 meq/day). Nevertheless, without regeneration of new HCO_3^- (excretion of acid), the plasma HCO_3^- concentration could not be maintained, and net acid retention would result.

51. Which two principal urinary buffers allow for net acid excretion (new HCO_3^- regeneration)?

Dibasic phosphate and ammonia. By accepting a proton, they become monobasic phosphate and ammonium ions, respectively, and are excreted in the urine. The phosphate is measured as titratable acid, and the ammonium is measured directly. Urinary excretion of these two substances minus urinary HCO_3^- excretion constitutes net acid excretion.

52. What are the four primary acid-base disturbances? How are they characterized?

Metabolic acidosis, metabolic alkalosis, respiratory acidosis, and **respiratory alkalosis.**

In the steady-state maintenance of normal acid-base balance, the addition of H^+ to the body fluids is balanced by their excretion, such that the H^+ concentration of the ECF remains relatively constant at 40 nM (40×10^{-9} M, or pH = 7.40). An imbalance in this process that leads to a net increase in $[H^+]$ is called **acidosis. Alkalosis** refers to an imbalance that leads to a net decrease in $[H^+]$.

53. What is meant by metabolic and respiratory when referring to these acid-base disturbances?

Metabolic and respiratory are terms used to describe how the imbalance occurred. Describing a disorder as ***metabolic*** infers that the imbalance leading to the change in H^+ occurred either because of addition of nonvolatile acid or base or because of a gain or loss of available buffer (HCO_3^-). HCO_3^- as a buffer reduces the concentration of free H^+ in solution. Referring to an acid-base disorder as ***respiratory*** infers that the net change in $[H^+]$ occurred secondary to a disturbance in ventilation that resulted in either a net increase or decrease in CO_2 gas in the ECF.

- **Metabolic acidosis** means there has been a net increase in $[H^+]$ as a result of a net gain in nonvolatile acid or from a net loss of HCO_3^- buffer.
- **Respiratory acidosis** means that there has been a net increase in $[H^+]$ as a result of decreased ventilation, leading to CO_2 retention.
- **Metabolic alkalosis** denotes a net decrease in $[H+]$ that occurs as a result of gain of HCO_3^- or loss of acid.
- **Respiratory alkalosis** means that there has been a net decrease in $[H^+]$ because of increased ventilation leading to decreased CO_2.

Note that these disorders refer to the imbalance that leads to the directional change in $[H^+]$ and do not denote what the final $[H^+]$, PCO_2, and $[HCO_3^-]$ will be. Two important facts should be kept in mind: (1) there are compensatory changes that occur in response to these disorders, and (2) more than one acid-base disturbance may occur simultaneously, such that the final parameters measured depend not only on the algebraic sum of the different disorders but also on their respective compensatory responses.

54. How are the four primary acid-base disorders diagnosed?

Relationships Between HCO_3^- and $PaCO_2$ in Simple Acid-Base Disorders

CONDITION	PRIMARY DISTURBANCE	PREDICTED RESPONSE
Metabolic acidosis	$\downarrow HCO_3^-$	$\Delta PaCO_2 (\downarrow) = 1{-}1.4\ \Delta HCO_3^-$*
Metabolic alkalosis	$\uparrow HCO_3^-$	$\Delta PaCO_2 (\uparrow) = 0.4{-}0.9\ \Delta HCO_3^-$*
Respiratory acidosis	$\uparrow PaCO_2$	Acute: $\Delta > HCO_3^- (\uparrow) = 0.1\ \Delta PaCO_2$
		Chronic: $\Delta HCO_3^- (\uparrow) = 0.25{-}0.55\ \Delta PaCO_2$
Respiratory alkalosis	$\downarrow PaCO_2$	Acute: $\Delta HCO_3^- (\downarrow) = 0.2{-}0.25\ \Delta PaCO_2$
		Chronic: $\Delta HCO_3^- (\downarrow) = 0.4{-}0.5\ \Delta PaCO_2$

*After at least 12 to 24 hours.
Hamm L, Jacobsen HR: Mixed acid-base disorders. In Kokko JP, Tannen KL (eds): Fluids and Electrolytes, 2nd ed. Philadelphia, W.B. Saunders, 1990, p 487.

55. What are secondary acid-base disturbances?

The phrase *secondary acid-base disturbance* is actually a misnomer. More correctly stated, these are compensatory physiologic responses to the cardinal acid-base disturbances. They usually alleviate the change in H+ concentration and therefore the pH that otherwise would occur. This can be seen more clearly by examining the mass-action equation defining the relationship of H+, HCO₃⁻, and the PaCO₂:

$$[H^+] = \frac{PaCO_2}{[HCO_3^-]} \times 24$$

This equation is derived from the more familiar Henderson-Hasselbalch equation. One can see that in the setting of metabolic acidosis, in which there is a primary decrease in [HCO₃⁻], the [H⁺] increases. It is also evident that the increase in [H⁺] in this setting can be alleviated by concomitantly decreasing the PaCO₂, which is exactly what occurs as a result of a ***physiologic*** increase in ventilation. This situation is properly described as metabolic acidosis with a directionally appropriate respiratory response. It is incorrect to describe the condition as primary metabolic acidosis with secondary respiratory alkalosis; to say that a patient has respiratory alkalosis is to say that a patient has ***pathologic*** hypoventilation, which is not this case in this situation. There are tables and formulas that can be used to calculate the expected respiratory response to a given degree of metabolic acidosis.

If the decrease in PaCO₂ in response to the degree of metabolic acidosis is exactly what we would have predicted from the formulas, then the patient is said to have one acid-base disorder: metabolic acidosis. In contrast, if the measured decrease in PaCO₂ is more than that predicted for the degree of metabolic acidosis, then the patient has an ***additional*** (not secondary) acid-base disorder: respiratory alkalosis in addition to metabolic acidosis. In other words, the patient has a **mixed disorder,** which is actually very common. If the measured PaCO₂ is higher than predicted, then the patient has an additional respiratory acidosis.

56. What is a respiratory acidosis?

Respiratory acidosis is a drop in the pH (acidosis) caused by alveolar hypoventilation. The alveolar hypoventilation leads to a rate of excretion of CO₂ that is less than its metabolic production. This net gain in CO₂ causes a rise in the PaCO₂. The lungs may be subject to diffuse hypoventilation (global alveolar hypoventilation), or only parts of the lungs may be involved (regional alveolar hypoventilation). As can be seen in the Henderson-Hasselbalch equation, any increase in the PaCO₂, if not accompanied by an increase in [HCO₃⁻], leads to a measurable drop in the pH.

57. How do you treat respiratory acidosis?

Treatment is aimed at the correction of the cause of the hypoventilation. This may involve the treatment of airway obstruction or, in respiratory failure, even mechanical ventilation.

58. What is a respiratory alkalosis?

Respiratory alkalosis, the opposite of respiratory acidosis, is a rise in pH (alkalosis). It is due to alveolar hyperventilation, which in turn leads to an increase in the excretion of CO₂ and a drop in the PaCO₂.

59. What are the causes of respiratory alkalosis?

Causes of Respiratory Alkalosis

1. CNS stimulation of ventilation:
    a. Physiologic (voluntary, anxiety, fear, fever, pregnancy)
    b. Pathologic (intracranial hemorrhage, stroke, tumors, brainstem lesions, salicylates)
2. Peripheral stimulation of ventilation:
    a. Reflex hyperventilation due to abnormal lung or chest wall
       mechanics (pulmonary emboli, myopathies, interstitial lung diseases)
    b. Arterial hypoxemia, high altitudes
    c. Pain
    d. Congestive heart failure, shock of any etiology
    e. Hypothermia
3. Hyperventilation with mechanical ventilation
4. Others:
    a. Severe liver disease
    b. Uremia

60. Are the plasma electrolytes alone (Na^+, K^+, Cl^-, and HCO_3^-) sufficient to determine a patient's acid-base status?

No. Remember that the regulatory systems of the body work to maintain the pH (or [H^+]), and that pH is a function of the ratio of $PaCO_2$ and [HCO_3^-]. The pH is not determined by the absolute value of $PaCO_2$ or [HCO_3^-] alone.

Thus, a set of plasma electrolytes demonstrating a normal [HCO_3^-] does not necessarily indicate a normal acid-base status. Furthermore, a low [HCO_3^-] and high [Cl^-] could represent either a metabolic acidosis (probably a nonanion gap acidosis) or a chronic respiratory alkalosis with an appropriate metabolic response (renal lowering of [HCO_3^-] as a response to the chronically low $PaCO_2$). This is an attempt to maintain a more normal pH.

Likewise, a high [HCO_3^-] with low [Cl^-] may represent a metabolic alkalosis or a chronic respiratory acidosis with an appropriate metabolic response (renal increase in [HCO_3^-] in response to chronically high $PaCO_2$) in an attempt to maintain a more normal pH. Note that without an accompanying pH and $PaCO_2$, one cannot tell if an abnormal [HCO_3^-] is due to a metabolic cause (a metabolic acidosis or alkalosis) or to a metabolic response to a primary respiratory disorder. This illustrates the importance of obtaining ABGs (with a pH and $PaCO_2$) in addition to a [HCO_3^-] to properly assess a patient's acid-base status.

61. What is meant by the anion gap?

The anion gap represents the difference between the routinely measured cations and anions in the plasma. It is usually calculated as follows:

$$\text{Anion gap} = [Na^+] - [Cl^-] + [HCO_3^-]$$

Since electroneutrality is always maintained in solution, there is no actual anion "gap". This gap is composed predominantly of negatively charged proteins in plasma and averages 12 ± 3 meq/l. An increase is most commonly caused by addition of an acid salt (H^+A^-), which reduces plasma HCO_3^- concentration by titration. Electroneutrality is maintained in the face of the reduced plasma HCO_3^- concentration by the accompanying anion. Since the anion is not measured routinely in the electrolyte profile, the routine measurement would reveal only decreased HCO_3^- concentration. With plasma Na^+ and Cl^- remaining unchanged, this reduced HCO_3^- concentration leads to an increased anion gap. Note that the anion gap would not change if the added acid were HCl. Other circumstances that can increase the anion gap include increased protein concentration and alkalemia, which increase the net negative charge on plasma proteins. The presence of a large quantity of cationic (positively charged) proteins, as with multiple myeloma, can reduce the anion gap.

62. What is the conceptual difference between an anion-gap and a non-anion-gap metabolic acidosis?

An anion gap acidosis is caused by the addition of a nonvolatile acid to the ECF. Examples include diabetic ketoacidosis, lactic acidosis, and uremic acidosis. A non-anion-gap acidosis commonly (but not exclusively) represents a loss of HCO_3^-. Examples include lower GI losses from diarrhea and urinary losses due to renal tubular acidosis. Therefore, when approaching a patient with an anion-gap acidosis, one should look for the source and identity of the acid gained. By contrast, when evaluating a patient with a non-anion-gap acidosis, one should begin by looking for the source of the HCO_3^- loss.

63. What are the causes of anion-gap metabolic acidosis?

The mnemonic **KUSMAL** can be used to remember the differential diagnosis of anion-gap metabolic acidosis.

K—Ketones (diabetic, alcohol, starvation)
U—Uremia
S—Salicylates
M—Methyl alcohol
A—Acid poisoning (ethylene glycol, paraldehyde)
L—Lactate (circulatory/respiratory failure, sepsis, liver disease, tumors, toxins)

Morganroth ML: An analytical approach in the diagnosis of acid-base disorders. J Crit Illness 5:138–150, 1990.

64. What is the significance of plasma osmolal gap? How does it help in the evaluation of a patient with metabolic acidosis?

The plasma osmolal gap is the difference between the measured and calculated plasma osmolality. Plasma osmolal gap of >25 mOsm/kg suggests, in a patient with anion-gap metabolic acidosis, the possibility of ingestion of methanol or ethylene glycol. Isopropyl alcohol and ethanol increase the osmolal gap but not the anion gap, since acetone is not an anion.

65. What are the common causes of a non–anion-gap metabolic acidosis?

Causes of a Non–anion-Gap Metabolic Acidosis

Associated with K⁺ loss	Drugs
Diarrhea	Acetazolamide
Renal tubular acidosis (proximal or distal)	Amphotericin B
Interstitial nephritis	Amiloride
Early renal failure	Spironolactone
Urinary tract obstruction	Toluene ingestion
Post-hypocapnia	**Urethral diversions**
Infusions of HCl (HCl, arginine HCl, lysine HCl)	Ureterosigmoidostomy
	Dual bladder
	Ileal ureter

Toto RD: Metabolic acid-base disorders. In Kokko UP, Tanner RL (eds): Fluids and Electrolytes, 2nd ed. Philadelphia, W.B. Saunders, 1990, p 326.

66. How is the urine anion gap useful in the evaluation of metabolic acidosis?

Measuring urine electrolytes and calculating the urine anion gap is useful diagnostically in the evaluation of some cases of hyperchloremic metabolic acidosis.

$$\text{Urine anion gap} = \text{Unmeasured cations} - \text{unmeasured anions}$$
$$= (Na^+ + K^+) - Cl^-$$

In normal subjects excreting 20–40 meq of NH_4^+/l, the urine anion gap is positive or near zero. On the other hand, in metabolic acidosis, the $NH4^+$ excretion increases if the renal acidification mechanisms are intact. Consequently, urinary Cl^- excretion also increases to maintain electroneutrality. Urinary Cl^- therefore exceeds cation ($K^+ + Na^+$) excretion, and the urine anion gap is negative (often -20 to $> ^-50$ meq\l. On the other hand, in acidosis where the renal acidification mechanisms are impaired (as in renal failure and renal tubular acidosis), the urine anion gap remains positive, as in normal subjects.

Battle DC et al: The use of the urine anion gap in the diagnosis of hyperchloremic metabolic acidosis. N Engl J Med 318:594, 1988.

67. In which two situations should the urine anion gap not be used?

1. In **ketoacidosis,** the excretion of ketoacids neutralize the increased excretion of NH_4^+ cations, decreasing the negativity of anion gap.

2. In **hypovolemia,** the avid proximal Na^+ reabsorption causes decreased distal Na^+ delivery resulting in a defect in acidification. The Cl^- reabsorption that accompanies Na^+ prevents NH_4Cl excretion, and the urine anion gap remains positive.

68. What causes a decreased anion gap?

Certain disorders are associated with an anion gap that is lower than normal. This can be due to an increase in **unmeasured cations** like (K^+, Ca^{++}, or Mg^{++}), the addition of **abnormal cations** (lithium), or an increase in **cationic immunoglobulins** (plasma cell dyscrasias). It can also be decreased by loss of unmeasured anions such as albumin (serum hypoalbuminemia) or if the effective negative charge (on albumin) is decreased by severe acidosis.

69. What is renal tubular acidosis (RTA)?

This term refers to a disorder of tubular function in which the kidney has a compromised ability to excrete acid and/or recover filtered HCO_3^- in the setting of higher than normal [H⁺] in the ECF. The laboratory presentation is that of a non-anion gap metabolic acidosis.

70. Describe the four types of RTA.

   Type I RTA (distal or classic RTA) is characterized by reduced net proton secretion by the distal nephron in the setting of systemic acidemia. Since the distal nephron is largely responsible for net acid excretion, patients with this disorder have continuous net acid retention (less net acid excretion than net acid production) and are therefore *not* in net acid balance. The diagnosis is made by demonstrating an inappropriately alkaline urine (pH > 5.5) in the setting of an acidemic serum (pH < 7.36) and by excluding the presence of drugs that alkalinize the urine (acetazolamide) or urea-splitting bacteria in the urine that can *increase* the urinary pH.

   Type II RTA (proximal RTA) is characterized by a reduced capacity for HCO_3^- recovery by the proximal tubule but intact distal nephron function. These patients waste HCO_3^- in the urine until the ECF concentration of HCO_3^- is reduced to a level such that the reduced filtered load of HCO_3^- (GFR × plasma HCO_3^-) can now be more completely resorbed and the urine becomes nearly bicarbonate free. The reduction in plasma HCO_3^- concentration results in an increase in $[H^+]$. However, in the steady-state condition of low plasma HCO_3^-, these patients can excrete an appropriately acid urine (pH < 5.5) because distal nephron function is intact, and they are thus in acid balance (amount of acid excreted equals amount of acid produced), unlike the situation described for type I.

   Type III RTA represents a variant of type I, and the term has been abandoned.

   Type IV RTA is characterized by reduced aldosterone effect on the renal tubules, which may result in insufficient secretion of acid necessary to maintain normal acid-base status. These patients nevertheless can excrete an appropriately acid urine in the face of acidemic stress. Unlike the other types of RTA, type IV RTA is commonly associated with hyperkalemia due to a coexisting reduction in K^+ secretion. This disorder is commonly seen in patients with hyporenin-hypoaldosteronism but is also seen in isolated aldosterone deficiency and resistance.

71. How are the common types of renal tubular acidosis managed?

   Type I (distal) RTA: Alkali is given in amounts necessary (usually 1–2 meq/kg/day) to correct the acidosis and to buffer the acid being retained. K^+ supplements are commonly required at the initiation of treatment but usually not in the steady-state treatment once the acidosis has been corrected.

   Type II (proximal) RTA: Alkali is not usually required in adults, because they do not have net acid retention and have only mild acidemia. But because the chronic acidemia inhibits bone growth in children, they must be treated with large amounts of alkali (10–20 meq/kg/day) as well as large K^+ supplements (the increased urinary HCO_3^- losses are accompanied by accelerated urinary K^+ losses).

   Type IV RTA: The clinically mild degrees of acidemia rarely require alkali treatment. Hyperkalemia is more commonly a clinical concern and dictates whether mineralocorticoid replacements with synthetic steroids are required.

72. What is lactic acidosis?

   Lactic acidosis is due to the accumulation of lactic acid, the end product of glycolysis. This accumulation leads to a depletion of the body's buffers and a drop in pH. Lactate, being an unmeasured anion, is one of the causes of an increased anion-gap acidosis.

73. List eight basic causes of lactic acidosis.

   1. **Cellular hypoxia:** Oxygen is required for the oxidative phosphorylation of the lactic acid produced by glycolysis. Anything interfering with the available cellular supply of O_2 or its utilization will lead to the accumulation of lactic acid. This category includes respiratory failure, circulatory failure, and CO poisoning.

   2. **Decreased hepatic utilization of lactic acid:** Seen in advanced hepatocellular insufficiency of any cause.

   3. **Cyanide poisoning:** CN causes increased lactic acid production because it blocks oxidative phosphorylation, leading to increased glycolysis, decreased utilization of lactic acid, and therefore lactic acid accumulation.

4. **Alcohol consumption:** Alcohol causes a modest increase in lactic acid production. In association with caloric depletion, the lactic acidosis can be severe.

5. **Neoplasms with a large tumor burden:** Neoplasms can lead to increased production of lactic acid, even with sufficient O_2, since the tumor cells can have higher rates of glycolysis than normal cells.

6. **Diabetic ketoacidosis (DKA):** DKA is associated with increased lactic acid levels even in the absence of shock or other etiologies.

7. **Lactic acidosis X:** This is a condition in which severe lactic acidosis occurs without obvious cause.

8. **Factitious lactic acidosis:** When blood is stored for prolonged periods of time, the red and white cells generate lactic acid in the tube as it is stored. It is most commonly seen in patients with high WBC counts.

74. What is metabolic alkalosis?

Metabolic alkalosis is a disorder characterized by a directional decrease in [H^+] from metabolic causes. It results from addition of excess HCO_3^- or alkali or loss of acid. Note that a low Cl^- and a high HCO_3^- concentration can result from both metabolic alkalosis as well as from a metabolic response to a respiratory acidosis. However, the pH and $PaCO_2$ help to differentiate these two disorders.

75. What are the common causes of metabolic alkalosis?

Chloride-Responsive (Urine Cl^-] < 10 meq/l)	Chloride-Resistant (Urine Cl^- > 20 meq/l)
Gastric fluid loss	Primary aldosteronism
Postdiuretic therapy	Primary reninism
Posthypercapnia	Hyperglucocorticoidism
Congenital chloride diarrhea	Hypercalcemia
	Potassium depletion
	Liddle's syndrome
	Bartter's syndrome
	Chloruretic diuretics

Toto RD: Metabolic acid-base disorders. In Kokko UP, Tannen RL (eds): Fluids and Electrolytes, 2nd ed. Philadelphia, W.B. Saunders, 1990, p 356.

Those forms of alkalosis responsive to chloride salt administration are generally associated with ECF fluid volume depletion and low urinary Cl^- concentration in spot urine tests, whereas the Cl^--unresponsive alkaloses are associated with ECF volume expansion and urine Cl^- > 20 meq/l.

76. Which is the commonest acid-base disturbance seen in cirrhosis?

Primary **respiratory alkalosis** due to centrally mediated hyperventilation is the most common acid-base disturbance in patients with severe hepatic disease, especially with superimposed encephalopathy. The exact etiology is unclear but may be related to the hormonal imbalance associated with liver failure. Estrogens and progesterone have been implicated, a situation somewhat similar to that seen in pregnancy.

77. How do you diagnose a mixed acid-base disorder?

Sometimes two or more primary acid-base disturbances are seen in the same patient, usually in critical care units. The steps in diagnosis are as follows:

1. Define the primary disturbance and the compensatory process involved. The primary disturbance is identified by the direction of the changes in pH, HCO_3^-, and $PaCO_2$ levels.

2. Determine if the pulmonary or renal compensation is appropriate (see Question 54). Two facts must be kept in mind while making these interpretations. First, adequate compensation takes 12–24 hrs to occur, and second, "overcompensation" never occurs in primary acid-base disturbances.

3. Consider the patient's history and clinical presentation to formulate a differential diagnosis.

- In combined **metabolic and respiratory acidosis,** even though the HCO_3^- and $PaCO_2$ may not be changed, pH is distinctly lower.
- In combined **metabolic acidosis** and **metabolic alkalosis,** the pH and HCO_3^- can be lower, normal, or higher, but an elevated anion gap with a high or normal HCO_3^- suggests the diagnosis.
- A combined **metabolic alkalosis** and **respiratory acidosis** (which can be seen in patients with ARDS or COPD who are vomiting) causes higher HCO_3^- level than predicted compensation for a given high $PaCO_2$.

In general, the underlying clinical condition gives clues to the possible mixed acid-base disturbance, which can then be defined using the nomograms of expected compensation.

Narins R, Emmett M: Simple and mixed acid-base disorders: A practical approach. Medicine 59:161–187, 1980.

78. In what situations are potentially fatal mixed acid-base disorders commonly encountered?

In general, combined respiratory and metabolic acidosis or metabolic and respiratory alkalosis can result in pH changes that are fatal. Some of the common examples are:

1. An alcoholic with ketoacidosis (metabolic acidosis) may have superimposed vomiting from gastritis (metabolic alkalosis) and hyperventilation associated with withdrawal (respiratory alkalosis).

2. A combination of metabolic acidosis and respiratory alkalosis is seen typically in patients with sepsis, salicylate intoxication, and severe liver disease.

3. Metabolic acidosis can coexist with metabolic alkalosis in patients with renal failure or with alcoholic or diabetic ketoacidosis (acidosis) who are vomiting or having gastric suction (alkalosis).

4. Vomiting in a pregnant female or liver failure causes a mixture of respiratory and metabolic alkalosis.

CALCIUM, PHOSPHATE, AND MAGNESIUM METABOLISM

79. How is calcium distributed in the body? In the serum?

A 70-kg man has approx. 1000 gm of calcium in his body. Of this, bone contains 99%, whereas the ECF and ICF contain only 1%. Furthermore, only about 1% of skeletal calcium is freely exchangeable with ECF calcium.

The routine measurement for serum calcium (normal = 9–10 mg/ml = 4.5–5.0 meq/l = 2.25–2.5 mM/l) measures total calcium. Approx. 40% of this is protein-bound, 5–10% is complexed to other substances (e.g., phosphate, sulfate), and 50% is ionized.

80. Why is it important to recognize the differences between ionized and protein-bound calcium?

It is the ionized fraction of calcium that determines the activity of this electrolyte in cellular and membrane function. It is possible to vary the concentration of total calcium without changing the ionized fraction by changing the protein concentration. By contrast, it is also possible to vary the ionized fraction without changing the total concentration by changing serum pH. Increasing serum pH decreases the ionized fraction of calcium and vice versa.

81. What are the major sites of calcium resorption in the nephron?

About 50% of the filtered calcium is resorbed in the proximal tubule, and most of the remainder (about 40% of the total) is reabsorbed in the loop of Henle, primarily the ascending limb of the loop of Henle. A small amount of calcium is resorbed in the distal convoluted tubule and an even smaller amount in the collecting tubule.

82. What are the major hormones involved in calcium metabolism?

Parathyroid hormone (PTH), vitamin D, and calcitonin.

PTH is secreted in response to a decrease in serum calcium and promotes calcium resorption from bone, because it enhances renal resorption of calcium and excretion of phosphate. Low serum calcium concentration stimulates 1-hydroxylation of 25-hydroxyvitamin D by the kidney to form 1,25-dihydroxyvitamin D (the active form of vitamin D). This hormone promotes calcium resorption from the gut and mineralization of bone. Increases in serum calcium lead to increased secretion of calcitonin. This hormone inhibits bone reabsorption and 1-hydroxylation of 25-hydroxyvitamin D and thereby ameliorates hypercalcemia.

83. Name some factors that affect renal calcium excretion.

With some exceptions, renal calcium handling varies directly with renal Na$^+$ handling. Therefore, renal calcium excretion is increased by saline diuresis, loop diuretics, and volume expansion. In contrast, renal calcium excretion is decreased in volume depletion and other states associated with renal salt retention. One notable exception to this general rule is that the natriuresis associated with thiazide diuretics is accompanied by decreased, rather than increased, urinary calcium excretion.

84. What are pseudohypocalcemia and pseudohypercalcemia?

These terms refer to an alteration of the total calcium concentration in the setting of a normal ionized fraction. Since the ionized fraction is normal, these patients are asymptomatic. Abnormalities in the concentration of serum proteins are a common cause of these disorders.

85. How do you correct the total serum calcium level for changes in the serum albumin?

Hypoalbuminemia causes a decrease in the total serum calcium level without a change in the level of ionized calcium. For each decrease of 1.0 g/dl in serum albumin, one should expect a drop in the total serum calcium of approx. 0.8 mg/dl.

86. What are some common causes of true hypocalcemia?

Hypoparathyroidism (usually following thyroid or parathyroid surgery)
Vitamin D deficiency
Magnesium depletion (usually at levels < 0.8 meq/l)
Liver disease (decreased synthesis of 25-hydroxyvitamin D)
Renal disease (hyperphosphatemia and decreased synthesis of 1,25-dihydroxyvitamin D)
Acute pancreatitis
Tumor lysis syndrome
Rhabdomyolysis

87. What are some common causes of true hypercalcemia?

Primary hyperparathyroidism (approx. 50% of cases), malignancy, use of thiazide diuretics, vitamin D excess, hyper- and hypothyroidism, granulomatous disorders, immobilization, and milk-alkali syndrome.

88. What are the signs and symptoms of hypocalcemia?

The symptoms are dependent on the magnitude of the decrease in serum calcium, the rate of the drop, and its duration. The symptoms of hypocalcemia are due to the resultant decrease in the excitation threshold of neural tissue. This causes an increase in excitability, repetitive responses to a single stimulus, reduced accommodation, or even continuous activity of neural tissue. The varied symptoms and signs include:

Signs and Symptoms of Hypocalcemia

Tetany and paresthesia	QT interval prolongation on the ECG
Altered mental status (lethargy to coma)	Increased intracranial pressure
Seizures	Lenticular cataracts

89. What are Trousseau's and Chvostek's signs?

Both are indications of the latent tetany caused by hypocalcemia. Of the two signs, Trousseau's is more specific and reliable.

1. **Trousseau's sign:** A sphygmomanometer is placed on the arm and inflated to greater than systolic blood pressure and left in place for at least 2 minutes. A positive response is carpal spasm of the ipsilateral arm. Relaxation takes 5–10 sec after the pressure is released.

2. **Chvostek's sign:** Tapping the facial nerve between the corner of the mouth and the zygomatic arch produces twitching of the ipsilateral facial muscle, especially the angle of the mouth. This sign may be seen in 10–25% of normal adult patients.

90. What are the symptoms and signs of hypercalcemia?

Symptoms include weakness, constipation, nausea, anorexia, polyuria, polydipsia, and pruritus. Severe hypercalcemia may present with progressive CNS symptoms of lethargy, depression, obtundation, coma, and seizures. Rapid onset is more likely to be symptomatic than a slowly progressive level, regardless of the ultimate level at presentation.

91. Describe the appropriate treatment for hypercalcemia.

Treatment depends on the calcium level and symptoms of the patient. Acute, symptomatic hypercalcemia should be treated aggressively, first with saline infusion to expedite calcium excretion. Most patients with hypercalcemia are significantly volume-depleted as a result of the osmotic diuresis related to the hypercalciuria.

1. **Normal saline** should be given at a rapid rate, 300 ml/hr or more, with KCl and possibly magnesium added to the solution depending on measured blood values. After the patient is volume-repleted, furosemide may be given to promote calciuresis. Care must be taken to keep input equal to or greater than output, to avoid making the patient hypovolemic again.

2. **Mithramycin** is effective when the patient cannot tolerate large fluid loads due to congestive heart failure or third-space losses or if there is an inadequate response to IV volume replacement. It should be given at a dose of 15 μg/kg (i.e., 1–2 mg) IVSS for one dose. The dose can be repeated if necessary, but doses more frequent than every 3–7 days have been associated with renal and hepatic toxicity. Mithramycin can also cause a coagulopathy, which can lead to serious bleeding complications.

3. **Calcitonin** is useful for decreasing serum calcium and has the added advantage of rapid onset of action. It may be given in the presence of renal insufficiency, thrombocytopenia, or when mithramycin is contraindicated. Its disadvantage is that rapid resistance often develops, probably related to the development of antibodies. This resistance can sometimes be delayed by concomitant administration of prednisone.

4. **Bisphosphonates** inhibit osteoclast activity and are effective with those cancers in which this mechanism is present. They are given as IV infusion over 5 days or as oral tablets.

Less significant levels of hypercalcemia can be treated with other agents, such as glucocorticoids (prednisone, 20–40 mg/day), phosphates (1–6 g/day), prostaglandin inhibitors (aspirin and NSAIDs), or oral bisphosphonates. All of these agents are less effective but may suffice for chronic maintenance.

Bilizekian JP: Management of acute hypercalcemia. N Engl J Med 326:1196–1203, 1992.

92. What are the major sites of phosphate resorption in the nephron?

Phosphate is resorbed predominantly in the proximal tubule, with small amounts being absorbed in the distal tubule.

93. What factors increase excretion of urinary phosphate?

PTH
Alkalosis
Saline diuresis
Ketoacidosis
Increased dietary phosphate intake

94. What factors can lower serum phosphate by shifting this ion into cells?

Insulin, glucose (by stimulating insulin secretion), and alkalosis.

95. In which clinical situations can hypophosphatemia develop?
1. **Decreased dietary intake:**
   a. Decreased intestinal absorption due to vitamin D deficiency, malabsorption, steator-rhea, secretory diarrhea, vomiting, or phosphate binders
   b. Alcoholism
2. **Shifts from serum into cells:**
   a. Respiratory alkalosis as seen in sepsis, heat stroke, hepatic coma, salicylate poisoning, gout, etc.
   b. Recovery from hypothermia
   c. Hormonal effects of insulin, glucagon, androgens, etc. (recovery from diabetic ke-toacidosis)
   d. Carbohydrate administration (hyperalimentation, fructose or glucose infusions)
3. **Increased excretion into urine:**
   a. Hyperparathyroidism
   b. Renal tubule defects as in aldosteronism, SIADH, mineralocorticoid administration, diuretics, corticosteroids
   c. Hypomagnesemia
4. **Spurious**
   a. Mannitol infusion

96. What are the main disturbances thought to be responsible for the abnormalities of calcium and phosphate metabolism seen with progressive renal disease?

Patients with progressive renal disease develop hyperphosphatemia, hypocalcemia, and secondary hyperparathyroidism. They are also at risk of developing at least two kinds of bone disease. The main disturbances that contribute to these abnormalities are:

1. A rise in inorganic phosphate concentration in the serum due to poor renal excretion. This leads to a decrease in serum calcium concentration and stimulation of PTH secretion. The increased PTH secretion leads to increased bone resorption and osteitis fibrosa cystica.

2. Resistance to the action of vitamin D. One function of this hormone is to promote calcium resorption from the gut. Decreased gut resorption of calcium exacerbates the hypocalcemia and reduces available calcium for bone mineralization.

3. Defective synthesis of 1,25-dihydroxyvitamin D (the active form of this hormone). Reduced levels of 1,25-dihydroxyvitamin D results in defective bone mineralization (osteomalacia in adults, rickets in children).

97. How does magnesium depletion affect calcium and phosphate metabolism?

Magnesium depletion results in decreased secretion and end-organ responsiveness of PTH. This leads to functional hypoparathyroidism and the resultant effects on the serum level and urinary excretion of calcium and phosphate. This disorder can be corrected with magnesium repletion.

98. What are the major nephron sites for magnesium resorption?

Magnesium is resorbed predominantly in the thick ascending limb of the loop of Henle, with a smaller amount being resorbed in the proximal tubule.

99. What are some common causes of magnesium deficiency?
- Dietary insufficiency (decreased intake, protein-calorie malnutrition, prolonged IV feeding)
- Intestinal malabsorption
- Chronic loss of GI fluids
- Diuretics

- Other drugs (gentamicin, cisplatin, pentamidine, cyclosporine)
- Alcoholism
- Hyperparathyroidism
- Lactation

100. What is the milk-alkali syndrome?

The presence of hypercalcemia, increased BUN and creatinine, increased serum phosphate, and metabolic alkalosis in a patient ingesting large quantities of milk and calcium carbonate-containing antacids. The patients usually present with nausea, vomiting, anorexia, weakness, polydipsia, and polyuria. If it continues, metastatic calcification can occur, leading to mental status changes, nephrocalcinosis, band keratopathy, pruritus, and myalgias. The treatment is withdrawal of the milk and antacid.

101. What electrolyte abnormalities are seen in HIV infection?

Apart from the main proteinuric syndrome caused by focal sclerosis (so-called HIV nephropathy), a variety of electrolyte disorders are commonly seen in patients with HIV. Asymptomatic **hyperkalemia** is a common manifestation. The hyperkalemia may be due to many possible causes, including hyporenin-hypoaldosteronism, adrenal insufficiency, drugs such as pentamidine and trimethoprim-sulfamethoxazole, and even isolated hypoaldosternism. **Hyponatremia** is frequently caused by hypovolemia, adrenal insufficiency, and SIADH due to associated pulmonary or cerebral diseases. Other electrolyte abnormalities include hypocalcemia, hypomagnesemia, and hypouricemia. Hypercalcemia has been seen in association with lymphomas and cytomegalovirus infection.

Glassock RJ, Cohen AH, Danovitch G: Human immunodeficiency virus (HIV) infection and the kidney. Ann Intern Med 112:35, 1990.

102. What are the common electrolyte abnormalities seen in alcoholics?

Hypokalemia is seen in one-half of hospitalized, withdrawing alcoholics. This does not necessarily mean a total body K^+ deficit. Respiratory alkalosis, inadequate dietary intake, and GI losses (vomiting, diarrhea) are the common etiologic factors for hypokalemia. Withdrawal as well as severe liver disease can cause respiratory alkalosis in alcoholics.

Hypophosphatemia (<2.5 mg/dl) is a common finding in hospitalized severe alcoholics, noted in more than half (50%) of patients in some series. The common predisposing factors are respiratory alkalosis, decreased dietary intake, transcellular shifts due to glucose administration, and rarely, associated proximal tubular injury leading to phosphate wasting.

Chronic alcoholism is the most common cause of **hypomagnesemia** in the USA. It is seen in alcoholics who are withdrawing and more commonly in those who had withdrawal seizures. GI losses, cellular uptake, dietary deficiencies, and possibly lipolysis leading to fatty acid-magnesium precipitation are the possible causes.

Hyponatremia sometimes is seen in beer-drinkers who ingest large quantities of beer, which is virtually solute-free. When this free-water volume exceeds the excretory capacity of the kidney, hyponatremia results.

BIBLIOGRAPHY

1. Brenner BM, Rector FC (eds): The Kidney, 5th ed. Philadelphia, W.B. Saunders, 1996.
2. Rose BD: Clinical Physiology of Acid-Base and Fluid and Electrolyte Disorders, 4th ed. New York, McGraw Hill, 1994.
3. Schrier RW (ed): Renal and electrolyte disorders, 4th ed. Boston, Little, Brown & Co., 1992.
4. Seldin DW, Giebisch G (eds): The Regulation of Acid-Base Balance. New York, Raven Press, 1992.
5. Bennett JC, et al (eds): Cecil Textbook of Medicine, 20th ed. Philadelphia, W.B. Saunders, 1996.

9. HEMATOLOGY

Mark M. Udden, M.D.

Blood is the originating cause of all men's diseases.
The Talmud
Baba Nathra, III.58a

The blood is the life.
The Bible
Deuteronomy 12:23

HYPOPROLIFERATIVE ANEMIAS

1. What are the two most helpful laboratory investigations in the initial evaluation of anemia?

The reticulocyte count and peripheral blood film. The peripheral blood film will demonstrate important abnormalities of red blood cell (RBC) shape, size, or hemoglobinization. In addition, an impression of the white blood cell (WBC) count and platelet count can be obtained. RBCs must also be examined for the presence of inclusions (such as Howell-Jolly bodies).

2. What are reticulocytes and why count them?

Reticulocytes are young RBCs newly released from the marrow, which can be detected by their lacy network of RNA. If the reticulocyte count is high, then blood loss or hemolysis is likely to be the cause of anemia. If the reticulocyte count is low, a primary marrow disorder (hypoproliferative anemia) should be considered.

Physiologic Classification of Anemia

RETICULOCYTE COUNT LOW	RETICULOCYTE COUNT HIGH
Hypoproliferative anemia	Blood loss
	Response to treatment of iron, folate, or B_{12} deficiency
	Hemolysis

Cavill I: The rejected reticulocyte. Br J Haematol 84:563–565, 1992.

The old method of determining the reticulocyte count relied on a manual count of 1000 cells stained with new methylene blue. Currently, it is usually determined by flow cytometric analysis of thiazole orange–stained cells or other automated analysis, which leads to greater reproducibility and allows a discrimination of mature and immature reticulocytes. The release of immature reticulocytes is often a sign of early marrow recovery after bone marrow transplantation or response to treatment in deficiency states.

3. How are the mean cell volume (MCV) and the red cell distribution width (RDW) used in the evaluation of anemias?

The complete blood count (CBC) now includes the MCV, and many clinical laboratories also determine an index of the heterogeneity of cell size, the RDW. In iron-deficiency anemia, for example, RBCs have been produced during periods of iron sufficiency and varying degrees of deficiency, so cell size in iron-deficiency anemia is more heterogeneous than that in thalassemia minor, in which the cells are all small. This results in a larger RDW for iron-deficiency anemia and a normal RDW for thalassemia.

241

Classification of Anemias Based on MCV and RDW

MCV LOW		MCV NORMAL		MCV HIGH	
RDW NORMAL	RDW HIGH	RDW NORMAL	RDW HIGH	RDW NORMAL	RDW HIGH
Chronic disease	Iron deficiency	Normal	Early or mixed nutritional deficiency	Aplastic anemia	Folate or vitamin B_{12} deficiency
Nonanemic heterozygous thalassemia	HbS-α or β thalassemia	Chronic disease			
	Hb H	Nonanemic hemoglobin or enzyme abnormality	Anemic abnormal hemoglobin		Sickle cell anemia ($\frac{1}{3}$ of cases)
Children			Myelofibrosis		Immune hemolytic anemia
		Splenectomy	Sideroblastic		
		CLL (except extreme high lymphocyte number)	Myelodysplasia		Cold agglutinins
					Preleukemia
		Acute blood loss			Newborn

Note: Chronic liver disease, chronic myelogenous leukemia, and cytotoxic chemotherapy may be associated with high or normal MCV and high or normal RDW. CLL = chronic lymphocytic leukemia.
Bessman JD: Automated Blood Counts and Differentials: A Practical Guide. Baltimore, Johns Hopkins University Press, 1986, p 11.

4. What are the causes of hypochromic microcytic anemias? How are iron studies used in their differentiation?

Hypochromic microcytic anemias are the most frequently encountered anemias in hospitalized and ambulatory patients. A working knowledge of these anemias and their laboratory diagnosis is essential to avoid wasting time and resources.

Causes of Hypochromic Microcytic Anemias

	NORMAL	IDA	ANEMIA OF CHRONIC DISEASE	SIDERO-BLASTIC ANEMIA	THALASSEMIA
Serum iron (μg/dl)	115 (70–180)	<	30 (15–65)	>180	Normal or elevated
TIBC (μg/ml)	340	>400	200	250	250
Transferrin saturation (%)	35 (25–50)	<16	15 (10–40)	80 (60–100)	Normal or elevated
Marrow hemosiderin	2+	0	3+	4+	2+ to 4+
Serum ferritin	Normal	Decreased	Slightly elevated	Elevated	Normal or elevated

IDA = iron-deficiency anemia; TIBC = total iron-binding capacity.

Note that a bone marrow examination in sideroblastic anemia shows increased iron stores and abnormal iron distribution in ringed sideroblasts. Both iron-deficiency anemia and anemia of chronic disease have a low transferrin saturation. In iron-deficiency anemia, the TIBC is often increased, whereas anemia of chronic disease is marked by an unusually low TIBC. Iron stores are usually normal in thalassemia-minor, although β-thalassemia major may be complicated by iron overload.

Massey AC: Microcytic anemia: Differential diagnosis and management of iron deficiency anemia. Med Clin North Am 76:549–566, 1992.

5. Summarize the symptoms and signs of iron deficiency.

Patients may have the symptoms of **anemia:** fatigue, dyspnea on exertion, and, in certain cases in which underlying cardiac disease exists, signs of congestive heart failure or angina. However, in many cases, the anemia develops insidiously and is well-tolerated. Iron deficiency is associated with **pica.** Adults may crave ice, starch, or even dirt. Iron-deficient children in older neighborhoods may eat lead-containing paint chips, leading to the association of iron deficiency and plumbism. Iron deficiency is also associated with **esophageal webs** (sometimes causing dysphagia), painless **stomatitis,** and spooning of the fingernails (**koilonychia**).

Moore DF, Jr, Sears DA: Pica, iron deficiency, and the medical history. Am J Med 97:390–393, 1994.

6. In the treatment of iron-deficiency anemia, how much iron should be administered, in what form, and for how long?

Iron is best given as ferrous sulfate in a formulation that does not include enteric coating. Typically, patients take 325 mg orally three times daily until the anemia corrects and for several months thereafter. This provides 60 mg of elemental iron per tablet, or 180 mg/day. Of this, 18–36 mg can be absorbed and utilized by an otherwise unimpaired marrow.

When a low serum ferritin value is used to make the diagnosis of iron deficiency, the ferritin can be checked to verify that iron stores have increased with therapy. In some instances, patients improve but do not fully correct their anemia. If the ferritin has normalized, another cause of anemia (i.e., coexistent thalassemia minor) should be sought. A useful guide to success is the occurrence of reticulocytosis about 10 days after initiation of iron therapy.

7. What are common causes of iron deficiency?

Diet, malabsorption, chronic blood loss, and chronic intravascular hemolysis. The last-mentioned disorder is usually seen in the rare stem cell disorder paroxysmal nocturnal hemoglobinuria or in patients with malfunctioning cardiac valves. Examination of a urine sediment stained for iron discloses iron-laden tubular cells (**hemosiderosis**).

Common Causes of Iron Deficiency

1. Chronic blood loss
   a. Gastrointestinal: gastritis, peptic ulcer disease, GI varices, GI malignancy, polyps, diverticulosis, telangiectasia (Osler-Weber-Rendu disease, scleroderma), angiodysplasia, long-distance running
   b. Menstrual loss and pregnancy
2. Dietary deficiency (infants)
3. Malabsorption: sprue, postgastrectomy patients
4. Other: chronic intravascular hemolysis, idiopathic pulmonary hemosiderosis, repetitive phlebotomy

8. What are the causes and consequences of iron overload?

Iron overload results from chronic administration of iron to non-iron-deficient persons, chronic transfusion therapy, and disorders associated with increased absorption of dietary iron (hemochromatosis, thalassemia intermedia or major, and certain refractory anemias such as sideroblastic anemia).

Although hereditary hemochromatosis, an autosomal recessive disorder, affects approx. 1 in 300 individuals, it is frequently missed. Many patients are diagnosed only after significant damage to heart or liver has occurred. Iron overload has many effects, including:

1. Cardiomyopathy, arrhythmias
2. Hepatic dysfunction and cirrhosis
3. Hepatoma
4. Endocrine dysfunction (hypothyroidism, hypogonadotrophic hypogonadism, hyperpigmentation, diabetes mellitus)
5. Arthropathy (chondrocalcinosis, synovial fluid containing calcium pyrophosphate or hydroxyapatite crystals)
6. Osteopenia and subcortical cysts
7. Peripheral neuropathy

9. How should iron overload be confirmed?

The **serum iron tests**—serum iron, TIBC, and ferritin—can be used to identify patients for further investigation for hemochromatosis. Elevated serum ferritin levels, however, can occur in a number of inflammatory conditions without iron overload. When hereditary hemochromatosis is identified, screening of relatives can detect young individuals at risk, who may then be saved considerable morbidity.

Olynyk JK, Bacon BR: Hereditary hemochromatosis: Detecting and correcting iron overload. Postgrad Med 96(5):151–165, 1994.

Lee MH, Means RT Jr: Extremely elevated serum ferritin levels in a university hospital: Associated diseases and clinical significance. Am J Med 98:566–571, 1995.

10. When is it appropriate to order a hemoglobin electrophoresis to evaluate hypochromic microcytic anemia?

This is best done when iron stores are established as being normal. The microcytic disorders that may be detected are β-thalassemia minor and the so-called thalassemic hemoglobinopathies (including hemoglobin [Hb] E in Asians). β-Thalassemia minor is marked by an increased Hb A_2 and sometimes increased fetal Hb. Iron deficiency results in a decreased pool of α-chains for which the β-chain of Hb A and the γ-chain of Hb A_2 must compete. β-chains are more successful, resulting in diminished Hb A_2 during iron deficiency. For this reason, a search for β-thalassemia may be thwarted when patients are also iron deficient.

Beutler E: The common anemias. JAMA 259:2433–2437, 1988.

11. Which diseases are usually associated with the anemia of chronic disease (ACD)?

ACD is typified by a low serum iron, low TIBC, and low percent saturation but increased iron stores, as evidenced by an increased ferritin. Traditionally, ACD is associated with inflammatory states, including malignancy, rheumatologic disease, and infection. However, a recent study of hospitalized patients shows that the laboratory pattern of ACD occurs in a significant number of anemic patients who do not have inflammatory conditions. These patients were severely ill with complications of diabetes, renal failure, and hypertension.

Cash JM, Sears DA: The anemia of chronic disease: Spectrum of associated disease in a series of unselected hospitalized patients. Am J Med 87:638, 1989.

12. What are the causes of macrocytosis?

Macrocytosis, or a large MCV, is not always associated with folate or vitamin B_{12} deficiency. Anemia with macro-ovalocytic RBCs (megaloblastic) is much more specific for folate or vitamin B_{12} deficiency.

Causes of Macrocytosis

Megaloblastic anemia (macro-ovalocytosis)	Sideroblastic anemia*
Alcoholism	Chronic obstructive pulmonary disease
Malignancy	Artifacts and idiopathic
Hemolysis (usually poorly compensated)	Pregnancy
Aplastic anemia	Liver disease
Hypothyroidism	
Refractory anemias (myelodysplasia)	

*Often marked by dual populations of RBCs—one hypochromic microcytic, and the other macrocytic.
Colon-Otero G, et al: A practical approach to the differential diagnosis and evaluation of the adult patient with macrocytic anemia. Med Clin North Am 76:581–596, 1992.

13. How are folate and vitamin B_{12} deficiency states recognized? How do they differ?

Common features of B_{12} and folate deficiency are those of megaloblastic anemia:

1. **Marrow:** Hyperplastic marrow demonstrating a markedly ineffective erythropoiesis; megaloblastic RBCs with open, granular nuclei, and mature cytoplasm or nuclear-cytoplasmic asynchrony; giant metamyelocytes.

2. **Peripheral blood:** Macro-ovalocytosis with occasional Howell-Jolly bodies and basophilic stippling; Hypersegmented neutrophils; variable degree of neutropenia and thrombocytopenia.

3. **Megaloblastic changes:** Affect rapidly proliferating cells of mouth, gut, small intestine, and cervix, showing immature-looking nuclei (indeed, some cervical Pap smears are mistakenly read as atypical or malignant).

Distinguishing Features of Folate vs B_{12} Deficiency

FEATURE	B_{12}	FOLATE
Neurologic disease	Subacute, combined systems	None, or associated with alcohol
Diet	Normal	Alcoholism, junk food, "tea and toast", no green leafy vegetables
Serum folate level	Normal	Low
RBC folate level	Low or normal	Low
Response to physiologic dose of folate (200 μg/d)	Absent*	Present
Urine formiminoglutamic acid	Absent	Increased
Serum methylmalonic acid	Increased	Normal
Homocysteine levels	Increased	Increased

*Pharmacologic dose of folate (1 mg/day) can correct the anemia but may exacerbate the neurologic symptoms. Babior BM: The megaloblastic anemias. In Williams WJ, et al (eds): Hematology, 5th ed. New York, McGraw-Hill, 1995.

14. What processes may interrupt B_{12} absorption?

Causes of B_{12} Deficiency

1. Pernicious anemia associated with gastric atrophy and loss of intrinsic factor due to an autoimmune-mediated attack on the gastric mucosa.
2. Postgastrectomy: After total gastrectomy, megaloblastic anemia develops 5–6 years later.
3. Disorders of the small intestine: ileal resection, Crohn's disease, sprue.
4. Competition with intestinal flora: blind-loop syndrome, fish tapeworm (*Diphyllobothrium latum*).
5. Pancreatic disease: deficiency of R-binders with chronic pancreatitis.
6. Dietary: strict vegetarians (no meat or eggs or milk), breastfed infants of strict vegetarians.

15. Describe the pattern of neurologic disease associated with B_{12} deficiency. Is the severity of anemia a good predictor of neurologic involvement?

B_{12} deficiency is associated with the findings of combined systems disease:
- Posterior column: paresthesia, disturbed vibratory sense, loss of proprioception
- Pyramidal: spastic weakness, hyperactive reflexes
- Cerebral: dementia, psychosis (megaloblastic madness), optic atrophy

Folate deficiency may be associated with peripheral neuropathy in alcoholics. Of interest is the lack of correlation between severity of anemia and neurologic manifestations of B_{12} deficiency. A recent study suggests that a significant minority of patients with peripheral neuropathy or other neurologic manifestations of B_{12} deficiency have a normal hematocrit and MCV, but low or low-normal B_{12} levels. It is possible that serum methylmalonic acidemia and homocystinemia are better indicators.

Lindebaum J, et al: Neuropsychiatric disorders caused by cobalamin deficiency in the absence of anemia or macrocytosis. N Engl J Med 318:1720, 1988.

16. Who should receive folate supplementation of their diet?
- The elderly, the poor, and alcoholics
- Patients receiving hyperalimentation or hemodialysis
- Premature infants, infants on synthetic diets, and children fed on goat's milk
- Patients with sprue or other small intestinal disease
- Pregnant women
- Persons with hemolysis and exfoliative dermatitis.

17. How much folate is required in pregnant women? Why?

Developmental anomalies of the fetal neural tube have been associated with poor folate intake early in pregnancy. For this reason, it has been recommended that women of child-bearing age consume 400 mg of folate per day. This recommendation is controversial because folate supplementation may mask symptoms of vitamin B_{12} deficiency.

Cziezel AE, Dudas I: Prevention of the first occurrence of neural-tube defects by periconceptional vitamin supplementation. N Engl J Med 327:1832–1835, 1992.

18. When are a bone marrow biopsy and aspirate indicated?

Bone marrow biopsy and aspiration are safely and easily performed and are particularly helpful in evaluating pancytopenia, thrombocytopenia, neutropenia, and hypoproliferative anemia. Because of the high prevalence of iron-deficiency anemia and anemia of chronic disease, a hypoproliferative (low reticulocyte count) anemia need not always require bone marrow biopsy if iron studies are consistent. The diagnosis of a sideroblastic anemia requires a bone marrow study to demonstrate the presence of ringed sideroblasts.

Indications for Bone Marrow Biopsy and Aspirate

1. Pancytopenia: myelodysplasia, aplastic anemia, myelophthisic states, hypersplenism, megaloblastic anemia
2. Anemia: sideroblastic anemia, refractory anemia, pure red cell aplasia
3. Staging of malignancy: Hodgkin's disease, leukemias, non-Hodgkin's lymphoma, small cell carcinoma of the lung, multiple myeloma
4. Thrombocytopenia: evaluation of idiopathic thrombocytopenic purpura
5. Neutropenia
6. Infectious diseases: typhoid, tuberculosis, pancytopenia seen in AIDS, brucellosis
7. Lipid-storage diseases

19. What are the diagnostic criteria for severe aplastic anemia?

Aplastic anemia is marked by peripheral pancytopenia and a hypocellular bone marrow aspirate. Commonly used criteria for severe aplastic anemia are:
- Marrow biopsy cellularity $< 25\%$
- Neutrophil counts $< 0.5 \times 10^9/l$
- Platelet counts $< 20 \times 10^9/l$
- Corrected reticulocyte count $< 1\%$

Patients meeting these criteria have a median survival of < 6 months, with only 20% surviving 1 year.

20. What is the best therapy for aplastic anemia in a young person?

For patients who are under age 40, a bone marrow transplantation (BMT) from an HLA-identical sibling is the current standard of care. Increasingly, HLA-identical but nonrelated donors may be used for such patients. For nontransfused patients, 80% long-term survival rates have been achieved with BMT, although this may be accompanied by disabling graft-versus-host disease in 10–20%.

Patients who do not have donors or who are otherwise unsuitable candidates for BMT have been successfully treated with immunosuppressive regimens. The most effective of these has been **antithymocyte globulin** (ATG), which produces remission rates of 40–60%. ATG or **antilymphocyte globulin** is administered via a central line in daily doses of 15–40 mg/kg for 4–10 days. Severe serum sickness and thrombocytopenia are consequences.

Patients frequently have partial responses, freeing them from infections or the need for transfusions. Unfortunately, relapses occur in 10%, and some patients, although clinically improved at first, develop myelodysplastic syndromes later. Recently, **cyclosporine A** has been employed in the treatment of aplastic anemia with good results.

Young NS, Barrett AJ: The treatment of severe acquired aplastic anemia. Blood 85:3367–3377, 1995.

21. Who should receive erythropoietin (EPO) therapy for anemia?

EPO deficiency regularly accompanies end-stage renal disease, and the resultant anemia is the principal indication for use of EPO. Recent studies suggest a role for EPO patients with AIDS-related anemia, particularly when they receive zidovudine. The anemia of chronic disease is associated with an inappropriately low EPO levels in some individuals with rheumatoid arthritis and with malignancy. EPO has also been used with success to improve the ability of patients to undergo autologous blood donation prior to surgery.

Erslev AJ: Erythropoietin. N Engl J Med 324:1939–1944, 1991.

22. Alcoholics admitted to the hospital are frequently anemic. Why?

Causes of Anemia in Alcoholics

Primary bone marrow toxicity of alcohol	Hemolytic anemia
Vacuolated marrow erythroid cells	Hypersplenism
Megaloblastic erythropoiesis due to folate deficiency	Spur cell anemia
Hypophosphatemia	Iron-deficiency due to hemorrhage
Sideroblastic anemia	

23. How should you evaluate anemia in the alcoholic?

Savage and Lindenbaum surveyed alcoholics and found that megaloblastic changes in the marrow were not usually associated with disorderly iron accumulation in the macrophages as is seen in anemia of chronic disorders. They emphasize the multifactorial nature of anemia and offer the following guide to workup:

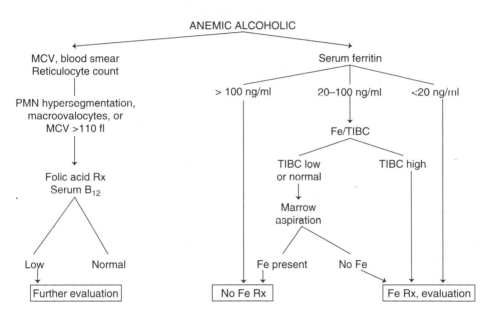

Diagnostic and therapeutic approach to anemia in alcoholics. (Adapted from Savage D, et al: Anemia in alcoholics. Medicine 65:322, 1986.)

HEMOLYTIC ANEMIAS

24. Patients with hemolytic anemia have shortened RBC survival. What are the laboratory features of hemolysis?

During hemolysis, the bone marrow responds to the premature destruction of RBCs by increasing its production of RBCs 7–8-fold. This expansion is marked by reticulocytosis. Other clues to accelerated RBC destruction are:

1. Indirect hyperbilirubinemia-acholuric jaundice (unconjugated bilirubin is not secreted in urine)
2. Hemoglobinuria
3. Fall of hemoglobin > 1 gm/7 days in the absence of bleeding or massive hematoma.

25. How is intravascular hemolysis distinguished from extravascular?

Laboratory Studies in Hemolysis

INTRAVASCULAR	EXTRA- AND INTRAVASCULAR
Hemoglobinemia	Increased reticulocyte count
Hemoglobinuria	Increased indirect, unconjugated bilirubin
Hemosiderinuria	Increased urobilinogen
Low serum haptoglobin	
Methemalbumin	
Low serum hemopexin	
Increased LDH	

Examples of intravascular hemolytic disorders include hemolytic transfusion reactions, paroxysmal nocturnal hemoglobinuria, march hemoglobinuria, and RBC fragmentation syndromes.

26. Name the three basic types of RBC defects that lead to hemolysis in the hereditary hemolytic anemias.

Membrane Disorders	*Hemoglobin Abnormalities*	*Enzymatic Defects*
Spherocytosis	Sickle cell anemia	G6PD deficiency
Elliptocytosis	Unstable hemoglobins	Pyruvate kinase
Stomatocytosis	Thalassemia	5'-nucleotidase
Cation transport		
Xerocytosis		

The RBC is extraordinarily adapted to a circulatory system that requires resistance to shear stresses in the arterioles and suppleness to negotiate small orifices in the spleen and capillaries.

27. Name some acquired hemolytic disorders.

Whereas hereditary disorders are examples of intracorpuscular defects, acquired hemolytic disorders typically result from extracorpuscular defects. These include autoimmune hemolytic anemia, fragmentation syndromes, malaria, hypersplenism, and physical agents such as heat, copper, and certain oxidants.

28. What are the complications of hereditary spherocytosis?

Aplastic crises (associated with parvovirus B19)	Pigment gallstones
Hemolytic crises	Splenomegaly
Megaloblastic crises (increased demand for folate)	Stasis ulcers

29. A patient presenting with life-long anemia and spherocytosis on the peripheral blood film probably has hereditary spherocytosis (HS). How do you confirm the diagnosis?

Patients with HS, usually an autosomal dominant disorder, may have affected siblings as well as an affected parent. But, as in other autosomal dominant disorders, there is a significant (10%) spontaneous mutation rate, so paternity need not be questioned when neither parent is affected.

A confirmatory test frequently obtained is the **osmotic fragility test**. The patient's blood is incubated in a series of tubes containing decreasing concentrations of saline. In increasing hypotonic media, RBCs swell until a critical hemolytic volume is reached, beyond which the RBC membrane ruptures. Since the RBC in HS is already a sphere, lysis occurs in media of relatively high osmotic strength. Osmotic fragility is therefore increased. Normal RBCs are underfilled spheres and can accommodate a lot of water before reaching their critical hemolytic volume.

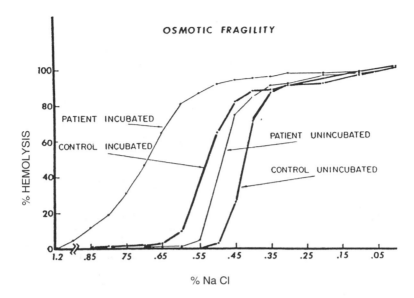

Osmotic fragility of unincubated and incubated RBCs from a normal individual and from a patient with hereditary spherocytosis. (From Rappaport S: Introduction to Hematology, 2nd ed. Philadelphia, J.B. Lippincott, 1987, p 135; with permission.)

30. What therapeutic interventions can be made in HS?

1. **Dietary:** Patients should receive dietary supplementation with folate.

2. **Splenectomy:** Older children and adults who have symptomatic anemia with ordinary viral illness or who have troublesome splenomegaly usually undergo splenectomy. Splenectomy prevents aplastic crises and gallstone formation, and many people who have adapted to mild anemia feel better. After splenectomy, there is increased risk for overwhelming pneumococcal bacteremia and greater morbidity and mortality from this and other encapsulated organisms. Risks are lessened by administration of pneumococcal vaccine. Decisions about attempts to cure HS by splenectomy should be individualized.

31. Describe the underlying membrane structural defects associated with hereditary spherocytosis.

HS is marked by decreased amounts of spectrin, the principal membrane protein found in erythrocytes. Spectrin has self-associative properties and forms a lattice with other RBC membrane proteins and actin. This supportive lattice on the inner aspect of the lipid bilayer gives the RBC its unique properties of strength and suppleness. Deficiency of spectrin correlates with the degree of hemolysis, changes in osmotic fragility, and response to splenectomy. The molecular mechanisms underlying HS include structural changes in spectrin itself, loss of ankyrin (a protein that links spectrin to the transmembrane protein band 3), and structural abnormalities of band 3. A deficiency of spectrin, for whatever reason, accounts for the decreased membrane surface area and spherocytosis.

32. What is hereditary elliptocytosis (HE)? What are its most important subsets?

HE includes a broad spectrum of disorders that result in an elliptical RBC shape and hemolysis.

1. Some families have a normal hematocrit and a mild reticulocytosis, or **mild common HE.**

2. Others have a more striking degree of hemolysis and anemia and more bizarre RBC morphology, which is **common HE with chronic hemolysis.**

3. Infants who have hemolytic HE at birth may later have striking hemolysis with bizarre RBCs and jaundice (**infantile poikilocytosis**).

4. A severe anemia accompanies the rare cases of **homozygous HE.**

5. **Hereditary pyropoikilocytosis** is another rare variant of HE in which the spectrin is abnormally sensitive to heat. The peripheral blood picture resembles that seen in hemolysis associated with severe burns. Most patients with HE and its variants have a structural abnormality of their spectrin protein which results in failure of this protein to self-associate into higher order tetramers and oligomers.

6. **Spherocytic elliptocytosis** is an unusual autosomal dominant disorder in which the elliptocytes are rounded. Spherocytes and an increased osmotic fragility are also found.

7. Resistance to malarial infection accompanies the **Melanesian** variant of HE. The central pallor in these cells is separated by a transverse ridge. This disorder is associated with an abnormal band 3 protein associated with membrane rigidity but only mild hemolysis.

33. What is the most common enzymatic defect in RBCs leading to hemolysis? How is it diagnosed?

Glucose-6-phosphate dehydrogenase (G6PD) deficiency. Hundreds of variants of this X-linked enzyme have been characterized. Because this is the first enzyme in the hexose monophosphate pathway, G6PD deficiency compromises the RBC's ability to regenerate NADPH from $NADP^+$. NADPH is necessary for the reduction of glutathione-containing disulfides (GSSG to GSH). The RBC as a carrier of oxygen is very vulnerable to oxidative attack when GSH is depleted. Oxidation results in precipitation of hemoglobin, which can be detected as Heinz bodies by supravital staining with crystal violet.

The diagnosis is established by measuring the enzymatic activity of G6PD.

34. How do patients with G6PD deficiency present?

Most patients are well until they come into contact with an oxidant drug. Some experience hemolysis with infections. Hepatitis in G6PD-deficient persons can result in spectacular jaundice. In the Mediterranean region, ingestion of fava beans can result in a severe hemolytic episode. It is important to identify any potential oxidant drugs such as nitrofurantoin, phenazopyridine (pyridium), primaquine, sulfacetamide, sulfamethoxazole, sulfanilamide, or sulfapyridine.

African-Americans have an increased prevalence (about 10% of men) of the type A−, which is unstable, losing G6PD activity as the RBC ages. During a hemolytic episode, the G6PD activity is normal because the young RBCs survive, while the older, deficient RBCs are lost. The deficiency is therefore not recognized until months later, when the patients no longer have a reticulocytosis.

Beutler E: Glucose-6-phosphate dehydrogenase deficiency. N Engl J Med 324:169–174, 1991.

35. Many abnormal hemoglobins with single amino acid changes are known. Of these, which sickle or participate in the sickling process during deoxygenation?

Sickle hemoglobin coexists with other β-chain variants to produce a spectrum of disorders from clinically insignificant conditions such as sickle trait to severe disease represented by homozygous SS.

Sickle Syndromes

SICKLE CELL DISEASE	SICKLE CELL TRAIT
SS (homozygous)	AS
Sβ-thalassemia	S-hereditary persistence
SC	of fetal hemoglobin
SD Los Angeles	
SO Arab	

36. What is the incidence of sickle hemoglobinopathies in births among African-Americans?

AS	8.0% (1 of 12)
SS	0.16%
AC	3.00%
SC	0.12%
SB_o	0.03%

Note that the incidence of $SB_0 + SC \cong$ that of SS. In adults, as many patients with sickle β-thalassemia or SC will be seen as homozygous S patients. Although SB_0 is clinically very similar to SS disease, SB_0 and SC patients are more likely to have palpable spleens and may experience splenic sequestration/infarctive crises as adults rather than in early childhood, as is the case in SS disease. Also, SC patients tend to have higher hematocrits: these patients may present with blindness due to retinopathy or aseptic necrosis of the hip.

37. Are any other ethnic groups at risk for sickle cell disease?

Sickle cell disease is usually thought of as a disease of blacks, but other ethnic groups originating from areas where malaria is or was prevalent also have the sickle gene. Consequently, Hispanics, Greeks, Turks, Arabs, and Veddoid Indians (Sri Lanka) have an increased incidence of sickle cell disease. In many of these groups, hemoglobin S is inherited with β-thalassemia to produce Sβ-thal. Interestingly, Arabs and Veddoid Indians have an increased proportion of F (fetal) hemoglobin that seems to alleviate the course of their disease.

Serjeant GR: Sickle Cell Disease, 2nd ed. New York, Oxford University Press, 1992, pp 16–28.

38. What are the main clinical manifestations of sickle hemoglobinopathies?

Hemolytic anemia
  Gallstones
  Increased folate needs
  Aplastic crises
  Indirect hyperbilirubinemia
  Increased LDH
Periodic vaso-occlusive disease ("crises")
  Pain crises
  Chest syndrome
  Abdominal pain
  Stroke
  Splenic infarct
  Splenic sequestration syndrome
  Multiorgan failure syndrome
  Priapism

Chronic end organ damage
  Retinopathy
  Aseptic necrosis of the hip
  Osteomyelitis
  Isosthenuria, hematuria, chronic renal
    failure
  Nephrotic syndrome
Hyposplenism
  Pneumococcal septicemia
  Increased morbidity with other encapsulated
    organisms
Reproductive
  High-risk pregnancy
  Impotence

39. Is there any morbidity truly associated with sickle trait?

Because 8% of African-Americans are heterozygous for sickle trait, this is an important question. The following abnormalities have been associated with sickle trait:

Splenic infarction at high altitude   Pulmonary embolism
Hyposthenuria   Glaucoma, anterior chamber bleeds
Hematuria   Sudden death following exertion
Bacteriuria and pyelonephritis in pregnancy Bacteremia in women

Sears DA: Sickle cell trait. In Embury SH, et al (eds): Sickle Cell Disease: Basic Principles and Clinical Practice. New York, Raven Press, 1994.

40. What are sickle crises?

Patients with sickle cell disease are susceptible to sudden, unheralded vaso-occlusive events that are called crises. The most common event is a simple pain crisis affecting the limbs, low back, chest, or abdomen. Sometimes, specific organs are affected by definite infarcts, including the bone and spleen (if splenic tissue has been preserved). The chest **syndrome** is marked by episodes of dyspnea, fever, pain, and the sudden appearance of an infiltrate on chest x-ray consistent with pneumonia. As often as not, no infection exists, but instead there is probably a sickle vaso-occlusion. Recent studies of the chest syndrome have emphasized the role of fat embolism from bone marrow infarcts and rib infarcts. Splinting while suffering a rib infarct may lead to hypoventilation and pulmonary vaso-occlusion. Incentive spirometry has been advocated to reduce the risk of chest syndrome in patients hospitalized with sickle crises and chest pain.

41. How are patients in a sickle crisis managed? How often do crises occur?

Patients with the chest syndrome often receive antibiotics and require oxygen. When hypoxemia continues despite oxygen therapy, exchange transfusions are helpful. The pathophysiology of the pain crisis is not well understood. It is interesting to note that most patients experience pain relatively infrequently—once every year or two. About 20% of patients, however, are troubled by more frequent crises and may visit the emergency room or hospital monthly. Why some homozygotes do poorly while others do relatively well is one of the mysteries of sickle cell disease. Similarly, it is not known what initiates crises or what mechanisms of spontaneous recovery act to terminate crises while patients are receiving only supportive care. The severity and duration of crises are variable. Stays for patients requiring hospitalization vary from 3–10 days.

Platt OS, et al: Pain in sickle cell disease: Rates and risk factors. N Engl J Med 325:11–16, 1991.

42. What are the routine health maintenance measures employed in patients with sickle cell anemia?

Now that many states routinely screen all births for hemoglobin S, practice guidelines for follow-up of parents and identified infants have been developed. Parents are taught to bring in their child when he or she is febrile and to examine for splenic enlargement. Penicillin prophylaxis is emphasized. Children should receive the polyvalent pneumococcal vaccine at age 2 years, *Haemophilus influenzae* type B vaccine, and hepatitis B immunization.

For adults, routine health maintenance includes genetic counseling about the risk of sickle cell disease in relatives or children. Patients are given folate supplementation and periodic ophthalmoscopic examinations. All adults should receive pneumococcal vaccine if they have not already been vaccinated. As patients get older, periodic review of renal function seems prudent.

43. Is pregnancy safe for women with sickle cell anemia?

With modern obstetric care, the risk of pregnancy for a woman with sickle cell disease has been greatly reduced. However, most obstetricians consider these pregnancies to be high risk and advocate close follow-up. Even so, the maternal mortality is < 2%, and the incidence of stillbirths and neonatal deaths is < 15%.

There is some controversy over the appropriate use of blood transfusions during prenancy. A recent study suggests that patients who receive prophylactic transfusions during pregnancy do no better than those who are transfused only when symptomatic. Many women with sickle cell disease are successful mothers. However, women who are often ill and who require frequent hospitalizations for control of pain may require a great deal of support from other family members if they are to have children. Women who do not wish to become pregnant can be placed on oral contraceptives.

Koshy M, et al: Prophylactic red cell transfusions in pregnant patients with sickle cell disease. N Engl J Med 319:1447, 1988.

44. Under what circumstances should RBC transfusion be considered in the treatment of sickle cell disease?

Indications for Transfusion in Sickle Cell Anemia

Strong indications	Relative indications
Aplastic crises	Before general anesthesia
Hypoxemia and chest syndrome	During pregnancy
CNS events, stroke	Priapism
Sequestration crises	Prior to arteriography
	Not indicated
	Management of typical pain crises

A national cooperative study found that simple transfusions to an arbitrary level of hemoglobin seemed to enable patients to undergo general anesthesia with no worse outcome than patients who had exchange transfusions. Because less blood was used, the conservative transfusion protocol was complicated less often by alloimmunization.

Vichinsky EP, et al: A comparison of conservative and aggressive transfusion regimens in the perioperative management of sickle cell disease. N Engl J Med 333:206–213, 1995.

45. What are the hazards of RBC transfusions in these patients?

Hazards include transmission of hepatitis, iron overload, and sensitization (which can be a significant problem). Delayed transfusion reactions occur in patients with a history of transfusions but with a negative crossmatch. After a few days, an anamnestic response occurs that results in hemolysis due to the sudden appearance of an IgG antibody. Delayed transfusion reactions usually involve Rh, Kidd, Kell, or Duffy antigens. In homozygous cases, delayed transfusion reactions can mimic a crisis and may result in death. Alloimmunization occurred in 30% of patients with sickle cell disease compared to 5% of a control group. Half of those alloimmunized had a recognizable delayed transfusion reaction.

46. A patient with sickle cell disease presents with a history of a viral syndrome, followed by dramatic worsening of the anemia. What entity needs to be strongly considered?

Aplastic crisis. Typically, patients have a flu-like illness, with or without an evanescent rash, fever, and myalgias, followed 5–10 days later by weakness and dyspnea. The patient presents with a sharply reduced hematocrit. A key finding is the nearly absolute absence of reticulocytes. This disorder is really a transient pure red cell aplasia. The platelet and WBC counts are usually unaffected. The bone marrow shows the absence of erythroid progenitors, except for a few "giant pronormoblasts."

This syndrome is most often caused by **parvovirus B19,** which seems to have a unique tropism for erythroid progenitors. In patients with hemolysis, parvovirus-induced aplasia is significant, because the duration of aplasia (5–10 days) coincides with the half-life of RBCs. Thus, cessation of RBC production for 10 days in a patient with a hematocrit of 22% and RBC lifespan of 9 days spells trouble. In these individuals, transfusions of packed RBCs are lifesaving. The 10-day cessation of erythropoiesis caused by the parvovirus goes unnoticed in a normal person with a hematocrit of 40% and an RBC lifespan of 120 days. The parvovirus may be the cause of fifth disease, arthritis, and spontaneous abortions.

Saarinen UM, et al: Human parvovirus B19-induced epidemic acute red cell aplasia in patients with hereditary hemolytic anemia. Blood 67:1411, 1986.

47. What treatment options are available for the patient with severe (> 3 crises/year) sickle cell anemia?

Perhaps the greatest therapeutic advance in sickle hemoglobinopathy was the recognition that certain chemotherapeutic agents could reverse the developmental "switch" from fetal to adult hemoglobin (Hb) synthesis. The rise in Hb F in each RBC suppresses sickling and offers the promise of reduced hemolysis and vaso-occlusive phenomena. A double-blinded trial of **hydroxyurea** was halted early when it was shown to reduce the rate of crises by about 40% and also to reduce the incidence of chest syndrome and the frequency of transfusions. Issues related to compliance with daily medications, frequent follow-up, and the potential for leukemogenesis have spurred the search for alternative agents that will increase Hb F production.

Bone marrow transplantation (BMT) has also been employed in the treatment of severe sickle cell disease with good results. This mode of therapy is controversial because of the morbidity and mortality associated with allogeneic BMT and graft-versus-host disease. The longevity enjoyed by most patients and the promise of regimens such as hydroxyurea cast doubt on the usefulness of BMT except for the sickest patients.

Charache S, et al: Effect of hydroxyurea on the frequency of painful crises in sickle cell anemia. N Engl J Med 332:317–322, 1995.

48. Which disorders result in decreased α-chain production? Why are they less severe than disorders of β-chain production?

Thalassemia minor is a frequent cause of microcytic hypochromic anemia. It is due to an imbalance of α- and β-chain production. The genetic information for the α-chain of hemoglobin is organized as two adjacent genes on chromosome 16. Thus, normal individuals have four copies of the gene for α hemoglobin. In α-thalassemias, deletions of one or more of these genes are present and result in a deficiency of α-chains and an excess of β-chains.

Deletion of a single gene is silent, but deletion of two genes is noticed as a microcytic mild anemia, with a normal hemoglobin electrophoresis. About 30% of African-Americans are heterozygous for a single-gene deletion, so that α-thalassemia is found in about 2.0% of individuals. Asians have a much higher incidence of a chromosome 16 with two deleted α-genes and therefore are at risk for bearing children with only one or no functional α genes. Those with only one functional α-gene have a mild hemolytic anemia (Hb H disease). Hemolysis results from oxidative attack on the β_4 tetramers present in the RBCs of affected individuals.

Hydrops fetalis in association with a tetramer of γ-chains (hemoglobin Bart's) is the cause of death at birth of a fetus with four α-gene deletions.

In **β-thalassemia major,** the absence of β-chains results in the presence of α_{-4}, a tetrameric α-chain protein that is highly toxic to the RBC membrane. Developing RBCs perish in the marrow or limp out to live a short, withered existence in the circulation. Erythropoiesis is highly ineffective. There is tremendous expansion of the bone marrow and extramedullary hematopoiesis. Affected children are transfusion-dependent, and if not transfused aggressively, they develop pathologic fractures and significant growth retardation.

Kazazian HH Jr: The thalassemia syndromes: Molecular basis and prenatal diagnosis in 1990. Semin Hematol 27:209, 1990.

49. Is there an effective treatment for children with β-thalassemia major?

In the modern era, **aggressive transfusion therapy** has greatly improved the outlook for these children. Iron overload is the price for this therapy. Chelation with deferoxamine by continuous subcutaneous infusion with a pump has been effective in reducing iron burden and prevents the onset of cardiomyopathy. However, the expense and inconvenience of chelation therapy are burdensome to these individuals when they reach young adulthood. Noncompliance with subcutaneus chelation has led to the pursuit of an effective oral agent.

Children with thalassemia major have been successfully treated with BMT. In the very young, graft-versus-host disease is less frequent, and the mortality and morbidity seem to be acceptable. After restoration of normal hematopoiesis, iron overload can be aggressively treated by phlebotomy.

Lucarelli G, et al: Marrow transplantation in patients with thalassemia responsive to iron chelation therapy. N Engl J Med 329:840, 1993.

50. A 20-year-old woman with a history of two previous laparotomies for abdominal pain presents with confusion, fever, tachycardia, abdominal pain, and peripheral neuropathy. Her mother had a similar history and died at a young age. What disorder do you suspect? How do you make a diagnosis?

The history is strongly suggestive of **porphyria,** acute intermittent type (AIP), which results from a deficiency of porphobilinogen deaminase. Physicians must be aware of two unfortunate facts about porphyria: Many people carry a diagnosis that is not founded upon adequate testing, while many others with the disease are unrecognized. Hence, before embarking on specific therapy, laboratory studies must be obtained to confirm the diagnosis.

Clinical Features of AIP

Autosomal dominant inheritance
Urine: δ-aminolevulinic acid, porphobilinogen, uroporphyrin
Symptoms/signs:
    Abdominal pain: fever, leukocytosis, vomiting, constipation
    Neurologic manifestations: peripheral neuropathy, paraplegia, Guillian-Barré, respiratory arrest, cranial
      nerve findings, psychosis, seizure, coma
    Other: hyponatremia, hypertension, tachycardia

Treatment includes carbohydrate infusions, hematin, β-blockers, and observation for respiratory compromise while obtaining appropriate lab studies to confirm the diagnosis. The patient should avoid barbiturates, anticonvulsants, estrogens, oral contraceptives, and alcohol.

Tefferi A, et al: Acute porphyrias: Diagnosis and management. Mayo Clin Proc 69:991–995, 1994.

51. A young man presents with symptomatic cyanosis. What is the most likely hematologic cause?

There are two likely possibilities:

1. **Congenital methemoglobinemia** due to an abnormal hemoglobin, M-hemoglobinopathy. These patients have congenital cyanosis that is transmitted as an autosomal dominant disorder. The M-hemoglobins are among the 400 or more human hemoglobin variants that have been reported in various parts of the world and are generally known by place names of first discovery, such as M-Boston, Saskatoon, Milwaukee, and Kochikuro. M-hemoglobins have been identified only rarely in blacks. These hemoglobins stabilize iron in its oxidized (FE^{+3}) state and have a muddy brown appearance.

2. **Methemoglobin reductase** (cytochrome b_5 reductase) deficiency, which is an autosomal recessive disorder. Cyanosis caused by hypoxemia requires at least 5 g/dl of deoxyhemoglobin to be noticeable, whereas only 1.5 g/dl of methemoglobin will be recognized.

Differential Diagnosis of Cyanosis

---

1. Hypoxemia
   a. Pulmonary disease
   b. Cardiac right-to-left shunting
   c. Shock, congestive heart failure
   d. Low oxygen affinity hemoglobin
2. Methemoglobinemia
   a. Congenital
      i. M-hemoglobin
      ii. Cytochrome b_5 reductase
   b. Acquired
      i. Drugs (dapsone, certain topical anesthetics)
      ii. Chemicals (well-water nitrates)
3. Sulfhemoglobinemia

Jaffe E: Methemoglobinemia in the differential diagnosis of cyanosis. Hosp Pract 20(12):92–110, 1985.

52. What disorder is associated with chronic intravascular hemolysis, anemia, iron-deficiency, and dark urine after waking from sleep?

Paroxysmal nocturnal hemoglobinuria (PNH). This is an acquired clonal or oligoclonal disorder that results in increased sensitivity to complement. Most patients have chronic hemolysis, hemoglobinuria, and hemosiderinuria without the paroxysmal nocturnal component. The sucrose hemolysis test is a useful screen for this disorder. An old, but favorite pimp question is to ask for the two disorders that result in a low leukocyte alkaline phosphatase score — chronic myelogenous leukemia and PNH.

PNH also has a close relationship to aplastic anemia, with some patients with aplastic anemia having a typical PNH defect, but producing few cells. PNH may arise after a hypoplastic event. The hemolytic disorder is complicated by unusual thrombi, including Budd-Chiari syndrome.

53. What is the cause of PNH on the molecular level?

The biochemical defect leading to increased complement lysis has been a hot topic for decades. New research has focused on abnormalities of the many proteins that are linked to the cellular membrane by a glycosylphosphatidylinositol anchor. These proteins are usually reduced or absent in PNH. Japanese investigators have identified abnormalities in an X-linked gene PIG-A (for phosphatidylinositol glycan class A) that apparently is responsible for PNH in the patients studied to date.

Hillmen P, et al: Natural history of paroxysmal nocturnal hemoglobinuria. N Engl J Med 333:1253–1258, 1995.

54. Compare the laboratory and clinical features of warm and cold antibody-mediated immune hemolytic anemias.

Warm vs. Cold Antibody Autoimmune Hemolytic Anemia

	WARM	COLD
Antibody	IgG	IgM
Complement	±	+
Spontaneous agglutination	–	+++
Active temperature	37°C	4°C
Antigen	Rh(pan)	I,i
Response to therapy with:		
Steroids	Good	Poor
Splenectomy	Good	Poor
Gloves, warmth	None	Good

Cold agglutinin disease may be a self-limited disorder brought on by Mycoplasma infection (usually anti-I) or infectious mononucleosis (usually anti-i). Chronic cold agglutination disease may be an idiopathic syndrome or associated with a lymphoproliferative disorder. In contrast, warm autoimmune hemolytic anemia is associated with lupus, chronic lymphocytic leukemia, Hodgkin's disease, non-Hodgkin's lymphomas, and certain drugs.

55. How is the Coombs' test used to evaluate autoimmune hemolytic anemia?

The Coombs' test is used to detect antibodies present on RBCs (direct Coombs' or direct antiglobulin test positive) or in plasma. In the **direct test,** the patient's RBCs are washed and incubated with an antiglobulin serum (rabbit or other species) and then examined for agglutination. In the **indirect test,** the patient's serum is reacted with a panel of RBCs bearing antigens of interest. Antibodies, if present in the patient's sera, bind to the RBCs bearing the relevant antigen. The panel cells are washed to reduce nonspecific binding, then incubated with an antiglobulin serum to detect agglutination. The antiglobulin reagent is necessary because antibodies attached to RBCs are usually IgG in low numbers and cannot ordinarily cross-link to agglutinate. The antiglobulin serum bridges these antibodies, favoring agglutination.

In autoimmune hemolytic anemia, the direct test is usually positive, indicating the presence of an autoantibody on the RBCs. The indirect test, indicating the presence of that same antibody in serum, may also be positive. Persons who have been exposed to blood or who have had a miscarriage or abortion may develop antibodies to certain antigens present on the transfused RBCs that do not exist on their native RBCs. Later, these individuals will have a positive indirect Coombs' test and negative direct Coombs' test.

56. What are the possible causes of fragmented RBCs on a peripheral smear from a patient with a hemolytic anemia?

Fragmentation hemolysis is characterized by the appearance of schistocytes, helmet cells, burr cells (echinocytes), and spherocytes. The hemolysis is intravascular and can be associated with a wide variety of conditions.

Fragmentation Syndromes

Macroangiopathic	
Valve hemolysis	Extracorporeal circulation
Endocardial cushion defect repair	
Microangiopathic*	
Cavernous hemangiomas	Malignant hypertension
Thrombotic thrombocytopenic purpura (TTP)	Scleroderma
Hemolytic uremic syndrome	Disseminated carcinomatosis
Eclampsia/pre-eclampsia	Disseminated intravascular coagulation (DIC)

*Thrombocytopenia often present.

57. What important syndrome is characterized by the triad of thrombocytopenia, fragmentation hemolysis, and fluctuating neurological signs?

Thrombotic thrombocytopenic purpura (TTP). TTP is perhaps the most spectacular of the fragmentation syndromes. Patients may present with seizures, coma, paresis, or more subtle neurologic signs and thrombocytopenia. Although the cause(s) is unknown, treatment with steroids, plasma exchange, or plasma infusion appears to be effective. The mortality is 20–50%. Some patients (20–30%) pursue a relapsing course. During remissions of their illness, unusually large multimers of von Willebrand factor have been found in the plasma, which disappear during relapse.

58. How does hemolytic uremic syndrome (HUS) differ from TTP?

In HUS, renal failure is the predominant organ syndrome associated with thrombocytopenia and fragmentation hemolysis. Recently, HUS has been observed to follow infection with *Escherichia coli* O157:H7, a newly arising contaminant of undercooked meat. This *E. coli* serotype elaborates a shiga-like toxin that may participate in the genesis of the syndrome.

LEUKOCYTES

59. What constitutes the lower limit for the absolute neutrophil count?

For adults, the level below which neutropenia is a consideration is 1.8×10^9/liter (1800/mm^3). African-Americans have a lower mean neutrophil count, which may be encountered during routine exams. These persons, however, do not have an increased incidence of infections, nor do they have increased severity of infectious diseases. When the neutrophil count is $< 0.5 \times 10^9$/liter (500/mm^3), neutropenia is severe, and there is a greater propensity for compromised response to infection.

60. What are the causes of neutropenia?

Causes of Neutropenia

DECREASED PRODUCTION

Drug-induced—alkylating agents, antimetabolites, antibiotics, phenothiazines, tranquilizers, certain diuretics, anti-inflammatory agents, antithyroid drugs, others
Hematologic diseases—idiopathic, cyclic neutropenia. Chèdiak-Higashi syndrome, aplastic anemia, infantile genetic disorders
Tumor invasion, myelofibrosis
Nutritional deficiency—vitamin B$_{12}$, folate (esp. alcoholics)
Infection—tuberculosis, typhoid fever, brucellosis, tularemia, measles, dengue, mononucleosis, malaria, viral hepatitis, leishmaniasis, AIDS

PERIPHERAL DESTRUCTION

Antineutrophil antibodies and/or splenic or lung (alveolar macrophage) trapping
Autoimmune disorders—Felty's syndrome, rheumatoid arthritis, SLE
Drugs as haptens—aminopyrine, α-methyl dopa, phenylbutazone, mercurial diuretics, some phenothiazines
Wegener's granulomatosis

PERIPHERAL POOLING (TRANSIENT NEUTROPENIA)

Overwhelming bacterial infection (gram-neg. septicemia)
Hemodialysis
Cardiopulmonary bypass

Gatlin JI: Quantitative and qualitative disorders of phagocytes. In Isselbacher KJ, et al (eds): Harrison's Principle of Internal Medicine, 13th ed. New York, McGraw-Hill, 1994, p 329.

61. Which drugs commonly cause neutropenia?

The cytotoxic chemotherapeutic agents (including alkylating agents and antimetabolites) as well as immunosuppressive drugs are obvious choices, but other drugs such as phenothiazines, antithyroid drugs, or chloramphenicol may cause neutropenia in a dose-dependent fashion by inhibiting cell replication. Immune-related neutropenia may be seen with penicillins, cephalosporins, and other agents. The more common agents associated with idiosyncratic neutropenia are shown below:

Some Noncytotoxic Drugs Associated with Neutropenia

Analgesics/anti-inflammatory agents	Antibiotics	Others
Indomethacin	Chloramphenicol	Phenytoin
Para-aminophenol derivatives	Penicillins	Cimetidine
Acetaminophen	Sulfonamides	Captopril
Phenacetin	Cephalosporins	Chlorpropamide
Pyrazolone derivatives	Phenothiazines	
Aminopyrine	Antithyroid drugs	
Dipyrone		
Oxyphenbutazone		
Phenylbutazone		

The International Agranulocytosis and Aplastic Anemia Study: Risks of agranulocytosis and aplastic anemia. JAMA 256:1749, 1986.

62. What is the significance of finding myelocytes, metamyelocytes, and nucleated RBCs in the peripheral blood?

Leukoerythroblastosis, or the presence of immature WBCs and nucleated RBCs, is often associated with a malignancy that has metastasized to the bone marrow. Numerous other, less serious conditions are also effect leukoerythroblastosis, albeit sometimes transiently:

Malignancies	**Nonmalignant Conditions**
Solid tumors	Hemolysis—including sickle cell disease
Prostate	Thrombocytopenic purpura
Breast	Infancy
GI	GI bleeding
Lymphoma	Renal transplants
Myelofibrosis	Septicemia
Leukemia	Chronic lung disease
Preleukemia	Myocardial infarction
	Liver disease

63. Describe the features of lymphocytosis caused by infections.

When infections (usually viral) cause lymphocytosis, the lymphocyte morphology is unusual or atypical. Thus, infection with the Epstein-Barr virus (EBV) or cytomegalovirus (CMV) can cause an infectious mononucleosis syndrome of fever, sore throat, lymphadenopathy, hepatosplenomegaly, and, in the case of EBV, an increased titer of the heterophile antibody. An acute lymphocytosis may be associated with primary infection with HIV-1.

In EBV infection, B cells are penetrated by the virus, eliciting a polyclonal T-cell response manifested in the peripheral blood as atypical lymphocytosis. Cold agglutinin disease may also occur in EBV virus disease. These IgM antibodies are usually directed against the i antigen. These disorders are usually self-limited. CMV, toxoplasmosis, or less commonly, EBV infection during the first trimester of pregnancy has been associated with serious developmental defects in the newborn.

Causes of Heterophile-Negative Mononucleosis

Cytomegalovirus	Herpes simplex II
HIV-1	*Toxoplasma*
Adenovirus	Rubella

MYELOPROLIFERATIVE DISORDERS

64. Polycythemia is frequently encountered by internists. Before you embark on a long and expensive workup, what two steps are necessary?

There is no point in pursuing a workup of polycythemia without demonstrating that:

1. The RBC mass is increased, *and*
2. Hypoxemia is not present as a cause of secondary erythrocytosis.

Many patients who are receiving diuretics have an increased hematocrit, but typically they also have a decreased plasma volume and normal RBC mass. Some patients who are not on diuretics (usually smokers) have so-called "stress erythrocytosis," with normal RBC mass and reduced plasma volume. Patients with chronic lung disease or congenital heart disease resulting in significant left-to-right shunts are also polycythemic.

Djulbegovic B, et al: A new algorithm for the diagnosis of polycythemia. Am Fam Physician 44:113–120, 1991.

65. List the major and minor criteria widely used to diagnose polycythemia vera (PCV).

The Polycythemia Study Group has developed the following guidelines to establish a diagnosis of PCV:

Category A (Major Criteria)	**Category B (minor criteria)**

1. Increased red cell mass
  Males: > 36 ml/kg
  Females: > 32 ml/kg
	1. Thrombocytosis: platelets $> 400 \times 10^9/l$

2. Normal SaO_2 ($\geq 90\%$)	2. Leukocytosis: WBC $> 12 \times 10^9/l$
3. Splenomegaly	3. Elevated leukocyte alkaline phosphatase (LAP)
	4. Elevated B_{12} level (> 900 pg/ml) or unbound B_{12} binding capacity (≥ 2200 pg/ml)

A diagnosis of PCV is supported by finding either (1) all three criteria of category A or (2) increased RBC mass, normal SaO_2 and two of the criteria in category B.

Although these criteria are useful, important causes of secondary polycythemia need to be considered. Carboxyhemoglobin should be measured if the patient is a heavy smoker, and in certain families, a high-affinity hemoglobin may be identified by determining the P_{50} (oxygen half-saturation pressure). Several kindreds have alterations in the gene for the erythropoietin receptor, resulting in familial erythrocytosis. A neoplasm producing ectopic erythropoietin also may result in erythrocytosis. Typically, these are obvious, but CT scans or liver scans may be necessary to evaluate the possibility of an occult neoplasm of the kidney or liver. In PCV the erythropoietin level is usually low or normal, whereas in secondary conditions, erythropoietin levels are increased.

Berlin NI: Diagnosis and classification of the polycythemias. Semin Hematol 12:339–351, 1975.

66. Once the diagnosis of PCV is established, how are patients treated? What are the expected complications of therapy?

Treatment of PCV is important, since untreated patients are uncomfortable and at risk for life-threatening thrombotic events. Initially, phlebotomy of 500 ml of blood every other day as tolerated is undertaken until the hematocrit is reduced to a normal range. Some patients are not well-controlled and require myelosuppressive therapy with hydroxyurea, alkylating agents, or ablation with the isotope [32]P. As phlebotomy proceeds, patients develop iron deficiency, which reduces the rate at which phlebotomy is necessary for control of the disease.

In an important Polycythemia Vera Study Group publication, treatment with phlebotomy, ^{32}P, or chlorambucil was compared. Treatment with phlebotomy alone was associated with an increased incidence of stroke and other thrombotic events, whereas treatment with chlorambucil or ^{32}P was associated with a high incidence of transformation into acute leukemia. Therefore, patients who are over age 70 or those who have had previous thrombotic events may do better with hydroxyurea and occasional phlebotomy, whereas phlebotomy alone usually suffices for younger patients.

Berk PD, et al: Therapeutic recommendations in polycythemia vera based on Polycythemia Study Group protocols. Semin Hematol 23:132–143, 1986.

67. What is the typical cytogenetic abnormality found in chronic myelogenous leukemia (CML)? Are there any other hematologic malignancies that share this finding?

The cytogenetic marker of CML is the **9:22 translocation,** in which portions of the long arms of chromosomes 9 and 22 are exchanged, resulting in a shortened 22 or **Philadelphia chromosome** (Ph[1]). This balanced translocation is now known to result in the juxtaposition of an oncogene c-*abl* originating on 9 with genes in the breakpoint cluster region (*bcr*) of 22. Cell lines established from CML cells express a new mRNA, which reflects the chimeric gene produced by the fusion of the *bcr* and c-*abl* genes. From this mRNA, a unique tyrosine phosphoprotein kinase, P210 *bcr-abl,* is translated, which may act to phosphorylate tyrosine residues in important cellular proteins. A small minority of CML patients have normal cytogenetics but have the c-*abl/bcr* translocation when studied at the molecular level.

Some patients with acute lymphoblastic leukemia (ALL) also have 9:22 translocations. Although some of these may have been lymphoblastic transformations of CML, most are thought to be de novo leukemias with subtle differences in the location of the c-*abl* translocation into the *bcr* region of 22.

Kantarjian HM, et al: Chronic myelogenous leukemia: A concise update. Blood 82:691–703, 1993.

68. How is CML differentiated from a leukemoid reaction?

Occasionally patients who have an inflammatory disease, infection, or cancer have a leukocytosis up to, but usually not over, 50×10^9/liter. In some instances, the cause may not be apparent and CML is a consideration. These two entities may be differentiated by considering the characteristics outlined below:

CML Compared to Leukemoid Reaction

	CML	LEUKEMOID REACTION
Juvenile neutrophils (metamyelocytes, myelocytes, etc.)	+	
Basophilia	+	−
Eosinophilia	+	−
Marrow fibrosis	+/−	−
Splenomegaly	+/−	−
Leukocyte alkaline phosphatase	Low	Increased
Philadelphia chromosome	+	−

+ = present; − = absent.

69. What is the prognosis of CML?

Despite control of symptoms with agents such as hydroxyurea or busulfan, CML uniformly transforms into an acute leukemia that is typically poorly responsive to chemotherapy. The median survival of patients ranges from 39–47 months. After the first year, the risk of transformation into blast phase is about 20% per year. Thus, a minority of patients have long survivals of 10–25 years with CML.

70. Describe the clinical and laboratory features of acceleration of CML into blast phase.

Certain clinical events herald the transformation of CML from chronic to blast phase. These include an enlarging spleen (with splenic infarcts), increased basophilia and eosinophilia, fever, fibrosis in the marrow, and resistance to alkylators or hydroxyurea. In many instances, an accelerated phase (marked by an increased percentage of blasts and promyelocytes) occurs before frank leukemia.

In about two-thirds of cases of transformation into acute leukemia, there is the appearance of a new cytogenic abnormality in addition to the Philadelphia chromosome. These new cytogenetic abnormalities suggest that the Ph[1] clone evolves into a more malignant cell. Four typical chromosomal changes are seen in the setting of transformation: (1) a second Ph[1] chromosome, (2) trisomy 8, (3) isochromosome 17, (4) trisomy 19. Interestingly, the phenotype of a leukemic cell in the blast crisis of CML is variable. While most patients have blasts with the characteristics of myeloid cells, about a third have cells that are lymphoid in character. Less often, the cells have features of erythroblastic leukemia or megakaryocytic leukemia.

71. Compare the roles of interferon and bone marrow transplantation (BMT) in the treatment of CML.

Recent studies have shown the usefulness of α-interferon in the treatment of CML in the chronic phase, particularly for those patients who have thrombocytosis as a manifestation of CML. Treatment with α-interferon can result in loss of the cytogenic abnormality, as a significant number of patients had no Ph[1] chromosomes detected in mitotic figures obtained from bone marrow aspirate after treatment. Whether this form of therapy delays the onset of blast crises is not known.

BMT is the only therapy at present that offers a hope of cure for CML. Although the peritransplant mortality is significant, the long-term outlook is better for young patients who have CML and an HLA-identical sibling. Patients should undergo BMT during chronic phase, because once patients reach blast crises, their outlook is poorer.

Kantarjian HM, et al: Prolonged survival in chronic myelogenous leukemia after cytogenetic response to interferon-α therapy. Ann Intern Med 122:254–261, 1995.

72. Patients presenting with large spleens, fibrotic marrows, and the presence of teardrop shaped erythrocytes on the peripheral blood film have what myeloproliferative disorder?

Myelofibrosis, or agnogenic myeloid metaplasia. This myeloproliferative disease is marked by splenomegaly, tear-drop RBCs, fibrotic marrow, and immature erythroid and myeloid cells in peripheral blood (leukoerythroblastic blood picture). Extramedullary hematopoiesis is usually present in the liver and spleen. Patients may have neutrophilia, thrombocytosis, and anemia, but other patients, typically with massively enlarged spleens, may be cytopenic instead. Patients with enlarged spleens and neutrophilia resemble patients with CML. Determination of the presence of Ph[1] chromosome may distinguish the two.

The fibroblast proliferation that is typically present in the marrows of these patients is polyclonal and appears to be fostered by fibroblast growth factors released by abnormal megakaryocytes. Patients may be troubled by bone pain and often have radiographic evidence of osteosclerosis. Massive splenomegaly may lead to portal hypertension and varices. Treatment is largely supportive and ineffective. As in other myeloproliferative diseases, transformation into acute leukemia has been observed in some patients.

Hasselbalch H: Idiopathic myelofibrosis: A clinical study of 80 patients. Am J Hematol 34:291–300, 1990.

73. Patients without massive splenomegaly may have platelet counts above 1,000,000/μl ("platelet millionaires"). What myeloproliferative disease do these patients have?

Patients may become platelet millionaires for a variety of reasons. Occasionally patients with severe **iron deficiency** and concurrent hemorrhage or inflammatory disease have platelet counts of $> 1,000,000/\mu l$. Once iron deficiency is corrected or the inflammatory disorder resolves, platelet counts return to normal levels.

Another myeloproliferative disorder, **essential thrombocythemia,** needs to be considered when the platelet count rises above 600,000/μl, although a count $> 1,000,000/\mu l$ is the rule. In this disorder, there is also evidence for clonal proliferation. Physical exam may show modest splenic enlargement and purpura. Patients are often troubled by hemorrhage due to poorly functioning platelets. Purpura, epistaxis, and gingival bleeding are typical manifestations, and these may be exacerbated by aspirin use. Erythromelalgia, characterized by a localized burning pain and warmth of the distal extremities, is commonly seen. Dramatic relief is obtained with small doses of aspirin. Also seen are neurologic manifestations such as dizziness, seizures, and transient ischemic attacks.

Tefferi A, et al: Issues in the diagnosis and management of essential thrombocythemia. Mayo Clin Proc 69:651–655, 1994.

74. What are the causes of thrombocytosis?

Causes of Thrombocytosis

REACTIVE	MYELOPROLIFERATIVE DISORDERS
Malignancy	Essential thrombocythemia
Iron deficiency	Polycythemia vera (PCV)
Splenectomy	CML (Ph[1]+)
Inflammatory bowel disease	Myelofibrosis
Infection	Myelodysplastic syndromes
Collagen-vascular diseases	

Iron studies, collagen vascular screen, and cytogenetic studies of the bone marrow aspirate are helpful in differentiating these disorders. PCV may present as essential thrombocythemia and iron deficiency with chronic GI blood loss. When the iron deficiency is corrected, the erythrocytosis of PCV will be manifest.

Buss DH, et al: Occurrence, etiology, and clinical significance of extreme thrombocytosis: A study of 280 cases. Am J Med 96:247–253, 1994.

75. What is the most likely complication in a patient with a myeloproliferative disease who presents with a swollen, hot ankle?

Patients with myeloproliferative syndromes (PCV, CML, myelofibrosis, essential thrombocythemia) may develop hyperuricemia and gout. Thus, arthritis in such patients should be investigated thoroughly, including arthrocentesis and examination for intracellular, negatively-birefringent crystals under polarized light.

ACUTE MYELOGENOUS LEUKEMIA (AML)

76. Which cytogenetic abnormalities have been described in AML?

At least 90% of patients with AML have cytogenetic abnormalities. Some of these, when detected, indicate a relatively good prognosis, and others bode ill. Interestingly, specific morphologic variants of AML have been linked to characteristic cytogenetic abnormalities, as shown in the table.

Cytogenetics Abnormalities in AML

CYTOGENETIC ABNORMALITY	LEUKEMIA TYPE	PROGNOSIS
Trisomy 8	M2	Average
t(8;21)	M2 with splenomegaly, chloromas, Auer rods	Good
t(15;17)	M3, many promyelocytes, DIC	Average
inv 16	M4 with abnormal eosinophils	Good
t(9;11)	M5, monocytic leukemia	Average
t(6;9)	M2 with increased basophils	Average
t(4;11)	Biphenotypic leukemia lymphoid and monocytic phenotype	Poor
5q-, 7-, 5-, 7-	Therapy-related leukemia	Poor

Yunis JJ, et al: High resolution chromosomes as an independent prognostic indicator in adult acute nonlymphocytic leukemia. N Engl J Med 311:812–818, 1984.

Koeffler HP: Syndromes of acute nonlymphocytic leukemia. Ann Intern Med 107:748–758, 1987.

77. How is AML classified and how do the subtypes differ in natural history and complications?

The diagnosis of AML M1–M5 requires a cellular bone marrow aspirate with blasts representing > 30% of all nucleated WBCs. If erythroblasts comprise > 50% of the nucleated bone marrow cells, erythroleukemia (M6) is present. If the marrow is cellular but blasts account for

$<$ 30% of the nucleated RBCs, myelodysplasia is present. Peroxidase stain is important in the definition of AML, in practice, the blasts are peroxidase (or Sudan black)-positive in AML and peroxidase-negative in acute lymphoblastic leukemia (ALL).

French-American-British (FAB) Classification of AML

TYPE	DESCRIPTION	CRITERIA
M1	Myeloblastic leukemia without maturation	$>3\%$ of blasts are peroxidase-positive. A few granules, Auer rods, or both; one or more distinct nucleoli; no further maturation
M2	Myeloblastic leukemia with maturation	$>50\%$ of marrow cells are myeloblasts and promyelocytes. Myelocytes, metamyelocytes, and mature granulocytes are seen; eosinophilia may predominate in some cases
M3	Hypergranular promyelocytic leukemia	Majority of cells are abnormal promyelocytes, reniform (kidney-shaped) nuclei, bundles of Auer rods; also some have closely packed bright pink or purple granules
M4	Myelomonocytic leukemia	$>20\%$ of bone marrow, peripheral blood nucleated cells, or both are promonocytes and monocytes; an eosinopholic variant is also recognized
M5	Monocytic leukemia (M5a = poorly differentiated) (M5b = differentiated)	Granulocyte component $<10\%$ of marrow cells, monocytoid cells have a fluoride-sensitive esterase reaction cytochemically
M6	Erythroleukemia	$>50\%$ of cells are erythroblasts; myeloblasts represent $>30\%$ of nonerythroid nucleated cells
M7	Megakaryoblastic	$>30\%$ of marrow cells are blasts; platelets peroxidase-positive on electron microscopy, or blasts react with antiplatelet monoclonal antibodies; marrow fibrosis is prominent; cytoplasmic budding is also a feature

Bennett JM, et al: Proposal for the classificiation of the acute leukemias. Br J Hematol 33:451, 1976.

78. How does the presentation and treatment of acute promyelocytic leukemia (APL) differ from other AML subtypes?

Patients with APL present with lower WBC counts but may have a normal count when first examined. Careful attention to the morphology of the circulating WBCs discloses the presence of the hypergranular blasts or blasts with multiple Auer rods. Less frequently the blasts are hypogranular. A significant hemorrhagic diathesis may complicate either the presentation or the treatment of APL with standard AML chemotherapy. A picture resembling disseminated intravascular coagulation (DIC) is characteristic and may be accompanied by CNS bleeding, which is sometimes fatal. Patients may require intensive support with platelets, fresh frozen plasma, and cryoprecipitate. In the past, heparin has been used to abrogate the consumptive coagulopathy.

79. What gene rearrangement defines APL?

The 15:17 translocation, which involves a rearrangement of a receptor for retinoic acid (retinoic acid receptor-α, or RAR-α). Administration of all-*trans* retinoic acid (ATRA) results in maturation of the promyelocyte to a granulocyte, such that complete morphologic and cytogenetic remission can be attained without the hemorrhagic diathesis. Although these remissions are short-lived, the combination of ATRA and chemotherapy seems to be the best way to treat patients with APL. ATRA does have side effects, the most important of which is the retinoic-acid syndrome of capillary leak, pulmonary infiltrates, and hypoxemia.

The reverse transcriptase polymerase chain reactions (rt-PCR) now allow the detection of minimal disease at the level of the gene rearrangement—a much more sensitive way to assess the presence of leukemic cells than counting blasts in the marrow or screening the karyotypes of marrow cells for the 15:17 translocation. The presence of the PML-RAR-α gene rearrangement detected by rt-PCR may predict relapse.

Tallman MS, et al: Acute promyelocytic leukemia: A paradigm for differentiation therapy with retinoic acid. Blood Rev 8:70–78, 1994.

80. What are the main causes of death in AML?

Infection, hemorrhage from thrombocytopenia, or resistant disease. Refractoriness to platelet transfusions is a significant problem that develops in patients who become sensitized to donor platelets. The use of filters to remove contaminating lymphocytes appears to reduce this complication of transfusion support. Resistance to chemotherapy may be related to changes the leukemic cells which affect the ability of drugs to enter the cell. The multidrug resistance phenotype is conferred by enhanced expression of a membrane protein, p-glycoprotein, which actively pumps a wide variety of chemotherapeutic agents out of the cell. Expression of this protein at diagnosis may confer a worse prognosis. Currently, there is great interest in the use of p-glycoprotein inhibitors, such as cyclosporine and verapamil, during chemotherapy to circumvent resistance to induction chemotherapy.

Ross DD, et al: Enhancement of daunorubicin accumulation, retention, and cytotoxicity by verapamil or cyclosporin A in blast cells from patients with previously untreated acute myeloid leukemia. Blood 82:1288–1299, 1993.

81. Which are the most frequent organisms causing infection during induction-chemotherapy-induced bone marrow aplasia?

Patients receiving induction chemotherapy usually endure a period of absolute granulocytopenia (leukocyte nadir) at a time when there have been breakdowns of important barriers to infection. These breakdowns include mucositis throughout the GI tract and the presence of chronic indwelling venous catheters.

Organisms Causing Infection in AML

BACTERIAL	FUNGI
Pseudomonas aeruginosa	Candida sp.
Escherichia coli	Aspergillus
Staphylococcus aureus	Phycomycetes
Klebsiella aerobacter	
Proteus vulgaris	
Bacteroides sp.	
α-Hemolytic streptococci	
Staphylococcus epidermidis	

Antibiotic therapy is usually designed to cover the bacterial pathogens on this list. If after a period of adequate treatment the patient remains febrile, amphotericin is usually begun. Controversy still rages over the need for reverse isolation, enteric sterilization with antibiotics, or other prophylactic measures that could be taken to reduce infection.

82. What proportion of AML patients attain complete remission? How many survive 5 years or more?

In the Toronto Leukemia Study, the complete remission (CR) rate among 272 patients with AML ranged from 43.8–85.3%, depending on the exclusion criteria used. The lower remission rate occurred in patients who were elderly (> age 70), had an antecedent myelodysplastic syndrome, or had partial treatment. A younger patient with no previous hematologic disorder had a 70–85% chance of attaining a CR which may last for 11–16 months on average. Of those who attain CR, 20% are durable for > 5 years.

More recently, the Cancer and Leukemia Group B found that younger patients (<40 years) had a 75% CR rate and a 4-year disease-free survival of 32%, whereas older patients had CR and disease-free rates of 47% and 14%, respectively. During induction chemotherapy, the younger patients died because they had disease resistant to two courses of therapy, but the older patients died more often during treatment-induced hypoplasia. Growth factors such as G-CSF and GM-CSF have been used to stimulate granulopoiesis after chemotherapy, but with mixed results.

Mayer RJ, et al: Intensive postremission chemotherapy in adults with acute myeloid leukemia. N Engl J Med 331:896–903, 1994.

83. Young patients with AML in first remission are usually evaluated or considered for BMT. Do syngeneic (identical twin) transplants or allogeneic (HLA-identical) transplants fare better after BMT?

Patients in remission who are age 40 or younger and have HLA-identical siblings are usually evaluated for BMT. In comparisons of BMT versus maintenance or other forms of post-induction chemotherapy, patients receiving transplants seem to have an advantage. This may be due to the intensity of the preoperative regimen for BMT, which includes lethal doses of chemotherapy, often in conjunction with total body irradiation. However, studies of identical-twin donor-recipient pairs indicate that the recipients have a higher relapse rate than HLA-identical sibling transplants. These studies indicate that there is an important "graft-versus-leukemia" effect of allogeneic BMT. The relatively recent recognition of "good prognosis" cytogenetic abnormalities has led some centers to treat patients having 8:21, 15:17 translocations or inv (16) with intensive chemotherapy alone. In these patients, BMT is reserved for relapse.

Appelbaum FR, et al: Chemotherapy vs marrow transplantation for adults with acute nonlymphocytic leukemia: A five-year follow-up. Blood 72:179–84, 1988.

84. What are the most important causes of death in patients undergoing BMT?

BMT is a challenging mode of therapy. After conditioning, patients become pancytopenic during the 3 weeks or so that is required for engraftment. During that time, they are prone to **infectious complications** similar to those experienced by patients undergoing remission-induction chemotherapy for AML. These patients are treated prophylactically with antibiotics and transfusions of RBCs and platelets. Blood products must be irradiated to prevent **graft-versus-host disease** from lymphocytes in the donor units. After engraftment, interstitial pneumonitis is a frequent complication, with a high mortality rate. Some of these deaths are due to infectious agents such as CMV. Recently, a severe form of **veno-occlusive disease** of **the liver** has emerged as a cause of morbidity and mortality post-BMT.

85. Describe the clinical findings in graft-versus-host disease (GvHD).

One consequence of engraftment is the potential for GvHD, which is caused by T cells from the donor. GvHD may be either acute or chronic. **Acute GvHD** arises during the first 100 days after transplant, with donor T lymphocytes targeting the host skin, liver, and GI tract. Patients may have mild skin rashes or more severe disease resulting in toxic epidermal necrolysis. Diarrhea and transient elevation of liver enzymes may occur and, in some patients, are more severe, resulting in massive diarrhea and liver failure. Immunologic competence is also delayed by GvHD, so that patients are susceptible to new infections, including those mediated by encapsulated organisms such as pneumococci.

Chronic GvHD results in the same organ involvement, but in addition, there are features of a scleroderma-like illness. Dry eyes, dry mouth, myasthenia, bronchiolitis, and infections are also observed.

ACUTE LYMPHOBLASTIC LEUKEMIA (ALL)

86. Can ALL be reliably differentiated from AML (M1) by examination of the peripheral blood smear only?

No. Although hematologists can sometimes distinguish between these two entities by looking at the morphology of the blasts, there is a very high rate of discordance with the results of special studies. Flow cytometry is now frequently used to show typical lymphoid markers in ALL and myeloid markers in AML. Some patients with leukemia show evidence of both types of markers and are called biphenotypic.

Distinguishing Cytologic Features of ALL and AML

WRIGHT'S STAIN MORPHOLOGY	AML	ALL
Cytoplasm	More abundant	Scanty
Granules	Sometimes present	Absent
Nucleoli	3–5 distinct	1–3, often indistinct
Auer rods	May be present	Absent
STAINING CHARACTERISTICS		
Peroxidase or Sudan black	+	−
Periodic acid–Schiff	+/−	+

87. What are the indicators of a poor prognosis in adults with ALL?

ALL has a 50% cure rate in young children, but in adults, the outlook is much worse. Certain features at presentation of ALL in adults confer a poorer prognosis and may suggest the need for very aggressive therapy. Adults are more likely than children to show:
- Unfavorable chromosomal abnormalities, such as Ph[1] and 8:14 translocation
- Biphenotypic disease and other than early pre-B immunophenotype
- Leukocytosis at presentation
- Multidrug resistance
- Mediastinal mass

Copelan EA, McGuire EA: The biology and treatment of acute lymphoblastic leukemia in adults. Blood 85: 1151–1168, 1995.

LYMPHOPROLIFERATIVE DISEASE

88. What is the most common leukemia of adults?

Chronic lymphocytic leukemia (CLL). This disorder is a neoplastic growth of lymphocytes, most often B lymphocytes. Patients are often elderly, and CLL is detected during examination for other problems. Lymphadenopathy and splenomegaly are also relatively frequent. Some patients present only with an elevated WBC count, comprised of lymphocytes with a normal morphology.

89. What are the diagnostic criteria for CLL?

1. Sustained lymphocyte count $\geq 10 \times 10^9$/liter. Morphology should be "typical."
2. Bone marrow involvement (> 30% lymphocytes)
3. B-cell immunophenotypes (typically weak expression of membrane immunoglobulin, CD5 expression, and rosette formation with mouse erythrocytes)

To make a diagnosis of CLL, criterion 1 should be satisfied along with either criterion 2 or 3. If criterion 1 is not satisfied (lymphocyte count $< 10 \times 10^9$/liter), then criteria 2 *and* 3 must be present.

International Workshop on Chronic Lymphocytic Leukemia: Chronic lymphocytic leukemia: Recommendations for diagnosis, staging, and response criteria. Ann Intern Med 110:236–238, 1989.

90. Patients with CLL are typically staged to determine prognosis and therapy. What are the current staging systems?

Many patients with CLL present with limited disease and live without trouble from their leukemia. Since most are elderly, death from other causes is most likely. Patients with more advanced disease, however, do less well, and unfortunately, chemotherapy has not improved survival. Treatment is usually given to patients who have anemia, thrombocytopenia, or bulky lymphadenopathy. Two staging systems have been in use for CLL:

Rai Staging System for CLL

STAGE	CLINICAL FEATURES	SURVIVAL*
0	Lymphocytosis in blood and bone marrow only	>120 mos
I	Lymphocytosis and enlarged lymph nodes	95
II	Lymphocytosis plus hepatomegaly, splenomegaly, or both	72
III	Lymphocytosis and anemia (hemoglobin < 110 g/l)	30
IV	Lymphocytosis and thrombocytopenia (platelets <100 × 10⁹/l)	30

*Weighted median survival was derived from 8 series that involved a total of 952 patients.

Binet Staging System for Chronic Lymphocytic Leukemia

STAGE	CLINICAL FEATURES	SURVIVAL*
A	Hemoglobin > 100 g/l; platelets > 100 × 10⁹/l and < 3 areas involved†	>120 mos
B	Hemoglobin > 100 g/l; platelets ≥ 100 × 10⁹/l and > 3 areas involved†	61
C	Hemoglobin < 100 g/l *or* platelets < 100 × 10⁹/l Or both (independent of the areas involved)	32

*Weighted median survival was derived from 8 series that involved a total of 1117 patients.
†Cervical, axillary, and inguinal lymph nodes (whether unilateral or bilateral); spleen; and liver.
International Workshop on Chronic Lymphocytic Leukemia: Chronic lymphocytic leukemia: Recommendations for diagnosis, staging, and response criteria. Ann Intern Med 110:236–238, 1989.

91. What are the complications of CLL?
- Autoimmune phenomena (warm antibody autoimmune hemolytic anemia, immune thrombocytopenia, neutropenia)
- Pure red cell aplasia
- Hypogammaglobulinemia
- Transformation into a large cell lymphoma with poor prognosis (Richter's syndrome)

Rozman C, Montserrat E: Chronic lymphocytic leukemia. N Engl J Med 333:1052–1057, 1995.

92. Which lymphoproliferative disorder is associated with pancytopenia, splenomegaly, absence of lymphadenopathy, and circulating lymphoid cells with multiple projections?

Hairy cell leukemia (HCL). Although an uncommon malignancy (2% of all leukemias), HCL receives a lot of attention because of the advances in its treatment and the unusual infections observed in the course of the disease. HCL is an important consideration in the workup of individuals who present with pancytopenia. Although the bone marrow aspirate is often scanty, characteristic "hairy" lymphs may be observed. The biopsy may show a diffusely involved marrow with mononuclear cells situated in a network of fibrosis. Some patients have had presentations as aplastic anemia.

Although hairy cells may be present in the marrow, the biopsy picture is one of profound hypocellularity. The hairy cell is a B lymphocyte with an immunophenotype consistent with a cell between a CLL-lymphocyte and a plasma cell. Hairy cells also possess the Tac antigen (CD25), a receptor for interleukin-2, usually seen on activated T cells. The distinctive cytochemical feature of the hairy cell is a tartrate-resistant acid phosphatase activity.

In the past many patients improved after splenectomy. Interferon has been used successfully in alleviating this disorder, but recent trials show that the most effective agent is the purine analog 2-chlorodeoxyadenosine.

93. What infectious complications are seen in HCL?

The course of HCL is marked by an increased incidence of infections with atypical mycobacteria or fungi, such as *Histoplasma* and *Cryptococcus*. There may also be an increased incidence of bacterial infections and perhaps legionellosis. Factors contributing to the occurrence of atypical mycobacterial and fungal infections in these patients may be their decreased neutrophils, absolute monocytopenia, and inability to form granuloma normally.

Westbrook CA, Golde DW: Clinical problems in hairy cell leukemia: Diagnosis and management. Semin Oncol 11:514, 1984.

HODGKIN'S AND NON-HODGKIN'S LYMPHOMAS

94. What are the common presentations of Hodgkin's disease?

Most patients often present with lymphadenopathy, in the neck or axilla, with lymph nodes that are nontender, rubbery, and discrete. Sometimes these nodes wax and wane in size until attention is sought. Important symptoms that figure into the staging of Hodgkin's disease are fever, weight loss (> 10% of body weight), and night sweats. Some patients are troubled by pruritus. Hodgkin's disease tends to originate in central lymph nodes, so that some patients present with mediastinal lymphadenopathy.

95. How does Hodgkin's disease spread? How does this pattern affect staging?

Hodgkin's disease is thought to spread from a unifocal site to contiguous lymph nodes. There may be early hematogenous dissemination to the spleen, with subsequent spread to the splenic hilar and retroperitoneal nodes as well as the liver. If large tumor masses develop, there may be extension into adjacent organs.

It is important to remember that the spleen is often significantly involved in the absence of palpable splenomegaly. Hence, many centers recommend staging laparotomy to avoid missing splenic and hepatic disease. The importance of staging in Hodgkin's disease is to determine the extent of disease and thereby decide on therapy.

Ann Arbor Staging of Hodgkin's Disease

STAGE	SUB-STAGE	INVOLVEMENT
I	I	Single lymph node
	IE	Single extralymphatic organ
II	II	$\geq$ lymph nodes on same side of diaphragm
	IIE	With localized extralymphatic site
III	III	Lymph nodes above and below diaphragm
	IIIE	With localized extralymphatic site
	IIIS	With isolated splenic site
	IIISE	With both extralymphatic and splenic sites
IV	IV	Disseminated or diffuse involvement of one or more extralymphatic sites
	IVA	Asymptomatic
	IVB	Fever, sweats, weight loss > 10% body

Aisenberg A: The staging and treatment of Hodgkin's disease. N Engl J Med 299:1228, 1978.

96. What are the histologic subtypes of Hodgkin's disease? Which carry the worst prognosis?

Nodular sclerosis	35%
Mixed cellularity	33%
Lymphocyte predominant	16%
Lymphocyte depletion	16%

Nodular sclerosis more frequently affects women, whereas the other three types more often affect males. While staging generally determines the outlook, histologic subtype is also important. Nodular-sclerosing and lymphocyte-predominant disease tend to present with limited disease. Lymphocyte-depletion is associated with more advanced disease, retroperitoneal involvement, and presentation in older adults.

97. What is the classic cell seen in the lymph nodes of patients with Hodgkin's disease?

The **Reed-Sternberg (RS) cell.** This is a large cell with two nuclei, each possessing a distinct nucleolus. RS cells are plentiful in mixed-cellularity and lymphocyte-depletion Hodgkin's disease, but rarer in nodular-sclerosis and lymphocyte-predominant disease, being overwhelmed by reactive lymphocytes, PMNs, and eosinophils. In nodular sclerosis, there is retraction of the cells surrounding the RS cell during fixation, producing the **lacunar cell.** Also present are bands of fibrosis.

The pathology of Hodgkin's disease is not straight-forward—there is diagnostic confusion with the newly recognized entities T-cell-rich B-cell lymphoma and peripheral T-cell lymphomas.

Banks PM. The pathology of Hodgkin's disease. Semin Oncol 17:683–695, 1990.

98. When should patients with Hodgkin's disease undergo staging laparotomy?

Patients must first undergo a comprehensive clinical staging evaluation before surgical staging is contemplated. The key elements in the clinical staging are as follows:

- **Detailed history**
- **Detailed physical exam,** with attention to lymph node areas, spleen, and liver
- **Laboratory:** CBC, ESR, alkaline phosphatase, renal and liver function tests
- **Radiology:** PA and lateral views of chest, abdominal and chest CT, bilateral lower-extremity lymphanigiogram
- **Bone marrow aspirate and biopsy**

Once this evaluation is complete, the need for surgical staging with laparotomy can be considered. There is no need for staging laparotomy if disseminated or diffuse extralymphatic involvement is found, unless the results would change therapy. In centers where treatment includes chemotherapy for limited disease, then the need for laparotomy is less apparent. Unfortunately, staging laparotomy carries a high morbidity from pulmonary emboli, subphrenic abscesses, stress ulcers, and wound infections.

Urba WJ, Longo DL: Hodgkin's disease. N Engl J Med 326:678–687, 1992.

99. In patients cured of Hodgkin's disease, what are the late sequelae of therapy?

The most important of the late sequelae consist of myelodysplasia, leukemia, and non-Hodgkin's lymphoma occurring 3–10 years after therapy. Certain complications of the high-dose irradiation given to patients are also evident: acute radiation pneumonitis with fever, cough, and shortness of breath. Cardiac effects of irradiation include pericarditis, pericardial effusions, and pericardial fibrosis. There may be an acceleration of coronary artery disease. Neurologic effects of irradiation include Lhermitte's syndrome (paresthesia produced by flexion of the neck).

Bookman MA, Longo DL: Concomitant illness in patients treated for Hodgkin's disease. Cancer Treat Rev 13:77, 1986.

100. How does the pattern of lymph node involvement in non-Hodgkin's lymphoma (diffuse versus nodular) correlate with the pace of disease progression?

In nodular lymphomas, the neoplastic lymphocytes congregate into aggregates that superficially resemble germinal centers. Lymphomas of this type generally pursue an indolent course. Diffuse lymphomas tend to behave in a more aggressive manner. Other adverse prognostic factors include older age, elevated lactate dehydrogenase, two or more extranodal sites, T-cell phenotype, and masses >10 cm.

101. How often do lymphoma patients have bone marrow involvement?

Bone marrow involvement is extremely common in non-Hodgkin's lymphoma, whereas it is relatively uncommon in Hodgkin's disease. Diffuse well-differentiated lymphocytic lymphoma is associated with bone marrow involvement 100% of the time. Small, cleaved-cell lymphomas, follicular and diffuse types, are associated with bone marrow involvement 40–50% of the time. Large-cell or histiocytic lymphomas are less likely to spread to the marrow (15% incidence). When bone marrow involvement occurs in large cell lymphoma, there is a greater risk for CNS disease.

102. In Africa, Denis P. Burkitt described an aggressive neoplasm that bears his name. What are the salient clinical features of this lymphoma?

Burkitt's lymphoma results from a proliferation of B lymphocytes with a striking appearance. They present as round or oval cells with abundant basophilic cytoplasm-containing vacuoles that stain positively for fat. The tissue is replaced with a monotonous infiltrate of cells with interspersed macrophages, giving a "starry sky" appearance. When the presentation is that of a leukemia, it is classified as L3 in the FAB scheme. These cells proliferate rapidly and have a potential doubling time of 24 hours.

In African Burkitt's, patients present with large extranodal tumors of the jaws, abdominal viscera (including kidney), and ovaries and retroperitoneum. In American Burkitt's, patients present with intra-abdominal tumors arising from the ileocecal region or mesenteric lymph nodes. In Africa, the disease is associated with Epstein-Barr virus, but this is less often true in American cases.

103. What characteristic cytogenetic abnormalities are seen in Burkitt's lymphoma?

A t(8;14) translocation is recognized in all cases. The proto-oncogene c-*myc* is located on chromosome 8 and usually becomes translocated to the locus of the heavy-chain immunoglobulin gene. This results in the activation of c-*myc*. Burkitt's is now classified as a subset of small non-cleaved-cell lymphoma (SNCL). SNCL is a frequent neoplasm diagnosed in association with HIV infection and has a predilection for CNS and bone marrow involvement.

Mashal RD, Canellos GP: Small non-cleaved cell lymphoma in adults. Am J Hematol 38:40–47, 1991.

104. When should patients with non-Hodgkin's lymphoma receive chemotherapy or radiotherapy?

In an evaluation of patients with favorable histology and stage III or IV disease, it was found that deferral of treatment until patients became symptomatic did not adversely affect survival. In fact, during the course of nontreatment, spontaneous regression was frequently observed. In patients, the median time to treatment was 31 months. Thus, in the absence of curative chemotherapy for indolent lymphomas, deferral of treatment is a reasonable course, provided patients are followed closely.

PLASMA CELL DYSCRASIAS

105. Which disorders are associated with the presence of a serum monoclonal immunoglobulin paraprotein?

Monoclonal immunoglobulins are detected frequently as a result of the routine availability of serum protein determinations and electrophoresis. The disorders associated with a secondary monoclonal gammopathy are shown in the table. These have to be distinguished from the monoclonal gammopathy associated with multiple myeloma, benign monoclonal gammopathy of uncertain significance, solitary plasmacytoma, amyloidosis, lymphoma, and Waldenström's macroglobulinemia.

Disorders Associated with Monoclonal Gammopathy

Collagen vascular diseases (SLE, scleroderma, Sjögren's disease, rheumatoid arthritis)	Hepatitis, cirrhosis
Crohn's disease	Infectious disease (tuberculosis, subacute bacterial endocarditis, AIDS, purpura fulminans)
Skin disease (pyoderma gangrenosum, psoriasis, scleromyxedema, urticaria)	Myeloproliferative diseases
	Post-BMT
Gaucher's disease	Cryoglobulinemia

Lichtman MA: Essential and secondary monoclonal gammopathies. In Williams WJ, et al (eds): Hematology, 5th ed. New York, McGraw-Hill, 1995, pp 1104–1108.

106. How do you differentiate multiple myeloma (MM) from benign monoclonal gammopathy (BMG)?

Differentiation of Multiple Myeloma from Benign Monoclonal Gammopathy

	MM	BMG
M-protein	>3.5 g/dl	<3.5 g/dl
IgG IgA	>2.0 g/dl	<2.0 g/dl
Anemia or other cytopenia	Usually present	Absent
Urine protein	>500 mg/24 hr	<500 mg/24 hr
Bones	Lytic lesions or osteoporosis	Normal
Marrow plasma cells	>10%	<10%
Serum β_2-microglobulin	>3.0 mg/l	<3.0 mg/l
Calcium	Elevated in 30%	Normal
Creatinine	± elevation	Normal
Change in monoclonal protein with time	Increases	No change

The discovery of a monoclonal protein on serum protein electrophoresis should be followed by a careful workup for MM. Patients who have a small serum spike, normal CBC, no proteinuria, and no lytic lesions, hypercalcemia, or renal dysfunction are usually followed with periodic serum protein electrophoresis. Patients meeting some of the criteria for MM, but showing no progression with follow-up, are described as having indolent MM. These patients generally do not have anemia or lytic bone lesions.

107. What are the common complications of multiple myeloma?

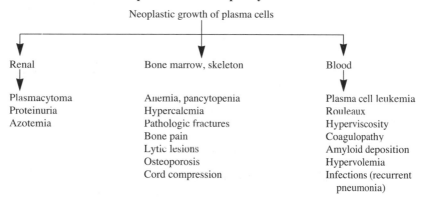

Neoplastic growth of plasma cells

Renal	Bone marrow, skeleton	Blood
Plasmacytoma	Anemia, pancytopenia	Plasma cell leukemia
Proteinuria	Hypercalcemia	Rouleaux
Azotemia	Pathologic fractures	Hyperviscosity
	Bone pain	Coagulopathy
	Lytic lesions	Amyloid deposition
	Osteoporosis	Hypervolemia
	Cord compression	Infections (recurrent pneumonia)

108. What are the renal manifestations of multiple myeloma?
Myeloma kidney
 Dense tubular casts and progressive azotemia
 Hyperviscosity
Renal tubular dysfunction
 Isosthenuria
 Renal tubular acidosis
 Adult Fanconi syndrome
Glomerulonephritis
Urate nephropathy
Pyelonephritis
Dye-nephropathy
Hypercalcemia renal damage
Plasma cell infiltration
Amyloid kidney
Nephrotic syndrome

109. Describe the clinical manifestations of Waldenström's macroglobulinemia.
Waldenström's macroglobulinemia is a B-cell disorder of proliferating plasmacytoid lymphs that produce an IgM monoclonal protein. Patients frequently have hepatosplenomegaly, lymphadenopathy, and bone marrow involvement. The elderly are affected most often. Neurologic disease, including peripheral neuropathy and cerebellar dysfunction, is also seen. A prominent feature is retinopathy with large sausage-shaped, dilated retinal veins. Bleeding and purpura are also

commonly seen. Of particular importance is the recognition of the hyperviscosity syndrome, which can also occur in MM. This syndrome can respond dramatically to plasmapheresis, because IgM does not have a large extravascular distribution.

Dimopoulos MA, Alexanian R: Waldenstrom's macroglobulinemia. Blood 83: 1452–1459, 1994.

110. Outline the manifestations of the hyperviscosity syndrome.

Hyperviscosity Syndrome

Global CNS dysfunction and stupor
Retinopathy
Retinal hemorrhages
Papilledema
Hypervolemia, congestive heart failure
Headache, vertigo, ataxia
Stroke
Coagulopathy

111. Patients with the λ-light-chain type of MM are prone to develop amyloidosis. What are the clinical and laboratory clues to the presence of this systemic disorder?

Amyloid is a lardaceous substance that accumulates in the tissues of patients with a variety of disorders, including MM. In MM, the amyloid is comprised of light chains, most often λ arranged in a β-pleated sheet. When stained with Congo red and viewed under polarized light, amyloid shows an apple-green birefringence. Patients may develop purpura from skin involvement, hepatosplenomegaly, macroglossia, orthostatic hypotension, congestive heart failure, malabsorption, nephrotic syndrome, peripheral neuropathy, and carpal tunnel syndrome. Interestingly, the consequences of amyloid include an acquired factor X deficiency, resulting in a prolonged PT and PTT and functional hyposplenism. The latter results in the presence of Howell-Jolly bodies, even though the spleen is present.

Gertz MA, Kyle RA: Primary systemic amyloidosis—a diagnostic primer. Mayo Clin Proc 64:1505–1519,1989.

HEMOSTASIS

112. Define the primary and secondary phases of hemostasis.

Hemostasis is a complicated process with several components, all of which must work well for normal hemostasis to occur. The two overlapping phases of the formation of a clot or hemostatic plug are:

(1) **primary hemostasis**—The ruptured vessel wall interacts with platelets that must adhere and aggregate to form the basis of the clot; and (2) **secondary hemostasis**—The clotting factors circulating in the blood activate each other in a cascade that results in the activation of thrombin and the deposition of fibrin around the platelet plug.

113. How do the disorders of primary and secondary hemostasis differ in clinical presentations?

	Primary	*Secondary*
Onset	Immediate	Delayed, hours after trauma
Sites, type of lesion	Mucosa, GI, GU, skin (purpura, petechiae)	Joints, retroperitoneum, muscles, hematuria, hematomas
Components involved	Vessel wall, platelet adhesion	Generation of fibrin from fibrinogen
Typical disorder	von Willebrand disease	Hemophilia A (factor VIII deficiency)

Schafer AI: Approach to bleeding. In Loscalzo J, Schafer AI (eds): Thrombosis and Hemorrhage. Boston, Blackwell, 1994, pp 407–422.

114. What conditions are associated with immune thrombocytopenias?

1. Collagen-vascular diseases (systemic lupus erythematosus)
2. Impaired immunity (Bruton's agammaglobulinemia, IV drug users, HIV-1 infection)
3. Lymphoid neoplasias (Hodgkin's disease, non-Hodgkin's lymphoma, CLL)
4. Drug-induced (quinine, quinidine, hydrochlorothiazide, gold, heparin)
5. Others (thyrotoxicosis, sarcoidosis, antithymocyte globulin, solid tumors, anaphylaxis)
6. Isoimmune (post-transfusion purpura, fetal-maternal isoimmunization)

115. Describe idiopathic thrombocytopenic purpura (ITP).

ITP, an autoantibody arises (usually IgG) that interacts with the patient's own platelets. Sometimes, these antibodies interact with specific antigens related to functional proteins; platelets coated with the auto-IgG are then sequestered and removed by macrophages in the spleen, liver, and bone marrow. Production of megakaryocytes as judged by a bone marrow aspirate appears to be normal. However, recent studies indicate that megakaryocytopoiesis is, in fact, suboptimal for the degree of peripheral destruction. Thus, megakaryocytes may be affected by the autoantibody of ITP. ITP implies no known cause and is a diagnosis of exclusion. ITP occurs early in HIV infection, often before typical AIDS-defining illness.

George JN, et al: Chronic idiopathic thrombocytopenic purpura. N Engl J Med 331, 1207–1211, 1994.

116. What disorders are associated with nonimmune destruction of platelets?

Thrombocytopenia can occur with a wide variety of disorders of hematopoiesis. Of most concern are those situations that result in the increased peripheral destruction of platelets. Some of these conditions may have immune components.

Conditions Resulting in Increased Platelet Destruction

Infections	Microangiopathic disease
Sepsis, gram-negative or gram-positive	DIC
	Thrombotic thrombocytopenic purpura
Viral, rickettsial	Eclampsia, preeclampsia
Histoplasmosis	Burns
Malaria	Cavernous hemangiomas
Typhoid, brucellosis	Kasabach-Merritt syndrome
Hypersplenism	Extracorporeal circulation, hypothermia
	Massive transfusion

117. Name the most common hereditary disorder resulting in a prolonged bleeding time.

von Willebrand's disease, an autosomal dominant disorder, results from several abnormalities in the production of a large, multimeric adhesive protein, von Willebrand factor (vWF). Classic vWF (type 1) disease results from decreased release of vWF from the endothelial cell. vWF is also synthesized by megakaryocytes and is a constituent of the α-granules of platelets. Decreased presence of vWF at the site of endothelial damage results in impairment of platelet adhesion and consequently poor primary hemostasis.

Patients with von Willebrand's disease have problems with epistaxis, hematuria, menorrhagia, GI bleeding, and bleeding after trauma. In classic type I disease, the platelet count is normal, but the bleeding time is prolonged. Factor VIII activity is also reduced in the plasma of patients with type 1 von Willebrand's disease. The reduction of vWF seems to shorten the circulating life of factor VIII. The pathophysiology of von Willebrand's disease has rapidly advanced so that now multiple types are recognized.

Bloom AL: Von Willebrand factor: Clinical features of inherited and acquired disorders. Mayo Clin Proc 66:743–751, 1991.

118. What are the hereditary disorders of platelet function?

Because von Willebrand disease is associated with platelet dysfunction, it is often considered with disorders resulting from congenital structural abnormalities of the platelet. These bleeding disorders are identified by a prolonged bleeding time and abnormal functional behavior in platelet aggregation tests. Three of these disorders are described below:

Hereditary Disorders Resulting in Platelet Dysfunction

	VON WILLEBRAND'S DISEASE	BERNARD-SOULIER SYNDROME	GLANZMANN'S THROMBASTHENIA
Defect	Reduced or abnormal factor VIII:vWF	Absence of plate gp Ib, a receptor for vWF	Absence of platelet gp IIb, IIIa, a receptor for vWF and fibrinogen
Inheritance	Autosomal dominant	Autosomal recessive	Autosomal recessive
Platelet appearance	Normal	Macrothrombocytes	Normal
Aggregometry			
Ristocetin	Decreased	Decreased	Normal
ADP	Normal	Normal	Decreased
Collagen	Normal	Normal	Decreased

gp = glycoprotein

119. What conditions result in an acquired platelet defect?

The biggest offender in this category is **aspirin**. Platelet cyclooxygenase is irreversibly inhibited by low doses of aspirin. As a result, the platelet has lifelong impaired function. Aspirin exacerbates the bleeding tendencies associated with von Willebrand's disease and other platelet disorders and by itself can produce prolongation of the bleeding time. It is important to note that the bleeding time does not predict the risk of hemorrhage in an individual patient. The potential benefit of this aspirin effect is to reduce platelet activity in critical areas, such as a stenosed coronary artery. The typical finding in platelet aggregometry with aspirin-treated platelets is the absence of the secondary wave of aggregation produced by ADP.

Another important acquired disorder of platelet function is that associated with **uremia**. Although the pathogenesis of this mild hemostatic defect is poorly understood, it appears that the administration of the vasopressin analog desmopressin increases vWF and shortens the bleeding time.

George JN, Shattil SJ: The clinical importance of acquired abnormalities of platelet function. N Engl J Med 324:27–39, 1991.

120. What two factor deficiencies result in hemophilia? What is their pattern of inheritance?

Hemophilia results from a deficiency of factor VIII (hemophilia A) or factor IX (hemophilia B). These are X-linked disorders, and the family history of an affected boy will reveal affected maternal uncles and cousins. Patients may have mild or severe disease. Severe disease requires frequent administration of factor VIII or IX concentrates. In the past, hemophilia was a crippling disorder because of the frequency of hemarthroses and arthritis that ensued. Prophylactic administration of factor VIII concentrate after trauma has reduced the incidence of complications dramatically.

Hoyer LW: Hemophilia A. N Engl J Med 330:38–47, 994.

121. How necessary is a preoperative measurement of the PT and PTT in a patient without a history of bleeding?

Although physicians order a preop or prebiopsy prothrombin time (PT) and partial thromboplastin time (PTT) routinely, the value of these tests as screens for coagulation defects has been disputed. In recent studies, no advantage was seen in performing these tests on the asymptomatic patient. The low prevalence of clinically important, yet unsuspected bleeding disorders results in more false-positive tests than true-positives. However, both tests are indicated in the symptomatic patient and in the monitoring of warfarin (via PT) or heparin (via PTT) administration.

Suchman AL, Griner PA: Diagnostic uses of the activated partial thromboplastin time and prothrombin time. Ann Intern Med 104:810–816, 1986.

122. What questions regarding bleeding problems need to be asked in the history?

The patient interview should include questions regarding personal or family history of bleeding problems, including prolonged bleeding after dental extraction, injury, or surgical procedure. Patients should be asked about frequent nosebleeds, menorrhagia, melena, and bruising. A history of liver disease, obvious malnutrition, or malabsorption syndrome should also be sought. Although irrelevant to the PT and PTT, a recent history of aspirin ingestion needs to be sought. The physical exam should include an inspection of the skin and mucosa for purpura or petechiae, hematomas, and ecchymotic lesions.

123. What hereditary disorders result in a prolonged PTT without bleeding?

When routine preoperative screening PT and PTT tests are obtained, occasional patients have a dramatic, reproducible prolongation of the PTT, but no historical or physical findings to suggest a hemostatic disorder. Familial disorders causing this phenomenon are:

1. Hereditary deficiency of factor XII (Hageman factor) and
2. Deficiency of factors in the contact activation system that activates XII, including Fletcher factor (prekallikrein) and Fitzgerald factor (high-MW kininogen).

These disorders produce an interesting in-vitro phenomenon that does not seem to result in any hemorrhagic tendency. In fact, Mr. Hageman, the first person recognized to be deficient in factor XII, died of pulmonary embolism.

124. What is the lupus anticoagulant? What is its relationship to the anti-phospholipid syndrome?

The **lupus anticoagulant** (LA) is an autoantibody that binds to the phospholipid component required in the formation of the prothrombin activation complex. Its presence on the phospholipid disrupts the association between factor Xa, prothrombin, factor V, and calcium, leading to an abnormally long PTT (and sometimes PT). The name is truly a misnomer since in vivo it is not an anticoagulant, nor does it only occur in lupus patients. There is a high but incomplete level of concordance with other known phospholipid antibodies, such as anticardiolipin antibodies.

The term **anti-phospholipid antibody syndrome** refers to patients with anti-phospholipid antibodies that may or may not behave in vitro as typical LAs. The presence of the LA or anti-phospholipid antibodies may also be associated with thrombotic disease and should be sought when a young person presents with a stroke.

Roubey RAS: Autoantibodies to phospholipid-binding plasma proteins: A new view of lupus anticoagulants and other "antiphospholipid" antibodies. Blood 84:2854–2867, 1994.

125. What are the causes of disseminated intravascular coagulation (DIC)?

Infections
- Viral (epidemic hemorrhagic fevers, herpes, rubella)
- Rickettsial (Rocky Mountain spotted fever)
- Bacterial (gram-negative sepsis, meningococcemia)
- Fungal (histoplasmosis)
- Protozoan (malaria)

Neoplasms
- Carcinomas (prostate, pancreas, breast, lung, ovary)
- Acute promyelocytic leukemia

Vascular disease
- Cavernous hemangiomas (Kasabach-Merritt syndrome)
- Aneurysms

Collagen-vascular disease
- Vasculitis
- Polyarteritis
- Systemic lupus erythematosus

Obstetric complications
- Abruptio placentae
- Septic abortion
- Amniotic fluid embolism
- Intrauterine fetal death
- Saline-, urea-induced abortions
- Eclampsia
- Hemolytic transfusion reactions
- Hypothermia-rewarming
- Shock
- Cocaine-induced rhabdomyolysis
- Use of factor IX concentrates

Colman RW, et al: Disseminated intravascular coagulation. Annu Rev Med 30:359, 1979.

126. When DIC is present, which coagulation tests are abnormal?

DIC occurs when there is inappropriate activation of thrombin and disseminated clotting, which in turn is associated with increased fibrinolysis. During this process, multiple coagulation factors are consumed. Byproducts of thrombin and plasmin activity circulate as well. As endothelial cell damage occurs, there is consumption of platelets and, in some instances, fragmentation of RBCs, resulting in significant intravascular hemolysis. Although DIC is often a hemorrhagic condition, certain patients present with thrombotic complications: digital ischemia, decreased mentation, migrating thrombophlebitis, and renal involvement.

Laboratory Findings in DIC

Peripheral blood smear	Platelets↓
	Red cell fragmentation
PT, PTT	Both ↑
Fibrinogen	↓
Fibrin degradation products	↑
D-dimers	↑
Platelet count	↓

127. How does the bleeding diathesis associated with liver disease resemble DIC?

The liver may not be the seat of the soul, but it is definitely the site of production of all clotting factors (except von Willebrand factor). Severe liver disease compromises hemostasis in a number of ways. Most readily detected is a decrease in the activity of the vitamin K-dependent factors II, VII, IX, and X. Patients with severe liver disease will have a prolonged PT and PTT that does not improve after the administration of vitamin K.

Low fibrinogen levels are also seen. They also elaborate a poorly functioning fibrinogen. Dysfibrinogenemia produces prolongation of the PT, PTT, and thrombin time. With the onset of cirrhosis and portal hypertension, splenomegaly and a reduced platelet count occur. The liver is also an important organ of clearance of plasminogen activators, so that increased fibrin degradation products may be measured. Thus, the laboratory abnormalities in severe liver disease may mimic DIC.

128. Patients receiving certain antibiotics develop prolongation of the PT and PTT. Which antibiotics and why?

Certain β-lactam antibiotics are known to reduce the prothrombin level. This characteristic is associated with a methylthiotetrazole substitution that appears to inhibit microsomal carboxylase activity, which in turn results in decreased γ-carboxylation of the vitamin K-dependent factors. Antibiotics in general may reduce vitamin K levels by destroying the bacterial flora of the gut, which also provide vitamin K. Thus, the combination of prolonged reduced feeding and antibiotic administration is associated with vitamin K deficiency and a bleeding diathesis. When β-lactam antibiotics with the methylthiotetrazole substitution are administered, the inhibition of the vitamin K-dependent carboxylase results in the more rapid onset of a bleeding diathesis.

Platelet function can be impaired by several antibiotics, such as carbenicillin or ticarcillin. Platelet function also may be affected by some of the β-lactam antibiotics (e.g., moxalactam), prolonging the bleeding time. Presumably, antibiotics interact with the platelet membrane to block receptor-mediated aggregation. Unfortunately, some patients who receive the β-lactam antibiotics experience a "double whammy" of hypoprothrombinemia and platelet dysfunction. Bleeding may be avoided by concomitant administration of vitamin K and using the lowest antibiotic dose possible. The patient who develops bleeding while receiving this antibiotic may benefit from platelet transfusions.

129. Which congenital disorders are associated with an increased incidence of deep venous thromboembolism (DVT)?

The occurrence of DVT in a young person, a family history of thrombosis, thrombosis at unusual sites (such as mesenteric vein), or recurrent thrombosis without precipitating factors suggests that a patient has a hypercoagulable state. Activated protein C inhibits coagulation by inactivating factors Va and VIIIa. A mutation in factor V (V_{Leiden}), arg506 to gly, results in resistance of Va to the activated protein C (APC). APC resistance has a remarkably high prevalence in certain populations and may account for 30% of the patients thought to have a congenital or hereditary susceptibility to thrombosis ("thrombophilia"). Patients with these disorders need careful evaluation and family screening. Symptomatic individuals are cautiously managed with coumarin anticoagulation.

Primary Hereditary Factors Associated with Hypercoagulability*

FACTOR	PERCENT
Antithrombin III deficiency	3%
Protein C deficiency	10%
Activated protein C resistance	30%
Protein S deficiency	12%
Plasminogen deficiency	1%
Dysfibrinogenemia	1%
tPA deficiency	1%
PAI-I excess	2%
Heparin cofactor II	1%

*It should be noted that about 65–70% of the causes of hereditary thrombotic disease are still unknown.

Dahlback B: Inherited thrombophilia: Resistance to activated protein C as a pathogenic factor of venous thromboembolism. Blood 85:607–614, 1995.

130. What serious complication can occur with anticoagulation therapy in patients with congenital hypercoagulable states?

Proteins C and S are vitamin K-dependent anticoagulant proteins. When patients are placed on warfarin for treatment of DVT, the goal of therapy is to reduce the activity of procoagulant factors (VII included). This is monitored by following the PT, which detects early changes in the activity of factor VII. When coumarin therapy is initiated, particularly when started at high doses or in patients with a congenital deficiency, the levels of protein C may drop precipitously before the onset of anticoagulation due to decreased factor VII activity. A consequence of this is a serious disorder, coumarin skin necrosis.

131. What are the acquired causes of hypercoaguability?

Secondary Hypercoagulable States

Abnormalities of coagulation and fibrinolysis	Abnormalities of blood vessels and rheology
Malignancy	Conditions promoting venous stasis (immobilization,
Pregnancy	obesity, advanced age, postoperative state)
Use of oral contraceptives	Artificial surfaces
Infusion of prothrombin complex concentrates	Vasculitis and chronic occlusive arterial disease
Nephrotic syndrome	Homocystinuria
Abnormalities of platelets	Hyperviscosity (polycythemia, leukemia, sickle cell
Myeloproliferative disorders	disease, leukoagglutination, increased serum vis-
Paroxysmal nocturnal hemoglobinuria	cosity)
Hyperlipidemia	Thrombotic thrombocytopenic purpura
Diabetes mellitus	
Heparin-induced thrombocytopenia	

From Schafer AI: The hypercoagulable states. Ann Intern Med 102:814, 1985, p 818; with permission.

BIBLIOGRAPHY

1. Loscalzo J, Schafer AI (eds): Thrombosis and Hemorrhage. Boston, Blackwell, 1994.
2. Williams WJ, et al (eds): Hematology, 5th ed. New York, McGraw-Hill, 1995.
3. Wood ME, Bunn PA Jr (eds): Hematology/Oncology Secrets, Philadelphia, Hanley & Belfus, 1994.

10. PULMONARY MEDICINE

Sheila Goodnight-White, M.D.

A medical chest specialist is long-winded about the shortwinded.
Kenneth T. Bird

DIAPHRAGM, n. A muscular partition separating disorders of the chest from disorders of the bowels.
Ambrose Bierce (1842–1914?)
The Devil's Dictionary

PHYSIOLOGY

1. What are the five basic mechanisms of hypoxemia?

Hypoxemia is usually defined as a $PaO_2 < 60$ mm Hg. There are five basic pathophysiologic mechanisms that can cause hypoxemia:

1. **Decreased PIO_2** ($PIO_2 = FIO_2 \times (P_{atm} - PH_2O)$): Any condition that leads to a decrease in the oxygen content of inspired gas can lead to hypoxemia. This can be expressed as a decrease in the FIO_2 (fraction of inspired gas made up of oxygen) or significant changes in barometric pressure (P_{atm}). Situations leading to this problem include high altitude, flying in a non-pressurized airplane cabin, or rebreathing expired gases (as in a paper bag or closed space).

2. **Hypoventilation:** Any condition that interferes with the normal movement of gas in and out of the alveoli, leading to an elevation in $PaCO_2$, leads to hypoxemia. Examples include choking, COPD (chronic obstructive pulmonary disease), asthma, respiratory muscle paralysis, and CNS impairment.

3. **Diffusion abnormality:** Any condition that interferes with the normal diffusion of oxygen from the alveolar space into the capillaries can lead to hypoxemia. For example, all causes of diffuse interstitial pulmonary fibrosis.

4. **Ventilation-perfusion (V/Q) abnormalities:** Any condition that leads to a mismatching of ventilation and perfusion can cause hypoxemia. Most pulmonary disorders are associated with some degree of V/Q mismatching. This is the most common cause of hypoxemia and is responsive to oxygen therapy.

5. **Shunt:** Any condition that leads to perfusion of nonventilated tissue can lead to hypoxemia. A shunt is an absolute mismatching of ventilation and perfusion in which there is perfusion of alveoli with absolutely no ventilation. Examples include pulmonary arteriovenous (AV) fistulae, intracardiac shunts, and conditions in which there is perfusion of alveoli that are filled with pus, fluid, or other substances (pneumonia, pulmonary edema, intrapulmonary hemorrhage). Hypoxemia secondary to shunting is refractory to oxygen therapy.

2. How can the five basic mechanisms of hypoxemia be differentiated?

The values of PaO_2, $PaCO_2$, alveolar arterial oxygen ($A–aO_2$) gradient, and the response to breathing 100% oxygen can be used to separate the basic causes of hypoxemia:

Differentiation of the Causes of Hypoxemia

MECHANISM	PaO$_2$	PaCO$_2$	A–aO$_2$ GRADIENT	RESPONSE TO 100% O$_2$
PIO$_2$	↓	↔ or ↓	→	N/A
Hypoventilation	↓	↑	→	N/A
Diffusion abnormality	↓	↔ or ↓	↑	Yes
V/Q mismatch	↓	↔ or ↓	↑	Yes
Shunt	↓	↔ or ↓	↑	No

↓ = decreased, ↔ = normal, ↑ = increased, N/A = not applicable.

3. What is the alveolar–arterial oxygen gradient (PA-aO$_2$)?

The PA-aO$_2$ is the difference in the partial pressure of oxygen between the alveolar air (PaO$_2$) and arterial blood (PaO$_2$):

$$PA\text{-}aO_2 = PAO_2 - PaO_2$$

A normal PA-aO$_2$ is 10–15 mm Hg in a patient breathing room air. In conditions that interfere with oxygen exchange between the alveoli and pulmonary capillaries, the PA-aO$_2$ increases.

4. How do you calculate a patient's PA-aO$_2$?

It can be calculated by estimating the alveolar PO$_2$ (PaO$_2$) using a simplified form of the alveolar air equation, and then subtracting from that estimate the measured value of the arterial PO$_2$ (PaO$_2$):

$$PAO_2 = PIO_2 - (PaCO_2/RQ)$$

The PIO$_2$ is the partial pressure of oxygen in the inspired gas and is calculated as follows:

$$PIO_2 = FIO_2 \times (P_{atm} - PH_2O)$$

RQ is the respiratory quotient (usually assumed to be 0.8), FIO$_2$ is the fraction of the inspired gas that is oxygen (21% in room air), P$_{atm}$ is the atmospheric pressure (760 mm Hg at sea level), and PH$_2$O is the vapor pressure of water (assumed to be 47 mm Hg). Therefore, in a patient breathing room air with a PaO$_2$ of 94 mm Hg and PaCO$_2$ of 40 mm Hg, the PAO$_2$ would be:

$$PAO_2 = 0.21 (760{-}47) - 40/0.8 = 150{-}50 = 100 \text{ mm Hg}$$

Therefore, the PA-aO$_2$ would be:

$$PA\text{-}aO_2 = PAO_2 - PaO_2 = 100{-}94 = 6 \text{ mm Hg (within normal limits)}$$

5. Does the PA-aO$_2$ increase with age?

Yes. An age-adjusted normal PA-aO$_2$ can be estimated: 2.5 + 0.21 × age. Thus, a healthy 70-year-old would be expected to have a PA-aO$_2$ of approx. 17 mm Hg. Of course, this is only an approximation, and there may be a great deal of individual variation.

6. How is the RQ used in the alveolar air equation? What factors affect its value?

The RQ is the ratio of CO$_2$ produced per unit of O$_2$ consumed at the cellular level. It ranges from 0.7 when fatty acids are the substrate to 1.0 when carbohydrates are the substrate. Usually, a value of 0.8 can be used, which reflects the normal mixture of substrates. The RQ increases toward 1.0 with increasing exercise because of the greater contribution of the high RQ of actively contracting muscles.

7. What is the oxyhemoglobin equilibrium curve? What does it demonstrate?

The oxyhemoglobin equilibrium curve (or dissociation curve) is a plot of the hemoglobin percent saturation (SaO$_2$) against the PaO$_2$. It demonstrates the binding reaction of hemoglobin and oxygen.

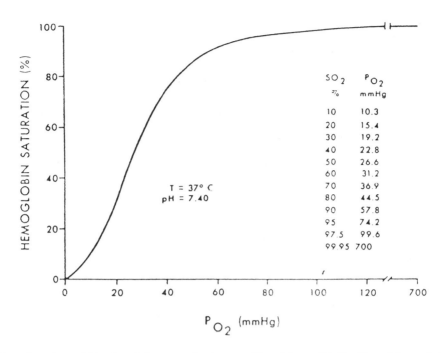

Normal oxyhemoglobin dissociation curve for humans. (From Murray JF: The Normal Lung, 2nd ed. Philadelphia, W.B. Saunders, 1986, p 174; with permission.)

The sigmoid-shaped curve shows that the binding (or releasing) of oxygen and hemoglobin is not a linear relationship (as is the case with dissolved oxygen). Oxygen is readily released at the lower range of PaO_2 values but very tightly held at the upper range of PaO_2 values—i.e., the affinity of hemoglobin for oxygen increases as more oxygen molecules bind to it. This enables the oxygen content of blood to remain high at high PaO_2 levels, but still allows hemoglobin to release oxygen readily as the PaO_2 drops below 60 mm Hg (the "steep" part of the curve).

8. How do you calculate the oxygen content of blood (CaO_2)?

CaO_2 includes the oxygen bound to hemoglobin, represented by hemoglobin (Hb) and the percent saturation (SaO_2), and the oxygen dissolved in solution in the plasma, represented by PaO_2. It can be calculated as follows:

$$CaO_2 = O_2 \text{ bound to Hb} + O_2 \text{ dissolved in plasma}$$

$$= (134 \times Hb \times SaO_2) + (PaO_2 \times 0.003)$$

The normal value is 16–20 ml/100 ml of blood.

The vast majority (> 99%) of the oxygen content of blood is that which is bound to hemoglobin. Only a very minor part of the total is dissolved oxygen (that which is measured by PaO_2). The obvious clinical importance of this fact is that any therapy that raises the PaO_2 while allowing a patient to remain anemic will have minimal effect on the oxygen-carrying capacity of the blood.

9. What is the P_{50}?

P_{50} is the PaO_2 that corresponds to a hemoglobin saturation (SaO_2) of 50% under conditions of standard temperature (37°C) and pH (7.40). Normally it is 26.6 mm Hg. It is a measure of the affinity of hemoglobin for oxygen. A higher P_{50} represents less hemoglobin affinity for oxygen, and vice versa. The P_{50} varies with conditions that shift the oxyhemoglobin equilibrium curve.

10. Clinicians refer to a shift of the oxyhemoglobin equilibrium curve to the left or right. What does this mean?

Since the curve represents the affinity of hemoglobin for oxygen over the range of PaO_2, a shift in the curve in either direction represents a change in that affinity. A shift of the curve to the **left** represents an **increase** in the affinity of hemoglobin for oxygen, meaning that oxygen is taken up more readily and released less readily for any given PaO_2. Conversely, a shift in the curve to the **right** represents a **decrease** in the affinity, meaning that oxygen is taken up less readily and released more readily.

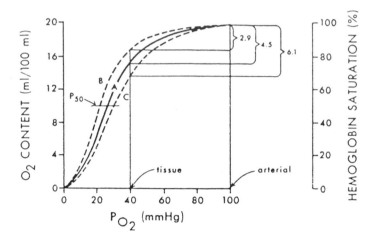

Effects of increases and decreases in O_2 affinity on the amount of O_2 available at the PO_2 values prevailing in arterial blood and tissues. Curve A = normal blood; B = blood with increased affinity (decreased P_{50}); C = blood with decreased affinity (increased P_{50}). (From Murray JF: The Normal Lung, 2nd ed. Philadelphia, W. B. Saunders, 1986, p 175; with permission.)

11. What factors can shift the oxyhemoglobin equilibrium curve?

Factors Influencing the Oxyhemoglobin Equilibrium Curve

SHIFT TO THE LEFT ($\uparrow$ HB/O_2 AFFINITY)	SHIFT TO THE RIGHT ($\downarrow$ HB/O_2 AFFINITY)
Hypothermia	Hyperthermia/fever
Alkalosis	Acidosis
Hypocapnia	Hypercapnia
$\downarrow$ 2,3 = DPG	$\uparrow$ 2,3 = DPG
$\uparrow$ Carboxyhemoglobin	$\downarrow$ Carboxyhemoglobin
Hemoglobin F, Chesapeake	Hemoglobin E,
Yakima, Ranier	Seattle, Kansas

DGP = diphosphoglycerate.

12. If the dissolved oxygen content of blood, measured by the PaO_2, is so small compared to the oxygen bound to hemoglobin, why do we measure the PaO_2 and follow it as we treat patients?

The oxyhemoglobin equilibrium curve answers this question. The PaO_2, although directly measuring only a tiny fraction of the total oxygen content of blood, is related to the total oxygen content through the dissociation curve. As the PaO_2 drops below 60 mm Hg, the curve is very steep, whereas at a $PaO_2 > 60$ mm Hg, the curve is flat. A drop of PaO_2 from 100 to 60 mm Hg (a drop of 40 mm Hg) represents a drop of SaO_2 from 99% to 90%, a loss of only 9% of the blood's total oxygen content. However, a further drop of 40 mm Hg, from a PaO_2 of 60 to 20 mm Hg, represents a drop in SaO_2 from 90% to about 30%, or a loss of 60% of the blood's total oxygen content. Therapeutic guidelines call for maintaining the PaO_2 above 60 mm Hg. Below this level, small decreases in PaO_2 are accompanied by very large drops in the SaO_2 and therefore very large drops in the total oxygen content of blood.

13. When is oxygen toxic?

Oxygen toxicity is an iatrogenic disease caused by prolonged administration of high concentrations of supplemental oxygen. Initially, it is manifested by an acute exudative phase, consisting of a decrease in vital capacity (within 6 hrs), interstitial and alveolar edema, decreased lung compliance, decreased diffusion capacity, and an increased $A–aO_2$ gradient. The chronic proliferative phase has also been seen in humans and animals on prolonged oxygen therapy.

14. What is the goal of oxygen therapy?

Because of oxygen toxicity, use of high concentrations of therapeutic oxygen ($>60\%$) should be limited to a short duration (<24 hours) if possible. The goal of oxygen therapy should be to use the minimum oxygen concentration needed to maintain the PaO_2 just over 60 mm Hg. Attempts to increase the PaO_2 further will not result in significant increases in the oxygen content of blood, but will increase the risk of oxygen toxicity.

DIAGNOSTIC TECHNIQUES

15. What are the indications for bronchoscopy?
Diagnostic uses:
- Evaluation of indeterminate lung lesions (abnormal chest film)
- Assessment of airway patency, including problems associated with endotracheal tubes, wheeze, and stridor
- Investigation of unexplained symptoms (cough, hemoptysis, stridor, etc.) or unexplained findings (recurrent laryngeal nerve paralysis, recent diaphragmatic paralysis)
- Evaluation of suspicious or malignant sputum cytology
- Preoperative staging of cancer
- Bronchoalveolar lavage for interstitial lung disease
- Specimen collection for selective cultures/suspected infection
- Determination of the extent of injury secondary to burns, inhalation, etc.

Therapeutic uses:
- Removal of mucous plugs/secretions, foreign bodies
- Assistance with difficult endotracheal intubations
- Treatment of endobronchial neoplasms

Prakash UBS, et al: Bronchoscopy in North America: The ACCP survey. Chest 100:1668–1675, 1991.

16. What are the contraindications and complications of fiberoptic bronchoscopy?

Although there are no *absolute* contraindications to bronchoscopy, sound clinical judgment should guide any decision concerning use of an invasive procedure with potential risk for morbidity and mortality. Well-trained and experienced bronchoscopists, supervision, and consideration of potentially high-risk patients (uremia, thrombocytopenia, pulmonary hypertension, bleeding diathesis) will reduce risk.

In a large series of over 24,000 cases, mortality was 0.01% and complications 0.08%. In 4,273 consecutive flexible bronchoscopies reviewed in another large study, the rate of major complications (significant hemorrhage, pneumothorax, respiratory failure, etc.) was 0.5% and the rate of minor complications (syncope, epistaxis, bronchospasm, etc.) was 0.8%. Complications resulting from fiberoptic bronchoscopy include reaction to topical anesthetic, trauma, laryngospasm, bronchospasm, hypoventilation, pneumothorax, hemorrhage, cardiac arrhythmia, myocardial infarction, hypoxemia, ruptured lung abscess with flooding of airways, and postbronchoscopy fever/infection.

Pue CA, Pacht ER: Complications of fiberoptic bronchoscopy at a university hospital. Chest 107:430–432, 1995.

17. Which conditions place patients at increased risk during bronchoscopy?

Bleeding diathesis	Inability to cooperate with the exam
Hypoxia	Cardiac arrhythmias
Unstable asthma	Recent myocardial infarction
Acute hypercapnia	Partial tracheal obstruction
Hepatitis	Uremia
Lung abscess	Immunosuppression
Superior vena cava syndrome	Respiratory failure requiring mechanical ventilation

18. What is the most common clinical use of pulmonary function tests (PFTs)?

Abnormalities detected by PFTs are usually categorized as obstructive or restrictive. By far the most common use of PFTs is the evaluation of **obstructive airway disease.** Causes of an obstructive ventilatory defect include emphysema, bronchitis, asthma, bronchiolitis, and upper airway obstruction (tumors, foreign bodies, stenosis, and edema). Obstruction is defined as a decrease in forced expiratory flow rates. The FEV_1 (forced expiratory volume in 1 sec) and FEV_1/FVC (forced vital capacity) are both reduced. Other supporting data include increased residual volume and increased airway resistance.

19. What are the lung volumes and capacities measured with PFTs?

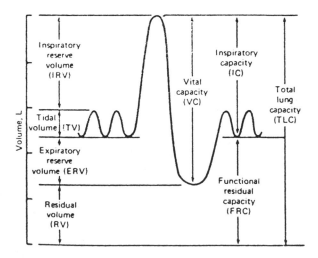

Residual volume (RV)—Volume of air remaining in lungs after maximum expiration

Expiratory reserve volume (ERV)—Maximum volume of air expired from resting end-expiratory level

Tidal volume (TV)—Volume of air inspired or expired with each breath during quiet breathing (The symbol TV is traditionally used for tidal volume to indicate a subdivision of static lung volume. However, the symbol VT is used for tidal volume in formulas for gas exchange.)

Inspiratory reserve volume (IRV)—Maximum volume of air inspired from volume resting end-inspiratory level

Inspiratory capacity (IC)—(sum of IRV and TV)

Vital capacity (VC)—Maximum volume of air expired from maximum inspiration

Inspiratory vital capacity (IVC)—Maximum volume of air inspired from maximum expiratory level

Functional residual capacity (FRC)—Volume of air remaining in lungs at the end-expiratory level (sum of RV and ERV)

Total lung capacity (TLC)—Volume of air in the lungs after maximum inspiration (sum of all volume compartments)

The term *capacity* is applied to a subdivision composed of two or more *volumes*. (From Fishman AP: Pulmonary Disease and Disorders. New York, McGraw-Hill, 1980, p 1752, with permission.)

20. What are common causes of a restrictive ventilatory defect?

- Interstitial lung disease (fibrosis, pneumoconiosis, edema)
- Chest wall disease (kyphoscoliosis, neuromuscular disease)
- Space-occupying lesions (tumors, cysts)
- Pleural disease (effusion, pneumothorax)
- Extrathoracic conditions (obesity, ascites, pregnancy)

21. What are the PFT findings suggestive of a restrictive ventilatory defect?

Decreased vital capacity, normal expiratory flow rates, and normal maximum voluntary ventilation. Supporting data confirming a restrictive defect are a decreased total lung capacity (TLC), decreased lung compliance, and decreased diffusion of carbon monoxide (DL_{CO}).

22. Which test can help differentiate the etiology of an obstructive ventilatory defect secondary to emphysema versus chronic bronchitis?

The finding of an obstructive pattern associated with a normal single-breath DL_{CO} argues against emphysema, whereas an obstructive defect with a decreased DL_{CO} suggests the presence of anatomic emphysema with a concomitant loss of alveolar capillary bed.

American Thoracic Society: Standards for the diagnosis and care of patients with chronic obstructive pulmonary disease. Am J Respir Crit Care Med 152(pt 2):S77–S120, 1995.

PLEURAL EFFUSION

23. What are the two basic types of pleural effusion?

A pleural effusion represents an increase in fluid in the pleural space, which may be due to increased hydrostatic pressure, decreased oncotic pressure, decreased pleural space pressure (lung collapse), obstruction of lymphatic drainage, or increased permeability. A **transudative** effusion is classically associated with volume overload states, such as congestive heart failure, nephrotic syndrome, and cirrhosis. An **exudative** effusion is a protein-rich effusion secondary to inflammation of the pleura or failure of lymphatic protein removal. Exudates occur in neoplasms, infection, and various collagen vascular diseases.

24. What findings on physical examination are suggestive of a pleural effusion?

Small effusions (< 500 ml) frequently have minimal findings. Larger effusions demonstrate dullness to percussion, diminished breath sounds, and reduced tactile and vocal fremitus over the involved hemithorax. Large effusions (>1500 ml), with concomitant atelectasis, demonstrate bronchial breath sounds, egophony (a sound on auscultation like the bleating of a goat), and inspiratory lag. Pleural friction rubs may be noted in the early stages or as the effusion resolves.

25. Which diagnostic tests are used to distinguish transudative from exudative pleural effusions? What are Light's criteria?

Thoracentesis (percutaneous removal of pleural fluid) is used to obtain pleural fluid for analysis. An exudative pleural effusion meets one or more of the following criteria, whereas a transudative meets none (Light's criteria):

a. Pleural fluid protein/serum protein ratio >0.5

b. Pleural fluid LDH/serum LDH >0.6

c. Pleural fluid LDH > two-thirds the upper limit of normal for serum

Other tests that may be helpful include pleural fluid glucose, pH, cell count, and WBC differential, amylase, Gram stain, special stains as indicated, and culture. Pleural glucose <60% of the serum valve suggests infection, rheumatoid arthritis, or neoplasm. A pH < 7.30 suggests empyema/infection. An elevated amylase in a left-sided pleural effusion may be secondary to pancreatitis. Pleural fluid WBC counts and differentials are usually of limited value, but lymphocyte predominance may suggest tuberculosis. Cytologic examination is indicated if a neoplasm is suspected.

26. Which radiologic test should be performed in a patient with suspected pleural effusion?

A small amount of pleural fluid can be detected as the obliteration of the posterior part of the diaphragm on lateral chest x-ray (CXR). When a larger amount of fluid is present, the lateral costophrenic angle on the posteroanterior radiograph is blunted. When pleural fluid is suspected, lateral decubitus films should be obtained to detect free fluid gravitating to the dependent side and accumulating between the chest wall and lung. The amount of fluid present can be roughly quantitated by measuring the distance between the inner border of the chest wall and the outer border of the lung. When this distance is < 10 mm, the amount of fluid present is small, and usually a diagnostic thoracentesis should be performed under ultrasonographic guidance.

27. What is an empyema?

Empyema describes the presence of infected liquid or frank pus in the pleural space. It may result from infection of a contiguous structure, instrumentation of the pleural space, or hematogenous spread of infection. The diagnosis is made by examination of the pleural fluid obtained from thoracentesis. An empyema should be suspected when the pleural fluid has a high WBC count, with predominantly PMNs, high protein (>3 g/dl), low glucose (<40 mg/dl), high LDH (>600 mg/dl), and low pH (<7.2). A Gram stain and culture of the pleural fluid may reveal the causative organism.

28. What other procedures are available if routine diagnostic pleural fluid analysis fails to diagnose an exudative effusion?

In approx. 20% of all exudative pleural effusions, no diagnosis will be made. In patients with a suspected neoplasm or tuberculous pleural effusion, a closed-needle biopsy of the parietal pleura may establish the diagnosis. Although the overall yield from pleural fluid cytology is slightly higher, needle biopsy of the pleura will be positive in 40% of patients with malignant pleural disease. When tuberculous pleuritis is suspected, a portion of the biopsy should be sent for culture. The initial biopsy is positive for granuloma in 50–80% of patients. Combining results of pleural fluid culture and biopsy has a diagnostic sensitivity of 90% for tuberculosis. Other procedures to be considered are:

- Bronchoscopy if the patient has a parenchymal abnormality on CXR or CT scan
- Thoracoscopy which allows direct visualization of the pleural surface and guided biopsy
- Open pleural biopsy

Prakash UBS, et al: Comparison of needle biopsy with cytologic analysis for the evaluation of pleural effusion: Analysis of 414 cases. Mayo Clin Proc 60:158–164, 1985.

Emerson DA, et al: Tuberculous pleurisy. Can Med Assoc J 126:493–495, 1982.

HEMOPTYSIS

29. What is hemoptysis? What is its differential diagnosis?

Hemoptysis can be defined as blood in the sputum and includes the full range of bloody sputum, from blood streaks to frank blood. In addition to history and physical examination, all patients should have a CXR. Further diagnostic procedures should be guided by the findings of these studies.

Differential Diagnosis of Hemoptysis

Pulmonary Vasculature	**Pulmonary Parenchyma**
Vasculitis	Trauma
Wegener's granulomatosis	Foreign body
Goodpasture's syndrome	Bronchitis
Arteriovenous malformation	Neoplasm
Bleeding diathesis	Tuberculosis
Pulmonary embolus with infarction	Pneumonia
Pulmonary hypertension	Abscess
	Bronchiectasis
Oropharynx	
Trauma	**Cardiac**
Gum bleeding	Mitral stenosis
Palate bleeding	Left ventricular failure
	Trauma
Other	
Factitious	

Adelman M, et al: Cryptogenic hemoptysis: Clinical features, bronchoscopy findings and natural history in 67 patients. Ann Intern Med 102:829–834, 1985.

30. What is massive hemoptysis?

Massive hemoptysis implies copious bleeding and has been defined as the expectoration of > 600 ml of blood in a 24-hour period. This potentially lethal and alarming clinical situation requires expeditious evaluation, close observation, and possible surgical intervention.

PNEUMOTHORAX

31. Which population of patients is most likely to experience a primary spontaneous pneumothorax? In which patients is a secondary spontaneous pneumothorax most often seen?

Primary spontaneous pneumothorax, occurring in patients with no history of pulmonary disease, is believed to result from spontaneous rupture of a subpleural emphysematous bleb. Primary spontaneous pneumothorax has a peak incidence at 20–30 years of age, is more common in smokers and exsmokers, has a 4:1 male to female ratio, and is most often seen in tall, thin individuals. **Secondary spontaneous pneumothorax,** occurring in patients with underlying pulmonary disease, is most often seen with COPD.

32. What is the likelihood that spontaneous pneumothorax will recur?

Recurrence rates for both primary and secondary spontaneous pneumothorax are similar. Recurrence rates range from 10–50%, and approx. 60% of those patients will have a third recurrence. After three episodes, the recurrence rate exceeds 85%. Therefore, repeated spontaneous pneumothorax should be treated by pleurodesis or surgical intervention, including parietal pleurectomy.

33. What are the causes of pneumothorax?

Spontaneous pneumothorax, although not common, should be considered in any patient with a history of underlying lung disease and unexplained clinical decompensation. Causes of pneumothorax secondary to underlying lung disease include COPD, asthma, lung abscess, adult respiratory distress syndrome (ARDS), neoplasm, Marfan syndrome, sarcoidosis, cystic fibrosis, tuberculosis, and eosinophilic granuloma. Pneumothorax may be iatrogenic (following thoracentesis or transbronchial biopsy, or secondary to barotrauma, etc.) or traumatic. Catamenial pneumothorax is rare and occurs in females at the time of menstruation.

34. How does pneumothorax present clinically?

Spontaneous pneumothorax usually occurs at rest. Pleuritic chest pain and dyspnea of acute onset are the most common complaints. The acute pleuritic pain, which is localized to the side of the pneumothorax, may become more of a dull ache with time. Symptoms, especially dyspnea, are more pronounced in patients with underlying pulmonary disease. Findings on physical exam include sinus tachycardia, reduced breath sounds, reduced tactile fremitus, hyperresonance, and reduced chest wall excursion on the ipsilateral side. Findings maybe subtle with small pneumothoraces.

35. What is a tension pneumothorax?

Tension pneumothorax is due to unidirectional flow of air into the pleural space from which it cannot escape. Tension pneumothorax develops when intrapleural pressure exceeds atmospheric pressure during expiration, causing collapse of the involved lung, shift of the mediastinum, and potentially acute deterioration in cardiopulmonary status.

36. When should the diagnosis of tension pneumothorax be suspected?

Tension pneumothorax is a medical emergency and requires prompt relief of the positive pleural pressure. It is usually heralded by sudden deterioration in cardiopulmonary status. It should be suspected:

1. In any patient with a history of pneumothorax
2. After a procedure known to cause pneumothorax
3. In patients receiving mechanical ventilation
4. During cardiopulmonary resuscitation, if it is difficult to ventilate the patient or if there is electromechanical dissociation

On physical exam, tension pneumothorax should be suspected if the patient has signs of a significant pneumothorax (no tactile fremitus, markedly decreased or absent breath sounds, and hyperresonance on percussion), cardiopulmonary compromise (rapid pulse, hypotension, cyanosis, electromechanical dissociation), and possibly a shift of the trachea away from the involved side.

37. What is Hamman's sign?

Mediastinal emphysema or pneumomediastinum can be detected on auscultation by the presence of a mediastinal "crunch" coinciding with cardiac systole and diastole. It is named after the American physician, Louis Hamman (1877–1946).

Collins RK: Hamman's crunch: an adventitious sound. J Fam Pract 38:284–286, 1994.

INFECTIONS

38. What is the most common cause of community-acquired pneumonia?

Pneumococcus, which accounts for about 60% of cases needing hospitalization. Other causes include *Mycoplasma, Legionella, Haemophilus influenzae,* atypical organisms, and viruses. However, the incidence varies depending on the community and the patient population. Staphylococci and gram-negative rods are uncommon causes.

39. Which community-acquired pneumonias are seen more commonly in the alcoholic patient?

As in the nonalcoholic patient, pneumococcal pneumonia is the most frequent. Although they are still at risk for the usual pathogens, alcoholics have higher incidence of pneumonia due to gram-negative organisms (including *Klebsiella pneumoniae* and *Haemophilus influenzae*), anaerobic pneumonia secondary to aspiration, and *Staphylococcus aureus.*

40. What clinical manifestations and laboratory tests are helpful in diagnosing pneumonia?

1. **History**

Fever	Cough productive of	Malaise
Dyspnea	yellow-green or bloody	Pleuritic pain
Abdominal pain	sputum	

2. **Physical Examination**

Fever	Tachycardia	Tachypnea
Cyanosis (if severe pneumonia)		

3. **Lungs Auscultation**
   Crackles   Egophony   Pectoriloquy
   Dullness to percussion
      (if pleural effusion present)
4. **Laboratory tests**
   Sputum Gram stain and culture
   Elevated WBC count
5. **Chest x-ray**
   CXR showing consolidation
      and/or pleural effusion

41. What are the predisposing factors for developing pneumococcal pneumonia?

Severe underlying illness such as multiple myeloma, lymphoma, and leukemia
Cirrhosis and renal failure
Poorly controlled diabetes mellitus
Sickle cell anemia
Post-splenectomy
Elderly age

42. Which factors determine the prognosis of pneumococcal pneumonia?

The mortality associated with pneumococcal pneumonia ranges from 6% to 19% in hospitalized patients without complications. Prognosis is worsened by the presence of the following:

Underlying illnesses

Alcoholism	Bronchiectasis
COPD	Hemoglobin SS and SC disease
Congestive heart failure	Bronchogenic carcinoma
Diabetes mellitus	Multiple myeloma

Other factors

Hypogammaglobulinemia	Bacteremia
Age > 60 yrs	Delay in onset of therapy
Multilobar involvement	Pneumococcal serotype 3
Leukopenia	Extrapulmonary involvement

Munson MA: Pneumococcal infections. JAMA 246:1942, 1981.

43. What are the common risk factors for the development of anaerobic pneumonia? Which bronchopulmonary segments are most commonly involved?

Approx. 25% of patients with anaerobic pneumonia report a history of transient loss of consciousness, especially seizures or alcohol-related loss of consciousness. Other predisposing factors include poor oral hygiene, dysphagia, endobronchial obstruction, and any risk factor for aspiration.

The posterior segment of the right upper lobe and superior segment of the right lower lobe are the most commonly involved, followed by the posterior segment of the left upper lobe and the superior segment of the left lower lobes. Individuals usually aspirate while in the supine position, and in this position, these are the dependent segments. The right lung is more frequently involved than the left, because the right mainstem bronchus comes off at a less acute angle than the left.

44. Which risk factors predispose for the development of nosocomial pneumonia?

Risk factors for the development of hospital-acquired pneumonia include:
- Increased severity of underlying illness
- Previous hospitalization
- Indwelling urethral catheters
- Presence of intravascular catheters
- Intubation (esp. prolonged intubation)
- Recent thoracic or upper abdominal surgery
- Use of broad-spectrum antibiotics (increased risk of superinfection).

45. Which organisms most commonly cause nosocomial pneumonia?

Nosocomial pneumonia, pneumonia occurring >48 hours after admission, is most commonly caused by gram-negative organisms, including *Pseudomonas aeruginosa, Klebsiella pneumoniae, Escherichia coli,* and *Enterobacter* sp. *Staphylococcus aureus,* including methicillin-resistant organisms, *Streptococcus pneumoniae,* anaerobes, *Candida,* and polymicrobial infections are also common. Mortality from nosocomial pneumonia remains high (30–50%) despite antimicrobial therapy.

Culver DH, et al: Nosocomial infections in adult and pediatric intensive care units in the United States: National Nosocomial Infections, Surveillance System. Am J Med, 91(3B): 185S, 1991.

46. What three radiographic patterns of pulmonary infiltrates are observed in immunocompromised patients?

Patterns of Pulmonary Infiltrates in Immunocompromised Patients

PATTERN	COMMON CAUSES	LESS COMMON CAUSES
Diffuse	*Pneumocystis* Cytomegalovirus Pulmonary edema NIP Drug-induced Lymphangitic carcinomatosis	*Cryptococcus* *Aspergillus* *Candida* Hemorrhage Leukemic involvement Varicella-zoster virus Leukoagglutinin reaction
Nodular or cavitary	*Cryptococcus* *Nocardia* Bacterial lung abscess Neoplasm *Aspergillus*	*Legionella* Septic emboli *Pneumocystis*
Segmental/lobar	Bacteria, including *Nocardia* *Cryptococcus* Mucormycosis NIP Pulmonary emboli	Tuberculosis Viral *Legionella* Radiation pneumonitis *Pneumocystis* Mixed infection

NIP=nonspecific interstitial pneumonitis
From Young, LS: The lung and immunosuppressive disease. In Murray JF, et al (eds): Textbook of Respiratory Medicine. Philadelphia, W.B. Saunders, 1988, p 1935, with permission.

47. Which pathogens cause lower respiratory tract infections in HIV-infected patients?

Pathogen	Well-Recognized	Unusual
Bacteria	*Streptococcus pneumoniae* *Haemophilus influenzae*	Many species
Mycobacteria	*Mycobacterium tuberculosis* *M. avium* *M. kansasii*	Many species
Fungi	*Pneumocystis carinii** *Cryptococcus neoformans* *Histoplasma capsulatum* *Coccidioides immitis*	*Aspergillus* *Candida*
Protozoa	None*	*Toxoplasma gondii* *Cryptosporidium*
Viruses	None	Cytomegalovirus Varicella-zoster Herpes simplex Epstein-Barr virus

**P. carinii* has been reclassified as a fungus.
Modified from Zurlo JJ: Respiratory Infections and AIDS. In Bone RC, et al (eds): Pulmonary & Critical Care Medicine. St Louis, Mosby-Year Book, 1993, sect J, ch 3, p 2.

TUBERCULOSIS

48. What symptoms are associated with tuberculosis (TB)?
The symptoms associated with TB are often nonspecific. Common complaints include productive cough, weight loss, weakness, anorexia, night sweats, and generalized malaise. These nonspecific symptoms are most often subacute or chronic (>8 wks) in duration. Both fever, present in one-third to one-half of the patients, and hemoptysis correlate with cavitary disease and positive sputum smears.

49. Describe the common anatomic distribution of CXR changes in postprimary (reactivation) TB. What is the differential diagnosis?
In postprimary TB, CXR abnormalities are predominantly located in the **apical and posterior segments of the upper lobes** (85%). Although the anterior segment of the upper lobes may be affected, a lesion found *only* in the anterior segment suggests a diagnosis other than TB (i.e., malignancy). The superior segments of the lower lobe account for approx. 10%, and the remainder of the lower lobe, < 7%. The right lung is more often affected than the left.

The differential diagnosis of upper lobe infiltrates with or without cavitation includes atypical mycobacterial infections, silicosis, pneumonia, malignancy, pulmonary infarct, ankylosing spondylitis, actinomycosis, fungal infections, and nocardia infection.

50. What specific factors are associated with an increased risk for developing TB?
Medical High Risk (increased susceptibility)

Silicosis	Postgastrectomy
Chronic renal failure	Diabetes mellitus
Alcoholism	HIV infection
Weight loss	Steroids
Malignancy	Immunosuppressive therapy

High Risk of Exposure

Foreign-born	Elderly in nursing home
Low socioeconomic status	Physicians
Prisoners	Hospital employees
Black, Hispanic, Native American	

51. How is active *Mycobacterium tuberculosis* infection diagnosed?
Because many months of medical therapy are required to adequately treat TB, a definitive diagnosis by culture is recommended. A negative tuberculin skin test (PPD) in a patient who does not have an underlying disease (a patient who is not anergic) or overwhelming TB infection makes the diagnosis of TB unlikely. A positive PPD without CXR changes also makes the diagnosis of *active pulmonary* TB unlikely and reflects previous exposure. A positive PPD and typical CXR findings or response to antituberculous medications may provide a presumptive diagnosis of TB, which should be verified by culture if at all possible.

52. What are the clinical problems associated with the treatment of TB?
1. **Drug resistance.** Primary resistance (resistant organisms present in the initial infection) is increasing in the U.S. and is most common for isoniazid (INH). Resistance to both isoniazid and rifampin has been reported. Primary drug resistance can vary with location and ethnic background and is higher in foreign-born patients. Secondary drug resistance develops during treatment.

2. **Noncompliance.** Multiple drug regimens are given over an extended period of time (6 months or more), and this may lead to failure to successfully complete therapy. Supervised biweekly home therapy can help ensure compliance and is now highly recommended.

3. **Medication side effects.** Hepatotoxicity, the most important side effect, is seen in 2–5% of patients treated. It occurs most frequently with INH therapy, less frequently with rifampin, and rarely with pyrazinamide (PZA). Other side effects include retrobulbar optic neuritis, hyper-

uricemia, thrombocytopenia (ethambutol), hyperglycemia (rifampin), and peripheral neuropathy (INH).

O'Brien RJ: Drug-resistant tuberculosis: Etiology, management, and prevention. Semin Respir Infect 9(2):104–112, 1994.

53. How do you monitor for adverse drug reactions during TB therapy?

Before therapy is started, baseline liver function tests (INH, rifampin, PZA); CBC with platelets, BUN, creatinine, and calcium (INH, rifampin); uric acid (PZA, ethambutol); and visual acuity (ethambutol) should be performed.

For persons with liver disease/alcoholism or older age 35, liver function tests should be performed periodically and symptoms monitored. Patients receiving INH should be questioned monthly regarding potential symptoms. All patients should be fully informed of potential complications of therapy.

American Thoracic Society/Centers for Disease Control: Treatment of tuberculosis and tuberculosis infection in adults and children. Annu Rev Respir Dis 134:355–363, 1986.

54. Why is multidrug therapy used in the treatment of TB?

Work done by Canetti over 30 years ago established the large numbers of organisms found in tuberculous cavities. Spontaneous resistance develops in 1 in 100,000–1,000,000 organisms. Therefore, single-drug therapy may lead to the selection of resistant organisms and treatment failure.

55. Which groups of individuals are candidates for isoniazid chemoprophylaxis?

Chemoprophylaxis is a misleading term; INH or any other antimicrobial agent has little effect on an infection in which microbial multiplication is minimal or absent. What is actually taking place is treatment of a potentially subclinical but active infection. The following is a list of candidates for INH prophylaxis (300 mg/day for 1 yr):

1. Persons of any age should receive INH if they:
   a. Are positive for antibody to HIV or suspected to be HIV-positive and have a tuberculin skin test (TST) of ≥5 mm of induration.
   b. Are close contacts of newly-diagnosed TB cases and have a TST of ≥ 5 mm of induration.
   c. Have an abnormal CXR with fibrotic lesions suggesting old TB and have a TST of ≥ 5 mm of induration.
   d. Are IV drug abusers, negative for HIV, and have a TST of ≥ 10 mm of induration.
   e. Have a medical condition that increases risk of TB (e.g., silicosis, gastrectomy, jejunoileal bypass, weight loss of ≥ 10% or more of IBW, chronic renal failure, diabetes mellitus, high-dose corticosteroid use, immunosuppression, leukemia, lymphoma, or malignancy) and have a TST of ≥ 10 mm of induration.
2. Persons < 35 years of age should receive INH if they have a TST of ≥ 10 mm of induration and:
   a. Are born in a high-prevalence country.
   b. Are in a medically underserved population (especially blacks, Hispanics, and native Americans).
3. Recent converters (within the past 2 yrs):
   a. With a TST of ≥ 10 mm of induration and age < 35 yrs.
   b. With a TST of ≥ 15 mm of induration and age > 35 yrs.
4. All persons < 35 years of age who are likely to have a low incidence of TB but have a TST of ≥ 15 mm of induration.

Centers for Disease Control: Screening for tuberculosis and tuberculosis infections in high-risk populations, and the use of preventive therapy for tuberculosis infection in the United States: Recommendations of the Advisory Council for the Elimination of Tuberculosis. MMWR 39(RR-8):1–12, 1990.

56. Which infectious agents can mimic TB?

Fungal infections, especially histoplasmosis and coccidioidomycosis, can mimic pulmonary TB. Histoplasmosis has similar presenting symptoms and CXR findings and should be considered in any differential where TB is considered. Lymph node involvement is more common with histoplasmosis than TB. Complications secondary to lymph node and mediastinal involvement include fibrosing mediastinitis (rare), pericarditis (rare), esophageal encroachment, superior vena cava syndrome, and tracheal/airway encroachment.

Nocardia, a gram-positive, aerobic, partially acid-fast organism, can mimic pulmonary TB. Symptoms include fever, night sweats, and productive cough. CXR findings with cavitation are frequent. Previously, nocardiosis was viewed as infection by a primary pulmonary pathogen. It is now more frequently recognized as an opportunistic infection in patients with underlying disease, such as pulmonary alveolar proteinosis. Most strains are susceptible to sulfonamides.

57. What are the mechanisms of hemorrhage from the site of previous pulmonary TB?
- Reactivation of TB
- Bronchiectasis
- "Scar carcinoma" (adenocarcinoma)
- Erosion of a vessel by a broncholith (calcified lymph node)
- Fungal infection (usually aspergillosis) in the cavity
- Rasmussen's aneurysm (terminal pulmonary artery)

NEOPLASTIC DISEASE

58. Which CXR and clinical criteria can help distinguish between a benign and malignant pulmonary nodule?

A pulmonary nodule can be described as a rounded lesion measuring < 3 cm at maximum diameter on a CXR. Although no single or group of characteristics can definitely predict the nature of a solitary pulmonary nodule, the following chart can be useful:

Differentiation of Benign and Malignant Solitary Pulmonary Nodules

FACTORS	BENIGN	MALIGNANT
Clinical		
Age	< 40 yrs (except hamartoma)	> 45 yrs
Sex	Female	Male
Symptoms	Absent	Present
Past History	Lives in area of high granuloma incidence, exposure to TB, mineral oil medication	Diagnosis of primary lesion elsewhere
Skin tests	Positive, usually with specific infectious organisms	Negative or positive
Roentgenographic		
Size	Small (<2 cm in diameter)	Large (>2 cm in diameter)
Location	No predilection (except for TB [upper lobes])	Predominantly upper lobes (except for lung metastases)
Definition & contour	Margins well-defined and smooth	Margins ill-defined, lobulated, umbilicated
Calcification	Almost pathognomonic of a benign lesion, particularly if of a laminated, multiple punctuate, or "popcorn" variety	Very rare, may be eccentric (scar carcinoma)
Satellite lesions	More common	Less common
Serial studies with no change over 2 years	Almost diagnostic of a benign lesion	Most unlikely
Doubling time	< 30 or >490 days	30–490 days

From Frazer RG, et al: Diagnosis of Diseases of the Chest, 3rd ed. Philadelphia, W.B. Saunders, 1989, p 1390; with permission.

59. How should you follow up an abnormal CXR?

Evaluation is directed by the patient's symptoms. If there is evidence of infection, treatment should begin before further evaluation. If the CXR is still abnormal after treatment or reveals an obvious mass, tissue diagnosis is imperative. This may be obtained by expectorated sputum, bronchoscopy with biopsy, or percutaneous fine-needle aspiration and cytology. Once the tissue diagnosis is established, treatment plans can be made.

If the abnormality is a solitary pulmonary nodule, the accompanying algorithm may be used:

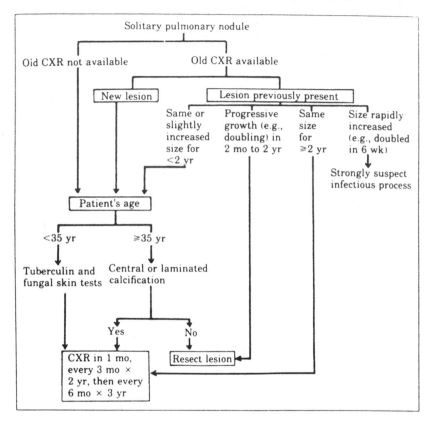

From Casciato DA, Lowitz BB: Manual of Clinical Oncology, 2nd ed. Boston, Little Brown, 1988, p 120; with permission.

60. What are the four most common histologic types of lung cancer?

Squamous cell carcinoma, adenocarcinoma, small cell carcinoma, and large cell undifferentiated carcinoma. Lung cancer is slightly more frequent in the right lung, in the upper lobes, and in the anterior segment. Both squamous and small cell carcinomas occur more commonly in a central location, whereas adenocarcinoma usually develops more peripherally. All major cell types have been associated with cigarette smoking.

Lung Malignancies and Associated Clinical Syndromes

TYPE	RELATIVE INCIDENCE	MAJOR LOCATION	ASSOCIATED CLINICAL SYNDROMES
Non-small lung cancer	70%		
Adenocarcinoma	30–35%	Peripheral	Hypertrophic osteoarthropathy
Bronchioloalveolar cell carcinoma	10%	Peripheral	Voluminous watery sputum
Squamous	25–30%	Central	Hypercalcemia
Large cell	15%	Peripheral	Gynecomastia, galactorrhea
Small cell lung cancer	20–25%	Central	Paraneoplastic syndromes

61. What are the symptoms and location of a Pancoast tumor?

First described by Henry Khunrath Pancoast, a Philadelphia radiologist, in 1932, this tumor is located in the extreme apex of the upper lobe of the lung. This type of tumor represents approx. 4% of all lung cancers. Although the tumor may be of various cell types, the most common is squamous cell carcinoma. Pancoast's original criteria included the following characteristics: arm/shoulder pain, Horner's syndrome, destruction of bone, and atrophy of the hand muscles.

62. Name the most common *pulmonary* complications of lung cancer.

Pulmonary complications include atelectasis, postobstructive pneumonia secondary to endobronchial obstruction, hemoptysis, pleural effusion, and respiratory failure. Symptoms may include cough, wheezing, stridor, chest pain, and hemoptysis.

63. What is Eaton-Lambert syndrome (ELS)?

ELS is a paraneoplastic myopathy, meaning it is associated with a malignancy but not secondary to the direct effects of the tumor or its metastases. This syndrome is most often seen with small cell carcinoma. Clinically, it resembles myasthenia gravis (MG), but it can be distinguished by careful neurologic examination and electromyography (EMG). Unlike MG, ELS involves proximal muscle groups, includes muscular strength *increases* with repetitive stimulation, has little response to neostigmine challenge, and demonstrates increased muscular response to repetitive stimulation on EMG tracings.

64. What symptoms and x-ray changes are associated with hypertrophic pulmonary osteoarthropathy (HPO)?

HPO is one of the many varied paraneoplastic syndromes. It is more often associated with squamous cell carcinoma. The patient complains of a deep burning pain, usually in the distal extremity. There is usually clubbing of the fingers and/or toes, periostitis of the long bones, and occasionally polyarthritis. The most commonly involved bones are the tibia, fibula, humerus, radius, and ulna. The x-ray of the extremity reveals subperiosteal new bone formation. The etiology is unknown, and the abnormalities resolve with treatment of the primary tumor.

Rassam JW, et al: Incidence of paramalignant disorders in bronchogenic carcinoma. Thorax 30:86, 1975.

65. Which tumors commonly metastasize to the lung?

Lung cancer itself	Genitourinary (renal, prostate, bladder)
Colorectal carcinoma	Breast cancer
Thyroid cancer	Testicular cancer
Ovarian cancer	Melanoma
Pancreatic/hepatic	Gastric
Head and neck	Sarcoma

Endobronchial metastasis occur most commonly in renal cell carcinoma, melanoma, and breast carcinoma.

PULMONARY THROMBOEMBOLISM

66. What are the predisposing factors for the development of pulmonary emboli (PE)?

- Injury or surgery of the pelvis and lower extremities
- Previous history of deep venous thrombosis (DVT)
- Prolonged general anesthesia
- Burns
- Pregnancy and postpartum period
- Right ventricular failure
- Immobility
- Age
- Obesity
- Cancer
- Estrogen-containing medications (high-dose)
- Coagulation disorders (including deficiency of protein C, antithrombin III, or protein S)
- Activated protein C resistance, dysfibrinogenemia
- Antiphospholid antibodies/lupus anticoagulant

Clagett GP, et al: Fourth ACCP Consensus Conference on Antithrombotic Therapy: Prevention of venous thromboembolism. Chest 108:312S–334S, 1995.

67. What is the mortality rate for PE?

PEs cause approx. 50,000 deaths/year. The mortality rate is 10%, and < 30% are diagnosed antemortem.

68. What CXR findings are associated with PE?

Commonly, the interpretation of the CXR of a patient with acute PE is "normal," although subtle nonspecific abnormalities are generally found. These subtle findings include differences in diameters of vessels that should be similar in size, abrupt cutoff of a vessel when followed distally, increased radiolucency in some areas, and regional oligemia (Westermark's sign).

69. What are the findings associated with pulmonary infarction?

Approx. 1 in 10 PE result in pulmonary infarction. Pleuritic chest pain, hemoptysis, and low-grade fever are present when infarction has occurred. Pulmonary infarction is classically described as a wedge-shaped infiltrate that abuts the pleura (Hampton's hump). It is often associated with a small pleural effusion that is usually exudative and may be hemorrhagic.

70. How is the diagnosis of PE established?

It is impossible to diagnose PE on clinical grounds alone, and therefore further testing is needed. The ventilation-perfusion (V/Q scan) lung scan, although highly sensitive, is nonspecific,

In patients who are clinically stable, the following may be used:

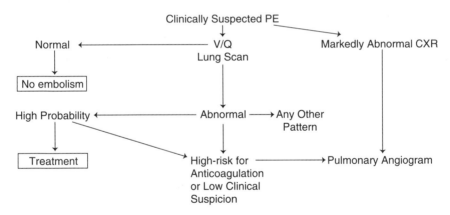

In patients whose V/Q scans are other than normal or high probability, an alternative approach is used:

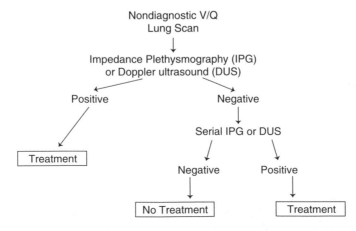

and interpretation is difficult in the patient with underlying pulmonary disease. Pulmonary angiography is the only established means to demonstrate the embolus itself, but the procedure is not without risk. Therefore, the tests used to establish the diagnosis depends on the clinical situation and information obtained in less invasive testing.

Adapted from Mitzner WA: Pulmonary circulation: General principles and diagnostic approach. In Bone RC (ed): Pulmonary and Critical Care Medicine. St. Louis, Mosby, 1993, Ch 3, vol 2, pp 17–18.

71. Name two types of nonthrombotic PE.

Fat emboli and **amniotic fluid emboli**. The pulmonary vasculature filters the venous circulation and is exposed to nonthrombotic emboli. Fat embolism usually follows bone trauma or fracture, and its symptoms begin 12–36 hours following the event. Clinical manifestations include altered mental status, respiratory decompensation, anemia, thrombocytopenia, and petechiae. Amniotic fluid embolism is secondary to entrance of amniotic fluid into the venous circulation, with resulting shock and DIC.

OBSTRUCTIVE AIRWAY DISEASE

72. What are the causes of chronic obstructive pulmonary disease (COPD)?

Cigarette smoking has a primary role in most cases of COPD, but the disease does not have a single cause. Pulmonary function declines normally with aging, and patients who experience a rate of loss that significantly exceeds the norm are classified as having COPD. Contributing factors include:

1. **Cigarette smoking:** There is a dose-related risk (usually expressed in pack-years) of cigarette/tobacco smoking and COPD, although there is great individual variation. Not all smokers develop COPD, even those with a high-dose history.

2. **Air pollution:** Although difficult to measure, there is an association between COPD and air pollution, especially sulfur dioxide and particulate matter.

3. **Mucosal hypersecretion and bronchial infection:** Both have been associated with COPD, but the causal relation is uncertain.

4. **Sex and race:** The higher prevalence of COPD in men is due to sex-related differences in cigarette smoking. Some studies have suggested that white males may be more susceptible than black males.

5. **Allergic factors:** Patients with a history of allergic disorders may be at higher risk, but the role is probably minor.

6. **Hereditary factors:** Certainly, the hereditary deficiency of α_1-antitrypsin is associated with diffuse emphysema, and there may be other contributing genetic factors.

7. **Sociologic factors:** The association of COPD with lower socioeconomic groups is probably due to differences in cigarette smoking, occupational factors, and air pollution.

8. **Occupational factors:** Occupations that are at increased risk include coal mining, fire fighting, grain handling, and copper smelting (sulfur dioxide exposure). Occupational exposures that increase risk include poison gas (mustard gas), granite dust, carbon black, cotton (byssinosis), hemp, and toluene diisocyanate.

Niewoehner DE: Clinical aspects of chronic airflow obstruction. In Baum GL, Wolinsky E (eds): Textbook of Pulmonary Diseases, 4th ed. Boston, Little, Brown, 1989.

73. Define chronic bronchitis.

Chronic bronchitis is defined by its symptoms, which include a productive cough on most mornings for 3 or more consecutive months for 2 or more consecutive years.

74. Define emphysema.

Unlike chronic bronchitis, which is described in terms of symptoms, emphysema is an anatomic/structural term. Emphysema is an abnormal enlargement of air-containing space distal to the terminal bronchioles accompanied by destruction of alveolar tissue.

75. What are the key aspects in the clinical evaluation of a patient with COPD?

HISTORY

* Smoking: age at initiation, quantity smoked per day, still smoking (if not, date of cessation)
* Environmental factors: may disclose important risk factors
* Cough (chronic, productive): frequency and duration, productive (esp. on awakening), presence of blood
* Wheezing
* Dyspnea
* Acute chest illnesses: frequency, productive cough, wheezing, dyspnea, fever

PHYSICAL EXAMINATION

* Chest
    Airflow obstruction evidenced by:
        Wheezing during auscultation on slow or forced breathing
        Prolonged forced expiratory phase
    Severe emphysema indicated by:
        Overdistention of lungs in stable state, low diaphragmatic position
        Decreased intensity of breath and heart sounds
    Severe disease suggested by:
        Pursed-lip breathing
        Use of accessory respiratory muscles
        Indrawing of lower interspaces
* Other: Unusual positions to relieve dyspnea at rest, digital clubbing (suggests lung cancer or bronchiectasis), mild dependent edema (may be seen in absence of right heart failure)

LABORATORY

* CXR: diagnostic only of severe emphysema but essential to exclude other lung disease
* Spirometry (pre- and post-bronchodilator): essential to confirm presence or reversibility of airflow obstruction, quantify maximum level of ventilatory function
* Lung volumes: FVC only, except in special instances (e.g., presence of giant bullae)
* DL_{CO}: unnecessary except in special instances (e.g., dyspnea out of proportion to severity of airflow limitation)
* ABGs: not needed in stage I airflow obstruction (FEV_1 >50% predicted); essential in stages II and III (FEV_1 < 50% predicted) and in very severe airflow obstruction, major monitoring tool

American Thoracic Society: Standards for the diagnosis & care of patients with chronic obstructive pulmonary disease. Am J Respir Crit Care Med 152:S77–S120, 1995.

76. What radiographic changes are associated with COPD?

The CXR findings are secondary to overdistension of the lungs. These findings include a low flat diaphragm, increased retrosternal airspace (on lateral x-ray), and an elongated, narrow heart shadow. Bullae, which appear as rounded radiolucent areas > 1 cm in diameter, are occasionally seen and reflect emphysematous changes.

77. Describe the findings of pulmonary function tests (PFTs) in patients with COPD.

The early signs, symptoms, and radiographic changes of COPD are variable and nonspecific, and therefore, PFTs are important in the diagnosis of COPD. Patients will show evidence of airway obstruction, such as decreased VC and expiratory flow rates (i.e., FEV_1 or $FEF_{25-75\%}$). There will also be evidence of lung hyperinflation and air trapping, manifested by increases in RV, FRC, and TLC. There is generally a response to bronchodilators which, although variable, is usually only about 15–20% over the prebronchodilator values.

78. Pink puffers and blue bloaters—what are these?

These are the two distinct clinical patterns of gas exchange abnormalities seen among patients with advanced COPD. In most patients, however, there is significant overlap of features.

"Pink puffers" tend to be thin and dyspneic but maintain relatively normal PaO_2 and $PaCO_2$ levels. They breathe with hyperinflated lungs and fast, shallow respirations. They remain relatively free of cor pulmonale. The pathophysiology seems to be that of severe emphysema, and their symptoms are largely the result of the loss of lung elastic recoil, with relatively little intrinsic airways disease.

"Blue bloaters," tend to be overweight, with minimal dyspnea but significant coughing and sputum production. They suffer from cor pulmonale, respiratory infections, and chronic CO_2 retention. Although they usually have some degree of emphysema, the pathophysiology is that of significant small and large airway inflammation, and the symptoms are largely due to the intrinsic airway disease.

Both patterns are usually a result of long-term cigarette smoking. The reason for the two different presentations is not clearly defined.

79. What complications are associated with COPD?

COPD is characterized by frequent exacerbations and decompensation. The exacerbations can be induced by upper respiratory tract infections, pneumonia, medical noncompliance, and environmental changes (temperature, allergens, irritants, etc.). Complications include sleep disturbances due to nocturnal desaturation, acute and chronic respiratory failure, chronic cor pulmonale, spontaneous pneumothorax, and impairment of pulmonary function secondary to large bullae.

80. What is cor pulmonale?

Cor pulmonale, or pulmonary heart disease, is right-sided congestive heart failure that is caused by an increase in pulmonary vascular resistance (pulmonary hypertension) due to intrinsic lung disease. It can be caused by pulmonary parenchymal diseases such as COPD, sarcoidosis, pneumoconiosis, and restrictive lung disease. It can also be caused by pulmonary vascular diseases such as primary pulmonary hypertension, recurrent pulmonary embolism, or scleroderma. It is a major cause of morbidity and mortality in COPD.

81. What is the prognosis of severe COPD? How is the severity staged?

Prognosis is based on age, severity of hypoxemia, presence of hypercapnea, and severity of airflow obstruction (FEV_1). Of these, the most relevant is FEV_1. An $FEV_1 < 0.75$ liters has a 1-year mortality of 30% and a 10-year mortality of 95%.

The severity of COPD is staged on the basis of airflow obstruction:

Stage I—$FEV_1 \geq 50\%$ predicted

Stage II—FEV_1 35–49% predicted

Stage III—$FEV_1 < 35\%$ predicted

Hodgkin JE. Prognosis in chronic obstructive pulmonary disease. Clin Chest 11:555–569, 1990.

82. How is COPD treated?

1. **Removal of risk factors:** The most important component is the cessation of smoking and removal of any other risk factors (i.e., environmental and occupational).

2. **Bronchodilators:** Although the airway obstruction is largely fixed, with only a small reversible component, most patients experience a small improvement in symptoms with the use of bronchodilator therapy.

3. **Corticosteroids:** Patients who are most likely to respond include those with recurrent attacks of wheezing and a relatively significant response to inhaled bronchodilators (FEV_1 increase >20%). Because of the risk of side effects, the lowest possible dose should be used, preferably inhaled steroids (if needed chronically) or an alternate-day oral regimen.

4. **Diuretics:** Indicated for the symptomatic relief of the symptoms of cor pulmonale.

5. **Vasodilators:** Long-term vasodilator therapy can decrease the pulmonary hypertension in patients with COPD, but it is not certain that this improves morbidity or mortality.

6. **Antibiotic therapy:** If indicated, broad-spectrum agents should be used (preferably the least expensive agent or an agent that the patient has tolerated well in the past).

7. **Continuous O₂ therapy:** In patients for whom it is indicated, long-term O_2 therapy decreases the morbidity and mortality of COPD.

8. **Phlebotomy:** In the past, this procedure was commonly performed in patients with COPD and a secondary erythrocytosis. At present, with the advent of long-term O_2 therapy, phlebotomy is rarely necessary.

83. Which classes of bronchodilator drugs are available for therapy for the obstructive airway diseases?

1. **Anticholinergic agents:** These agents, which can be given parenterally or via inhalation, compete with acetylcholine at its receptors. The currently available congener, ipratropium bromide (Atrovent), is available for inhalational use and causes far fewer systemic side effects than atropine. It also has an extended duration of action over that of atropine.

2. **β-Adrenergic agonists:** These agents, available for oral, parenteral, or inhalational use, produce bronchodilation by directly stimulating the β_2 receptors on the bronchial smooth muscle cell. Epinephrine was the first available agent, but newer agents offer increased duration of action and increased β_2 selectivity. Oral agents should be reserved for patients unable to use inhaled agents.

3. **Methylxanthines:** These agents, available for oral or parenteral use, include aminophylline, theophylline, and related compounds. To achieve maximal benefit from theophylline and to minimize toxic effects, the serum level must be maintained within the therapeutic range of 10–20 g/ml.

Following is a typical regimen for treating COPD:

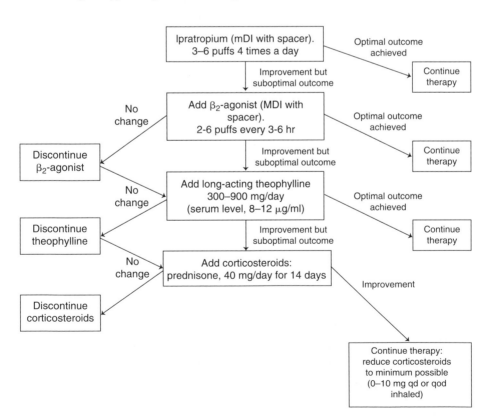

Adapted from Ferguson GT, Cherniack RM: Management of chronic obstructive pulmonary disease. N Engl J Med 328:1017–1022, 1993.

84. Why is theophylline beneficial in patients with COPD?

Theophylline is classified as a bronchodilator. However, since patients with COPD may have a very small reversible component to their obstruction, the significance of theophylline's bronchodilatory effects in COPD is questionable. A variety of other beneficial actions have been attributed to theophylline, including:

- Increased mucociliary clearance
- Increased respiratory drive
- Improved cardiovascular function
- Increased diaphragmatic contractility
- Decreased dyspnea
- Improved exercise capacity

85. Are there toxic effects of theophylline therapy?

Theophylline's toxic effects occur with increasing frequency as the serum level exceeds 20 µg/ml, although they can be seen even within the therapeutic range of 10–20 µg/ml. Whereas the serious toxicities (especially seizures and cardiac arrhythmias) are usually not seen until the serum levels rise above 30 µg/ml, they can be seen at lower serum levels and are often not preceded by any less severe sign of toxicity. The common toxic effects are:

1. **GI:** Nausea, vomiting, diarrhea and abdominal pain
2. **Cardiac:** Various arrhythmias (including sinus tachycardia, multifocal atrial tachycardia, extrasystoles)
3. **Neurologic:** Headache, nervousness, insomnia, tremor, seizures

86. What factors affect the clearance of theophylline?

Clearance of theophylline is mainly through hepatic oxidation and demethylation, with hepatic metabolites and unmetabolized theophylline excreted in the urine. Any increase or decrease in theophylline clearance will necessitate increasing or decreasing the maintenance dose to maintain therapeutic serum levels.

Factors Affecting Theophylline Clearance and Dosage Requirements

	INCREASE CLEARANCE (LARGER DOSAGE REQUIRED)*	DECREASE CLEARANCE (SMALLER DOSAGE REQUIRED)
Major change (26–50%)	Cigarette smoking Phenytoin Rifampin Isoproterenol IV Phenobarbital Carbamazepine Aminoglutethimide	Hepatic insufficiency Heart failure Cor pulmonale Viral pneumonia Cimetidine Mexiletine Ciprofloxacin, other quinolones Allopurinol Erythromycin Influenza vaccination Triacetyloleandomycin (TAO) Propranolol Oral contraceptives
Lesser change (10–25%)†	Low-carbohydrate, high-protein diet Charcoaled food Isoniazid Ketoconazole	Verapamil Nifedipine Tetracycline Hydrocortisone Aluminum hydroxide Magnesium hydroxide Thiabendazole

*Serum levels must be used for guidance when increasing dosage.
†Data supporting these changes are less well-documented.

American Thoracic Society: Standards for diagnosis and care of patients with chronic obstructive pulmonary disease. Am J Respir Crit Care Med 152(5):S87, 1995.

87. When should antibiotics be given to a patient presenting with an acute exacerbation of COPD?

- Increasing dyspnea
- Increased sputum production
- Purulent sputum

Anthonisen NR, et at: Antibiotic therapy in exacerbations of COPD. Ann Intern Med 106:196–204, 1987.

88. What are the criteria for continuous low-flow oxygen therapy?

The role of O_2 therapy was largely established in the early 1980s by the Nocturnal Oxygen Therapy trial in the U.S. and by the Medical Research Council trial in Great Britain. O_2 therapy is indicated for any one of the following conditions:

1. A patient at rest and on an optimal medical regimen whose PaO_2 is <55 mm Hg.
2. A patient at rest and on an optimal medical regimen whose PaO_2 is >55 mm Hg, if there is evidence of hypoxic end-organ dysfunction manifested by one or more of the following:
- Cor pulmonale
- Secondary erythrocytosis
- Secondary pulmonary hypertension
- Impaired mentation
3. A patient whose PaO_2 drops below 55 mm Hg on exercise and who has evidence of significant improvement in one or more of the following with O_2 therapy:
- Exercise duration
- Exercise performance or capacity
4. A patient whose PaO_2 drops below 55 mm Hg during sleep and has evidence of one or more of the following:
- Hypoxic organ dysfunction
- Disturbed sleep pattern
- Significant cardiac dysrhythmia

89. Does the cessation of smoking have an effect on patients with COPD?

Yes. The morbidity and mortality associated with COPD are reduced, there is small but significant improvement in objective tests of pulmonary function and subjective symptom severity, and pulmonary function reverts to the normal, age-related levels seen in nonsmokers once COPD patients stop smoking. These benefits are more dramatic in patients with mild COPD than in those with more advanced disease.

90. What are the poor prognostic signs in an acute exacerbation of asthma?

- Pulse rate > 100/min
- Pulsus parodoxus > 10 mm Hg
- PEFR < 16% of predicted
- $PaCO_2$ > 45 mm Hg
- Retraction of sternocleidomastoid muscles
- FEV_1 < 600 ml before treatment
- FEV_1 < 1600 ml after treatment

91. What is bronchiectasis?

Bronchiectasis is a fixed dilatation of bronchi due to destructive changes in the elastic and muscular layers of the bronchial wall. It was a more common disease prior to the advent of appropriate antibiotic therapy for pulmonary infection. Currently, it is seen in patients with a history of gram-negative pulmonary infection or chronic pulmonary inflammatory condition, immunodeficiency state, cystic fibrosis, and occasionally asthma. Patients usually present with a chronic cough productive of large quantities of foul, often blood-tinged sputum. The diagnosis is made with contrast bronchoscopy or CT scan.

INTERSTITIAL LUNG DISEASE

92. How are the interstitial lung diseases (ILD) classified?

ILD refers to a heterogeneous group of diseases with similar clinical and x-ray abnormalities. The CXR shows varying degrees of fibrotic changes (usually widespread). The most common symptoms include dyspnea and dry cough. PFTs reveal a restrictive defect. There are over 100 causes of ILD, and these are often classified according to *known* versus *unknown* etiology.

Classification of ILD

Idiopathic Fibrotic Diseases	
Idiopathic pulmonary fibrosis	Lymphocytic interstitial pneumonitis
Acute interstitial pneumonitis	Bronchiolitis obliterans organizing pneumonia (BOOP)
Connective Tissue Diseases	
SLE	Rheumatoid arthritis
Scleroderma	Ankylosing spondylitis
Sjögren's syndrome	Others less commonly
Primary Diseases	
Sarcoidosis	ARDS
Lymphangitic carcinoma	Eosinophilic granulomatosis
Systemic vasculitides	Alveolar microlithiasis
Lymphangioleiomyomatosis	Neurofibromatosis
Eosinophilic pneumonia	Other rare diseases
Drug-Related	
Oxygen	Radiation
Chemotherapy	Antiarrhythmic agents (amiodarone, others)
Antibiotics (macrodantin, others)	
Narcotics (morphine, cocaine, others)	Anti-inflammatory agents (aspirin, gold, others)
Occupational	
Pneumoconiosis	Hypersensitivity pneumonitis

Schwartz MI, King TE: Interstitial Lung Disease, 2nd ed. St. Louis, Mosby, 1993.

93. How can the ILDs be classified according to clinical findings?

ILD and Associated Findings

ILD associated with spontaneous pneumothorax	
Eosinophilic granuloma	Neurofibromatosis
Lymphangioleiomyomatosis	Tuberous sclerosis
ILD associated with increased lung volumes	
Eosinophilic granuloma	Neurofibromatosis
Tuberous sclerosis	Chronic hypersensitivity pneumonitis
Sarcoidosis	
ILD associated with upper lobe predominance	
Ankylosing spondylitis	Berylliosis
Eosinophilic granuloma	Neurofibromatosis
Silicosis	Chronic sarcoidosis
ILD associated with lymphadenopathy	
Sarcoidosis	Berylliosis
Lymphoma	Lymphangitic carcinoma

Crystal RG, et al: Interstitial lung disease of unknown etiology: Disorders characterized by chronic inflammation of the lower respiratory tract. N Engl J Med 310:154, 1984.

Stokes LT, et al: Lungs and connective tissue disorders. In Murray J. Nadel J (eds): Textbook of Respiratory Medicine. Philadelphia, W.B. Saunders, 1988, pp 1462–1485.

94. What is Hamman-Rich syndrome?

In 1944, Hamman and Rich first described rapidly progressive and fatal pulmonary fibrosis for which no etiology could be identified. This term is used only for rapidly progressive ILD of unknown etiology.

Hamman L, Rich AR: Acute diffuse interstitial fibrosis of the lungs. Bull Johns Hopkins Hosp 74:177–212, 1944.

95. What clinical characteristics are seen in patients with rheumatoid arthritis and ILD?

Rheumatoid arthritis may be associated with interstitial pulmonary changes. The condition is more common in men, rarely precedes joint disease, and may be associated with cutaneous nodules. The most common pulmonary complication is pleural effusion.

96. How prevalent is sarcoidosis?

Sarcoidosis is a multisystem disorder of unknown etiology that has a prevalence of approx. 20 cases/100,000. Although it may occur at any age, patients are usually 20–40 years of age. Females have a slightly higher prevalence, and in the U.S., sarcoidosis is more common in blacks than whites, with a 10:1 ratio. Many organs may be involved, but the lung is the organ most frequently involved (> 90%)—hence sarcoidosis appears in this chapter.

97. What CXR abnormalities are observed in sarcoidosis?

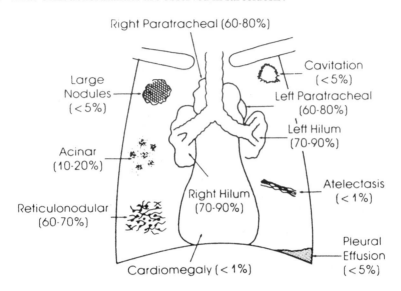

From Crystal RG: Sarcoidosis. In Isselbacher KJ, et al (eds): Harrison's Principles of Internal Medicine, 13th ed. New York, McGraw-Hill, 1994, p 1682; with permission.

98. How is sarcoidosis staged by CXR?

About 90% of patients have an abnormality on CXR sometime during the course of the disease. The following categories represent CXR patterns and are not "stages" of the disease, as is usually understood. However, patients with stage I disease are more likely to have reversible sarcoidosis.

Stage	CXR Findings
0	Clear (< 10%)
I	Bilateral hilar adenopathy (25–40%)
II	Bilateral hilar adenopathy with pulmonary infiltrate (25–50%)
III	Pulmonary infiltrate without adenopathy (<15%)

99. What are the clinical and laboratory abnormalities associated with sarcoidosis?

Because sarcoidosis is a multisystem disease, clinical manifestations can be nonspecific, and approx. 20% of patients are symptomatic. When symptomatic, patients complain of malaise, fever, weight loss, or symptoms referable to the specific organ involved.

Laboratory abnormalities are also nonspecific and include increased ESR, hyperglobulinemia, increased ACE activity, and occasionally hypercalcemia and/or hypercalciuria.

100. How is the diagnosis of sarcoidosis established?

The diagnosis rests upon the combination of history, radiographic, and histologic findings. The typical pathologic finding is the **noncaseating granuloma.** This pathologic finding, in conjunction with the appropriate clinical picture and lack of infectious etiology (TB, fungal, etc.), establishes the diagnosis. Although any involved organ may be biopsied for pathologic changes, transbronchial lung biopsy is positive in about 90% of the cases.

101. Which organs, in addition to the lung, are most frequently involved in sarcoidosis?

The lymph nodes (> 75%), skin (25%), eyes (25%), and musculoskeletal system (arthralgias). Although the bone marrow, spleen, and liver are frequently involved, this finding is usually not clinically significant. Skin manifestations include erythema nodosum and plaques. Ocular manifestations include both anterior and posterior uveitis and can lead to blindness. CNS and cardiac involvement are present in approx. 5%.

102. Which patients with sarcoidosis should be treated?

Sarcoidosis is usually a self-limited disease, with 30–50% of cases spontaneously remitting, 20–30% remaining stable, and 30% demonstrating progression. Because therapeutic intervention is not without side effects, close observation of patients who are asymptomatic and without organ dysfunction is warranted. Therapy should be initiated in patients with significant systemic organ impairment (lung, eyes, heart, CNS, or extensive skin lesions) or evidence of hypercalcemia or hypercalciuria. Corticosteroids are considered the first line of therapy.

103. What is Goodpasture's syndrome?

Goodpasture's syndrome usually refers to a combination of glomerulonephritis and diffuse pulmonary hemorrhage associated with development of anti-glomerular basement membrane (anti-GBM) antibodies and, less frequently, anti-pulmonary basement membrane antibodies. Some use the eponym more broadly to refer to all diseases characterized by glomerulonephritis and pulmonary hemorrhage.

104. Which diagnostic tests can help differentiate Goodpasture's syndrome from other pulmonary-renal syndromes?

Anti-GBM antibodies can be demonstrated in serum, renal tissue, and, less frequently, pulmonary tissue. Immunofluorescent staining of tissue reveals a *linear* pattern of deposition of IgG.

Goodpasture's syndrome is predominantly a disease of young adults (mean age, 21 years) and is more common in males. The typical initial presentation is hemoptysis, but rarely renal involvement will present first. The differential diagnosis includes other pulmonary-renal syndromes, including vasculitis, Wegener's granulomatosis, polyarteritis nodosa, uremia with pulmonary edema, and immune complex disease (SLE).

ADULT RESPIRATORY DISTRESS SYNDROME (ARDS)

105. What are the hallmarks of ARDS?

The term ARDS is applied to diverse etiologies of lung injury in which there is an initial noxious event, followed by an interval of normal lung function, and then progressive and rapid hypoxemia and diffuse pulmonary infiltrates. The incidence of ARDS is estimated to be > 150,000 cases/year. The overall mortality remains 40–60% despite ICU intervention.

106. Can cardiogenic pulmonary edema be distinguished from noncardiogenic pulmonary edema based on clinical and radiographic findings?

No. The two conditions can be differentiated by measurement of the pulmonary capillary wedge pressure (PCWP), which reflects left ventricular (LV) filling pressures (normally 6–12 mm Hg). The PCWP is elevated in cardiogenic pulmonary edema, reflecting the elevated LV filling pressures, but it is normal in ARDS, because LV filling pressures are normal since the defect is at the alveolocapillary membrane.

107. Name some of the known causes of ARDS.

The etiologies of ARDS are diverse and include:

Shock (hemodynamic, septic, hypovolemic)	Immunologic disorders	Trauma
	Hematologic disorders	CNS disease
Diffuse pulmonary infection	(DIC, transfusion, car-	Uremia
Exposure to drugs or toxins	diopulmonary bypass)	Aspiration
Pancreatitis		

108. What are the complications of ARDS?

LV failure, secondary bacterial infection, DIC, pulmonary oxygen toxicity, barotrauma secondary to mechanical ventilation (pneumothorax, pneumomediastinum), and multisystem organ failure.

109. What is the prognosis of ARDS? How is the syndrome managed?

Despite the increased understanding of the pathophysiology of ARDS, the mortality rate remains high (40–60%). The prognosis at the time of diagnosis depends on a variety of factors: acute underlying diagnosis, etiology of ARDS, severity of illness, physiologic reserve, and comorbidity and preexisting conditions.

Management involves ruling out treatable causes of respiratory failure, treating underlying disease processes, maintaining $PaO_2 > 55$ mm Hg, supporting hemodynamics and nutritional status, and avoiding complications.

ENVIRONMENTAL LUNG DISEASE

110. What is pneumoconiosis?

The term is derived from Greek *pneumo,* lung, and *konis,* dust. It currently refers to an accumulation of inorganic dust in the lungs and the consequences of the tissue's response to the presence of the dust. The most common pneumoconioses are silicosis, asbestosis, and coalworker's pneumoconiosis (black lung).

111. What are the CXR abnormalities and clinical complications associated with silicosis?

Silicosis is a pulmonary disease secondary to the inhalation of quartz or silica dust. Occupations leading to potential exposure include mining, quarrying, sandblasting, pottery/stoneware production, and tunnelling. The disease is characterized by focal pulmonary fibrosis that has a tendency to occur first in the upper lobes. Enlargement of the hilar lymph nodes and eggshell calcifications are suggestive.

Complications silicosis include spontaneous pneumothorax, cor pulmonale, and infection with mycobacteria (TB and atypical mycobacteria) and fungi, increased frequency of connective tissue disorders, and possibly an increased risk of lung cancer.

112. What is Caplan's syndrome?

Caplan's syndrome, or rheumatoid pneumoconiosis, refers to the association of rheumatoid arthritis and nodules on CXR in patients with coalworker's pneumoconiosis. This has been associated with risk for pneumothorax.

113. Is asbesto exposure associated with any clinical problems?

Asbestosis (bibasilar predominant pulmonary fibrosis), pleural plaques, pleural effusions, and malignancies are associated with a history of asbestos exposure. Asbestosis is a fibrotic disease of the lung and visceral pleura. The CXR shows interstitial fibrosis beginning usually at the bases and progressing upward. There is usually no hilar adenopathy. Asbestos exposure increases the risk of malignancy, including lung cancer, GI cancer, and mesothelioma. There is no associated increase of infection or collagen vascular diseases.

114. Which tests are useful in diagnosing mesothelioma?

Because generous biopsy specimens are needed to diagnose mesothelioma, diagnosis is usually made following open thoracotomy. Periodic acid-Schiff (PAS) stain, immunoperoxidase staining for carcinoembryonic antigen (CEA) and keratin, and electron microscopy are useful in differentiating mesothelioma from adenocarcinoma. Mesothelioma lacks PAS-positive vacuoles and has weak staining with CEA antigen.

Antman KH, et al: Benign and malignant mesothelioma. Clin Chest Med 6:141–152, 1985.

MEDIASTINUM

115. Name the three major compartments of the mediastinum viewed on lateral CXR.

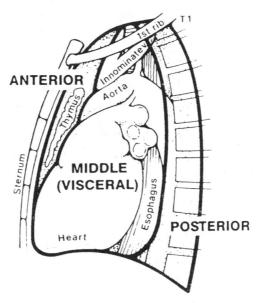

By convention, the mediastinum is divided into anterior, middle, and posterior compartments, according to its appearance on the lateral CXR. From Shields TW: Chest wall, pleura, mediastinum and diaphragm. In James EC, et al (eds): Basic Surgical Practice. Philadelphia, Hanley & Belfus, 1987, p 179; with permission.

116. What are their components?

Anterior mediastinum: Consists of everything forward of and superior to the heart shadow, which includes:

Thymus gland

Aortic arch and major branches

Substernal extension of the thyroid
  or parathyroid glands

Innominate veins

Lymphatic vessels and lymph nodes

Middle mediastinum: Extends from anterior heart border to the anterior ventral border, and includes:

Heart and pericardium

Trachea and mainstem bronchi

Pulmonary hila

Lymph nodes

Phrenic and vagus nerves

Posterior mediastinum: Occupies the space within the margins of the vertebrae on lateral film, including:

Esophagus

Descending aorta

Azygous and hemiazygous veins

Areolar connective tissue

Thoracic duct and lymph nodes

Vagus nerves and sympathetic chains

Pierson, DJ: Disorders of the mediastinum. In Murray JF, Nadel JA (eds): Textbook of Respiratory Medicine. Philadelphia. W.B. Saunders, 1988, p 1782.

117. What is the most common mediastinal tumor in the adult? In which compartment does it occur?

Thymic tumors are the most common tumors in the adult, of which thymoma is the most common. The tumors are usually located in the anterior mediastinum and are often quite large (80% > 5 cm). The mean age at presentation is 40–60 years, and two-thirds are symptomatic (cough, pain, rarely fever).

118. What systemic syndromes may be associated with thymoma?

Approx. 35% of patients will have myasthenia gravis (MG), although the majority of patients with MG do not have thymoma. Other syndromes include erythrocyte aplasia, collagen vascular disease (lupus, rheumatoid arthritis, dermatomyositis), polycythemia/pancytopenia, and Cushing's syndrome.

119. What are the presenting signs and symptoms of superior vena cava obstruction?

The patient may complain of headache, chest pain, cough (sometimes associated with syncope or headache), lacrimation, and periorbital/facial edema. Symptoms are present in most patients for 2–4 weeks prior to hospitalization. Physical findings include neck vein distention; edema, plethora, and cyanosis of the face; tachypnea; edema of the upper extremities; paralysis of the vocal cords; and distention of retinal veins or veins beneath the tongue. Veins of the upper extremities do not empty when lifted above the level of the heart.

THE DIAPHRAGM

120. Name the three major diaphragmatic hernias.

Herniation of abdominal contents into the chest can occur through a region of congenital defect or weakness. **Hiatal hernias** (via the esophageal hiatus), with displacement of the stomach into the posterior mediastinum, are the most common. **Herniation via the retrosternal foramen of Morgagni** is often asymptomatic and appears as an abnormal shadow frequently on the right heart border. **Herniation via the posterolateral foramen of Bochdalek** is more common in infancy.

121. What are the causes of elevation of a hemidiaphragm on CXR?

Normally, the right hemidiaphragm is several centimeters higher than the left because of displacement upward by the liver. Elevation of a hemidiaphragm may be secondary to:
- Unilateral diaphragmatic paralysis
- Displacement secondary to intraabdominal masses or ascites
- Loss of lung volume on the affected side
- Eventration of the diaphragm (a rare, congenital disorder)
- Subpulmonic effusion

122. What are the most common causes of unilateral diaphragmatic paralysis?

Each diaphragm is innervated by a phrenic nerve originating from the third, fourth, and fifth cervical roots. Paralysis results from disruption of this nerve. The most common causes include invasion by bronchogenic carcinoma, thoracic trauma, surgical resection or disruption, and possibly postviral neuropathy. Slightly more than one-half of the cases remain unexplained. Occasionally, recovery occurs. Unilateral diaphragmatic paralysis is usually asymptomatic.

123. How is the "sniff" test useful in evaluating unilateral diaphragmatic paralysis?

The diagnosis of unilateral diaphragmatic paralysis is suggested by elevation of one hemidiaphragm on CXR. Under fluoroscopy, this diagnosis can be confirmed by asking the patient to "sniff," which rapidly increases intraabdominal pressure, lowers intrathoracic pressure, and causes an upward (paradoxical) movement of the affected diaphragm.

VENTILATORY SUPPORT

124. List the indications for initiation of mechanical ventilation.
Absolute indications:

Apnea   Administration of paralyzing agents

Clinical examination alone:

Ineffectual respiratory efforts   Inspiratory muscle fatigue

ABG values plus clinical evaluation:

Hypoxemia not corrected by other means   Progressive hypercarbia with acidosis

Johanson WG Jr, et al: Critical care. In Murray JF, Nadel JA (eds): Textbook of Respiratory Medicine. Philadelphia, W.B. Saunders, 1988, p 1994.

125. Which physiologic guidelines should be used to evaluate the need for ventilatory support in respiratory failure?

Guidelines for Ventilatory Support in Respiratory Failure

PARAMETER	READING	PARAMETER	READING
Respiratory rate	> 35/min	$PaCO_2$	> 55 mm Hg
Vital capacity	< 15 ml/kg	$A–aO_2$ gradient	> 450 mm Hg
FEV_1	< 10 ml/kg	PaO_2	< 70 mm Hg with oxygen
Inspiratory force	< 25 cm H_2O	V_D/V_T	> 0.60

Johanson WG Jr, Peters JI: Critical care. In Murray JF, Nadel JA (eds): Textbook of Respiratory Medicine. Philadelphia, W.B. Saunders, 1988, p 1994.

126. What are the complications of endotracheal intubation?

Immediate	Delayed	Late
Difficult intubation	Self-extubation	Tracheomalacia
Local trauma	Infections (tracheobron-	Tracheal perforation
Malposition of endotra-	chitis, pneumonia)	Laryngeal dysfunction
cheal tube	Mucosal edema, denudation	Subglottic/tracheal stenosis

Johanson WG Jr, Peters JI: Critical care. In Murray JF, Nadel JA (eds): Textbook of Respiratory Medicine. Philadelphia, W.B. Saunders, 1988, p 1979.

APNEA SYNDROMES

127. How do you differentiate central apnea and obstructive sleep apnea?
Apnea refers to a pause in respiration of > 10 sec. Both central sleep apnea (CSA) and obstructive sleep apnea (OSA) result in cessation of respirations (apnea) but are differentiated by a lack of respiratory effort in CSA versus continued but *ineffective* respiratory effort in OSA.

Clinical Characteristics of Patients with Sleep Apnea

CSA	OSA	
Normal body habitus	Commonly obese	Sexual dysfunction
Insomnia, hypersomnia rare	Daytime hypersomnia	Morning headache
Awaken during sleep	Rarely awaken during sleep	Nocturnal enuresis
Snoring mild and intermittent	Loud snoring	
Depression	Intellectual deterioration	
Minimal sexual dysfunction		

White DP: Central sleep apnea. Med Clin North Am 69:1208, 1985.

128. What underlying mechanisms explain the events occurring during obstructive sleep apnea?

UNDERLYING MECHANISMS   PRIMARY EVENTS

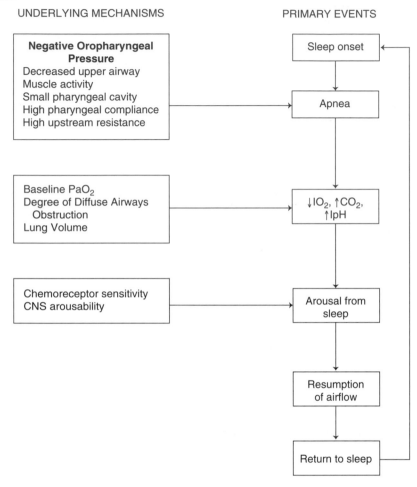

The primary sequence of events in patients with OSA and the pathogenetic mechanisms that contribute to these events. (From Bradley TD, Phillipson EA: Pathogenesis and pathophysiology of obstructive sleep apnea syndrome. Med Clin North Am 69:1170, 1985; with permission.)

BIBLIOGRAPHY

1. Baum GL, Wolinsky E (eds): Textbook of Pulmonary Diseases, 5th ed. Boston, Little, Brown, 1994.
2. Bone RC, et al (eds): Pulmonary and Critical Care Medicine, St. Louis, Mosby Yearbook, 1993.
3. Fishman AP: Pulmonary Diseases and Disorders, 2nd ed. New York, McGraw-Hill, 1992.
4. Guenter CA, Welch MH (eds): Pulmonary Medicine. 2nd ed. Philadelphia, J.B. Lippincott, 1982.
5. Murray JF, Nadel JA (eds): Textbook of Respiratory Medicine. 2nd ed. Philadelphia, W.B. Saunders, 1994.
6. Parsons PE, Heffner JE (eds): Pulmonary/Respiratory Therapy Secrets. Philadelphia, Hanley & Belfus, 1997.

11. RHEUMATOLOGY

Richard A. Rubin, M.D.

The wolf, I'm afraid, is inside tearing up the place.
Flannery O'Connor (1925–1964)
Novelist, sufferer of SLE (Letter)

Screw up the vise as tightly as possible—you have rheumatism; give it another turn, and that is gout.
Anonymous

1. Give an operational definition for rheumatic diseases.
Rheumatic diseases are syndromes of pain and/or inflammation in articular or periarticular tissues.

2. What is a "joint mouse"?
Osteocartilaginous bodies within a joint are often termed joint mice or loose bodies and occur commonly in osteoarthritis. They are felt to arise when bits of articular cartilage and subchondral bone break off the surface and enter into the joint. There may be proliferation and deposition of new bone on these fragments.

3. What is chondromalacia patella?
Chondromalacia is a softening and degeneration of articular cartilage. In the patella, it is often associated with meniscal disease, knee laxity, or recurrent trauma. Typically, pain is associated with activity, characteristically descending stairs.
Moskowitz RW: Clinical and laboratory findings in osteoarthritis. In McCarty DJ, Koopman WJ (eds): Arthritis and Allied Conditions, 12th ed. Philadelphia, Lea & Febiger, 1993, pp 1735–1760.

4. How do bunions occur?
A bunion (hallux valgus) is a deviation of the proximal phalanx of the great toe toward the fibular side of the foot. It can be caused by biomechanical factors (tight and pointy-toed shoes that push the proximal phalanx across the other toes), inflammatory disease (gout or rheumatoid arthritis), or abnormal alignment (usually congenital) at the first metatarsal-cuneiform joint. If the cuneiform is abnormal, the first metatarsal may deviate excessively toward the midline (a primary *varus* deformity), which will lead to a *valgus* deformity (lateral deviation) of the great toe when the abnormal foot is placed into standard shoes.

5. What conditions are associated with avascular necrosis (AVN) of bone?
Trauma (femoral head fractures)	Gaucher's disease
Hemoglobinopathies	Pregnancy
Exogenous or endogenous overproduction of glucocorticoids	Systemic lupus erythematosus (SLE)
	Kidney transplantation
Alcoholism	Lymphoproliferative diseases

6. What mechanisms contribute to bone loss with the use of glucocorticoids?
Use of glucocorticoids is a cornerstone of treatment of many rheumatic diseases, but one of its most concerning toxicities is accelerated bone loss. Corticosteroids have been shown to decrease intestinal absorption of calcium, increase urinary calcium excretion, and inhibit osteoblast

function. Calcium loss from trabecular bone is greater than that from cortical bone, although the mechanism for this difference is not known.

Sambrook PN, et al: Corticosteroid osteoporosis. Br J Rheum 34:8–12, 1995.

7. Which clinical syndromes are associated with complement deficiencies?

Rheumatic Diseases Associated with Complement Deficiencies

PROTEIN	DISEASE
C1q	Glomerulonephritis and poikiloderma congenita
C1r	Glomerulonephritis, lupus-like syndrome
C1s	Lupus-like syndrome
C1INH	Discoid lupus, SLE, lupus-like syndrome
C4	SLE, Sjögren's syndrome
C2	SLE, discoid lupus, polymyositis, Henoch-Schönlein purpura, Hodgkin's disease, vasculitis, glomerulonephritis, common variable hypogammaglobulinemia
C3	Vasculitis, lupus-like syndrome, glomerulonephritis
C5	SLE, *Neisseria* infection
C6	*Neisseria* infection
C7	SLE, rheumatoid arthritis, Raynaud's phenomenon and sclerodactyly, vasculitis, *Neisseria* infection
C8	SLE, *Neisseria* infection
C9	*Neisseria* infection

Ruddy S: Complement deficiencies and rheumatic diseases. In Kelly WN, et al (eds): Textbook of Rheumatology, 4th ed. Philadelphia, W.B. Saunders, 1993, pp 1283–1289.

DIAGNOSIS

8. How much synovial fluid is present in the normal knee?

Detection of a joint effusion is important in the evaluation of patients with articular symptoms. The knee normally has up to 4 ml of fluid.

9. Which studies should generally be performed on synovial fluid after arthrocentesis?

Important information can be gained by evaluating joint fluid with selected tests. Gram stain and bacterial culture may confirm the presence of an infective agent. In the right clinical setting, similar procedures for mycobacteria or fungi are important. A WBC count with differential is one of the best indicators of the degree of inflammation. Evaluation for crystals by polarized light microscopy may cinch the diagnosis. Although a good deal has been written about various other tests—glucose, complement, rheumatoid factor, antinuclear antibodies (ANA), lactate dehydrogenase, protein—they add little diagnostic information.

10. What are the "string" and "mucin clot" tests?

The primary component of joint fluid is hyaluronic acid. It is quite viscous and thus will make a "string" when expressed from a syringe as a single drop. Dilute acetic acid causes hyaluronate and protein to clump and fall to the bottom of a test tube (producing the famous "mucin clot"). Inflammatory mediators cause fragmentation of the hyaluronate–protein, rendering it unable to form a good mucin clot.

Basically, these tests provide a crude bedside estimate of the level of synovial inflammation. Since the wet prep and a total synovial fluid WBC give more objective data, the mucin clot and string tests are primarily of historic interest. It is also probably true that when done in the traditional manner at the bedside, these tests violate OSHA and CLIA regulations for the handling of body fluids.

Schumacher HR Jr: Synovial fluid analysis and synovial biopsy. In Kelly WN, et al (eds): Textbook of Rheumatology, 4th ed. Philadelphia, W.B. Saunders, 1993, pp 562–578.

11. Straight leg raising is a useful diagnostic maneuver in what common condition?

The straight leg raising test is designed to reproduce back pain secondary to nerve root compression. The leg is lifted by the calcaneus with the knee remaining straight. Bringing the heel across the other leg may increase the sensitivity of this maneuver.

12. What clinical features help to distinguish neurogenic from arterial claudication?

Progressive leg or back pain with walking can occur because of either arterial insufficiency or nerve compression, but distinguishing between these entities can be difficult. Absence of pedal pulses suggests arterial disease, although one study reported this sign in 9% of patients with spinal stenosis. Patients with arterial insufficiency can often get relief of pain simply by pausing or slowing their pace. Patients with nerve compression rarely get relief unless they sit or lie down. Neurologic signs such as weakness, abnormal reflexes, and abnormal EMG/NCV are present in spinal stenosis but absent in arterial disease.

O'Duffy JD, Ebersold MJ: Spinal stenosis. In McCarty DJ, Koopman WJ (eds): Arthritis and Allied Conditions, 12th ed. Philadelphia, Lea & Febiger, 1993, pp 1601–1608.

13. What is onychodystrophy and with which diseases is it associated?

Separation of the nail plate, usually beginning at the free margin and progressing proximally, is called onychodystrophy. Both systemic and local processes are associated with this physical examination finding, including hypo- and hyperthyroidism, pregnancy, syphilis, trauma (particularly clawing), psoriasis, SLE, atopic dermatitis, eczema, use of solvents (including nail hardeners), and mycotic, pyogenic, or viral infections.

Domonkos AN, et al: Diseases of the skin appendages. In Andrews' Diseases of the Skin: Clinical Dermatology, 7th ed. Philadelphia, W.B. Saunders, 1982, pp 930–984.

14. Which rheumatic syndromes have been associated with uveitis?

Ankylosing spondylitis	Juvenile rheumatoid arthritis
Reiter's syndrome	Sjögren's syndrome
Psoriasis	Sarcoidosis
Inflammatory bowel disease	Behçet's disease
Kawasaki disease	Relapsing polychondritis

Rosenbaum JT: Uveitis. In McCarty DJ (ed): Arthritis and Allied Conditions, 11th ed. Philadelphia: Lea & Febiger, 1989, pp 1563–1568.

15. Which diseases are associated with soft tissue calcification?

Soft tissue calcification detected by plain roentgenograms can be an important clue in the diagnosis of rheumatic conditions. A partial list includes:

Calcific tendinitis	Neuropathic arthropathy
Chondrocalcinosis	Parathyroid disease
Dermatomyositis	Renal osteodystrophy
Diabetes	Sarcoidosis
Ehlers-Danlos syndrome	Scleroderma
Neoplasia	Trauma

Resnick D, Niwayama G: Soft tissues. In Resnick D, Niwayama G (eds): Diagnosis of Bone and Joint Disorders, 2nd ed. Philadelphia, W.B. Saunders, 1988, pp 4171–4294.

16. Which conditions commonly mimic systemic necrotizing vasculitis?

Bacterial endocarditis, atrial myxoma, and multiple cholesterol embolization syndrome have many of the same presenting signs and symptoms as systemic vasculitis.

17. What is the differential diagnosis of subcutaneous nodules?

Subcutaneous nodules are found in rheumatoid arthritis, rheumatic fever, and SLE. Additionally, gouty tophi, synovial cysts, and xanthomas can sometimes appear as subcutaneous nodules.

18. What are Gottron's papules?

Patches of erythematous scaly plaques on knuckles in patients with dermatomyositis.

RHEUMATOID ARTHRITIS

19. Give an operational definition for rheumatoid arthritis (RA).

RA is a *systemic* disease characterized clinically and pathologically by inflammation of diarthrodial joints. Although often accompanied by a variety of extra-articular manifestations, arthritis represents the major expression of the disorder, and currently we must rely on the characteristics of this expression to recognize the disorder.

20. Is there an HLA association with RA?

Approximately 93% of patients with RA have either the HLA-DR4 or -DR1 antigens. Exactly how these molecules confer increased susceptibility to the disease is unclear, but it is an area of active research.

McDermott M, McDevitt H: Immunogenetics of rheumatic diseases. Bull Rheum Dis 38(1):1–10, 1989.

21. Is there uniformity in the onset of RA?

Although some interesting patterns and observations of onset of RA have been described, these are of little diagnostic usefulness. For example, patients have been documented to develop RA twice as commonly in the months between October and March as between March and October. Most patients have an insidious onset of their disease. Generalized achiness and nonspecific symptoms may be followed by joint pain and swelling. Up to 15% of patients may have an abrupt onset of their disease, with the explosive development of intense, symmetrical, articular, stiffness, pain, and swelling. Occasionally, patients may suffer intermittent attacks involving single or multiple joints that gradually quiet, leaving them asymptomatic for prolonged periods. Hench coined the term "palindromic rheumatism" for this mode of presentation.

22. What is "gelling"?

Gelling describes the achiness and stiffness that occurs in RA patients after a period of inactivity.

23. How does pannus develop?

The synovium is a primary target for the inflammatory process in RA. In established disease, an infiltrate of mononuclear cells, primarily T lymphocytes, is seen. Additionally, activated macrophages and later plasma cells are present. Synoviocytes become hyperplastic. Grossly, the synovium becomes boggy and edematous with villous projections. This congested proliferative synovium is called **pannus.** Destruction of the joint occurs not only from the direct effect of the invading granulation tissue (pannus), but also from the degradative enzymes of the synovial fluid.

24. What are the mechanisms by which the classic swan neck and boutonnière deformities occur?

The **swan neck deformity** describes flexion at the metacarpophalangeal (MCP) and distal interphalangeal (DIP) joints with extension at the proximal interphalangeal (PIP) joints. This results from inflammation and subsequent contraction of interosseous and flexor muscles and tendons. Also contributing is the synovitis and destruction leading to MCP subluxation. There is flexion at the MCP, leading to exaggerated pull on the extensor tendon of the PIP. The flexion at the DIP is caused because the pull of the flexor tendon overcomes the pull of the extensor tendon.

Flexion contracture at the PIP with extension of the DIP is referred to as the **boutonnière deformity.** The pathogenesis of this deformity is thought to relate to an injury of the extensor tendon. If it becomes lengthened or torn, the flexor tendons are unopposed. The altered mechanics and location of the joint lead to functional shortening of the lateral tendons and hyperextension of the DIP joint.

25. What is the mechanism for the development of cocked-up toes in RA?

Inflammation of the metatarsophalangeal (MTP) joints in RA can often lead to subluxation of the metatarsal heads, leading to collapse of the arch of the foot. A claw-like or cocking up appearance of the toes follows.

McCarty DJ: Clinical picture of RA. In McCarty DJ, Koopman WJ (eds): Arthritis and Allied Conditions, 12th ed. Philadelphia, Lea & Febiger, 1993, pp 781–809.

26. What are rheumatoid factors (RF)? Which conditions are associated with their presence in the circulation?

RFs are antibodies (usually IgM) directed at the Fc portion of the IgG molecule. The presence of RF is not specific for RA, as patients with other rheumatic conditions, including SLE and Sjögren's syndrome, may have circulating RF. Viral, parasitic, and other infectious diseases including mononucleosis, hepatitis, malaria, tuberculosis, and bacterial endocarditis may be associated with these antibodies.

Carson DA: Rheumatoid factor. In Kelly WN, et al (eds): Textbook of Rheumatology, 4th ed. Philadelphia, W.B. Saunders, 1993, pp 155–163.

27. How many RA patients have no circulating RF detectable?

Up to 25% of patients with clinical RA have no circulating RF. In addition, it may take as long as 2 years for the RF to become detectable in those who ultimately do become seropositive. Thus, just when it would be most helpful diagnostically, RF is least likely to be present. The titer has little prognostic value in an individual patient, and remeasuring it provides little added information.

28. How many patients with RA test positive for antinuclear antibodies (ANA)?

Up to 25% of patients with established RA have circulating ANA. Patients with RA and Sjögren's syndrome often have positive anti-Ro antibodies. Patients with positive ANA are often considered to have a poorer prognosis.

29. Does RA confer an increased mortality?

For many years, it was felt that although RA was a painful and destructive condition, it had no influence on mortality. Recent studies have shown that patients with RA die an average of 10–15 years before a similar population without disease. Cause of death, interestingly enough, is not substantially different from that for the general population (cardiovascular disease and cancer leading the list). Predictors of early mortality of RA include older age, the presence of concomitant cardiovascular disease, high number of involved joints, fewer years of formal education, and poor functional status.

Pincus T, Callahan LF: Early mortality in RA predicted by poor clinical status. Bull Rheum Dis 41(4):1–4, 1992.

30. How has the general approach to the treatment of RA changed over the past decade? Why?

In the past, it was felt that *not* all RA was severe and required aggressive interventions. Treatment was instituted with the least toxic but also least efficacious medications. Medication would then be increased in a stepwise fashion as the disease flared or did not respond to treatment. Unfortunately, it may take 6 months to learn if a disease-modifying antirheumatic drug (DMARD) has failed, and considerable joint damage can be done in this period. The patient is left with early articular damage that will likely predispose to deformity and mechanical problems even if the disease is subsequently successfully controlled.

Data also have been accumulated on patient outcome when treated with this approach. Unfortunately, the likelihood of progressive deformity, disability, decline in the quality of life, and even increased mortality have been documented. Therefore, many rheumatologists now recommend earlier initiation of DMARDs and a more aggressive approach to the management of disease.

31. How is the functional capacity of RA patients classified?

- **Class I:** No restrictions, able to perform normal activities
- **Class II:** Moderate restriction, but able to perform normal activities.
- **Class III:** Marked restriction, inability to perform most duties of the patient's usual occupation or self-care.
- **Class IV:** Incapacitation or confinement to a wheelchair.

32. What classification scheme is available to describe the progression of RA?

Stage I: Early
- No destructive changes on x-ray examination
- X-ray evidence of osteoporosis acceptable

Stage II: Moderate
- X-ray evidence of osteoporosis with or without slight subchondral bone destruction; slight cartilage destruction may be present
- No joint deformities, although limitation of joint mobility may be present
- Adjacent muscle atrophy
- Extra-articular soft tissue lesions such as nodules or tenosynovitis may be present

Stage III: Severe
- X-ray evidence of cartilage and bone destruction in addition to osteoporosis
- Joint deformity such as subluxation, ulnar deviation, or hyperextension without fibrosis or bony ankylosis
- Extra-articular soft tissue lesions such as nodules or tenosynovitis may be present

Stage IV: Terminal
- Bony or fibrous ankylosis
- Criteria of Stage III

33. Which factors suggest an aggressive disease course in RA?

High titer RF, positive ANA, and nodules.

34. Do patients with RA develop gout with increased, decreased, or the same frequency as the general population?

There is a negative association between RA and gout.

35. How does pregnancy affect RA?

Signs and symptoms of RA quiet in approx. 70% of women during pregnancy. There are no data to suggest RA has a detrimental effect on the fetus. However, an assessment of the arthritis should be undertaken prior to pregnancy if possible, since anesthesia and intubation can be problematic and even dangerous when cervical spine disease is present. Delivery can also be difficult if arthritis limits hip motion. Postpartum flares of disease occur in approx. 90% of women who experienced improvement.

Griffin J: Rheumatoid arthritis: Biological effects and management. In Scott JS, Bird HA (eds): Pregnancy, Autoimmunity and Connective Tissue Disorders. Oxford, Oxford University Press, 1990, pp 140–162.

36. List some of the extra-articular manifestations of RA.

As noted previously, although synovium is the major target of disease in RA, the disease can effect nonjoint areas. Some specific nonarticular manifestations of disease are:
- Nodules
- Vasculitis
- Cardiac disease
- Pulmonary involvement
- Eye involvement
- Felty's syndrome

37. What are rheumatoid nodules? Where are they found?

The classic rheumatoid nodule has a central area of necrosis surrounded by a rim of palisading fibroblasts surrounded by a collagenous capsule with perivascular collections of chronic inflammatory cells. They occur in 20–35% of RA patients and can be found at the elbow, wrist, soles, Achilles tendon, head, or sacrum. RF is usually present in patients with rheumatoid nodules.

38. What is the classic clinical setting for the development of vasculitis associated with RA?

The development of vasculitis in RA patients classically occurs in patients with long-standing disease and severe joint disease with destruction, high titer RF, and nodules. Men are affected more than women. There is generally associated fever.

Conn DL, et al: Vasculitis and related disorders. In Kelly WN, et al (eds): Textbook of Rheumatology, 4th ed. Philadelphia, W.B. Saunders, 1993, pp 1077–1102.

39. How does RA affect the heart?

Cardiac involvement in RA can take several forms and is considered one of the extra-articular manifestations of the disease. Even though **pericardial disease** is present in nearly half of RA patients at autopsy and up to a third studied by echocardiography, the clinical impact of pericardial inflammation is usually minimal. **Myocarditis** has also been demonstrated, and may be granulomatous with nodules present. **Conduction defects, coronary arteritis,** and **granulomatous aortitis** have also been described.

40. How does RA affect the lung?

Pulmonary disease is an extra-articular feature of RA that increases both morbidity and mortality. **Pleural disease** is a common postmortem finding, but it is less commonly clinically relevant. **Pneumonitis** and **interstitial fibrosis** are also known to occur in RA. **Nodules** can be present in the lung and only rarely precede the articular disease; they may be present individually or in clusters and occasionally cavitate. Rarely, **arteritis** can be present and, if so, often leads to pulmonary hypertension. Finally, **airway disease** has been described, typically as reduced maximal midexpiratory flow rate and maximal expiratory flow rate at 50% of functional capacity. In its most severe form, **bronchiolitis obliterans** can occur, with a uniformly unfavorable outcome.

In addition to the RA itself, the treating physician should also consider drug induced lung disease. Methotrexate, D-penicillamine, gold salts, and even sulfasalazine have been associated with the development of pulmonary complications.

Anaya JM, et al: Pulmonary involvement in rheumatoid arthritis. Semin Arthr Rheum 24(4):242–254, 1995.

41. What is the mechanism for low pleural glucose in pleural effusions of RA?

It appears to result from a defect of the transport of glucose into the fluid.

42. What ocular abnormalities occur in RA?

Episcleritis and scleritis.

43. Define Felty's syndrome.

Felty's syndrome describes the constellation of circulating neutropenia and splenomegaly in patients with established RA. There are generally recurrent infections as well.

44. Does Still's disease occur in adults? How is it diagnosed?

Still's disease is the eponym assigned to systemic-onset juvenile arthritis. It has been reported in adults as a seronegative polyarthropathy associated with sudden-onset high fever and chills, with evanescent rash on the trunk and extremities. Bony erosions are uncommon, although fusion of the carpal bones may occur.

Reginato AJ: Adult onset Still's disease. In: Schumacher HR Jr, et al (eds): Primer on the Rheumatic Diseases, 10th ed. Atlanta, Arthritis Foundation, 1993, pp 182–183.

45. How does aspirin's effects on platelets differ from those of other NSAIDs?

NSAIDs, including aspirin, decrease platelet aggregation by inhibiting the enzyme cyclooxygenase. Acetylated salicylates (such as aspirin) irreversibly destroy this enzyme, whereas other NSAIDs (including nonacetylated salicylates) allow the return of normal enzyme function once the drug level has dropped.

46. What are the common GI side effects of NSAIDs?

NSAIDs are some of the most commonly used medications in the U.S., being available over-the-counter as well as by prescription. Side effects from this class of medication are among the most common reported to the FDA. They include:

1. Dyspepsia.

2. Gastroduodenal ulcer disease. NSAIDs may contribute to the development of ulcer disease in several ways. First, as a direct irritant to the mucosa. Second, because gastric prostaglandins inhibit gastric acid secretion and provide for mucosal defense, NSAIDs predispose the gastroduodenal mucosa to injury by inhibiting the production of prostaglandins. This second effect is really a systemic chemical effect of the medication, occurring with NSAIDs administered parenterally or via suppository as well as orally. Ulcer complications are more common in those taking NSAIDS than in those with ulcers not taking these drugs.

3. Enteropathy. Especially with long-term NSAID use, low-grade blood and protein loss has been documented. The etiology is unknown, but it has been hypothesized that NSAIDS lead to increased intestinal permeability.

4. Colon injury ("colopathy"). Reports include exacerbations of inflammatory bowel and diverticular disease.

5. Hepatic toxicity. Up to 15% of patients taking NSAIDs may have reversible hepatocellular toxicity, usually manifested by elevations of serum transaminases. Very rarely, more fulminant hepatopathy can occur, and therefore regular review of serum transaminases should occur in these patients.

Lichtenstein DR, et al: Nonsteroidal anti-inflammatory drugs and the gastrointestinal tract: The double edged sword. Arthritis Rheum 38:5–18, 1995.

47. What are the common side effects of methotrexate (MTX) when used for the treatment of RA?

Because of its effectiveness and its relatively quick onset of action (4–6 weeks compared to 4–6 months for gold or hydroxychloroquine), MTX is becoming more widely used *earlier* in the treatment of RA. Reported toxicities include stomatitis, alopecia, bone marrow suppression, macrocytosis, liver damage, and pulmonary disease. The latter can be mild or potentially life-threatening (pneumonitis) and may begin as a benign but persistent cough. It does appear that preexisting lung disease (especially interstitial disease) may predispose to MTX pulmonary toxicity.

Liver toxicity most commonly takes the form of transient elevation of serum transaminases. These episodes do not correlate with the more disturbing complication of hepatic fibrosis. Although the risk of fibrosis is unknown, long-term studies have produced waning concern about the need for liver biopsy after prolonged treatment. The drug is immunosuppressive and herpetic outbreaks as well as infections such as *Pneumocystis carinii, Nocardia asteroides,* and cytomegalovirus have been reported. MTX is teratogenic and should not be given to women who are or may become pregnant. It produces chromatin abnormalities in sperm and should not be given to men within 9–12 months of conception. MTX should not be used with trimethoprim/sulfamethoxazole because of increased toxicity. When given in modest doses (1 mg PO daily), folic acid has been shown to reduce some of the troubling toxicities of MTX without impairing its efficacy.

Golden MR, et al: The relationship of preexisting lung disease to the development of methotrexate pneumonitis in patients with rheumatoid arthritis. J Rheumatol 22:1043–1047, 1995.

Kremer JM, Phelps CT: Long-term prospective study of the use of methotrexate in the treatment of rheumatoid arthritis: Update after a mean of 90 months. Arthritis Rheum 35:138–145, 1995.

Weinblatt ME, et al: Long-term prospective study of methotrexate in the treatment of rheumatoid arthritis: 84-month update. Arthritis Rheum 35:129–137, 1995

48. What are some of the newer treatments for RA?

Cyclosporin A has been shown in double-blind placebo-controlled trials to be useful in the treatment of RA. Its toxicity, especially hypertension and potentially irreversible renal insufficiency (the latter likely worsened by concomitant use of NSAIDs), make it very difficult to use. It is not yet approved by the FDA for use in RA.

Minocycline has likewise been shown to be better than placebo in the treatment of RA. Its success may not be due to its antimicrobial effect.

Finally, in a small trial, a statistically significant number of patients had a response to orally given **chicken type II collagen.** The study was undertaken to try to take advantage of the incompletely understood concept of "oral tolerance".

SJÖGREN'S SYNDROME

49. What is Sjögren's syndrome?

Sjögren's syndrome is an inflammatory disease of exocrine glands manifested primarily by dryness of the eyes and mouth. It can occur as an isolated entity (primary Sjögren's syndrome) or in association with another rheumatic disease, commonly RA or SLE (secondary Sjögren's syndrome).

50. Which glands are most commonly involved in Sjögren's syndrome?

Major and minor salivary glands as well as lacrimal glands are commonly involved. These include parotid and submandibular glands.

51. How does one document keratoconjunctivitis sicca?

Many believe that Sjögren's syndrome is underdiagnosed. The first step then is to ask the appropriate **historical questions.** Inquiries about eye grittiness or the ability to eat crackers without water have been suggested as nonleading ways to ask about dryness. The **Schirmer's test** can document diminished output of the lacrimal glands. Likewise, **biopsy of the salivary glands** (usually in the lower lip) showing the presence of infiltrating lymphocytes establishes the diagnosis.

Talal N: Sjögren's syndrome and connective tissue diseases association with other immunologic disorders. In McCarty DJ, Koopman WJ (eds): Arthritis and Allied Conditions, 12th ed. Philadelphia, Lea & Febiger, 1993, pp 1343–1356.

52. What percent of patients with primary Sjögren's syndrome subsequently develop a connective tissue syndrome?

If symptoms of an underlying connective tissue disease do not appear within 12 months of the keratoconjunctivitis sicca, then the chances are approx. 10% that it will appear later in life.

53. Are patients with Sjögren's syndrome at increased risk for certain malignancies?

Yes, non-Hodgkin's lymphoma. The lymphomas are usually B-cell-derived, and some patients may also have serum protein spikes. The diagnosis of tumor may be difficult, given that the nonmalignant lymphoid infiltration of lymphocytes can often simulate neoplasm (pseudolymphoma).

SYSTEMIC LUPUS ERYTHEMATOSUS (SLE)

54. What are the most common clinical and laboratory features of SLE?

Clinical and Laboratory Features of SLE

FEATURE	FREQUENCY	FEATURE	FREQUENCY
Positive ANA	97%	Leukopenia	46%
Arthritis/arthralgia	80%	Anemia	42%
Fever	48%	Myalgia	60%
Skin involvement	71%	Nephritis	42%
Low complement	51%	Pleurisy	44%
Elevated anti-dsDNA	46%	CNS symptoms	32%

Wallace DJ: The clinical presentation in SLE. In Wallace DJ, et al (eds): Dubois' Lupus Erythematosus, 4th ed. Baltimore, Williams & Wilkins, 1993, pp 317–321.

55. Describe the common skin manifestations of SLE.

The skin is a frequent target organ in SLE. The classic lesion of **acute lupus** is the malar (butterfly) rash. This rash consists of an area of redness across the cheeks, usually involving the bridge of the nose, and is often exacerbated by UV light (either artificial or sunlight). Atrophic dermal scarring does not develop with clearing of the rash.

Symmetric, superficial, nonscarring annular lesions of the shoulders, upper arms, and back are the classic lesions of **subacute cutaneous lupus**. Nonscarring **alopecia** often occurs concurrently. These patients may or may not have circulating anti-Ro antibodies. These lesions are very photosensitive.

The skin lesions of **discoid lupus** (chronic cutaneous lupus erythematosus) most commonly occur over the face and neck. These lesions eventually become hypopigmented and atrophic.

Sontheirmer RD: Clinical manifestations of cutaneous lupus erythematosus. In Wallace DJ, et al (eds): Dubois' Lupus Erythematosus, 4th ed. Philadelphia, Lea & Febiger, 1993, pp 285–301.

56. What is subacute cutaneous lupus (SCLE)?

Some consider this cutaneous eruption somewhere between chronic discoid lupus and acute cutaneous lupus. The lesions generally occur on the shoulders, upper chest, and neck and are symmetric and nonscarring. They can be annular or resemble psoriasis. Between 25–50% of patients have constitutional symptoms, and they may have circulating antibodies to Ro antigen. There is an association with HLA-DRW3.

McCauliffe DP, Sontheimer RD: Subacute cutaneous lupus erythematosus. In Wallace DJ, et al (eds): Dubois' Lupus Erythematosus, 4th ed. Philadelphia, Lea & Febiger, 1993, pp 302–309.

57. What is the relationship between discoid lupus and systemic lupus?

This is an area of some controversy. Approximately 25% of patients with classic discoid lesions may have constitutional symptoms but do not meet the ARA criteria for SLE. Approx. 10% of discoid lupus patients go on to develop SLE. These data are inexact, since early epidemiologic studies lumped SCLE and discoid lupus together in assessing risk for the development of systemic disease.

58. How commonly does SLE affect the GI tract?

There are many GI manifestations in SLE, and they may be present in up to 50% of patients. Anorexia, nausea, and vomiting are among the most common. Oral ulceration (most commonly buccal erosions) were identified in 40% of one group studied. Esophageal involvement, either as esophagitis, esophageal ulceration, or esophageal dysmotility have all been reported. The latter seems to correlate with the presence of Raynaud's phenomenon. Intestinal involvement results in abdominal pain, diarrhea, and occasionally hemorrhage. Intestinal ischemia may be present and may progress to infarction and perforation. Pneumatosis intestinalis in SLE is usually benign and transient but may represent an irreversible necrotizing enterocolitis. Additionally, pancreatitis and abdominal serositis are well-recognized. Abnormal liver functions likewise occur. A vasculitic process has been implicated in the pathogenesis of these GI manifestations.

Wallace DJ: Gastrointestinal manifestations and related liver and biliary disorders. In Wallace DJ, et al (eds): Dubois' Lupus Erythematosus, 4th ed. Philadelphia, Lea & Febiger, 1993, pp 410–417.

59. What is the most common pathologic abnormality found in patients with lupus CNS disease?

Commonly used designations such as "lupus cerebritis" suggest that CNS lesions in lupus patients are usually inflammatory. Small infarcts and hemorrhages are more commonly encountered than vasculitis.

Johnson RT, Richardson EP. The neurological manifestations of systemic lupus erythematosus. Medicine 47:337–369, 1968.

60. What is the LE cell and how does it relate to the ANA?

An LE cell is a PMN that has ingested the nucleus of a damaged cell. The destruction occurs secondary to an autoantibody directed toward nuclear components. Thus, the LE cell is really a manifestation of circulating ANA.

61. What conditions are associated with a positive ANA?

- Lupus
- Drug-induced lupus
- Rheumatoid arthritis
- Systemic sclerosis
- CREST syndrome
- Polymyositis
- Dermatomyositis
- Mixed connective tissue disease
- Chronic hepatitis
- Infectious mononucleosis

62. Is the ANA one antibody?

The detection of the LE cell really initiated the study of autoantibodies. With the development of immunofluorescent techniques, different staining patterns were discovered, and it became clear that many different nuclear antigens could elicit an antibody response. Thus, many antibodies can be classified as ANA. Detecting the specific antibody reaction requires more refined techniques.

Antinuclear Antibodies

ANTIGEN	ANTIBODY
Deoxyribose phosphate backbone of DNA	Anti-DNA (double-stranded or native)
Purine and pyrimidine bases	Anti-single-stranded DNA
H1, H2A, H2B, H3, H2A/H2B complex, H3/H4 complex	Anti-histones
DNA topoisomerase I	Anti-SCL-70
Histidyl tRNA transferase	Anti-Jo-1
Kinetochore	Anti-centromere
RNA polymerase I	Anti-nucleolar
Y^1–Y^5 RNA and protein	Anti-Ro
U1–6 RNA and protein	Anti-RNP (includes anti-Sm)

von Mühlen CA, et al: Autoantibodies in the diagnosis of systemic rheumatic diseases. Semin Arthritis Rheum 24:323–358, 1995.

63. Do ANA staining patterns detect specific ANAs that are present? What is their clinical relevance?

The fluorescence test for ANA is performed by incubating the patient's serum with a fixed monolayer of human larynx epithelioma cancer (HEp-2) cell lines. If ANAs are present in the patient's serum, they bind to the nuclear component of the substrate. Next, fluorescent anti-Ig is added which binds to antibodies (if present) in the test serum. With the fluorescent tag, the ANA can be directly visualized under fluorescent light.

Different patterns of staining occur, and although they may provide some information, they do not identify the specific antibody present, nor are they specific for a disease entity. For example, the rim or peripheral pattern (usually associated with antibodies directed against nuclear membrane proteins) may be obscured if another autoantibody (staining a homogeneous pattern) is present.

64. Why is it helpful to know the specific ANA present in a patient?

Although no laboratory test is absolutely diagnostic for a rheumatic disease, the presence of certain autoantibodies in the appropriate clinical setting can be helpful. Some common disease associations include:

Ro/SSA	SLE, neonatal lupus syndrome, subacute lupus, Sjögren's syndrome, RA
DS DNA	SLE
Sm	SLE
Jo-1	Polymyositis
Centromere	CREST syndrome
SCL-70	Systemic sclerosis

Craft J, et al: Antinuclear antibodies. In Kelly WN, et al (eds): Textbook of Rheumatology, 4th ed. Philadelphia, W.B. Saunders, 1993, pp 164–187.

65. Which drugs are commonly associated with the development of a positive ANA?

Historically, a clinical syndrome of arthritis, fever, rash, and positive ANA was seen in some patients after initiating antihypertensive treatment with the drug hydralazine. Since then, the development of circulating ANA (primarily to histones) has been demonstrated with many drugs, including procainamide, diphenylhydantoin, isoniazid, chlorpromazine, D-penicillamine, sulfasalazine, methyldopa, and quinidine, among others.

Fritzler MJ, Rubin RL: Drug-induced-lupus. In Wallace DJ, et al (eds): Dubois' Lupus Erythematosus, 4th ed. Philadelphia, Lea & Febiger, 1993, pp 442–453.

66. Does lupus nephritis recur in a transplanted kidney?

Disease activity in SLE often quiets with the onset of uremia and dialysis. Several studies note the ability to discontinue glucocorticoids without a return of extrarenal manifestations of disease once dialysis has been initiated. Although there are reports of subsequent disease exacerbations, kidney transplantation can usually be accomplished *without* a return of disease activity.

67. Discuss the interaction of pregnancy and SLE.

There has been a considerable evolution of thought regarding pregnancy in patients with SLE:

1. Fertility is unaffected by the disease—i.e., patients get pregnant just as readily as persons without lupus.

2. Although recent data suggest that pregnant lupus patients do not have disease flares more frequently than nonpregnant lupus patients, disease exacerbations during pregnancy can occur. Because these flares can be severe, patients with SLE should be considered as high risk. Active disease during the antecedent 3–6 months may increase the risk of a flare.

3. Preeclampsia occurs more frequently in the pregnant lupus patient. There is also increased risk of miscarriage, abortion, intrauterine growth delay, and prematurity in patients with SLE when compared to controls.

4. The Ro antibody crosses the placenta and is responsible for most of the neonatal lupus syndromes, including skin manifestations and congenital heart block.

Lochshin MD: Pregnancy does not cause systemic lupus erythematosus to worsen. Arthritis Rheum 32:665–670, 1989.

68. What is the role of cytotoxic therapy in the treatment of nephritis in lupus patients?

Cytotoxic agents, such as azathioprine and cyclophosphamide, are useful in the management of many rheumatic diseases. Because of their toxicity, they should be used in situations where careful clinical trials point to significant advantages. One clinical condition in which clinical trials using cytotoxic agents have shown an advantage is in patients with lupus nephritis. Patients with inflammatory renal lesions had slower progression to end-stage renal disease and diminished mortality when their regimens included cyclophosphamide.

69. What is the antiphospholipid antibody (APA) syndrome?

APA syndrome refers to the clinical syndrome made up of one or more of the following: multiple miscarriages, arterial or venous thrombosis, and thrombocytopenia in association with a laboratory finding of antibodies directed against phospholipids. These antibodies can be specific (such as anticardiolipin antibodies) or they can be identified by their effect on the clotting cascade (lupus anticoagulant). Common laboratory tests indicating the presence of antibodies to various phospholipids include a prolonged PTT, false-positive VDRL, or positive anticardiolipin antibodies. Another is the dilute Russell Viper Venom clotting time. APA syndrome can occur by itself (primary APA syndrome) or in association with an underlying connective tissue syndrome, primarily lupus (secondary APA syndrome).

70. How frequently do APAs occur in established SLE?

A biological false-positive serologic test for syphilis occurs in 10% of SLE patients. The lupus anticoagulant is reported present in 6–10% and anticardiolipin antibodies in 15–40%.

71. Which rheumatic conditions are characteristically associated with Raynaud's phenomenon?

Raynaud's phenomenon is the eponym given to the occurrence of color change (usually red, white, and blue) in the hands (or any distal part of the body) that is incited by intense emotion or exposure to cold. When one inquires about Raynaud's, it is sometimes difficult not to suggest a positive answer. Thus, one might ask, "While grocery shopping, do you notice any problems in the frozen food section?" or "If you look at your hands when you get cold, do they look any different to you?" Many conditions have Raynaud's phenomenon as part of their clinical presentation. A partial list might include:

- SLE
- CREST syndrome
- Drug-induced lupus
- Reflex sympathetic dystrophy
- Systemic sclerosis
- Idiopathic Raynaud's phenomenon
- Polymyositis
- Sjögren's syndrome
- Cold agglutinin disease

72. What factors predict the development of systemic sclerosis in a patient presenting with Raynaud's phenomenon?

Patients presenting with Raynaud's phenomenon are at increased risk to develop a rheumatic disease. Positive serology, abnormal nailbed capillaries, or abnormal pulmonary function studies suggest an increased risk for development of disease.

73. List the noncutaneous features of scleroderma.

Arthritis, inflammatory muscle disease, GI dysmotility with resulting malabsorption, pulmonary interstitial fibrosis with resulting pulmonary hypertension, and scleroderma renal crisis.

74. Which autoantibodies are associated with polymyositis?

A positive ANA is not uncommon. Specifically, anti Jo-1, is found in polymyositis patients, particularly those who have concomitant pulmonary fibrosis. The antigen has been found to be histidyl-tRNA synthetase.

75. What is Jaccoud's deformity?

Deformities of the hands that occur secondary to chronic inflammation of the joint capsule, ligaments, and tendons. The changes may mimic those of RA (ulnar deviation of the fingers, MCP joint subluxation). Erosions are not present, although after several recurrences, notches may be seen in x-rays on the ulnar side of the metacarpal heads. Early on, patients can correct these changes voluntarily. Although originally described in rheumatic fever, this disorder has been extended to include the arthropathy occurring in other conditions, most commonly SLE.

SPONDYLOARTHROPATHIES

76. What is a spondyloarthropathy? What diseases are usually so classified?

Spondyloarthropathies describe a group of diseases of uncertain etiology that have a predilection for inflammatory lesions of the spine and sacroiliac joints. In addition, they are characterized by the absence of RF or other autoantibodies. Other unifying features include peripheral oligoarthropathy, enthesopathy, extra-articular foci of inflammation, and an association with HLA-B27. Diseases classified as spondylarthropathies include:

Ankylosing spondylitis
Reiter's syndrome
Arthropathy of psoriasis
Arthropathy associated with inflammatory bowel disease
Arnett FC: Sero-negative spondyloarthropathies. Bull Rheum Dis 37(1):1–12, 1987.

77. Define enthesopathy.

The *enthesis* is the junction of ligament and bone. It is the site of inflammation in the spondyloarthropathies. In response to this inflammation, reactive new bone is formed. This process accounts for the formation of syndesmophytes in ankylosing spondylitis.

78. What possible mechanisms exist to explain the association of HLA-B27 with arthropathy?

The mechanism by which HLA-B27 predisposes to arthritis after urogenital or intestinal infection is unknown. Two hypotheses include:

1. B27 is directly involved in disease predisposition. It might act as a receptor for a microorganism, or it could be modified by an infecting microorganism to elicit an immune reaction against the new antigen. Or, B27 might resemble the microbial epitopes, and thus antibodies directed against the microorganism cross-react with host antigens (molecular mimicry).

2. Disease susceptibility could be conferred by a particular configuration of the T-cell receptor. Recent data using transgenic mice make a previous hypothesis—that a gene closely linked to HLA-B27 was the pathogenic culprit—very unlikely.

Careless DJ, Inman RD: Etiopathogenesis of reactive arthritis and ankylosing spondylitis. Curr Opin Rheum 7:290–298, 1995.

79. What are the principal clinical features of ankylosing spondylitis?

Ankylosing spondylitis is one of the few inflammatory arthropathies that occurs more commonly in men than in women. The disease begins in late adolescence, usually with gradually worsening low back pain and stiffness. The pain typically improves with activity and worsens with rest, leading to the commonly experienced symptom of night-time awakening with pain and stiffness that requires getting out of bed to stretch. Peripheral joints may be involved early on, mostly in the lower limbs. The disease is generally progressive, and extra-articular features may develop.

The peripheral arthropathy can occur in both sexes, although sacroiliac and spinal involvement is more prominent in men.

Gran JT: An epidemiological survey of the signs and symptoms of ankylosing spondylitis. Clin Rheum Dis 4:161, 1985.

80. Name the extra-articular features of ankylosing spondylitis.

Anterior uveitis, aortitis, and pulmonary fibrosis.

81. What is the difference between a syndesmophyte and an osteophyte?

Syndesmophytes are thin vertical outgrowths and represent calcifications of the annulus fibrosis. As syndesmophytes enlarge, ossification can involve adjacent anterior longitudinal and paravertebral connective tissue. Syndesmophytes predominate on the anterior and lateral aspects of the spine, particularly near the thoracolumbar junction, eventually bridging the disc space and connecting one vertebral body with its neighbor. **Osteophytes** are triangular and arise several millimeters from the discovertebral junction.

82. How is inflammation of the sacroiliac (SI) joint graded radiographically?

- Grade I: normal
- Grade II: sclerosis of bone adjacent to the SI joints
- Grade III: erosion at the SI joints
- Grade IV: bony fusion across the SI joints

Arnett FC: Seronegative spondyloarthropathies. Bull Rheum Dis 37(1):1–12, 1987.

83. What is reactive arthritis?

Reactive arthritis is an inflammatory arthropathy of at least 1 month's duration occurring after a bout of urethritis or dysentery. The mechanism for the development of the arthropathy is unclear.

84. What are the mucocutaneous manifestations of Reiter's syndrome?

Skin and mucous membranes are commonly involved in Reiter's syndrome. Small painless areas of desquamation on the tongue may not even be noticed by the patient. Circinate balanitis, conversely, is rarely missed by the patient. It primarily affects the glans penis and can range from small erythematous macules to larger areas of dry flaking skin. Keratoderma blennorrhagica is a thickening and keratinization of the skin that generally involves the feet, hands, and nails. The lesions resemble psoriasis both clinically and pathologically.

Fan PT, Yu TY: Reiter's syndrome. In Kelly WN, et al (eds): Textbook of Rheumatology, 4th ed. Philadelphia, W.B. Saunders, 1993, pp 961–973.

85. Are there radiographic manifestations of Reiter's syndrome?

Periostitis at areas of tendinous insertions, frank articular erosions, and syndesmophyte formation have all been documented radiographically in Reiter's syndrome.

86. What five patterns of arthritis are associated with psoriasis? What are their relative frequencies?

- DIP joints of hands and/or feet   8%
- Peripheral asymmetric oligoarthropathy   48%
- Symmetric polyarthritis resembling RA   18%
- Arthritis mutilans ("opera glass hands")   2%
- Sacroiliitis with or without higher levels of spinal involvement   24%

Arnett FC. Sero-negative spondyloarthropathies. Bull Rheum Dis 37(1):1–12, 1987.

87. What percentage of people with psoriasis suffer from an associated inflammatory arthritis?

Anywhere from 6–20% of people with cutaneous psoriasis develop an inflammatory arthropathy. In 80% of these, the arthritis develops after the skin disease is already present.

88. Discuss the two patterns of arthritis associated with inflammatory bowel disease (IBD)?

Approx. 20% of patients with IBD have a peripheral arthropathy. This arthropathy is often accompanied by fever, oral ulcers, and eye or skin lesions (erythema nodosum or pyoderma gangrenosum). The activity of this arthropathy usually parallels the gut disease, but occasionally the arthropathy precedes the bowel symptoms. There is no increased frequency of HLA-B27 phenotype among patients with IBD and peripheral arthritis.

Sacroiliitis and spondylitis occur in approx. 10% of IBD patients, and HLA-B27 is found more commonly in IBD patients with this form of arthropathy. This arthropathy is independent of bowel disease activity, so that successful treatment of bowel disease does not influence outcome of spondylitis.

Arnett FC: Seronegative spondyloarthropathies. Bull Rheum Dis 37(1):1–12 1987.

89. What is pyoderma gangrenosum?

Pyoderma gangrenosum is the term applied to skin lesions that begin as pustules or erythematous nodules and break down to form spreading ulcers with necrotic, undermined edges. It is associated with IBD but also occurs in chronic active hepatitis, seropositive RA (without evidence of vasculopathy), leukemia, and polycythemia vera. Differential diagnosis of the lesions includes necrotizing vasculitis, bacterial infection, and spider bites.

CRYSTAL ARTHROPATHY

90. What three principal crystals are associated with joint inflammation?

Urate (gout)

Calcium pyrophosphate ("pseudogout")

Hydroxyapatite

Dieppe P, Calvert P: Crystals and Joint Disease. London, Chapman and Hall, 1983.

91. How does the polarizing microscope work? Why is it important in the diagnosis of rheumatic diseases?

Use of a polarizing microscope allows the identification of specific etiologies in certain clinical syndromes. Its function is based on the relatively simple observation that crystals rotate light (they are birefringent). Polarized light passing through a crystal will no longer be parallel to light not passing through the crystal. If a second polarizer is added so that its axis is rotated 90° (extinction) to the light as it emerges from the first polarizer but before reaching the crystal, then the only light reaching the observer's eye will be the light that the crystal has rotated.

92. Where is chondrocalcinosis commonly demonstrated roentgenographically?

Chondrocalcinosis describes the radiographic appearance of calcium pyrophosphate crystals in the joint cartilages. They are generally punctate and linear densities in the articular cartilages:

- Menisci of knee
- Radiocarpal joints
- Annulus fibrosis of intervertebral discs
- Symphysis pubis

93. What is the most common pathogenic mechanism for the development of hyperuricemia in gout?

Hyperuricemia can develop secondary to overproduction or underexcretion of urate. 5–15% of gout patients are found to be urate overproducers. The remaining patients have decreased renal clearance of urate, accounting for their hyperuricemia. Although nonrenal mechanisms for the removal of urate are known (GI tract, for example), diminished clearance by these routes does not lead to hyperuricemia.

94. What are the four stages of gout?

Stage 1 consists of **asymptomatic hyperuricemia**. There is elevated serum urate without articular disease or nephrolithiasis. Not all patients with asymptomatic hyperuricemia go on to develop gout, but the higher the serum level, the greater the likelihood of developing articular disease. In most cases, 20–30 years of sustained hyperuricemia pass before an attack of nephrolithiasis or arthropathy.

Stage 2 is reached with the first attack of **acute articular disease**. It is exquisitely painful and usually occurs in a single joint. There may be associated fever, swelling, erythema, and skin sloughing. 50% of initial attacks occur as podagra, and 90% of patients with gout have podagra at some stage of disease, if not treated.

Stage 3 is the period between attacks, described as **intercritical gout.** Generally, patients are completely asymptomatic. However, 62% of patients will have a second attack of articular disease within 1 year of the first attack, 16% within 1–2 years, 11% within 2–5 years, 4% after 5–10 years, and 7% after >10 years.

Stage 4 is termed **chronic tophaceous gout** and occurs with the development of chronic arthritis with tissue deposition of urate. The principal determinant of the rate of urate deposition is the serum urate concentration.

Gutman AB: The past four decades of progress in the knowledge of gout with an assessment of present status. Arthritis and Rheum 16:431, 1973.

95. Do women get gout?

Gout is being recognized with increasing frequency in women. Some distinctions from gout as it occurs in men have been observed. The disease has its onset later in life. In fact, it appears to occur after menopause (not too surprising given the hormonal influences on urate metabolism) in women not receiving supplemental estrogens. Diuretic therapy and renal insufficiency are also independent risk factors in women as compared to men with gout. Alcohol is a significantly less common precipitating factor in women than in men.

OSTEOARTHRITIS

96. Is osteoarthritis a genetic disease?

The role played by genetic factors in rheumatic disease is an area of vigorous research. Clearly, an hereditary component exists for osteoarthritis. Perhaps the most recognized feature is the presence of Heberden's nodes in mothers and sisters. Recent studies have uncovered a mutation in a type II collagen gene (Arg519 to Cys) that predisposes to early osteoarthritis.

Pun YL, et al: Clinical correlations of osteoarthritis associated with a single-base mutation (arginine 519 to cysteine) in type II procollagen gene: A newly defined pathogenesis. Arthritis Rheum 37:264–269, 1994.

97. Compare the biochemical changes of the aged joint with the osteoarthritic joint?

Although age is the single most significant epidemiologic factor associated with OA, there are biochemical differences between an old joint and an osteoarthritic one. The major components of the joint are the bone and cartilage. The major components of the cartilage include the chondrocytes and the matrix (which in turn is composed of collagen, water, and proteoglycans).

	Aging	*Osteoarthritis*
Bone	Osteoporosis	Thickened cortices, osteophytes, subchondral cysts, remodeling
Chondrocyte activity	Normal	Increased
Collagen	Increased cross-linking of fibrils	Irregular weave Smaller fibrils
Water	Slight decrease	Significant increase
Proteoglycan	Normal total content	Decreased total proteoglycan component
	Decreased chondroitins	Increased chondroitins
	Increased keratin	Decreased keratin
	Normal aggregation	Decreased aggregation

Brandt KD, Fife RS: Aging in relation to the pathogenesis of osteoarthritis. Clin Rheum Dis 12:117–130, 1986.

98. What is the prevalence of osteoarthritis in the population?

The prevalence of osteoarthritis increases with age. But it also depends on which criteria are used to make the diagnosis. The prevalence of osteoarthritis by autopsy in persons over age 65 years is nearly 100%. Roentgenographic studies reveal a prevalence ranging from approx. 4% in patients aged 18–24 years to >85% in persons older than 75 years.

99. Describe the syndrome of spinal stenosis.

Progressive narrowing of the spinal canal leads to the syndrome of spinal stenosis. This occurs most commonly because of osteoarthritis of the lumbar or cervical spine. With cervical disease, patients typically present with pain and limitation of motion. Hyperreflexia is common. Other signs may include muscle weakness, spastic gait, and Babinski's sign. In the lumbar region, the clinical manifestations are mostly those of compression of the cauda equina, commonly claudication.

100. What is the difference between spondylolysis and spondylolisthesis?

Spondylolysis refers to an interruption of the pars interarticularis of the vertebra. **Spondylolisthesis** refers to displacement of one vertebra on another. The most common etiology of spondylolisthesis is bilateral spondylolysis. Severe osteoarthritis of the apophyseal joints can produce spondylolisthesis without spondylolysis.

101. What is the vacuum sign?

A radiographic sign of intervertebral osteochondrosis. These radiolucencies represent gas (nitrogen) that appears at the site of negative pressure produced by abnormal spaces or clefts. Clefts are produced by degeneration of intervertebral disc, especially the nucleus pulposus.

102. What is DISH?

Diffuse idiopathic skeletal hyperostosis, or DISH, is a syndrome characterized by extensive ossification of tendinous and ligamentous attachments to bone. Involvement of the spine with flowing calcification over the anterior longitudinal ligament is among the most common findings. Extraspinal manifestations are reported as well. Clinical symptoms are often mild and consist of morning stiffness and deep achiness of the affected portion.

The following radiographic features help to distinguish DISH from ankylosing spondylitis, degenerative spine disease, and spondylosis deformans:

1. Flowing calcification along the anterolateral aspect of at least four contiguous vertebral bodies.

2. Relative preservation of intervertebral disc height in the involved vertebral segment and the absence of extensive radiographic changes of "degenerative" disc disease (vacuum phenomena, vertebral body marginal sclerosis).

3. Absence of apophyseal joint ankylosis and sacroiliac joint erosion, sclerosis, and intra-articular osseous fusion.

103. List five classic radiographic findings of osteoarthritis.
1. Subchondral cyst formation
2. New bone formation (osteophytes)
3. Sclerosis of bone
4. Joint space narrowing
5. Lack of osteoporosis

INFECTIOUS ARTHRITIS

104. What is the mechanism for acute rheumatic fever?
Rheumatic fever occurs after a group A streptococcal pharyngitis (which may not be symptomatic). Data indicate that the immune response initiated against the bacteria plays an important role. These antibodies cross-react with human antigens, leading to a persistent autoimmune reaction and tissue destruction (molecular mimicry). Development of immune complexes has also been documented.

105. What common viral illnesses are associated with arthropathy?
Common viruses that have an associated arthropathy include hepatitis B, parvovirus B19, rubella, and HIV. Chronic hepatitis B with persistent circulating B antigen has been associated with polyarteritis nodosa. Hepatitis C has a dramatically high rate of occurrence in patients with mixed cryoglobulinemia, and this virus also has been documented in several cases of otherwise unexplained inflammatory polyarthropathy.

Active infection with parvovirus has been associated with a nondestructive RA-like picture, with RFs even documented in circulation. Interestingly, the arthropathy clears without any chronic or destructive sequelae.

Some rare viral infections strongly associated with arthropathy include the group A arboviruses (Ross River virus, chikungunya, o'ynong-nyong, sindbis, Mayaro). Common viral infections that occasionally produce arthropathy include mumps, smallpox (vaccinia), Epstein-Barr virus, cytomegalovirus, and enteroviruses (ECHO and coxsackievirus).

Naides SJ: Viral arthritis including HIV. Curr Opin Rheumatol 7:337–342, 1995.

106. What are the most common bacterial pathogens responsible for septic arthritis?
Septic arthritis is usually classified as gonococcal or nongonococcal. Of the nongonococcal bacteria causing joint infections, *Staphylococcus* remains most common. Species of *streptococcus* are the next most frequent when grouped together. Finally, gram-negative bacilli may cause 20–30% of septic joints.

107. Describe the common clinical manifestations of gonococcal arthritis.
Gonococcal arthritis occurs in approx. 0.1–0.5% of patients with gonorrhea. Clinical manifestations may differ from those of other bacterial arthropathies. Even under optimal conditions, joint fluids are culture-positive in <50% of cases. The arthropathy is commonly migratory and often accompanied by tenosynovitis. Skin lesions are often present, usually as a small macule or papule on a distal extremity.

108. Name the classic skin manifestation of Lyme disease.
Erythema chronicum migrans. This is an expanding erythematous ring with central clearing beginning at the sight of the tick bite. The *Borrelia* organism can be cultured from the margin of lesion. The rash is occasionally accompanied by flu-like symptoms.

Recently, *Borrelia* has been found in diffuse fasciitis. The disease caused by European ticks produce what is described as acrodermatitis chronica atrophicans.

Evans J: Lyme disease. Curr Opin Rheumatol 7:322–328, 1995.

109. Is the chronic arthritis of Lyme disease produced by active joint infection?

About 70% of untreated Lyme patients in the U.S. get arthritis. It may take the form of arthralgia, intermittent episodes of arthritis, or, in about 10% of patients, a chronic inflammatory synovitis. Treatment failure is associated with HLA-DR4. Some hypothesize that an autoimmune response is produced; others have suggested persistent infection. Data, including that using PCR technology, suggest acute arthritis is due to active infection, although viable organisms may not be necessary for the development of a chronic synovitis.

Evans J: Lyme disease. Curr Opin Rheumatol 7:322–328, 1995.

MISCELLANEOUS RHEUMATIC CONDITIONS

110. What are the muscles of the rotator cuff? What syndromes are associated with their malfunction?

The muscles of the rotator cuff include supraspinatus, infraspinatus, teres minor, and subscapularis, and disease of the rotator cuff is a common cause of shoulder pain. **Impingement syndrome** occurs when the supraspinatus tendon gets caught between the head of the humerus and the acromion, resulting in pain. The activity most likely to bring these structures into proximity (and thus cause pain) is overhead movement and internal rotation of the arm. Night pain is characteristic. If the tendon ruptures (rotator cuff tear) significant weakness may result. Impingement syndrome usually results from injury to the supraspinatus during repetitive elevation and forward motion of the arm. **Rotator cuff tendinitis** is often an acute problem and may be associated with calcification.

111. What are the most common causes of the neuropathic joint in the upper extremity?

Without sensation and proprioception as regulators of joint function, there is a gradual relaxation of supporting structure, abnormal mechanics, and ultimately joint destruction. Many diseases including congenital pain insensitivity, amyloidosis, diabetes mellitus, alcoholism, and tabes dorsalis can lead to neuroarthropathy. In the upper extremities, particularly the elbow, syringomyelia is a common cause of sensory abnormalities leading to arthropathy.

112. Describe the rheumatic manifestations of sarcoidosis.

Sarcoidosis is a systemic disease characterized by a noncaseating granulomatous reaction of unknown origin. Besides the lungs, involvement of the eyes, skin, and joints is not uncommon. Skin involvement, including erythema nodosum, occurs in approx. 30% of patients. Asymptomatic sarcoid granulomas have been found in muscle biopsy, and may occur in bones, appearing radiographically as cysts. Osteolysis has also been described.

Articular symptoms are present in most patients with acute sarcoidosis (hilar adenopathy, fever, erythema nodosum), often affecting the ankles and knees. This articular syndrome is usually self-limited, lasting up to 4 weeks. When the disease is less acute in onset, articular involvement is less common. It can, however, be recurring and protracted, although joint destruction is infrequent. The articular involvement may predate the pulmonary involvement or occur after 10 years of disease.

113. Which conditions are associated with Dupuytren's contracture?

Fibrosis and thickening of the palmar fascia can lead to the flexion contracture first described by Dupuytren. Associated diseases include diabetes mellitus, chronic liver disease, epilepsy, plantar fasciitis, carpal tunnel syndrome, RA, trauma to the hand, pulmonary tuberculosis, and alcoholism, to name a few.

114. Which conditions are associated with mononeuritis multiplex?

Mononeuritis multiplex is a peripheral neuropathy involving one or more nerves. It is sometimes difficult to distinguish from other mononeuropathies caused by local factors, such as trauma, compression (acoustic neuroma or peroneal palsy), and entrapment (carpal tunnel). Reported associations include diabetes mellitus, polyarteritis, SLE, RA, Lyme disease, Sjögren's syndrome, cryoglobulinemia, giant cell arteritis, scleroderma, leukemia, leprosy, AIDS, carcinoma, and lymphoma. One recent study found that even after extensive workup, almost half of all nondiabetic patients with EMG evidence of mononeuritis multiplex did not have an established diagnosis.

Hellmann CB, et al: Mononeuritis multiplex: The yield of evaluations for occult rheumatic disease. Medicine 67(3):145–153, 1988.

115. What are the characteristic features of Wegener's granulomatosis?

Wegener's granulomatosis is one of the systemic necrotizing vasculopathies. The organs primarily affected are the respiratory tract (upper and/or lower) and kidneys. Respiratory tract involvement can manifest as recurrent sinusitis, otitis media, tracheobronchial inflammation and erosions, or pneumonitis with cavitation. With the inflammatory process unchecked, a saddle-nose deformity can occur. Additional symptoms, such as arthritis, neuropathies, and eye inflammation, can occur. Laboratory data are generally nonspecific, but recently an antibody to cytoplasmic components of the PMN leukocyte (c-ANCA) has been associated with active disease.

116. What are anti-neutrophil cytoplasmic antibodies (ANCA)?

ANCAs are antibodies directed against enzymes found in azurophilic granules (proteinase-3 [PR-3] and myeloperoxidase). Immunofluorescence detects two principal staining patterns: a fine granular cytoplasmic staining (c-ANCA) and a perinuclear collection of antibody (p-ANCA). Despite the similar in vivo location of these enzymes, ethanol fixation produces an artifactual migration of the myeloperoxidase to a perinuclear location. There is no movement of the PR-3, which then produces the cytoplasmic staining pattern. Although artifactual, the staining distinction is useful.

The p-ANCA is most associated with a microscopic polyarteritis or a pauci-immune crescentic glomerulonephritis. The PR-3 ANCA (usually staining as c-ANCA) is more sensitive and specific for Wegener's granulomatosis. In fact, the antibody has often allowed earlier diagnosis and allowed description of what appears to be milder forms of the disease. There seems to be a correlation between disease activity and titers of c-ANCA in Wegener's patients.

Gross WL, Csernok E: Immunodiagnostic and pathologic aspects of antineutrophil cytoplasmic antibodies in vasculitis. Curr Opin Rheumatol 7:11–19, 1995.

117. Name the characteristic features of Churg-Strauss vasculitis.

The Churg-Strauss syndrome, one of the systemic necrotizing vasculopathies, is associated with **eosinophilia** (circulating or tissue infiltration) and late-in-life onset of **atopic disease** (asthma or allergic rhinitis). This disease has been hypothesized to represent an overlap between the hypereosinophilic syndromes and vasculitides.

118. What is fibromyalgia (FM)?

FM is a chronic nondestructive illness characterized by fatigue, generalized pain, sleep disturbance (sometimes termed "nonrestorative" sleep), and tender points in a characteristic distribution (see figure on next page). FM replaces the term *fibrositis* since no inflammatory process has been objectively documented. Patients may have only FM or may have concomitant diseases, such as RA, osteoarthritis, Lyme disease, and sleep apnea, to name a few. The disease is often mimicked by hypothyroidism.

In addition to the generalized achiness, patients may have associated irritable bowel syndrome, tension headaches, irritable bladder, and even a chronic cough. Sleep is disturbed by alpha intrusion into delta sleep as documented by EEG. Eighteen reproducible tender points have been established, and diagnosis of FM requires the presence of at least 11 of these.

Treatment is aimed at reconditioning muscles (slow but consistent physical training), restoration of more-normal sleep patterns (tricyclic antidepressants in low doses are often helpful), and pain control (generally using non-narcotic medications such as NSAIDs or acetaminophen and other techniques such as biofeedback).

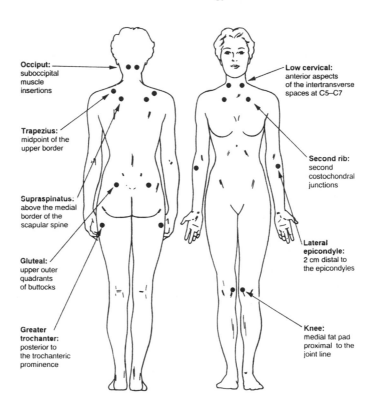

Location of tender points in fibromyalgia.

Wolfe F, et al: The American College of Rheumatology 1990 criteria for the classification of fibromyalgia: Report of the multicenter criteria committee. Arthritis Rheum 33:160–172, 1990.

Figure from Freundlich B, et al: The fibromyalgia syndrome. In Schumacher HR Jr, et al (eds): Primer on the Rheumatic Diseases, 10th ed. Atlanta, Arthritis Foundation, 1993, p 247; with permission.

BIBLIOGRAPHY

1. Kelly WN, et al (eds): Textbook of Rheumatology, 4th ed. Philadelphia, W.B. Saunders, 1993.
2. McCarty DJ, Koopman WJ (eds): Arthritis and Allied Conditions, 12th ed. Philadelphia, Lea & Febiger, 1993.
3. Resnick D, Niwayama G (eds): Diagnosis of Bone and Joint Disorders, 2nd ed. Philadelphia, W.B. Saunders, 1988.
4. Schumacher HR Jr, et al (eds): Primer on the Rheumatic Diseases, 10th ed. Atlanta, Arthritis Foundation, 1993.
5. Sheon RP, et al (eds): Soft Tissue Rheumatic Pain: Recognition, Management, Prevention, 2nd ed. Philadelphia, Lea & Febiger, 1987.
6. West SG (ed): Rheumatology Secrets. Philadelphia, Hanley & Belfus, 1997.

12. ALLERGY AND IMMUNOLOGY

Anthony J. Zollo, Jr., M.D.

Some men also have strange antipathies in their natures against that sort of food which others love and live upon. I have read of one that could not endure to eat either bread or flesh; of another that fell in a swooning fit at the smell of a rose. . .there are some who, if a cat accidentally come into the room, though they neither see it, nor are told it, will presently be in a sweat, and ready to die away.

Increase Mather
Remarkable Providence (1639–1723)

1. Name the two major limbs of the immune system and the principal components of each.

The two major limbs of the immune system are **humoral immunity** (HI) and **cellular** or **cell-mediated immunity** (CMI). Although this division has some usefulness, there are many interactions and areas of overlap between the two limbs. The humoral response is primarily mediated by antibodies produced by terminally differentiated B cells (plasma cells), but the complement system also plays an important role. HI serves as the principal host defense against bacterial infections and also functions in other important immune responses, such as antibody-dependent cellular cytotoxicity (ADCC).

The principal effector of CMI is the T cell, although macrophages and other cellular components are important participants. Intact CMI is critical for host defense against viral, fungal, and protozoan infections, and against development of malignancies, particularly of the lymphoreticular system. An important example of CMI is delayed-type hypersensitivity.

2. What is the major histocompatibility complex (MHC)?

The MHC is a cluster of genes (located on chromosome 6 in man) whose products play critical roles in regulation of immune recognition and responsiveness. In man, MHC genes code for class I (HLA-A, -B, -C), class II (HLA-DR, -DQ, -DP), and class III (complement components C2, C4, factor B) antigens, as well as a number of other molecules with important immunoregulatory properties, including tumor necrosis factor alpha and tumor necrosis factor beta (lymphotoxin).

3. What are B lymphocytes (B cells)?

B cells are derived from hematopoietic stem cells and are precursors of plasma cells, which are the antibody- or immunoglobulin-producing cells in the body. They are found primarily in the bone marrow, spleen, lymph nodes, and peripheral blood.

4. What is an antibody? What is its basic structure?

An antibody or immunoglobulin (Ig) molecule is a protein produced by B cells in response to antigen and has the ability to bind to the antigen that induced its formation. The basic Ig structure (see figure) consists of four polypeptide chains, two light and two heavy chains. The two heavy chains, and the light chains and heavy chains, are bound together by inter-chain disulfide bonds. The exception to this is IgA2, in which the light and heavy chains are not co-valently linked to each other. There are two types of light chains, kappa (κ) and lambda (λ), but all light chains of any individual Ig molecule are either kappa or lambda. The carboxy-terminal half is the constant region of the light chain (C_L) and heavy chain (C_H), and the amino-terminal half is the variable region (V_L and V_H). The heavy chain constant region contains three domains in IgG, IgD, and IgA, and four domains in IgE and IgM. These constant regions are responsible for the functional aspects of the Ig molecules (i.e., complement binding to the C_H2 region), whereas the light and heavy chain variable regions together determine antibody specificity and binding to antigen. IgG, IgD, and IgE are monomeric in form. IgM is pentameric, and IgA is either monomeric or polymeric (some serum and all secretory IgA are dimers). Some of the major characteristics and biologic functions of the five isotypes of Ig are shown in the table for question 6.

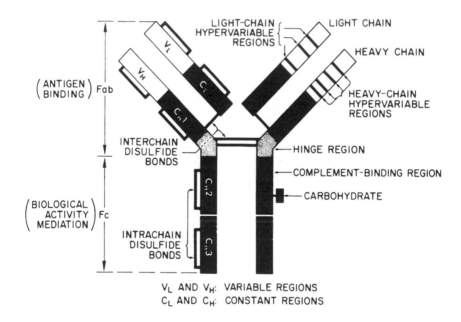

Structure of an Ig molecule. The figure is a schematic representation of an Ig molecule indicating the chain and domain structure of the molecule and the existence of hypervariable regions within variable regions of both H and L chains. Fab and Fc refer to fragments of the IgG molecule formed by papain cleavage. The former contains the V_H and C_H1 H chain regions and an intact L chain; the latter consists of C_H2 and C_H3 region of two H chains, linked to one another by disulfide bonds. (From Wasserman RL, Capra JD: Immunoglobulins. In Horowitz Ml, Pigman W (eds): The Glycoconjugates. New York, Academic Press, 1977, pp 323–348, with permission.)

5. What are the features of primary and secondary antibody responses?

A primary antibody response occurs following the first exposure to an antigen, while secondary antibody response occurs with the second and subsequent exposures. Major features of these two responses are illustrated at right.

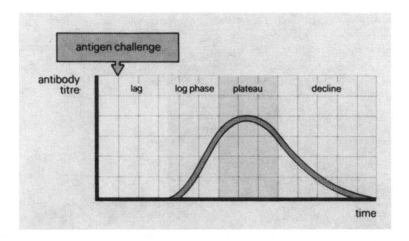

The four phases of a primary antibody response. Following antigen challenge the antibody response proceeds in four phases:

1. a lag phase when no antibody is detected;
2. a log phase when the antibody titer rises logarithmically;
3. a plateau phase during which the antibody titer stabilizes; and
4. a decline phase during which the antibody is cleared or catabolized.

From Roitt IM, et al: Immunology. New York, Gower Medical, 1985, Fig. 8.1, p 8.1, with permission.

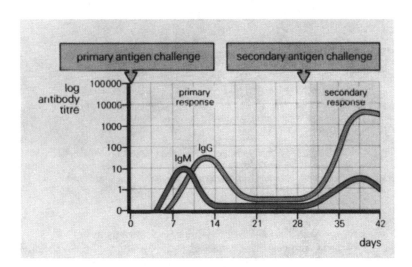

Primary and secondary antibody responses. In comparison with the antibody response following primary antivenin challenge, the antibody level following secondary antigenic challenge in a typical immune response:

1. appears more quickly and persists for longer;
2. attains a higher titer;
3. consists predominantly of IgG. In the primary response the appearance of IgG is preceded by IgM.

From Roitt IM, et al: Immunology. New York, Gower Medical, 1985, Fig. 8.2, p 8.1, with permission.

6. What are the physical and biologic properties of the different classes of immunoglobulin (Ig)?

Physical and Biologic Properties of Human Immunoglobulins*

PROPERTY	IgG	IgA	IgM	IgD	IgE
Molecular form	Monomer	Monomer, polymer	Pentamer	Monomer	Monomer
Subclass	IgG 1,2,3,4	IgA 1,2	None		
Molecular weight	150,000 for IgG 1,2,4 180,000 for IgG3	160,000	950,000	175,000	190,000
Serum level (mg/cc)	9,3,1,0.5	2.1	1.5	4	0.03
Serum half-life (days)	IgG 1,2,4:23 IgG 3:7	6	10	3	2
Complement fixation	IgG 1,2,3+ but IgG4−	−	+	−	−
Placental transfer	+	−	−	−	−
Other properties	Secondary response	Mucous secretions	Primary response, rheumatoid factor	Class switching	Allergy

*The plus and minus signs indicate whether the pathway exists (+) or not (−).
Modified from Samter M. et al (eds): Immunological Diseases, 4th ed. Boston, Little, Brown, 1988, p 44, with permission.

7. Summarize the functions of the complement system.

The complement system functions as part of humoral immunity and also promotes inflammatory reactions. Specific functions of the complement system are summarized in the figure below.

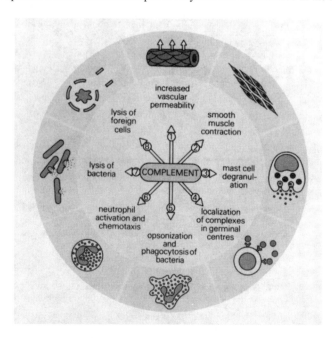

Summary of the actions of complement and its role in the acute inflammatory response. Note how the elements of the reactions are induced: increased vascular permeability (1) due to the action of C3a and CSa on smooth muscle (2) and mast cells (3) allows exudation of plasma protein. C3 facilitates both the localization of complexes in germinal centers (4) and the opsonization and phagocytosis of bacteria (5). Neutrophils, which are attracted to the area of inflammation by chemotaxis (6), phagocytose the opsonized microorganisms. The membrane attack complex, C5–9, is responsible for the lysis of bacteria (7) and other cells recognized as foreign (8). (From Roitt IM, et al: Immunology. New York, Gower Medical, 1989, Fig. 13–22, p 13.11, with permission.)

8. Compare the activation sequences of the classical and alternative complement pathways.

Classical complement pathway activation utilizes components C1–9. Activation of the alternative pathway also consumes C5–9 but not C1, 2, and 4. The classical and alternative pathways are diagrammed below.

An overview of the complement cascade showing the classical and the alternative pathways. The central position of C3 in both pathways is indicated. (From Samter M (ed): Immunological Diseases, 4th ed. Boston, Little, Brown, 1988, p 205, with permission.)

9. What factors cause activation of the classical complement pathway?

The classical pathway is principally activated by antibody-antigen (immune) complexes. A single IgM or two IgG molecules (IgG doublet) of IgG subclasses 1, 2, and 3, but not 4, bind C1, causing complement activation. Certain viruses, urate, and DNA also may activate the classical pathway.

10. What factors cause activation of the alternative complement pathway?

Substances that activate the alternative pathway include zymosan; cobra venom factor; bacterial lipopolysaccharide; aggregated IgG, M, A, and E; and cells that are free of sialic acid on their surface. Most bacteria, some parasites, and virtually all plant cells lack sialic acid. Some of the pathogenicity of encapsulated bacteria that have sialic acid as part of their capsule may be due to their ability to evade destruction by the alternative pathway.

11. What considerations limit the usefulness of serum complement levels in assessing the role of complement pathway activation in a disease process?

When interpreting serum complement levels (C3 and C4), one must realize that a normal level does not rule out either complement activation or complement-mediated tissue damage. In some diseases, complement synthesis is increased (i.e., acute inflammation), thereby potentially masking increased consumption. In addition, under certain conditions, complement may be extremely efficient at causing cell damage without lowering serum levels. Furthermore, serum complement levels do not necessarily reflect activity in other body compartments. For example, in rheumatoid arthritis, complement levels may be normal in serum but decreased in joint fluid. Finally, low serum complement levels may occur in hepatic failure due to decreased synthesis of complement components.

12. What patterns of serum C3 and C4 levels are seen with activation of the classical and alternative complement pathways? Name at least one disease associated with each pattern.

Serum Complement Levels in Disease

PATHWAY	C4	C3	DISEASE
Classical	↓	↓	Systemic lupus erythematosus, serum sickness
Classical (Fluid phase)	↓	N	Hereditary angioedema
Alternative	N	↓	Endotoxemia (gram negative sepsis)
Alternative (Fluid phase)	N	↓	Type II membranoproliferative glomerulonephritis (C3 nephritic factor)

↓ = Decreased, ↑ = Increased, N = Normal

13. What are the two major pathways of arachidonic acid metabolism? What effects do aspirin, NSAIDs, eicosapentaenoic acid (fish oil), and corticosteroids have on mediator production by these pathways?

Prostaglandins (PG) and thromboxanes are produced via the cyclooxygenase (CO) and leukotrienes (LT) by the lipoxygenase pathways of arachidonic acid metabolism. These eicosanoids exhibit an array of potent inflammatory and immunoregulatory properties. Aspirin and NSAIDs inhibit CO and, therefore, PG/thromboxane but not LT production. Eicosapentaenoic acid (fish oil) inhibits both PG/thromboxane and LT formation by preferential fatty acid substitution for arachidonic acid in the cell membranes of eicosanoid-producing cells. Corticosteroids also inhibit both PG/thromboxane and LT generation by stimulating production of the in-

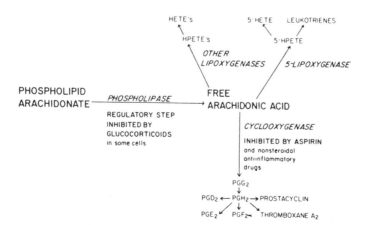

Sites of inhibition of arachidonic acid release and metabolism by pharmacologic agents. (From Wyngaarden JB, Smith LH: Cecil Textbook of Medicine, 17th ed. Philadelphia, W.B. Saunders, 1985, p 1240, with permission.)

tracellular protein, lipocortin, which inhibits the activity of phospholipase A. Specific lipoxyge-nase inhibitors are currently undergoing clinical trials.

14. What are alpha, beta, and gamma interferons (IFNs)?

Since their discovery, interferons have been divided into three classes, IFN-α, IFN-β, and IFN-γ. IFN-α and IFN-β were previously classified as Type I and IFN-γ as Type II. IFN-α comprises 20 or more subtypes, all of which have a high degree of homology. IFN-β has at least two subtypes. IFN-β_1 has only about a 34% sequence homology with IFN-α, but the biologic effects of both are similar. IFN-β_2 has been found to be "B cell differentiation factor-2," now named interleukin-6 (IL-6). It has essentially no homology with IFN-α. IFN-γ is unrelated to the other IFNs in either structure or function.

15. Which cells produce interferon and what are their major function(s)?

IFN-α is produced by leukocytes, fibroblasts (to a lesser degree), and many other cells. IFN-β_1 is produced by fibroblasts, leukocytes (to a lesser degree), and many other cells. Both IFN-α and IFN-β_1 function in the immunomodulation of antibody production, graft rejection, and delayed-type hypersensitivity (DTH) reactions. They can induce autoimmune and inflammatory reactions, and they play a role in antiviral, antibacterial, antifungal, and antitumor responses.

IFN-β_2 (IL-6) is produced by fibroblasts, T cells, monocytes, and endothelial cells, and has poor antiviral activity. It has also been called "B cell differentiation factor," because it stimulates the differentiation of mature B cells to immunoglobulin-secreting plasma cells. It also plays a role in early hematopoiesis and may be an important autocrine growth factor for multiple myeloma and other malignancies.

IFN-γ is produced by activated T lymphocytes, natural killer (NK) cells, and lymphokine-activated killer (LAK) cells. Its biologic effects include enhancing cytotoxic T cell and NK cell activity; induction of class II antigen expression on B cells, multiple antigen presenting cells, dendritic cells, endothelial cells, and fibroblasts; induction of IL-2 receptor expression on T cells; down-regulation of collagen synthesis; and inhibition of IL-4-induced IgE synthesis.

16. What is the bursa of Fabricius and which lymphoid organ is its equivalent in humans?

The bursa of Fabricius is the site of B cell development in the chicken *(Gallus domesticus)*. In humans, B cell maturation occurs primarily in the bone marrow.

17. Outline B cell ontogeny from stem cell to plasma cell.

Stem cell → Pre-B cell → Immature B → Mature B → Activated →
Secretory B → Plasma cell

18. What is the role of surface Ig on B cells?

Surface Ig serves as the antigen-binding site and as an activation receptor for B cells. Receptor function includes both signal transduction and participation in antigen processing and presentation for cognate interaction with T cells.

19. What are the major subtypes of T cells? Describe the principal function of each.

T cells function both as effectors and regulators of the immune response. Like B cells, they are derived from the embryonic hematopoietic stem cells. The major types of T cells are:

1. *CD4+ T cells:* These function primarily as helper/inducer T cells by providing soluble and cognate signals to B cells for stimulating antibody production. Antigen recognition is MHC class II restricted.

2. *CD8+ T cells:* These cells function as cytotoxic and suppressor T cells. Cytotoxic T cell function includes recognition and destruction of cells bearing antigen recognized as foreign. Examples include tumor cells, virally infected cells, and allogeneic cells. An example of suppressor cell function is inhibition of antibody synthesis by B cells. CD8+ T cell function is MHC class I restricted.

20. What is the CD nomenclature of phenotyping cells?

The CD (cluster designation) nomenclature is a system for the universal identification of cell surface antigens that have been defined by monoclonal antibodies. Some of the major CD markers are listed on the next page.

Characteristics of Cell Surface Markers

SURFACE MARKER	COMPOSITION	ALTERNATIVE NAMES	SITES OF EXPRESSION	COMMENTS
T cell receptor	43 kd glycoprotein, 40 kd glycoprotein	TCR, Ti	Thymocytes, T cells	Recognizes antigen
CD2	50 kd protein	LPA-2, T11, sheep red blood cell receptor	Thymocytes, T cells, NK cells (large granular lymphocytes)	Adhesion molecule that binds to LFA-3; anti-T11$_2$ is mitogenic
CD3	25 kd glycoprotein, 20 kd glycoprotein, 20 kd protein	T3, Leu-4	Thymocytes, T cells	Associated with T cell receptor; anti-CD3 is mitogenic
CD4	57 kd glycoprotein	T4, Leu-3	Thymocytes, CD4$^+$ T cells	Recognizes MHC class II antigens; anti-CD4 blocks helper T cell responses
CD8	32 kd glycoprotein	T8, Leu-2	Thymocytes, CD8$^+$ T cells	Recognizes MHC class I antigens; anti-CD8 blocks cytotoxic T cell responses
CD28	44 kd homodimer	Tp44	Mostly CD4$^+$ T cells, some CD8$^+$ cells	Ligand B7 on antigen-presenting cell binds to CD28 and gives second signal to activate lymphocyte
CD29	130 kd glycoprotein, 150 kd glycoprotein, 160 kd glycoprotein, 180 kd glycoprotein	4B4, fibronectin receptor	Thymocytes, T cells, B cells, granulocytes, monocytes	Present on helper-inducer T cells
CD45RO	180 kd glycoprotein	UCHL1	Memory T cells	See CD45RA
CD45RA	205 kd glycoprotein, 220 kd glycoprotein	2H4	Naive T cells	Role in signal transduction, tyrosine phosphatase
CD5	67 kd glycoprotein	T1, Leu-1	Thymocytes, T cells, B cells	Anti-CD5 partially augments T cell activation
CD20	35 kd phosphoprotein	B1	B cells	Commonly used B cell marker; anti-CD20 can activate or inhibit B cells
LFA-1	180 kd glycoprotein, 90 kd glycoprotein	—	Most leukocytes	Anti-LFA-1 inhibits cellular immune responses
CD56	135 kd heterodimer, 200 kd heterodimer	NKH1A, Leu-19	Nk cells	Promotes homotypic adhesion
CD16	50–70 kd phosphatidylinositol-linked transmembrane molecule	FcRIII	NK cells, granulocytes, macrophages	Low-affinity Fcγ receptor that plays a role in antibody-dependent cell-mediated cytotoxicity; activation of NK cells
B7	44 kd protein, 54 kd protein	BB1	B cells, macrophages	Ligand for CD28

From David J: Immunology. In: Dale DC, Federman DD (eds): Scientific American Medicine. New York, Scientific American, Inc., 1996, Section 6, Subsection I, Table 1, p 6, with permission.

21. What are the cytokines, their sites of production and major activities?

Cytokines and Their Biologic Activities*

CYTOKINES INTERLEUKIN	T	CELL SOURCE MACROPHAGES	OTHER	MAJOR ACTIVITIES
Interleukin-1α and β (IL-1α and β)		+	+	Fever; bone resorption; prostaglandin release; stimulate cytokine production by macrophages and T cells.
IL-1α		+		
IL-1β			+	Some
IL-2	+			Activates cytotoxic T cells and NK cells. Stimulates proliferation of T cells and NK cells. Stimulates differentiation of T cells and LAK cells. Costimulates proliferation of B cells and antibody secretion.
IL-3	+	+	+	Supports proliferation of mast cells and pre-B cells. Supports differentiation of stem cells.
IL-4	+		+	Activates resting B cells and macrophages. Induces IgG and IgE secretion in LPS-activated B cells. Stimulates proliferation of T cells and mast cells. Suppresses TNF-α, IL-1, IL-6 in monocytes.
IL-5	+			Induces IgA production and IgM secretion from LPS-activated B cells. Proliferation of eosinophils; supports differentiation of cytotoxic T cells.
IL-6	+	+	+	Induces antibody secretion; differentiation of cytotoxic T cells; proliferation of megakaryocytes. Promotes myeloma cell growth.
IL-7			Thymic strand cells	Proliferation and differentiation of pre-B cells. Proliferation of thymocytes.
IL-8		+		Neutrophil and T-cell chemotaxis.
IL-9	+			Growth of T-helper cell clones.
IL-10	+	−	+	Inhibits production of (IFN-γ and TNF-α) and B-cell growth and differentiation.
IL-11			+	Proliferation and development of B cells, macrophages, and megakaryocytes.
IL-12			B cells	Proliferation of activated T cell induction of IFN-γ.
Tumor necrosis factor-α (TNF-α) (cachectin)	+	+		Fever; shock; activates macrophages; stimulates PMN chemotoxin; angiogenesis, bone resorption; cytotoxic to many cells.
Tumor necrosis factor-β (TNF-β) (lymphotoxin)	+			Activates endothelial cells, granulocytes, and B cells. Inhibits angiogenesis; cytotoxic to many cells.
Interferon-γ (IFN-γ)	+		NK cells	Activated NK cells, cytotoxic T cells, endothelial cells, and macrophages. Has antitumor activity. Stimulates LAK activity; costimulates B-cell proliferation; inhibits T-cell proliferation.

*Plus and minus signs indicate whether pathway exists (+) or not (−).
From Bennett JC: Approach to the patient with immune diseases. In Bennett JC, Plum F (eds): Cecil Textbook of Medicine, 20th ed. Philadelphia, W.B. Saunders, 1996, Table 221–2, p 1395, with permission.

22. What is anergy? What is its clinical significance?

Anergy is the lack of delayed-type hypersensitivity (DTH) reactivity to a battery of common antigens following intradermal challenge. Its presence is a very sensitive reflection of depressed cell-mediated immunity (particularly T-cell function). Anergy may be temporary, such as in viral infections (measles), or prolonged, as in sarcoidosis, AIDS, and malignancies. The accurate assessment of anergy by DTH skin testing depends on a number of factors, including use of an appropriate battery of skin test reagents, proper reagent dilution and storage, injection technique (intradermal), and interpretation of results.

23. What are antigen-presenting cells (APCs)? What is their role in the immune response?

APCs are a heterogeneous population of cells that are capable of surface presentation of antigen to immune responder cells, resulting in immunostimulation. In most cases, it is obligatory that antigen be presented in close proximity to MHC molecules on the presenting cell. For example, CD4+ (helper) T cells will not recognize antigen on the surface of macrophages (an APC) unless it is presented in conjunction with MHC class II molecules. Viral and foreign tissue antigens are presented in association with class I MHC molecules and are recognized primarily by cytotoxic (CD8+) T cells. T cell antigen recognition requires intimate association between antigen and MHC molecules on the APC and the CD4 or CD8 and the CD3/T cell receptor complex on the T cell. This interaction leads to T cell activation and effector function with resultant immune responsiveness. APCs may have constitutive antigen-presenting capability or capability only after induction of MHC molecules on their surface, such as occurs with fibroblasts (Class I) and some types of macrophages (Class II). APCs include macrophages, Langerhans cells, dendritic cells, R cells, Kupffer cells, microglial cells, astrocytes, fibroblasts, and endothelial cells.

24. What is major basic protein (MBP)?

MBP is the principal protein of the cytoplasmic granules of eosinophils and has been localized to the crystalline core. It is also present in much smaller amounts in basophils.

Biologic Effects of Major Basic Protein

1.	Nonspecific toxicity to many parasites (including *Schistosoma mansoni, Trichinella spiralis,* and *Trypanosoma cruzi*).
2.	Toxicity to a wide variety of mammalian cells (including human cells).
3.	Stimulation of histamine release from basophils and mast cells.
4.	Neutralization of heparin. An example of the potential clinical significance of MBP is that MBP deposition by eosinophils may play an important role in the pathophysiology of asthma by causing desquamation of respiratory tract epithelium.

25. Describe the mechanism of immediate hypersensitivity reactions and give some clinical examples.

Type I, or immediate hypersensitivity, reactions are classic allergic reactions initiated by the binding of an antigen to IgE attached to the surface of mast cells or basophils. This results in cross-linkage of high-affinity IgE receptors, cell activation, and noncytolytic degranulation, with release of potent mediators (including histamine, prostaglandins, and leukotrienes). The reaction becomes clinically manifested within seconds to minutes and is almost always apparent within 1 hour. Clinical examples include anaphylaxis, allergic rhinitis (hay fever), food allergy, extrinsic (allergic) asthma, immediate drug allergy (such as to penicillin), and acute urticaria (hives).

26. What are the four types of hypersensitivity reactions?

The four classic types of hypersensitivity reactions, also referred to as the Coombs and Gell classification of immunologically mediated inflammation, are summarized at right.

Types of Immunologically Mediated Inflammation

TYPE OF INFLAMMATION	RECOGNITION COMPONENT	SOLUBLE MEDIATOR	INFLAMMATORY RESPONSE	DISEASE EXAMPLE
I. Reagenic, allergic	IgE	Basophil and mast cell products	Immediate flare and wheal, smooth muscle constriction	Atopy, anaphylaxis
II. Cytotoxic antibody	IgG, IgM	Complement	Lysis or phagocytosis of circulating antigens, acute inflammation in tissues	Autoimmune hemolytic anemia, thrombocytopenia associated with systemic lupus erythematosus
III. Immune complex	IgG, IgM	Complement, lipid mediators	Accumulation of polymorphonuclear leukocytes and macrophages	Rheumatoid arthritis, lupus erythematosus
IV. Delayed hypersensitivity	T lymphocytes	Cytokines	Mononuclear cell infiltrate	Tuberculosis, sarcoidosis, polymyositis, granulomatosis, vasculitis

From Wyngaarden JB, Smith LH : Cecil Textbook of Medicine, 18th ed. Philadelphia, W.B. Saunders, 1988, p 1989, with permission.

27. Describe the mechanism of delayed type hypersensitivity (DTH) reactions. What are the four major types?

Type IV, or DTH, reactions are a reflection of cell-mediated immunity and are primarily mediated by T cells. Unlike reaction types I–III, DTH can be transferred by T cells, but not by serum. When antigen-sensitized T cells are re-exposed to that specific antigen by antigen-presenting cells, T cell activation occurs, resulting in secretion of gamma interferon and multiple other cytokines. Monocyte/macrophage influx and activation occur, leading to release of an array of inflammatory mediators and cytokines. Chronic presence of antigen leads to continued lymphocyte and macrophage activation. This results in the characteristic pathologic changes, including granuloma formation and tissue destruction.

Key Features of the Four Types of Delayed Hypersensitivity Reactions

TYPE	INDUCING ANTIGEN	REACTION TIME	EXTERNAL SIGNS	HISTOLOGICAL APPEARANCE
Tuberculin	Tuberculin, typhoidin, abortin, leishmanial antigens	48 h	Indurated, painful skin swelling	Dermal reaction, lymphocyte and monocyte infiltration
Jones-Mote	Innocuous proteins such as ovalbumin	24 h	Slight skin thickening	Dermal reaction, lymphocyte and basophil infiltration
Contact	Urushiol, varnish, resins, nickel	48 h	Eczema	Epidermal reaction, lymphocyte and monocyte infiltration
Granulomatous	Persistent Ag or Ag-Ab complexes, talcum powder	4 weeks	Skin induration	Epithelioid cell granuloma formation, giant cells, macrophages, fibrosis, necrosis

Ab = antibody; Ag = antigen; h = hour.
From Klein J: Immunology. Oxford, Blackwell Scientific Publications, 1990, with permission.

28. Describe the mechanism of cytotoxic reactions and give some clinical examples.

Type II, or cytotoxic, reactions occur when antibody binds to specific antigens on circulating cells or in tissue. Antibody binding can lead to cytotoxicity by complement activation or interaction with Fc receptors on effector cells, such as neutrophils, macrophages, eosinophils, and natural killer (NK) cells. Examples include hemolytic disease of the newborn, autoimmune hemolytic anemia, and Goodpasture's syndrome.

29. Describe the mechanism of immune complex reactions and give some clinical examples.

Type III, or immune complex, reactions are caused by the formation of immune complexes (antigen and antibody bound together) and their deposition in tissue. The immune complexes may cause complement activation that results in neutrophil accumulation and tissue damage. Examples include the Arthus reaction and serum sickness (glomerulonephritis, endocarditis).

30. What is an Arthus reaction? When does it occur in a clinical setting?

Arthus reactions are caused by antigen-antibody complexes (immune complexes) and were first described by Nicolas-Maurice Arthus, a French physiologist, in 1903. The reaction is an acute, hemorrhagic, inflammatory skin lesion elicited in the dermis by injection of an antigen. It relies on high serum levels of complement-fixing antibodies, which lead to the formation of immune complexes in the blood vessel walls of the dermis and a localized vasculitis. It is dependent on both neutrophil and complement function. In humans, Arthus reactions have been reported after tetanus and diphtheria immunization, and in some diabetics after insulin injection.

31. What is an allergen?

An allergen is an antigen (usually a protein) that induces IgE synthesis and sensitization with IgE. The IgE response to an allergen is dependent on multiple factors including cellular (i.e., T and B cell) function, soluble mediators, and genetic factors.

32. What are the major differences between mast cells and basophils?

Comparison of Mast Cells and Basophils

PARAMETER	MAST CELL	BASOPHILS
Life span	? weeks to years	Days
Origin	Probably bone marrow	Bone marrow
Location	Tissues, noncirculating	Normally circulating, may egress into tissues under certain conditions
Size	8–20 μm	5–7 μm
Nucleus	Round to oval, may be indented	Multi-lobulated
Cytoplasmic granules	Smaller, more numerous, relatively homogeneous	Larger, fewer, variable in size
Ultrastructure	Scroll structure of granules, filopodia on cell surface	Scroll patterns absent, smooth cell surface
High affinity IgE receptor	Present	Present
Histamine release	+	+
Major arachidonic acid metabolites	PGD2, LTC4,* LTD4,* LTE4*	LTC4
Staining characteristics:		
Toluidine blue	+	+
Tryptase	+	−
Chloroacetate esterase	+	−

* = previously collectively referred to as slow-reacting substance of anaphylaxis (SRS-A), PG = prostaglandin, LT = leukotriene.

33. Are all mast cells alike?

No. Mast cell heterogeneity exists in both animals and man. This has been most extensively studied in the mouse, where there appear to be two major mast cell populations. These have been labelled mucosal mast cells (MMC) and connective tissue mast cells (CTMC). MMC are found principally at mucosal surfaces, whereas CTMC are found within connective tissue, lining blood vessels, and at serosal surfaces. They differ with respect to histamine content, degranulation to non-IgE stimuli, arachidonic acid metabolite production, and histochemical-staining characteristics caused by differences in proteoglycan content of their granules. MMC are dependent on the T cell cytokine interleukin-3 (IL-3). In contrast, expression of the CTMC phenotype is dependent on the presence of fibroblasts.

In man, there also appear to be two major mast cell populations, which are identified by differences in neutral protease content of their cytoplasmic granules. Both populations contain tryptase, but only one contains both tryptase and chymase. The **tryptase-only mast cells (MC^T)** are located primarily at mucosal surfaces, whereas the **tryptase and chymase-positive mast cells (MC^{TC})** are located primarily in connective tissue, lining blood vessels, and at serosal surfaces. The factors responsible for human mast cell growth remain to be clearly defined. Although human IL-3 appears to have some mast cell growth-promoting activity, its effect in man is less well defined. Whether an additional factor(s) is needed for human mast cell growth and differentiation remains to be determined. Of interest is that MC^T mast cells, but not MC^{TC} mast cells, appear to be T-lymphocyte dependent. This is suggested by a marked decrease in MC^T but not MC^{TC} mast cell numbers in the tissues of patients with severe T cell immunodeficiency disorders.

34. Which single procedure or test is most useful in the diagnosis of systemic mastocytosis?

A bone marrow biopsy is the procedure of choice because of its high sensitivity and specificity. A positive skin biopsy does not indicate internal organ involvement. Plasma histamine levels may be normal or elevated (although very high levels are highly suggestive of systemic disease). Bone scan findings are nonspecific. Hepatomegaly and splenomegaly may or may not be seen and are not diagnostic.

The bone marrow is characterized by prominent aggregates of mast cells in association with spicules, lymph tissue, or blood vessels. Eosinophils are often prominent, and variable degrees of fibrosis are present. If the diagnosis of systemic mastocytosis is suspected, the pathologist should be notified, since the standard bone marrow preparation involves decalcification, which results in poor staining of mast cell granules by metachromatic dyes such as toluidine blue. A Giemsa stain may be useful in identifying mast cells in these samples. It is emphasized that bone marrow *aspiration* without biopsy is insufficient to rule in or rule out systemic mastocytosis.

35. Which biologic functions are mediated via H_1, H_2, or a combination of H_1 and H_2 histamine receptors?

Biologic Effects of H_1 and H_2 Histamine Receptor Stimulation

H_1 RECEPTORS	H_2 RECEPTORS	H_1 AND H_2 RECEPTORS
Smooth muscle contraction	Gastric acid secretion	Hypotension
↑ vascular permeability	↑ cyclic AMP	Tachycardia
Pruritus	Mucous secretion	Flushing
Stimulation of prostaglandin synthesis	Inhibits basophil, but not mast cell histamine release	Headache
Tachycardia	↑ suppressor cell function	
↑ cyclic GMP production	↓ lymphocyte cytotoxicity	

↑ = increased, ↓ = decreased.

36. What is the reticuloendothelial system (RES)? What are its principal functions?

The RES (mononuclear/phagocyte system) comprises a heterogeneous population of fixed-tissue phagocytic cells throughout the body which are critical in the removal of particulate and soluble substances from the circulation and tissues. Substances removed include immune complexes, bacteria, toxins, and exogenous antigens. These molecules may be internalized by nonspecific endocytosis, nonimmune but receptor-mediated phagocytosis, or immunologic phagocytosis mediated by binding to Fc or complement receptors. Components of the RES include Kupffer cells of the liver, microglial cells of the brain, pulmonary alveolar macrophages, and macrophages in the bone marrow, lymph nodes, gut, and other tissues. Blockade of the RES is one postulated mechanism for prevention of platelet destruction by high-dose IV gamma globulin (IVGG) in idiopathic thrombocytopenic purpura (ITP). The binding of IgG-sensitized platelets to the IgG-Fc receptors on RES cells, particularly in the liver and spleen, leads to phagocytosis and platelet destruction in ITP. This IgG-Fc receptor mechanism may be "blocked" or overwhelmed by the infusion of high dose IVGG. IgG-Fc receptors are lost during phagocytosis and may take as long as several days to be re-expressed.

37. What maneuver elicits Darier's sign?

Darier's sign is the erythema and whealing that occurs following gentle stroking of the characteristic, reddish-brown skin lesions of urticaria pigmentosa. It is presumably caused by degranulation and mediator release from the large numbers of dermal mast cells in these patients.

38. What is the cold-agglutinin syndrome? How is it diagnosed?

The cold agglutinin syndrome is characterized by hemolytic anemia secondary to IgM antibodies, which cause increasing red blood cell (RBC) lysis with decreasing temperature. Agglutination of normal RBCs at 20°C occurs with serum from virtually all patients with the cold agglutinin syndrome. The direct Coombs test is typically positive for complement and negative for immunoglobulin. The cold agglutinin syndrome is typically idiopathic, with the presentation of hemolytic anemia in the sixth or seventh decade of life. These patients have a high titer of monoclonal IgM kappa antibody, with anti-I specificity. Despite the monoclonal nature of the antibody response, these patients typically do not develop multiple myeloma or Waldenstrom's macroglobulinemia.

Cold agglutinin syndrome may also occur in association with the lymphoproliferative disorders (i.e., non-Hodgkin's lymphoma), infections (*Mycoplasma* pneumonia, infectious mononucleosis), and rarely in connective tissue disorders (systemic lupus erythematosus [SLE]). With the lymphoproliferative disorders, the IgM is often monoclonal. The cold agglutinin in these disorders is often anti-I, but other antibodies may be present, particularly in infectious mononucleosis when anti-i is often found. Determination of antibody specificity is not necessary for either diagnosis, or as a prerequisite for blood transfusion.

39. Name some of the clinical characteristics of antibody deficiency disorders.

Antibody deficiency disorders, whether acquired or congenital, have several general characteristics that are manifestations of the defect in humoral-mediated immunity:

1. Recurrent infections with high-grade extracellular encapsulated pathogens.
2. Few problems with fungal or viral (except enteroviral) infections.
3. Chronic sinopulmonary disease.
4. Growth retardation is *not* a striking feature.
5. Low antibody levels measured in serum and secretions.
6. Patients may or may not lack B lymphocytes with surface immunoglobulins or complement receptors.
7. Absence of cortical follicles in lymph nodes and spleen in X-linked agammaglobulinemia.
8. Paucity of palpable lymphoid and nasopharyngeal tissue in X-linked agammaglobulinemia.
9. Compatible with survival to adulthood or for several years after onset except for those with persistent enterovirus infections, autoimmune disorders or malignancy.

(From Wyngaarden JB, Smith LH: Cecil Textbook of Medicine, 18th ed. Philadelphia, W.B. Saunders, 1988, p 1943, with permission.)

40. What are the features of some of the primary specific immunodeficiencies involving antibodies?

Primary Specific Immunodeficiencies Involving Antibodies

DESIGNATION	USUAL PHENOTYPIC EXPRESSION ANTIBODY DEFI-CIENCIES	CELLULAR ABNORMAL-ITIES	PRESUMED LEVEL OF BASIC CELLULAR DEFECT	KNOWN OR PRESUMED PATHO-GENETIC MECHANISM	INHERITANCE
X-linked agammaglobulinemia	All immunoglobulins	↓ B cells	Pre-B cells	Mutations in the gene for agammaglobulinemia tyrosine kinase (atk)	X-linked
Common variable immunodeficiency	All immunoglobulins	Faulty B cell maturation	B cells	Intrinsic B cell defect Underproduction of B cells ↓ Helper T cells Autoantibodies to B cells	Unknown
Selective IgA deficiency	IgA	↓ IgA plasma cells ± ↑ IgΛ⁺ B cells	Terminal differentiation of IgA⁺ cells impaired	Unknown	Usually unknown (autosomal recessive more common than autosomal dominant); frequent in families of patients with common variable immunodeficiency
Ig deficiencies, with increased IgM	IgG, IgA, and IgB	↓ IgG and IgA plasma cells ↑ IgM plasma cells ± ↑ IgM⁺ and IgG⁺ B cells	Failure of immunoglobulin class switching	Mutations in the gene for the CD40 ligand (X-linked form)	X-linked, autosomal recessive, or unknown
Selective deficiency of IgG subclass	One or more IgG isotypes	↓ Plasma cells ± ↓ T cells	Unknown	Unknown	Unknown
κ-Chain deficiency	IgG(κ)	↓ κ⁺ B cells	Unknown	Point mutation at 2p11	Autosomal recessive
Transient hypogammaglobulinemia of infancy	IgG and IgA	↓ Plasma cells B cells normal	Impaired terminal differentiation of B cells	↓ Helper T cells	Frequent in heterozygous individuals in families with various severe combined immunodeficiencies
Ig heavy-chain deficiency	IgG1, IgG2, IgG4, and, in some cases, IgE and IgA2	None	Chromosome deletion at 14q32	Unknown	Autosomal recessive

From David J: Immunology. In Dale DC, Federman DD (eds): Scientific American Medicine. New York, Scientific American, Inc., 1996, Section 6, Subsection VII, Table 5, p 19, with permission.

41. What is the most common immunoglobulin deficiency disorder?

Selective IgA deficiency has a frequency of approximately 1 in 500–700. Many patients are symptomatic, but some have recurrent infections, particularly of the respiratory tract. IgG2 deficiency sometimes accompanies IgA deficiency and these patients are particularly prone to infectious complications with encapsulated bacteria (such as *Haemophilus influenzae)* because IgG2 is the principal IgG antibody response against bacterial polysaccharide. In selective IgA deficiency, the serum IgA level is less than 5 mg/dl (0.05 mg/cc). IgA in secretions is almost always depressed as well. IgG and IgM levels are normal. The patients have an increased incidence of autoimmune disorders (including SLE and rheumatoid arthritis). Treatment is supportive unless frequent infections and IgG2 deficiency are present. In that case, IV gamma globulin (IVGG) may be helpful, but severe anaphylactoid reactions may occur due to the presence of anti-IgA antibodies, which may occur in as many as 50% of IgA-deficient patients.

42. What is the common variable immunodeficiency disease (CVID)?

CVID is a heterogeneous group of disorders characterized by hypogammaglobulinemia (total IgG < 250 mg/dl and usually total Ig < 350 mg/dl), decreased ability to produce antibody following antigenic challenge, and recurrent infections. It is apparent, however, that a significant number of patients whose serum IgG level is depressed but greater than 250 mg/dl may have a similar clinical presentation. The most common serum Ig pattern is panhypogammaglobulinemia with a deficiency of IgG, IgM, and IgA.

CVID usually presents in late childhood or early adulthood but may present at any age. Recurrent bacterial infections of the upper and lower respiratory tract with encapsulated bacteria (*Streptococcus pneumoniae, Haemophilus influenzae*, etc.) are common pathogens, and bronchiectasis may develop. Patients may also have defective cell-mediated immunity and may have mycobacterial, fungal, and protozoal (i.e., *Giardia lamblia*) infections.

Patients with CVID have an increased frequency of a number of autoimmune disorders, including pernicious anemia, Coombs-positive hemolytic anemia, autoimmune thrombocytopenia, and thyroiditis. GI disorders are common, including diarrhea, malabsorption, and nodular lymphoid hyperplasia of the small intestine. Finally, there is an increased incidence of malignancy, particularly of the lymphoreticular system and the GI tract.

43. Identify the principal immunologic defects in CVID.

The immunologic abnormality that affects most patients appears to be a defect in B cell maturation, in which the B cells cannot terminally differentiate into antibody-producing plasma cells. These patients generally have normal numbers of circulating, surface Ig-positive, B cells. Up to 20% of patients may have increased suppressor-cell activity causing decreased antibody production. Other T cell immunoregulatory defects have also been described. Depressed cell-mediated immunity, as demonstrated by cutaneous anergy, may be present in up to 30% of patients.

44. Is there a specific treatment for CVID?

The principal therapy for CVID is IV gamma globulin (IVGG) replacement and aggressive management of infections with appropriate antibiotics. IVGG is given every 3–4 weeks. The usual dose is 200 mg/kg and the infusion is given slowly over several hours. Adverse reactions consisting of pruritus, headache, and nausea usually resolve with slowing or stopping of the infusion. IVGG often dramatically decreases the frequency and severity of infections and may also alleviate some of the symptoms, such as arthralgias, that sometimes accompany CVID.

45. What are the clinical characteristics of disorders of cell-mediated immunity?

The manifestations of cellular immunodeficiency disorders, due to a partial or total defect in T cell function, include:

1. Recurrent infections with low-grade or opportunistic infectious agents, such as fungi, viruses, or protozoa (e.g., *Pneumocystis carinii).*

2. Delayed cutaneous anergy.

3. Accompanied by growth retardation, short life span, wasting, and diarrhea.

4. Susceptible to graft-versus-host disease (GVHD) if given fresh blood, plasma, or unmatched allogeneic bone marrow.

5. Fatal reactions from live virus (including BCG) vaccination.

6. High incidence of malignancy.

(From Wyngaarden JB, Smith LH (eds): Cecil Textbook of Medicine, 18th ed. Philadelphia, W.B. Saunders, 1988, p 1945, with permission.)

46. What are the primary specific immunodeficiencies involving cell-mediated immunity?

Classification of Primary Specific Immunodeficiencies Involving Cell-mediated Immunity

DESIGNATION	USUAL PHENOTYPIC EXPRESSION		PRESUMED LEVEL OF BASIC CELLULAR DEFECT	KNOWN OR PRESUMED PATHO-GENETIC MECHANISM	INHERI-TANCE	MAIN ASSOCIATED FEATURES
	FUNCTIONAL DEFI-CIENCIES	CELLULAR ABNOR-MALITIES				
Congenital thymic hypoplasia (DiGeorge's syndrome)	CMI, impaired antibody	↓ T cells	Thymus	Embryopathy of third and fourth pharyngeal pouch areas	Usually not familial	Hypoparathy-roidism Abnormal facies Cardiovascular abnormalities
Severe com-bined immun-odeficiency	CMI, antibody	↓ T cells, ↓ B cells	LSC	Unknown	Autosomal recessive or X-linked	—
Adenosine deam-inase (ADA) deficiency	CMI, antibody	↓ T cells, ± B cells	LSC or early T cells	Metabolic ef-fects of ADA deficiency	Autosomal recessive	—
Purine nucleo-side phospho-rylase (PNP) deficiency	CMI ± antibody	↓ T cells	T cells	Metabolic ef-fects of PNP deficiency	Autosomal recessive	Hypoplastic anemia
Reticular dysgenesis	CMI, anti-body, phagocytes	↓ T cells, ↓ B cells, ↓ phago-cytes	HSC	Unknown	Autosomal recessive	Neutropenia
Wiskott-Aldrich syndrome	Antibody to certain antigens (mainly polysaccha-rides), CMI (progressive)	↓ T cells, ↓ B cells (progres-sive)	Unknown	Defect in cell membrane glycoproteins	X-linked	Thrombocytope-nia Eczema Lymphoreticular cancers
Immunodefi-ciency with ataxia telan-glectasia	CMI, anti-body (partial)	↓ T cells, ↓ plasma cells (mainly those cells producing IgA, IgE, ± IgG)	Early T cells and defective terminal differen-tiation of B cells	Unknown Faulty thymic epithelium DNA repair defect	Autosomal recessive	Cerebellar ataxia Telangiectasia Chromosomal abnormalities Raised serum α-fetoprotein levels
MHC class II deficiency	CMI ± antibody	None	T cells, B cells, and antigen-present-ing cells	Defect of promoter-binding protein	Autosomal recessive	Intestinal mal-absorption
CD3 deficiency	CMI	None	Unknown	Defective transcription on CD3-ϵ or CD3-γ	Autosomal recessive	—
CD8 deficiency	CMI	↓ T cells	Early T cells	Defective maturation of CD8⁺ T cells	Autosomal recessive	—

CMI=cell-mediated immunity, LSC=lymphocytic stem cell, HSC=hematopoietic stem cell.
From David J: Immunology. In Dale DC, Federman DD (eds): Scientific American Medicine. New York, Sci-entific American, Inc., 1996, Section 6, Subsection VII, Table 7, p 22, with permission.

47. What are some of the secondary causes of hypogammaglobulinemia?

Causes of Secondary Hypogammaglobulinemia

CAUSE	MECHANISM
Drugs	Drugs
a. Anticonvulsants (esp. phenytoin)	a. Increased suppressor cell activity (any or all isotopes affected)
b. Cytotoxic agents	b. Decreased Ig production
Multiple myeloma	Decreased Ig production
Chronic lymphocytic leukemia	Decreased Ig production
Myotonic dystrophy	Selective hypercatabolism of IgG
Nephrotic syndrome	Ig loss in urine (particularly IgG)
Intestinal lymphangiectasia	Ig loss through GI tract, increased catabolism
Radiation therapy	Decreased Ig production

48. How is the radioallergosorbent test (RAST) performed?

The RAST is used for measurement of specific IgE antibody in serum. The test is only semi-quantitative. Purified allergen is coupled to a carrier (particles, paper discs, plastic wells) and incubated with the patient's serum. After washing, ^{125}I-labelled anti-IgE is added and radioactivity present on the immunoabsorbent material (carrier) is measured. The RAST is increasingly being converted to an ELISA system that uses enzymatic color change rather than radioactivity.

49. How does the RAST compare with skin testing in the diagnosis of allergy?

The RAST is less sensitive, and its correlation with some allergies is poorer than with skin testing. Furthermore, validity of the RAST is highly dependent on proper controls and interpretation of the results by the reporting laboratory. However, the RAST may be particularly useful in patients in whom skin testing performance or interpretation is compromised. This includes patients with extensive skin disease such as dermatographism, urticaria pigmentosa, and diffuse cutaneous mastocytosis. It may also be useful in patients receiving H_1 antihistamines and patients in whom skin testing is considered to carry a high risk of severe anaphylaxis. By itself, a positive RAST does not diagnose a specific allergy but should be used only in conjunction with the clinical history.

50. Describe the basic technique for performance of the enzyme-linked immumosorbent assay (ELISA).

The ELISA has, to a great extent, replaced the radioimmunoassay (RIA) in diagnostic testing. Compared to the RIA, the ELISA eliminates the radioactive hazards and has a sensitivity that is comparable or better (sensitivity of 1 ng or less, depending on the test substance and the various components used in the assay). The ELISA is typically performed in plastic, flat-bottomed, 96-well, microtiter plates. The basic ELISA procedure used to test for antibody against specific antigen is outlined below. The concentration of the substance to be measured is determined by comparing the optical density of the test samples against negative controls and a standard curve.

ELISA Test Procedure

1. Coat wells with antigen (by incubation of appropriate concentration of antigen in the wells)and then wash.	4. Add enzyme-linked anti-species immunoglobulin and incubate.
2. Add test sample and incubate.	5. Wash
3. Wash.	6. Add developing substrate and measure optical density

51. Which principal components of house dust have been implicated in causing allergic disease?

House dust is a frequent cause of allergic rhinitis and asthma. House dust is a mixture of variable amounts of antigens from dust mites, cockroaches, cats, dogs, pollens, molds and other environmental substances. Dust mites are often the most important source of offending allergen and are particularly prevalent in clothing, carpets, and mattresses. The principal mite in house dust is *Dematophagoides pteronyssimus* and the allergen is the mite feces. Dust mites thrive optimally at 25°C and 80% relative humidity. Human epidermal scales are a major substrate for dust mite growth. Efforts to minimize exposure to dust and to decrease favorable environments available for dust mite growth may be very beneficial for allergic patients. Treatment with antiallergic medications and, when necessary, immunotherapy (allergy shots) is an effective form of therapy.

52. What are the modes of therapy available for allergic rhinitis?
1. Avoidance of the offending allergens
2. Medical therapy
   a. H_1 antihistamines
   b. Sympathomimetics
   c. Cromolyn sodium
   d. Corticosteroids (nasal spray; systemic therapy only for severe acute exacerbations)
3. Allergen specific immunotherapy

53. What immunologic changes occur in patients who undergo allergen-specific immunotherapy?
Allergen-specific immunotherapy involves the subcutaneous injection of extracts of the specific allergens responsible for a patient's symptoms. Immunologic changes that have been reported in response to allergen-specific immunotherapy include:
1. Diminished seasonal increases of allergen-specific IgE
2. Increased allergen-specific IgG
3. Decreased basophil histamine release
4. Development of allergen-specific suppressor T cells

Despite these observations, the specific cause(s) for the effectiveness of immunotherapy remains to be precisely determined.

54. What is the mechanism of action of cromolyn?
Cromolyn sodium is available for use via inhalational, intranasal, and topical ophthalmic routes. It inhibits the degranulation of mast cells, thereby preventing the release of the mediators of immediate hypersensitivity. The mechanism by which this occurs is unknown, although inhibition of calcium influx is one of several proposed explanations. It has no intrinsic antihistamine, bronchodilator, or anti-inflammatory activity. Cromolyn is used as a prophylactic agent in patients with sufficiently frequent symptoms to justify continuous therapy, because it is most effective when administered prior to exposure to an allergen (i.e., prior to mast cell degranulation). Cromolyn inhibits both immediate hypersensitivity and late-phase reactions.

55. How would 2 weeks of treatment with H_1 antihistamines, H_2 antihistamines, or corticosteroids (CS) be expected to affect the results of allergy and delayed type hypersensitivity (DTH) skin testing?
Allergy skin testing is used to evaluate a patient for potential immediate hypersensitivity reactivity (a type I reaction) against a specific allergen. Thus, if a patient's mast cells have been sensitized with IgE antibody against the injected allergen, mast cell degranulation will occur, resulting in release of mediators such as histamine into the skin. The wheal and flare reaction of a positive skin test is primarily due to histamine stimulation of H_1 receptors. Thus, H_1 antihistamines would markedly inhibit positive skin test reactivity and must be discontinued for a period of time (depending on the antihistamine) prior to skin testing. H_2 antihistamines do not typically, but may occasionally, have significant effects on skin test reactivity. This emphasizes the importance of always using a histamine standard as a positive control when performing allergy skin testing. CS do not affect mast cell degranulation nor do they affect the biologic effects of histamine. Thus, CS do not alter allergy skin test results.

In contrast **DTH skin testing** is a type IV reaction and is a sensitive measurement of T-cell function. Histamine does not play a significant role in DTH, and antihistamines (both H_1 and H_2) do not affect DTH skin testing. However, corticosteroids may substantially depress cell-mediated responses, including T-cell function, so that DTH responsiveness may be profoundly depressed with CS treatment.

56. Which types of infections play a role in the exacerbation of asthma?

Strong evidence implicates upper respiratory infections (URI) caused by viruses and *Mycoplasma pneumoniae* as important causes of exacerbations of asthma. The association is especially pronounced in the pediatric age group. Respiratory syncytial virus (RSV) is an especially important offending organism. Other implicated viruses include parainfluenza, influenza A, and adenovirus. The severity of the exacerbation depends on multiple factors, including age, severity of the underlying asthma, concurrent medical problems, the site and severity of the infection, and the specific infectious agent. Bacterial infections of the respiratory tract, with the exception of chronic sinusitis, have not been commonly associated with exacerbations of asthma.

57. A 22-year-old patient complains of symptoms of asthma after playing basketball. What is a likely explanation?

The patient probably has exercise-induced asthma (EIA). Bronchoconstriction typically begins following cessation of exercise and is usually maximal 3–12 minutes later. The severity varies, but it is almost always short-lived. The diagnosis of EIA is confirmed by a decrease in the forced respiratory volume (FEV) following exercise or isocapnic hyperventilation, although the former is the preferred form of testing. The etiology of EIA is believed to be water loss from the bronchial mucosa, resulting in hyperosmolarity in the bronchial tissue. This has been demonstrated by prevention of EIA during exercise by means of air that is fully saturated with water vapor at body temperature. Water content of the inspired air is probably the single most important factor affecting bronchospasm, but level of ventilation achieved, temperature of the inspired air, and the interval since the previous episode of EIA are also contributing factors. The last factor is important because a refractory period usually occurs for as long as 2 hours following the previous episode. During this period a second challenge will invoke less than half of the initial airway response. The severity of EIA cannot be predicted by baseline pulmonary function tests (PFTs).

58. What treatment is available for prevention of exercise-induced asthma?

Inhaled beta agonists are the most effective treatment (90% or greater response rate). Approximately 60–70% of patients will respond to inhaled cromolyn alone. Some patients will require combination therapy and ipratropium bromide (an anticholinergic agent) may offer additional relief. Treatment should be administered by a hand-held nebulizer immediately before exercise. The protective effects of pharmacologic therapy may last for only 2 hours, even though in nonexercise related bronchospasm there may be continued benefits for an additional 2–4 hours. Inhaled corticosteroids, when taken over several weeks, may decrease both the severity of EIA and the doses of the other medications required for control. Finally, nasal breathing may attenuate EIA but it is not practical in strenuous exercise.

59. In a patient who complains of nocturnal worsening of asthma, what potential factors should be considered?

Considerable attention has been directed toward the role of circadian rhythms in nocturnal exacerbations of asthma (usually between 3 am and 7 am). Cortisol levels decrease, plasma histamine levels increase, and epinephrine levels decrease during the night. The decrease in plasma cortisol is not thought to be a major factor since administration of corticosteroids in the evening is ineffective in preventing nocturnal exacerbations. Plasma histamine levels do not correlate with changes in pulmonary function tests (PFTs). However, epinephrine levels do correlate, suggesting a possible important physiologic role.

Circadian changes in the airways themselves are also important. Both airway caliber and reactivity are affected, with an overall 5–10% decrease in flow rates in normal individuals, but up to a 50% decrease in asthmatics. Increased vagal tone, impaired mucociliary clearance, and airway cooling and drying have also been reported as contributing factors in nocturnal asthma. Gastroesophageal reflex disease (GERD) may also exacerbate asthma at night by microaspiration or reflex bronchoconstriction caused by stimulation of nerve endings by acid in the lower esophagus. GERD may be exacerbated by theophylline, which decreases lower esophageal sphincter tone.

The patient's pharmacologic regimen should be carefully examined and compliance assured. Longer-acting, inhaled beta agonists are useful. Theophylline absorption may be decreased at night, leading to lower serum levels. If necessary, the evening dose should be adjusted so that peak levels occur approximately 6 hours later. H_2 antihistamines may be helpful in some patients with GERD. Evening corticosteroids should not generally be given because of marked suppression of the adrenal axis and lack of demonstration of a beneficial effect. Patients who have an allergic component to their asthma and who are on maximal pharmacologic therapy should be considered for immunotherapy.

Potential environmental and dietary agents should be considered as exacerbating factors. For example, dust mites may cause immediate hypersensitivity reactions during the night. Allergen or irritant exposure several hours before going to sleep can also be important. The late-phase response that may occur following such exposure typically peaks 6–12 hours later and may cause severe prolonged bronchospasm. Finally nonasthmatic causes of wheezing such as cardiac disease should be considered as potential contributing factors. Nocturnal asthma is not related to any particular stage of sleep. The contribution of sleep "per se" is unclear but does not appear to be of major significance.

60. Why is it critical that nocturnal asthma be treated aggressively?

The importance of the treatment of nocturnal asthma cannot be overemphasized, since the majority of fatalities due to asthma occur during the early morning hours.

61. What are Charcot-Leyden crystals, Creola bodies, and Curschmann's spirals?

Charcot-Leyden crystals are composed of lysophospholipase, and their presence in tissue or secretions has been considered as specific for eosinophil activity. However, lysophospholipase is also found in basophils.

Creola bodies are clumps of epithelial cells and suggest a desquamating disease process.

Curschmann's spirals are mucus plugs composed of mucus, proteinaceous material, and inflammatory cells in a swirling, spiraling pattern. They usually conform to the configuration of the involved airways.

These findings may be seen alone or together as part of the clinical presentation of asthma. They are characteristically seen in patients who have died from status asthmatics.

62. What are the clinical manifestations of anaphylaxis?

Clinical Manifestations of Anaphylaxis

General	Flushing, sense of foreboding
Skin	Urticaria/angioedema, flushing, pruritus
Eyes	Lacrimation, pruritus
Upper respiratory tract	Sneezing, nasal pruritus, discharge and congestion, hoarseness, laryngeal edema, stridor
Lower respiratory tract	Bronchospasm, tachypnea, intercostal retractions, use of accessory muscles of respiration
Cardiovascular	Hypotension, tachycardia, arrhythmia
GI	Nausea, vomiting, abdominal pain, diarrhea
Neurologic	Headache, syncope, seizure

63. A 20-year-old patient presents with hypotension, wheezing, and urticaria 30 minutes after a bee sting. What is the appropriate treatment?

This presentation is that of systemic anaphylaxis, an immediate hypersensitivity reaction caused by mast cell/basophil release of multiple potent mediators, including histamine, prostaglandins, and leukotrienes, into tissues and the circulation. Prompt treatment is critical, and should be directed toward maintaining cardiovascular and pulmonary function. Initial treatment should be administration of epinephrine either by subcutaneous or intramuscular routes (0.3–0.5 cc of a 1:1000 dilution). In the face of cardiovascular collapse, IV epinephrine may be indicated. Other immediate steps include applying a tourniquet proximal to the site of allergen inoculation (for example, a bee sting or allergen injection in the forearm). If the anaphylaxis is due to oral intake of an allergen (such as food ingestion), a nasogastric (NG) tube may be inserted and residual gastric contents removed to prevent further antigen absorption. The patient's legs should be elevated, oxygen and airway support provided as needed, and IV fluids (such as normal saline) given for blood pressure support. Parenteral H_1 and H_2 antihistamines may also be administered. Inhaled beta-1 agonists can be given prophylactically or if bronchospasm is present. Repeat doses of medication such as epinephrine should be given as needed and vasopressor agents given when indicated. Although steroids will not alter the acute course of anaphylaxis, they may be given to attenuate a subsequent late phase response. The aggressiveness of the above outlined therapy depends on the severity of the anaphylaxis and the response to treatment.

64. What are the major distinguishing factors between Churg-Strauss syndrome (allergic angiitis and granulomatosis) and classic polyarteritis nodosa (PAN)?

Both of these diseases are systemic necrotizing vasculitides. It is important to recognize that some patients may have characteristics of both Churg-Strauss and PAN. These patients are classified as having polyangiitis overlap syndrome. Patients who fail corticosteroid therapy or who have fulminant disease should receive cytotoxic drug therapy.

Comparison of Churg-Strauss and PAN

	CHURG-STRAUSS	PAN
Pulmonary involvement	+	−
Histology	Necrotizing vasculitis with granulomas	Necrotizing vasculitis
Vessel involvement	Small-to-medium arteries	Medium muscular arteries; veins, venules with aneurysmal dilation
Asthma/atopic disease	+*	−
Eosinophilia (blood and/or tissue)	+	−
Association with serum hepatitis B surface antigen (HB_sAg)	−	+

* Often present for years before onset of vasculitis.

65. What does palpable purpura indicate?

Palpable purpura indicates cutaneous vasculitis.

66. What is the classic triad of Wegener's granulomatosis (WG)? Describe the clinical presentation and laboratory findings.

WG is a systemic necrotizing vasculopathy of unknown etiology. The classic triad includes (1) necrotizing granulomatous vasculitis of the upper respiratory tract and (2) lungs, in addition to (3) glomerulonephritis. Vasculitis of many other organs, including the skin, ears, eyes, joints, and central nervous system, may also be present. Vasculitis typically involves small arteries and veins. The glomerulonephritis is usually focal or crescentic without vasculitis or granulomas. Since the original description by Wegener in Germany in 1939, many more limited forms of the disease have been recognized.

The clinical presentation may include fever, chronic sinusitis, otitis media, cough, chest pain, hemoptysis, and arthralgias. Upper airway infections are common, with *Staphylococcus aureus* the most common pathogen. Such infections may mimic exacerbation or recurrence of disease following remission. With the inflammatory process unchecked, nasal septal perforation may occur, leading to a saddle-nose deformity.

Laboratory data are generally nonspecific, although recently an antibody to cytoplasmic components of the polymorphonuclear leukocyte (anti-neutrophil cytoplasmic antibody [ANCA]) has been associated with active disease. The erythrocyte sedimentation rate (ESR) is markedly elevated (often > 100 mm/hr) and is a sensitive indicator of disease activity. Mild anemia, leukocytosis, and an increase in serum IgG and IgA levels are commonly seen. Chest x-ray patterns include multiple nodules (which frequently cavitate), infiltrates, and solitary nodules. The mean age of onset is 40 years with a male predominance.

67. What is the treatment for WG?

Prior to the use of cytotoxic drugs, specifically cyclophosphamide, WG was an almost uniformly fatal disease, with a mean survival of 5 months. Corticosteroid therapy did not significantly alter the disease's outcome. However, treatment with cyclophosphamide results in complete remission in over 90% of patients. Combination treatment with corticosteroids and cyclophosphamide should be given initially to gain benefits from the rapid anti-inflammatory effects of the steroid while the cytotoxic actions of the cyclophosphamide are taking effect. Prednisone may be started at 1 mg/kg daily, maintained for 1 month, tapered to alternate day therapy, and then gradually discontinued, depending on the patient's response to the taper. Cyclophosphamide should be started at 2 mg/kg orally and continued for at least a year. If, at the end of the year, clinical remission has been obtained, the cyclophosphamide may be tapered and discontinued. The patient's hematologic parameters should be closely monitored for cyclophosphamide toxicity. The patient's WBC count should be maintained above 3,000/mm^3 with a neutrophil count above 1,000/mm^3 to lessen the risk of infectious complications. Other cytotoxic drugs, such as azathioprine, are less effective than cyclophosphamide in the treatment of WG.

68. What are the major differences between Wegener's granulomatosis and Goodpasture's syndrome?

Wegener's Granulomatosis Versus Goodpasture's Syndrome

	WEGENER'S	GOODPASTURE'S
Etiology	Unknown	Unknown, but hydrocarbon exposure increases risk
Patients	Male > female Fifth decade	Male >> female Young adults
Histopathology	Necrotizing granulomatous vasculitis of upper/lower respiratory tract	Linear deposition of IgG along basement membrane of lung and kidney demonstrated by immuno-fluorescence, vasculitis absent
Target organs	Lung > kidney May also affect: CNS, eyes, ears, joints, skin, heart, others	Kidney > lung
Primary symptoms	Chronic sinusitis/rhinitis, fever, weight loss, cough, chest pain, hemoptysis may occur.	Hemoptysis, dyspnea, easy fatigability
Typical chest x-ray findings	Pulmonary nodule(s) with or without cavitation	Diffuse bilateral infiltrates
Diagnosis	Clinical picture with biopsy showing necrotizing vasculitis with granulomas of small arteries and veins.	Demonstration of circulating or tissue-bound anti-basement membrane antibodies, pulmonary hemorrhage, glomerulonephritis
Treatment	Cyclophosphamide, corticosteroids	Plasmapheresis, corticosteroids, cyclophosphamide

69. What clinical and laboratory findings are most important in determining the cause of angioedema?

In a patient who presents with recurrent angioedema, a careful history is of the utmost importance. For example, allergic angioedema might be suggested by a temporal relationship to exposure to specific allergens (such as food). Cold urticaria/angioedema would be indicated by on-set following exposure to cold temperatures. A number of findings might indicate hereditary an-gioedema (HAE), including a positive family history, low C4 during and between attacks, and low antigenic or functional activity of C1 esterase inhibitor. The majority of angioedema cases are idiopathic, and an extensive evaluation fails to reveal a specific cause or associated underly-ing disease. The list of diseases reported to be associated with angioedema is exhaustive, but some of the most widely recognized are connective tissue diseases, malignancies, thyroid disease, and liver disease (such as hepatitis B).

70. What is the cause of angioedema in the hereditary angioedema syndrome (HAE)?

HAE is caused by deficiency of C1 esterase inhibitor enzyme (C1INH). Eighty-five percent of HAE patients have depressed serum levels of C1INH (by antigenic assay), whereas the re-maining 15% have normal enzyme levels but lack functional activity. The clinical presentation and inheritance patterns are similar for both groups. Decreased C1INH leads to unchecked acti-vation of the classical complement pathway and decreased inhibition of Hageman factor-depen-dent activation of the kinin and plasmin pathways. This results in increased generation of C2 kinin, bradykinin, and other putative molecules.

71. What are some of the most important clinical characteristics of hereditary angioedema (HAE)?

HAE is transmitted in an autosomal dominant pattern, although sporadic cases do occur. The age of onset is variable and the diagnosis can be hindered by a predilection for nonlaryngeal sites, such as the abdominal viscera. Inciting causes are not usually identified, although trauma, even if minor, can lead to attacks. Most patients have a high propensity for life-threatening laryngeal edema that is not characteristic of angioedema due to other causes. Urticaria, although commonly seen in association with other causes of angioedema, is not part of the HAE syndrome. Pain, not pruritus, is typical of HAE lesions. Patients typically have depressed serum C4 levels even when they are asymptomatic between attacks. Attenuated androgen (i.e., stanazolol) therapy dramati-cally decreases the severity and frequency of attacks. Androgens should be tapered to the lowest dose that adequately controls disease activity in order to minimize potential adverse effects such as virilization and hepatic toxicity.

72. How would you evaluate a previously healthy 26-year-old patient who presents with an 8-week history of daily urticaria?

Urticaria persisting for longer than 6 weeks is deemed chronic. A careful history should be obtained to determine whether the urticaria is related to the ingestion of a specific food or liquid, environmental exposure, animal exposure, physical condition (heat, cold, water, sunlight, pres-sure, exercise, etc.), or stress. The history should also seek to rule out symptoms suggestive of an underlying systemic disease. A careful medication history should also be obtained for the inges-tion of both prescription and over-the-counter medications (particularly aspirin and aspirin-con-taining compounds). A thorough physical examination should be performed to identify potential underlying illnesses, such as thyroid disease, malignancy, infection, and rheumatic diseases.

A chest x-ray usually should be obtained, particularly if the patient has not had one within 6 months. If the patient has poor dental health or findings suggestive of a dental abscess, dental x-rays may reveal the source of an occult infection. Screening laboratory tests should include a com-plete blood count (CBC) with white blood cell (WBC) count and differential, urinalysis, erythro-cyte sedimentation rate (ESR), antinuclear antibody (ANA) screen, and liver function tests. In patients over the age of 40, a serum protein electrophoresis should be obtained. Other tests that may be helpful include C3, C4, rheumatoid factor, stool for ova and parasites, thyroid function studies, hepatitis B surface antigen (HB_sAg), and cryoglobulins. Whether these and other tests for the evaluation for systemic diseases are obtained depends upon the degree of clinical suspicion based on the history, physical examination, and initial laboratory results. Tests for specific types of the physical urticarias can be performed as indicated.

Despite extensive evaluation, as many as 90% of the cases of chronic urticaria may be classified as idiopathic, since an etiology cannot be determined. Typical urticarial lesions do not usually require biopsy. However, in particularly severe, persistent cases, and especially when urticarial lesions are very painful (as opposed to pruritic), very erythematous, or persist longer than 24 hours, a biopsy may reveal urticarial vasculitis. Some of these cases are accompanied by hypocomplementemia and may require more aggressive medical therapy.

73. What is the usefulness of rheumatoid factors (RFs) in the diagnosis of rheumatoid arthritis (RA)?

RFs are autoantibodies (most commonly IgM) that react with the Fc portion of IgG. The presence of RF is not diagnostic of RA and may *not* be detected in approximately 20% of patients with this disease. When present, RF may be detected in blood, synovial fluid, and pleural fluid. The potential pathogenic significance of RF is indicated by the more aggressive joint and extra-articular disease (especially vasculitis) in patients with RA who have a high titer of RF.

RF is also found in a long list of other illnesses, including other systemic inflammatory diseases, malignancies, infectious diseases (such as tuberculosis, viral, subacute bacterial endocarditis), and sarcoidosis. Furthermore, RF can be detected in a small percentage of normal individuals, particularly in the elderly population.

74. What is the single best test for the diagnosis of Sjögren's syndrome?

Sjögren's disease is a chronic inflammatory disease of the exocrine glands characterized by keratoconjunctivitis sicca and xerostomia. The inflammatory infiltrate is comprised primarily of lymphocytes and plasma cells. Primary Sjögren's disease is exocrine gland disease alone, whereas secondary Sjögren's is the occurrence with another connective tissue disease, most commonly rheumatoid arthritis. Eye involvement may be confirmed by the Schirmer test (a measurement of tearing on filter paper with < 10 mm wetting in 5 minutes defining a positive test), rose bengal staining of the conjunctivae, or the finding of keratitis on slit lamp examination. Parotid salivary flow rates and salivary radionuclide scanning may be used to assess salivary gland function. Autoantibodies present include Ro(SS-A), La(SS-B), rheumatoid factor, and Epstein-Barr-related nuclear antigen (RANA). Although all of the above tests may be helpful in the evaluation of Sjögren's syndrome, biopsy of the labial minor salivary glands is the most specific diagnostic procedure available.

75. What is the Prausnitz-Kustner (P-K) reaction?

The P-K reaction was used in the past to demonstrate the passive transfer of reaginic (IgE) antibodies in humans. Serum was removed from an allergic individual and injected into the skin of a person known not to be allergic to the specific allergen being tested. Twenty-four hours later, the antigen (allergen) was injected intradermally into the sensitized skin and observed for a wheal and flare response. A positive response indicated passive transfer of IgE antibodies from the donor serum, which bound to the dermal mast cells in the recipient's skin, leading to an immediate hypersensitivity reaction.

76. What do the direct and indirect Coombs tests measure and what is the diagnostic usefulness of each?

Once the presence of hemolytic anemia has been confirmed, additional testing should be performed to determine whether an immune mechanism is causing the hemolysis. The direct Coombs test (direct anti-globulin test, or DAT) measures antibody or complement on the surface of the RBC. Titrations are performed to determine the degree of RBC sensitization.

Briefly, the test is performed by incubation of the patient's RBCs with anti-Ig or anti-C3 reagent. If surface-bound immunoglobulin or complement is present, then agglutination will occur with the appropriate antisera.

The indirect Coombs test (indirect antiglobulin test, or IAT) measures the presence of antibody in the patient's serum. The patient's serum is added to normal RBCs, and after incubation and washing, anti-Ig reagent is added. If the antibody from the patient's serum has bound to the

RBCs, agglutination will occur. The usefulness of the DAT and IAT in the diagnosis of autoimmune hemolytic anemia (AIHA) is outlined in the table.

Usefulness of the Coombs Test in Autoimmune Hemolytic Anemias

TYPE OF ANEMIA	RESULT OF DIRECT COOMBS TEST IgG, C3	RESULT OF INDIRECT COOMBS TEST	ANTIBODY SPECIFICITY	COMMENT
Autoimmune				
Warm antibody (most common type)	+ + (67%) + − (20%) − + (13%)	Majority + (57%)	Most often within Rh system	With SLE, DAT usually positive for both C3 and IgG
Cold agglutinin syndrome	− +	High titer at 4°C	Usually anti-I, but also anti-i, especially with infectious mononucleosis	Agglutinating activity up to 30°C in albumin; high titer (usually >500) at 4°C
Paroxysmal cold hemoglobinuria	− +	Biphasic hemolysin	anti-P	Donath-Landsteiner antibody
Drug-induced				
Alpha-methyldopa (Aldomet)	+ −	Similar to warm antibody AIHA	Usually within Rh system	IgG autoantibody directed against RBC surface antigen, DAT positivity is dose-dependent, occurs after 3–6 months of treatment, and may remain (+) for up to 2 years after stopping the drug. Hemolysis improves in 1–3 weeks after stopping.
Penicillin	+ − (mostly)	(−) unless testing with penicillin-coated RBCs	Reacts with penicillin-coated RBCs	Haptenic mechanism, penicillin binds to RBCs
Other drugs (such as quinidine)	− +	Negative unless drug, normal RBCs, and serum incubated together		Immune complex mechanism (innocent bystander), intravascular hemolysis with anti-drug antibody (usually IgM).

From McMillan R (ed): Immune cytopenias. In Methods in Hematology. Livingstone, 1983, p 30, with permission.

77. When does a food allergy occur? What can mimic a food allergy?

True food allergy occurs when ingested food antigens bind to IgE on the surface of intestinal mast cells, causing an immediate hypersensitivity reaction. Basophils may also participate if food antigens appear in the circulation. The diagnosis is complicated by a bewildering array of other factors that may cause adverse reactions to food and that mimic allergic reactions. These include reactions to food additives, preservatives, dyes, and toxins. GI disorders such as eosinophilic gastroenteritis, malabsorption syndromes, enzyme deficiencies, gluten-sensitive enteropathy, gallbladder disease, peptic ulcer disease, and scrombroid poisoning are among a long list of important, nonimmunologic causes of adverse food reactions. Finally, the psychological aspect may be important, particularly in patients who are convinced that allergy is the cause of their GI symptoms. A partial list of some of the foods that most commonly cause true food allergies are peanuts, true nuts, shellfish, eggs, and wheat. Cooking may destroy a food's allergenicity.

78. How is a food allergy diagnosed?

A careful history and physical examination should be performed to rule out other potential causes of adverse reactions to food. In an allergic reaction, symptoms should occur following each ingestion of the specific food. This and the resolution of symptoms with elimination of the food from the diet support a diagnosis of food allergy. The onset of symptoms may occur for up to 2 hours. The longer time until onset of symptoms with some GI reactions compared to typical (<1 hr) immediate hypersensitivity reactions may be due to the need for transport of the antigen into the GI tract, processing of antigen by digestion, and absorption into the intestinal mucosa. Symptoms of food allergy may be localized to the GI tract (including nausea, vomiting, diarrhea, bloating, and pain), or may be systemic (urticaria, angioedema, headache, wheezing, hypotension, and other symptoms of anaphylaxis).

Of the immunologic diagnostic procedures, skin testing is the most useful. By itself, a positive skin test is not diagnostic of food allergy and must be interpreted in the context of other clinical findings. A positive skin test in the presence of a positive clinical history is highly suggestive of specific food allergy, whereas a negative skin test suggests that allergy to that specific food is highly unlikely. The RAST may also be helpful, but its use should be limited to patients in whom skin testing cannot be properly performed and interpreted, or in those thought to be at particular risk of a severe anaphylactic reaction to skin testing.

A clinical diagnosis of food allergy can be confirmed by food challenge. If the challenge is negative, there is strong evidence against allergy to that specific food. Food challenge should be performed only in an appropriate medical setting, since life-threatening anaphylaxis may occur. The double-blinded, placebo-controlled food challenge is the ideal method for confirming food allergy. In some patients, such as those with a low probability of a positive reaction, an open challenge may be useful. If positive, then a double-blinded, placebo-controlled challenge may be necessary.

Bock SA: Double-blind, placebo-controlled food challenge (DBPCFC) as an office procedure: A manual. J Allergy Clin Immunol 82:986, 1988.

79. What is the treatment for food allergy?

The treatment for food allergy is avoidance. Treatment with antiallergic medications, such as antihistamines or oral cromolyn, cannot be expected to decrease the risk of life-threatening reactions. Anaphylaxis caused by food ingestion should be treated like any other anaphylactic reaction, except that nasogastric (NG) tube placement and lavage may be useful to remove residual food antigen. Immunotherapy has no place in the treatment of food allergy.

80. What is the difference between a drug allergy, drug intolerance, and an idiosyncratic drug reaction?

All three are types of adverse drug reactions. A true **drug allergy** is an **immunologically mediated** adverse reaction to a drug. It can occur with very small doses of the offending agent and accounts for only 54% of all adverse drug reactions. **Drug intolerance,** which also can occur with very small doses, is the result of an **undesirable pharmacologic effect** of the drug. An **idiosyncratic drug reaction** is based on an individual patient's **biochemical alterations** of a drug's metabolism.

81. What are the indications for skin testing for penicillin allergy?

Skin testing for penicillin allergy is indicated in patients with a possible or definite past history consistent with immediate hypersensitivity to penicillin and in whom penicillin therapy is indicated and effective alternative antibiotic therapy is not available. Penicillin sensitization occurs by the haptenation mechanism and may involve a number of structural components (or "determinants") of the penicillin molecule. The penicilloyl determinant is referred to as the major determinant, and the penicillin G, penicilloate, and penicilloate determinants are referred to as the minor determinants. This "major" and "minor" nomenclature refers only to abundance of breakdown product and does not indicate relative clinical importance, as the minor determinants are responsible for the majority of life-threatening anaphylactic reactions.

82. What is the "innocent bystander" mechanism of drug-induced hemolysis?

Some drugs (such as sulfonamides, phenothiazines, quinidine, and quinine) can cause an immune hemolytic anemia even though they do not bind to RBCs. These drugs, bound to plasma proteins, stimulate the formation of complement-fixing antibodies that activate the classical complement pathway. Generated C3b binds to the RBC, which leads to intravascular hemolysis of these "innocent bystanders."

83. Which class of medications should be used with particular caution in patients prone to develop anaphylaxis?

Beta blockers should be avoided whenever possible, because they may accentuate the severity of anaphylaxis and prolong its cardiovascular and pulmonary manifestations. They may also markedly decrease the effectiveness of epinephrine in reversing the life-threatening manifestations of anaphylaxis.

84. What is C3 nephritic factor?

C3 nephritic factor (C3NF) is an IgG3 antibody that binds to the C3 convertase (C3b,Bb) of the alternative pathway of complement. This results in stabilization of C3b,Bb, which prevents its inactivation and results in uncontrolled C3 cleavage and alternative pathway activation. C3NF is found in partial lipodystrophy, some patients with SLE, and in most patients with type II membranoproliferative glomerulonephritis. The pathologic significance of the antibody is unknown. The antibody level and degree of lowering of the serum C3 level do not correlate with the severity of tissue damage or with disease activity.

85. What is the mechanism of action of cyclosporine? What are its principal adverse effects?

Cyclosporine A inhibits the production of multiple cytokines, but its principal immunosuppressive effect appears to be mediated through inhibition of interleukin-2 (IL-2) production. The principal side effects are listed in the table below.

Principal Side Effects of Cyclosporine

Renal dysfunction	Central nervous system toxicity
Hypertension	Tremor
Hirsutism	Seizures
Hepatotoxicity	Hypomagnesemia
Gingival hyperplasia	

86. What are the serum half-lives and relative potencies of the following steroid preparations: prednisone, prednisolone, methylprednisolone, dexamethasone, hydrocortisone, and cortisone?

Relative Potencies and Effects of Common Glucocorticoids

PREPARATION	POTENCY RELATIVE TO HYDROCORTISONE	RELATIVE SODIUM-RETAINING POTENCY	APPROXIMATELY EQUIVALENT DOSE OF ACTION (MG)	DURATION
Hydrocortisone	1	1	20	Short
Cortisone	0.8	0.8	25	Short
Prednisolone	4	0.8	5	Intermediate
Prednisone	4	0.8	5	Intermediate
6α-Methylprednisolone	5	0.5	4	Intermediate
Triamcinolone	5	0	4	Intermediate
Dexamethasone	25	0	0.75	Long
Betamethasone	25	0	0.75	Long

From Schleimer RP: Glucocorticosteroids. In Middleton E, et al (eds): Allergy: Principles and Practice, 3rd ed. St. Louis, Mosby, 1988, p 742, with permission.

87. What are the effects of corticosteroids on circulating leukocytes?

Effects of Corticosteroids on Leukocytes

CELL TYPE	EFFECT ON NUMBERS	EFFECT ON FUNCTION	COMMENT
Neutrophil	Increase	Minimal effect on chemotaxis, phagocytosis, bactericidal activity	Decreased from circulation marginating pool, increased production and release from bone marrow, increased half-life in circulation
Lymphocytes	Decrease	Decreased proliferative response, inhibition of mediator production and release, altered helper and suppressor function	Greater effect on T cells than on B cells
Lymphocytes T cells	Decrease a. Helper/inducer (CD4)-decrease b. Cytotoxic/suppressor (CD8)—no change		
B cells	Minimal decrease or no change		
Monocytes	Decrease	Depressed chemotaxis, suppression of cytotoxic activity	Possible sequestration
Eosinophils	Decrease	Inhibition of mediator production and release	Possible sequestration
Basophils	Decrease	Inhibition of degranulation	Possible sequestration
NK cells	No effect	No effect	
Null cells	No effect	Unknown	

88. What is the recommended treatment for Guillain-Barré syndrome (GBS)?

The cause of GBS remains obscure and the principal therapy is supportive, particularly with regard to decreased respiratory function. Plasmapheresis, particularly when instituted within 7 days of the onset of symptoms, has been shown to be beneficial in acute GBS. Typically 6–10 plasmapheresis procedures are performed. Each procedure consists of the exchange of total plasma volume (usually 2–3 liters in an adult) with an albumin/saline/electrolyte solution. The frequency of procedures varies with the overall medical condition of the patient and the availability of venous access.

89. What is the Chinese restaurant syndrome?

It is a reaction to glutamate ingested as MSG (monosodium glutamate), a flavoring agent commonly used in Chinese cooking. It occurs within 15–30 minutes of ingestion and consists of a sensation of warmth and tightness on the face and anterior chest. It is occasionally confused with angina pectoris, but is benign and requires no therapy except avoidance of foods cooked with MSG.

Kwok RHN: Chinese restaurant syndrome. N Engl J Med 278:1122, 1968.

90. What is the triad of Kartagener's syndrome?

Originally described by Kartagener in 1904, the syndrome consists of the triad of situs inversus, bronchiectasis, and chronic sinusitis. It is an autosomal recessive disorder resulting in a defect of the cilia, which lack dynein arms. Patients also suffer from chronic sinopulmonary infections and sterility may occur in males (due to immotile spermatozoa).

Eliasson R. et al: The immotile cilia syndrome. N Engl J Med 297:1–6, 1977.

91. Chronic or recurrent meningococcemia and gonococcemia have been particularly associated with which host immune defects?

Deficiencies of the late components of complement (C6, C7, and C8) are the predominant defects associated with these disorders. Several reports of C3, C5, properdin, IgG2 subclass, and IgM deficiencies have also been reported with these syndromes.

Ross S, et al: Complement deficiency and infection: Epidemiology, pathogenesis and consequences of neisserial and other infections in an immune deficiency. Medicine 63:243–273, 1984.

92. A patient with a history of hypotension following an intravenous pyelogram (IVP) now requires a radiocontrast study. What procedure should be followed?

Systemic reactions to radiocontrast media administration occur in 1–2% of patients. The reaction may begin from just after the onset of the infusion to 30 minutes after its completion. Cardiovascular collapse results in death in approximately 1 in 50,000 test procedures. The cause is unknown, but it does not appear to be a true immediate hypersensitivity (IgE mediated) reaction. A method for detection of patients at risk is not available, and skin testing with contrast or iodine is of no value. A patient who experiences a reaction has approximately a 33% chance of having another reaction with repeated radiocontrast exposures. Management of patients who *require* the radiocontrast procedure includes careful evaluation and documentation of the essential nature of the procedure and obtaining informed consent from the parent and the family (especially with regard to the potentially fatal outcome). The presence of necessary personnel and supplies for emergency treatment, adequate patient hydration, and preprocedure medical prophylaxis are also necessary. The usual prophylactic regimen consists of steroids (usually prednisone 50 mg orally at 13, 7 and 1 hour before the procedure) and H_1 antihistamines (diphenhydramine, 50 mg parenterally or orally 1 hour before radiocontrast media administration). When not contraindicated, ephedrine, 25 mg orally, may offer additional benefit. The usefulness of H_2 antihistamines and/or ephedrine is controversial.

Reactions after prophylactic therapy are usually mild. However, it is important that the procedure be started at the scheduled time or the efficacy of the prophylaxis may be decreased. Newer, lower osmolality contrast media are much less likely to cause systemic reactions, but their high expense limits their routine use. Furthermore, in patients with a history of radiocontrast media reactions, nonionic media do not seem to offer significant protective advantage over medical prophylaxis.

Patterson R, et al: Drug allergy and protocols for the management of drug allergies. New England & Regional Allergy Proceedings 7(4):325–342, 1989.

93. What clinical conditions are associated with deficiencies of the various components of the complement system?

Diseases Associated with Inherited Complement Deficiencies

DEFICIENT COMPONENT	NUMBER OF REPORTED CASES	ASSOCIATED DISEASES
C1	31	Autoimmune diseases, SLE-like syndromes
C4	20	Autoimmune diseases, SLE-like syndromes
C2	109	Autoimmune diseases, SLE-like syndromes
C3	20	Bacterial infections; mild glomerulonephritis
C5	28	Gram-negative coccal infections
C6	76	Gram-negative coccal infections
C7	67	Gram-negative coccal infections
C8	68	Gram-negative coccal infections
C9	18	Gram-negative coccal infections
Properdin	70	Gram-negative coccal infections
Factor I	17	Bacterial infections
Factor H	13	Bacterial infections
Factor D	3	Bacterial infections
C4-binding protein	3	—
C1 Inhibitor	>100	Hereditary angioedema

From David J: Immunology. In Dale DC, Federman DD (eds): Scientific American Medicine. New York, Scientific American, Inc., 1996, Section 6, Subsection VII, Table 9, p 26, with permission.

94. Which diseases and relative risks are associated with the various HLA antigens?

Diseases Showing Positive HLA Antigen Association(s)

DISEASE	HLA ANTIGEN	RELATIVE RISK*
Rheumatic		
Ankylosing spondylitis	B27	69.1
Reiter's syndrome	B27	37.0
Acute anterior uveitis	B27	8.2
Reactive arthritis (*Yersinia, Salmonella,* gonococcus)	B27	18.0
Psoriatic arthritis, central	B27	10.7
	B38	9.1
Psoriatic arthritis, peripheral	B27	2.0
	B38	6.5
Juvenile rheumatoid arthritis	B27	3.9
Juvenile rheumatoid arthritis, pauciarticular	DR5	3.3
Rheumatoid arthritis	Dw4/DR4	3.8
Sjögren's syndrome	Dw3	5.7
Systemic lupus erythematosus	DR3	2.6
Gastrointestinal		
Gluten-sensitive enteropathy	DR3	11.6
Chronic active hepatitis	DR3	6.8
Ulcerative colitis	B5	3.8
IgA deficiency	DR3	13.0
Hemotologic		
Idiopathic hemochromatosis	A3	6.7
	B14	2.7
	A3, B14	90.0
Pernicious anemia	DR5	5.4
Hodgkin's disease (white)	DP3	2.0
Skin		
Dermatitis herpetiformis	DR3	17.3
Psoriasis vulgaris	Cw6	7.5
Psoriasis vulgaris (Japanese)	Cw6	8.5
Pemphigus vulgaris (Jewish)	DR4	14.6
	A26	4.8
Behçet's disease (white)	B5	3.8
Behçet's disease (Japanese)	B51	12.4
Endocrine		
Insulin-dependent diabetes mellitus (juvenile diabetes mellitus)	DR4	3.6
	DR3	4.8
	DR2	0.2
	BfF1†	15.0
Graves' disease	B8	2.5
	DR3	3.7
Graves' disease (Japanese)	B35	4.4
Addison's disease	Dw3	10.5
Subacute thyroiditis (de Quervain)	B35	13.7
Hashimoto's thyroiditis	DR5	3.2
Congenital adrenal hyperplasia	Bw47	15.4
Neurologic		
Myasthenia gravis (without thymoma)	B8	3.3
Multiple sclerosis	Dw2/DR2	6.0
Manic-depressive disorder	B16	2.3
Narcolepsy	DR2	130.0
Schizophrenia	A28	2.3
Renal		
Idiopathic membranous glomerulonephritis	DR3	5.7
Goodpasture's syndrome (anti-GBM)	DR2	15.9
Minimal change disease (steroid responsive)	DR7	4.2
IgA nephropathy (French, Japanese)	DR4	3.1
Gold/penicillamine nephropathy	DR3	14.0
Polycystic kidney disease	B5	2.6

continued

Diseases Showing Positive HLA Antigen Association(s)—Cont.

DISEASE	HLA ANTIGEN	RELATIVE RISK*
Infectious		
Tuberculoid leprosy (Asians)	B8	6.8
Paralytic polio	B16	4.3
Low vs high response to vaccinia virus	Cw3	12.7

$$*\text{Relative risk} = \frac{(\% \text{ antigen-positive patients}) (\% \text{ antigen-negative control subjects})}{(\% \text{ antigen-negative patients}) (\% \text{ antigen-positive control subjects})}$$

†BfF1 is an allele of the complement system that is HLA-linked but is not an antigen.
From David J: Immunology. In Dale DC, Federman DD (eds): Scientific American Medicine. New York, Scientific American, Inc., 1996, Section 6, Subsection V, Table 3, p 9, with permission.

95. What is the lupus band test?

It is a test that may be of value in questionable cases of SLE. It involves demonstration of granular deposition of C3 and IgG along the dermal-epidermal junction in a biopsy of normal skin. The test is most likely to be positive in hypocomplementemic patients. However, the test rarely correlates with renal involvement.

96. What percentage of patients with SLE have a negative antinuclear antibody test (ANA)?

Five percent or less of patients with SLE have been reported to be ANA negative. However, these patients have probably been tested using mouse kidney as the test substrate. This substrate will not readily detect antibody against Ro/SSA, ssDNA, Jo, and centromere. Antibodies against Ro and ssDNA are found in SLE. The HEp^{-2} cell line, which is now widely used as the substrate for ANA testing, will detect these antibodies. Virtually all SLE patients probably are ANA positive using this testing protocol.

97. What are the most common clinical manifestations of drug-induced lupus? Which organs are characteristically spared in this syndrome when compared to idiopathic SLE?

Hydralazine and procainamide are the most common causes of drug-induced lupus. Up to 50% of patients receiving these drugs may have a positive antinuclear antibody test (ANA), although fewer will actually develop symptoms. Slow acetylators of these drugs are particularly susceptible for developing clinical disease. Hydralazine-induced lupus is most commonly encountered when the total daily dose administered exceeds 400 mg, with 10–20% of these patients developing a lupus-like syndrome. Other causes include D-penicillamine, isoniazid, and phenytoin. The ANA pattern in drug-induced lupus is usually homogeneous or speckled and is caused by anti-histone antibodies. Antibodies to double-stranded DNA, often seen in SLE, are not found in drug-induced lupus.

Drug-induced lupus manifests many of the same symptoms as idiopathic SLE, although they are generally milder. However, lupus nephritis and cerebritis rarely, if ever, complicate the syndrome. Drug-induced lupus is more frequent in women than men and in those with HLA DR4 phenotype. Symptoms resolve shortly after discontinuation of the drug, although laboratory abnormalities may persist for months or years.

Clinical and Serologic Features of Drug-induced Lupus and Systemic Lupus Erythematosus

	DRUG-INDUCED LUPUS	IDIOPATHIC SLE		DRUG-INDUCED LUPUS	IDIOPATHIC SLE
Polyserositis	+	+	Nephritis	−	+
Arthritis	+	+	Cerebritis	−	+
Fever	+	+	Positive ANA	+	+
Rash	+	+	Positive anti-dsDNA	−	+
Photosensitivity	+	+	Reversible*	+	−
Hemolytic anemia	+	+			

* Within several months of drug discontinuation.
From Cush JJ, et al: Drug-induced lupus: Clinical spectrum and pathogenesis. Am J Med Sci 290:36, 1985, with permission.

98. A patient with SLE asks whether or not she should be vaccinated against measles. What is your recommendation?

The major live attenuated vaccines currently available are rubella (measles), poliomyelitis, BCG (bacille Calmette-Guérin), mumps, and yellow fever. Vaccinia (small pox) is no longer given. Live vaccines should not be administered to immunologically compromised patients, particularly those with depressed cell-mediated immunity (CMI), including SLE. Conditions in which live vaccination of patients should be avoided include:

1. Patients treated with primary immunodeficiency disorders (especially those with defective CMI such as severe combined immunodeficiency syndrome [SCID]).

2. Patients given immunosuppressive therapy (including corticosteroids, cytotoxic drugs, and radiation therapy).

3. Patients with malignancies, including leukemia, lymphoma, and Hodgkin's disease.

4. Patients with systemic immunoregulatory, inflammatory, or infectious diseases associated with defective CMI (such as SLE, diabetes mellitus, sarcoidosis, AIDS, and atopic dermatitis).

5. Children less than 1 year of age.

6. Patients with severe malnutrition or burns.

7. Live vaccines should not be given to pregnant women because of the potential harm to the fetus. The exception is yellow fever when the mother must travel to an endemic area. In this case, the risk of infection and detrimental effects without the vaccine are greater than that of receiving the immunization.

Also noteworthy, household contacts of immunocompromised patients should not receive oral live polio vaccine, since the live attenuated strain may revert back to the wild type in the GI tract and be spread by the fecal-oral route.

99. What is the Donath-Landsteiner antibody? In which disease is it found?

The Donath-Landsteiner antibody is an IgG cold-reacting antibody. It was described in patients with syphilis who developed paroxysmal cold hemoglobinuria (Donath Landsteiner hemolytic anemia) on exposure to cold temperatures. The clinical syndrome consists of paroxysmal chills, fever, headache, and diffuse pain in the abdomen, back, and legs, in addition to the hemoglobinuria.

100. What is erythema multiforme (EM)?

EM is an immunologic reaction of the skin and mucous membranes to a variety of antigenic stimuli, but no such stimulus can be identified in up to 50% of cases. The lesions may be localized or widespread, and consist of bullae, erythematous plaques, and epidermal cell necrosis. The lesions are usually bilaterally and symmetrically distributed on the extensor surfaces of the limbs, on the dorsal and volar aspects of the hands and feet, and on the trunk. The lesions, which resemble "targets" or "bull's eyes," are diagnostic. They appear as a central vesicle or dark purple papule, surrounded by a round, pale zone that is in turn surrounded by a round area of erythema.

101. What are the precipitating factors in EM?

Precipitating Factors in Erythema Multiforme

1. **Viral diseases:** Herpes simplex, hepatitis, influenza A, vaccinia, mumps
2. **Fungal diseases:** Dermatophytoses, histoplasmosis, coccidioidomycosis
3. **Bacterial diseases:** Hemolytic streptococcal infections, tuberculosis, leprosy, typhoid
4. **Collagen vascular disease:** Rheumatoid arthritis, SLE, dermatomyositis, allergic vasculitis, polyarteritis nodosa
5. **Malignant tumors:** Carcinoma, lymphoma after radiation therapy
6. **Hormonal changes:** Pregnancy, menstruation
7. **Drugs:** Penicillins, sulfonamides, barbiturates, salicylates, halogens, phenolphthalein
8. **Miscellaneous:** Rhus dermatitis, dental extractions, mycoplasma pneumonia infection

From Abel AE, Farber EM: Dermatology. In Dale DC, Federman DD (eds): Scientific American Medicine. New York, Scientific American Medicine Inc., 1990, Section 2 (Dermatology), Subsection IX, Table 2, p 9, with permission.

102. What is Stevens-Johnson syndrome?

Stevens-Johnson syndrome is a severe form of erythema multiforme associated with fulminant, disseminated, multi-system involvement. The patients appear toxic, with fever, chills, malaise, tachycardia, tachypnea, and prostration. Diffuse vesicular, bullous, and ulcerative lesions of the skin and mucous membranes develop and desquamate, leading to secondary infections, which in turn may lead to sepsis and even death. It is associated with all the causes of erythema multiforme.

103. Why is the Kviem test no longer performed?

The Kviem test was performed by intradermal injection of sarcoid spleen suspension into patients suspected of having sarcoidosis. The development of a skin reaction revealing noncaseating granulomas on biopsy was considered positive. However, the test lacked specificity, and availability of the reagent was poor. Because of these problems and the risk of transmission of infectious diseases, the test is no longer performed.

104. What is the significance of erythema nodosum (EN) in sarcoidosis?

EN is a favorable prognostic sign, indicating a low propensity for development of chronic disease.

105. Hepatitis B surface antigenemia is associated with which of the vasculitides?

Polyarteritis nodosa. It is seen in 40% of HB_SAg-positive patients. The severity of the vasculitis and hepatitis is not correlated.

106. What is the differential diagnosis of a positive blood test for rheumatoid factor?

Differential Diagnosis of a Positive Rheumatoid Factor

Rheumatological diseases:	Pulmonary diseases:
Rheumatoid arthritis	Bronchitis or asthma
Juvenile rheumatoid arthritis	Coal miner's disease
SLE	Asbestosis
Mixed connective tissue disease	Idiopathic pulmonary fibrosis
Behçet's syndrome	Sarcoidosis
Sjögren's syndrome	
	Other diseases:
Infectious diseases:	Cirrhosis
Syphilis	Myocardial infarction
Viral hepatitis	Neoplasms
Parasitic infections	Essential mixed cryoglobulinemia
Granulomatous disease	
Mononucleosis	**Healthy persons**—increases with age

From Coffey R, et al: Immunologic tests of value in diagnosis. I. Acute phase reactants and autoantibodies. Postgrad Med 70:164,1981, with permission.

107. An 18-year-old male presents with abdominal pain, bloody diarrhea, peripheral neuropathy, and demonstration of IgA deposition on biopsy of the GI tract. What is the most likely diagnosis?

The clinical presentation is characteristic of Henoch-Schonlein purpura (HSP), although the age of onset is typically younger. The disease is almost always limited to males. This type of hypersensitivity vasculitis principally involves the skin, joints, intestine, and kidney. The disease is usually self-limited, although chronic renal failure may rarely occur. A history of recent infection, usually of the upper respiratory tract, is often reported. Circulating IgA immune complexes are common. Serum IgA levels may be elevated and IgA deposition can be demonstrated in the affected tissues.

108. Is skin testing useful for the diagnosis of histoplasmosis?

Skin testing is rarely useful in the diagnosis of histoplasmosis and should be principally limited to epidemiologic surveys. A positive skin test indicates prior exposure and not necessarily active infection. Furthermore, the histoplasmin reagent often causes a significant rise in antibody titers, thereby complicating interpretation of subsequent serologic studies. A negative skin test is highly suggestive of the absence of disease (even during dissemination stages), unless the patient is anergic.

109. How do anticentromere antibodies help differentiate between the CREST syndrome and scleroderma?

The anticentromere antibody, which is found by antinuclear antibody (ANA) testing, is characteristic of CREST patients but is usually absent in patients with diffuse scleroderma.

110. Which other laboratory and clinical findings distinguish the CREST syndrome from diffuse scleroderma (progressive systemic sclerosis)?

Skin involvement is principally limited to the extremities, and internal organ involvement generally develops more slowly and is less severe than in diffuse scleroderma. Particularly noteworthy of the CREST syndrome (but not in diffuse scleroderma) is the development of pulmonary arterial hypertension in the absence of pulmonary fibrosis. Intimal proliferation of the small and medium-sized pulmonary arteries is prominent. Pulmonary hypertension may be progressive and is almost uniformly fatal. Biliary cirrhosis also may occur in the CREST syndrome but is uncommon in diffuse scleroderma.

111. In a patient who complains of fatigue with hair-combing and stair-climbing, what are the most likely diagnoses?

Diseases characterized by proximal muscle weakness, such as myasthenia gravis, Eaton-Lambert syndrome (myasthenic syndrome), polymyositis, dermatomyositis, and polymyalgia rheumatica.

112. Explain the importance of HLA and ABO typing in solid organ and bone marrow transplantation (BMT).

HLA compatibility of donor and recipient affects graft outcome in both solid organ transplantation (such as kidney, heart, lung, and liver) and BMT. HLA compatibility is not a major graft survival factor for first-time, nonvascularized corneal transplants. HLA incompatibility may lead to graft rejection and destruction in solid organ transplantation and to graft-versus-host disease in BMT. In graft rejection, the graft is attacked by the recipient's immune system. In contrast, with graft-versus-host disease, the immunocompetent cells from the donor attack the recipient. ABO blood typing is critical in solid organ transplants, because ABO antigens are expressed on tissue cells of the transplanted organ. Thus, transplantation of a donor kidney from a type A donor into a type O recipient could lead to hyperacute rejection and graft death.

113. What are the four types of graft rejection and their immunologic mechanisms?

Types of Graft Rejection

TYPE	ONSET	MAJOR EFFECTOR MECHANISMS
Hyperacute	Minutes to hours	Humoral: preformed cytotoxic antibody in the recipient against donor graft antigen(s) a. ABO system b. Anti-HLA class I
Accelerated	2–5 days	Cell-mediated: due to prior T cell sensitization against donor antigen(s)
Acute	7–28 days	a. Principally cell-mediated immunity: allogeneic reactivity by recipient T cells against donor antigen(s) b. Humoral immunity
Chronic	>3 months	a. Principally cell-mediated immunity allogeneic reactivity by recipient T cells against donor antigen(s) b. Humoral immunity

114. What are the targets of the responsible antibodies in the various autoimmune diseases?

Autoimmune Diseases

DISEASE	TARGET OF ANTIBODY
Organ-Specific Diseases	
Myasthenia gravis	Acetylcholine receptors
Graves' disease	Thyroid-stimulating hormone receptor
Thyroiditis	Thyroid
Insulin-resistant diabetes with acanthosis nigricans	Insulin receptor
Insulin-resistant diabetes with ataxia telangiectasia	Insulin receptor
Allergic rhinitis, asthma, and autoimmune abnormalities	Beta$_2$-adrenergic receptors
Juvenile insulin-dependent diabetes	Pancreative islet cells, insulin
Pernicious anemia	Gastric parietal cells, vitamin B$_{12}$ binding site of intrinsic factor
Addison's disease	Adrenal cells
Idiopathic hypoparathyroidism	Parathyroid cells
Spontaneous infertility	Sperm
Premature ovarian failure	Interstitial cells, corpus luteum cells
Pemphigus	Intercellular substance of skin and mucosa
Bullous pemphigoid	Basement membrane zone of skin and mucosa
Primary biliary cirrhosis	Mitochondria
Autoimmune hemolytic anemia	Erythrocytes
Idiopathic thrombocytopenic purpura	Platelets
Idiopathic neutropenia	Neutrophils
Vitiligo	Melanocytes
Osteosclerosis and Ménière's disease	Type II collagen
Chronic active hepatitis	Nuclei of hepatocytes
Systemic (Non-Organ-Specific) Diseases	
Goodpasture's syndrome	Basement membranes
Rheumatoid arthritis	γ-Globulin, Epstein-Barr virus-related antigens, types II and III collagen
Sjögren's syndrome	γ-Globulin, SS-A (Ro), SS-B (La)
Systemic lupus erythematosus	Nuclei, double-stranded DNA, single-stranded DNA, Sm, ribonucleoprotein, lymphocytes, erythrocytes, neurons, γ-globulin
Scleroderma	Nuclei, Scl-70, SS-A (Ro), SS-B (La), centromere
Polymyositis	Nuclei, Jo-1 PL-7, histadyl-tRNA synthetase, threonyl-tRNA synthetase, PM-1, Mi-2
Rheumatic fever	Myocardium, heart valves, choroid plexus

From David J: Immunology. In Dale DC, Federman DD (eds): Scientific American Medicine. New York, Scientific American, Inc., 1996, Section 6, Subsection VI, Table 1, p. 3, with permission.

115. What are the principal immunologic defects associated with recurrent bacterial infections?

The principal defects are antibody deficiency, complement deficiency, and defective neutrophil function. Infections in patients with antibody deficiencies are most commonly due to encapsulated organisms (i.e., *Hemophilus influenzae, Pneumococcus)*. Screening for antibody deficiency first includes determination of serum immunoglobulin levels (IgG, IgM, and IgA) and IgG subclass levels if subclass deficiency is suspected. Further evaluation may include measuring serum isohemagglutinin titers (these are IgM antibodies) and serum IgG antibody levels against protein (tetanus toxoid) and carbohydrate *(Pneumococcus* and/or *Hemophilus influenzae)* antigens before and after immunization in order to determine antibody response capability following specific antigen challenge.

Isolated C3 deficiency is associated with severe, recurrent pyogenic (particularly gram-negative) infections. Particularly noteworthy is the association of recurrent, disseminated *Neisseria* infections with terminal complement component deficiencies (except C9). Properidin deficiency may also be accompanied by recurrent pyogenic and *Neisseria* infections. Complement deficiency can be evaluated by obtaining a CH50 (or CH100) and by measuring levels of specific complement components when indicated.

Most defects of neutrophil function associated with recurrent infections occur in the pediatric age group. However, it is now recognized that some adults may have a variant of chronic granulomatous disease of childhood (CGD) in which the defect in respiratory burst is qualitatively less than in typical CGD. A nitroblue tetrazolium test can be performed to assess neutrophil respiratory burst in patients with a clinical history suggestive of CGD. These patients are particularly susceptible to catalase-positive organisms. Bacteria infections are typically caused by *Staphylococcus aureus*, *Escherichia coli* and *Serratia marcescens* and fungal infections by *Candida albicans*, *Aspergillus*, and *Nocardia*.

116. What causes rhinitis medicamentosa (RM)? How is it treated?

RM is caused by rebound vasodilation due to long-term use of topical vasoconstrictors (decongestants, cocaine). The nasal mucosa typically is reddened in appearance. Treatment consists of discontinuation of the offending drug and beginning therapy with topical intranasal or, for severe cases, oral corticosteroids.

117. What are the differentiating clinical and immunologic features of primary biliary cirrhosis and idiopathic sclerosing cholangitis?

Comparison of Primary Biliary Cirrhosis and Idiopathic Sclerosing Cholangitis

PARAMETER	BILIARY CIRRHOSIS	SCLEROSING CHOLANGITIS
Etiology	Unknown	Unknown
Sex	Middle-aged women	Men
HLA association	None	B8
Histology	Destructive, nonsuppurative cholangitis, cirrhosis	Fibrosis with obliteration of intra- and extrahepatic bile ducts
Cholangiography	Normal early, cirrhosis late	Narrowing and dilatation of intra- and extra-hepatic bile ducts causing "beaded appearance"
Associated diseases	CREST form of scleroderma, hypothyroidism, keratoconjunctivitis sicca	Ulcerative colitis, biliary cholangiocarcinoma
Autoantibodies	Antimitochondrial	None
Immunologic	Polyclonal hypergammaglobulinemia, particularly ↑ IgM (may be monomeric) and also ↑ IgA, anergy, ↓ NK, and T cell function	No major defects known
Treatment	Supportive, liver transplantation for end-stage disease	Supportive, liver transplantation for end-stage disease
Prognosis	Variable	Variable

↑ = increased, ↓ = decreased.

118. Name some diseases associated with elevation of the total serum IgE level.

Diseases Associated with Increased Total Serum IgE

Atopic (allergic) diseases:
  Allergic rhinitis
  Allergic asthma
  Allergic bronchopulmonary aspergillosis
Primary immunodeficiency disorders:
  Hyper IgE syndrome
  Wiskott-Aldrich syndrome
  Nezelhof's syndrome (cellular immunodeficiency with Ig's)
  Selective IgA deficiency (with concomitant atopic disease)

Infections:
  Parasitic infections
  Viral infections (infectious mononucleosis, others)
  Fungal infections (candidiasis, others)
Malignancies:
  Hodgkin's disease
  Bronchial carcinoma
  IgE myeloma

Acute graft-versus-host disease

Dermatologic disorders:
  Atopic dermatitis
  Bullous pemphigoid
  Others

In many of these diseases, IgE levels may be normal, mildly elevated, or markedly elevated. The clinical usefulness of measurement of total serum IgE is usually limited to diagnosis and monitoring of exacerbations, remissions, and/or treatment of allergic bronchopulmonary aspergillosis, parasitic infections, and immunodeficiency disorders.

BIBLIOGRAPHY

1. Klein J: Immunology. Oxford, Blackwell Scientific Publications, 1990.
2. Middleton E, et al (eds): Allergy: Principles and Practice, 4th ed. St. Louis, Mosby, 1993.
3. Paul WE (ed): Fundamental Immunology, 3rd ed. New York, Raven Press, 1994.
4. Roitt IM, et al: Immunology, 4th ed. St. Louis, Mosby, 1996.

13. AIDS AND HIV INFECTION

Christopher J. Lahart, M.D.

> *Dr. Rieux resolved to compile this chronical. . . to state quite simply what we learn in a time of pestilence: that there are more things to admire in men than to despise.*
>
> Albert Camus
> *The Plague, Pt. V, tr. by Stuart Gilbert*

> *He is the best physician who is the best inspirer of hope.*
>
> Samuel Taylor Coleridge
> *Table Talk*

1. HIV is a retrovirus. What is a retrovirus?

A retrovirus, a member of the Retroviridae family, is an RNA virus that contains an enzyme, reverse transcriptase, that is capable of transcribing DNA from the viral RNA. This process is the reverse of the normal DNA-to-RNA transcription, hence the name.

2. A patient tests positive for HIV. Does he have AIDS?

A positive HIV test indicates infection with HIV, but HIV infection is a wide spectrum of illness, and the vast majority of patients are not symptomatic. AIDS is a syndrome of explicitly defined conditions that represent severe immunosuppression and is the final band in this spectrum of illness. A diagnosis of AIDS is made when a person with HIV infection develops a malignancy, opportunistic infection, other symptomatic illness, or a decreased CD4-lymphocyte count that meets the diagnostic criteria for AIDS.

When a patient has tested positive for infection by HIV, a comprehensive history and physical examination are needed to identify symptoms and signs of immunosuppression and any comorbid conditions. A laboratory evaluation can help place the patient in a relative position on the spectrum.

CDC: 1993 revised classification system for HIV infection and expanded case surveillance definition for AIDS among adolescents and adults. MMWR 41(RR-17):1–19, 1992.

NATURAL HISTORY AND TRANSMISSION

3. How long is someone with HIV infectious?

For life. There may be periods of increased infectiousness, such as during the initial infection with its high levels of viremia and at the later stages of disease, but there is never a period of absolute noninfectiousness. This highlights the importance of changing high-risk behavior patterns. Such change must be consistent and permanent.

4. What is the risk of HIV transmission via a needlestick?

The average risk of transmission in a large group of health-care workers suffering percutaneous exposure to HIV is approx. 0.3%. However, each exposure needs to be evaluated individually. There is tremendous variation in the degree of exposure, which affects the likelihood of infection.

Tokars JI, et al: Surveillance of HIV infection and zidovudine use among health-care workers after occupational exposure to HIV-infected blood. Ann Intern Med 118:913–919, 1993.

5. What variables increase the risk of occupational exposure?

Exposure to a large volume of infectious material (or material with a high viral load), a deep injury, visible blood on the device causing the injury, prolonged contact with the infectious material, and the body area exposed (portal of entry) are all important factors. Mucosal splashes and exposure on *intact* skin are not routes of transmission (no transmission in > 12,500 exposures followed prospectively). Associated with increased risk are intramuscular injection, exposures via hollow needles (as opposed to suture needles, pins, etc.), and exposure to material from a viremic HIV-infected patient.

6. Does postexposure zidovudine therapy prevent infection?

No controlled trial has been performed and, most likely, none ever will be. However, a retrospective case-control study involving 31 exposed and infected health-care workers and 679 exposed, uninfected workers found that postexposure zidovudine reduced the risk of HIV infection by 79%. The study design is not the proper one for evaluating drug efficacy, but it does provide important information. Drug therapy must be part of a program that includes immediate availability of counseling as well as medication. Close follow-up needs to be provided, and confidentiality guaranteed.

CDC: Case-control study of HIV seroconversion in health-care workers after percutaneous exposure to HIV-infected blood—France, United Kingdom, and United States, January 1988–August 1994. MMWR 44(50):929–933, 1995.

7. Are heterosexuals at risk for HIV infection?

Most certainly. Although heterosexual contact does not appear to be an efficient transmitter of infection, it clearly does transmit HIV. In many developing countries, the *equal* incidence of AIDS in males and females provides evidence for heterosexual transmission. As of October 31, 1995, in the U.S., 7.7% of the first 500,000 AIDS cases (38,541 cases)—3% of male cases (12,049 cases) and 36% of female cases (23,633 cases) were attributed to heterosexual contact. If the temporal trends are examined, between 1981–87, 2.5% of cases were attributed to heterosexual contact; 1988–92, 6.1%; and, 1992–1995, 10.1%. About 50% of the cases of heterosexually acquired AIDS result from sexual contact with an intravenous drug user.

CDC: First 500,000 AIDS cases—United States, 1995. MMWR 44(46):849–853, 1995.

8. How much time elapses between infection with HIV and the diagnosis of AIDS?

This period is not easily defined. Studies of large patient cohorts indicate that 50% of HIV-positive patients will progress to AIDS in approx. 10 years. The rate of disease progression is not stable over this period, since few develop disease early on and proportionally more develop AIDS with each passing year. It is not certain at this time that 100% of HIV-infected individuals will develop AIDS.

Litson AR, et al: The natural history of human immunodeficiency virus infection. J Infect Dis 158:1360–1367, 1988.

9. What is a CD4+-lymphocyte count and why is it obtained?

A CD4+-lymphocyte count is a laboratory measurement of the number of CD4-postive (T4 or helper-inducer) lymphocytes present in peripheral blood. Since very early in the HIV epidemic, it has been known that one of the most problematic effects of HIV infection is the de-

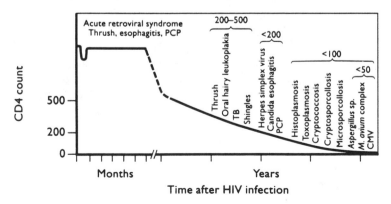

Onset of opportunistic infections with decreasing CD4+ count. (From Mildran D (ed): Atlas of Infectious Diseases: I. AIDS. Philadelphia, Current Medicine, 1995, p. 15.2; with permission.)

pletion of CD4+-lymphocytes. By measuring these cells, a clinician can attempt to place a patient in a general position on the spectrum of HIV-related illness. The CD4+-lymphocyte count is also used to determine the timing of various interventions, such as antiretroviral therapy or prophylaxis against *Pneumocystis carinii* pneumonia (PCP). Thus, it is of prognostic and therapeutic value.

10. Are any other laboratory tests of prognostic value?

Tests that measure HIV viral load by assaying for plasma HIV RNA have recently been demonstrated to be the single best indicator of prognosis in HIV infection. The first such test was licensed in June 1996, so clinical experience is short, but in a study using stored serum specimens in 181 patients, even a single plasma HIV RNA level was able to help predict clinical events occurring up to 10 years later. CD4+ lymphocyte counts are still necessary to estimate immediate risk for the development of opportunistic infections.

β2-Microglobulin, a marker of lymphoid activity, and neopterin, a product of T-cell-stimulated macrophages, both add some prognostic information in that higher levels of either are correlated to poorer outcomes.

1. Mellors JW, et al: Prognosis in HIV-1 infection predicted by the quality of virus in plasma. Science 272:1167-70, 1996.

2. O'Brien WA, et al: Changes in plasma HIV-1 RNA and CD4+ lymphocyte counts and the risk of progression to AIDS. N Engl J Med 334:426-31, 1996.

11. What is the prognosis for patients infected with HIV-1?

In a review of 32 follow-up studies, Cooper and Jeffers reported the following:

- From the time of seroconversion, 10–20% of HIV-infected individuals will progress to AIDS in 3–6 years.
- Once the patient has constitutional symptoms, herpes zoster, thrush, or a lowered CD4+-lymphocyte count, chances are > 40% of progressing to AIDS after 3 years of follow-up and > 50% after 5 years.

These data are from *untreated* patients. Prognosis can be modified by antiretroviral therapy and general medical support.

Cooper GS, Jeffers DJ: The clinical prognosis of HIV-1 infection: A review of 32 follow-up studies. J Gen Intern Med 3:525–532, 1988.

12. How has HIV contributed to overall mortality in the U.S.?

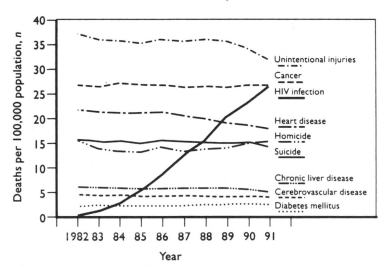

From Vermund SH: Rising HIV-mortality in young Americans. JAMA 269:3034–3035, 1993; with permission.

CDC: Update: Mortality attributable to HIV infection among persons aged 25–44 years - United States, 1994. MMWR 45(6):121–125, 1996.

In 1993, HIV infection became the leading cause of death among persons aged 25–44 years, accounting for 19% of all deaths in this age group. It became the most common cause of death for black men in 1991, for all men in 1992, and for white men in 1994, and also in 1994 it became the third most common cause of death in women. For the entire population across all age groups, HIV infection is the eighth leading cause of death.

13. Is AIDS invariably fatal?

Certainly a large majority of patients with AIDS die, but it is not yet clear whether all will die from this disease. The Centers for Disease Control and Prevention (CDC) report approx. 30% mortality 1 year after a diagnosis of AIDS, > 50% at 2 years, and > 75% at 3 years. Of the 501,310 AIDS cases reported to CDC through October 31, 1995, 62% have died.

DIAGNOSIS

14. Who should be tested for HIV?

Groups to Test for HIV Infection

Gay or bisexual males	Patients in tuberculosis (TB) clinics
Injecting drug users	Persons who received blood products from 1978–1985
Prostitutes	Anyone having sex with a member of a high-risk group
Patients in STD clinics	

A clinician should recommend HIV testing for any patient with a high index of suspicion for HIV infection. Several states now mandate that HIV testing be offered to pregnant women.

Additionally, the CDC recommends that hospitals with an HIV prevalence rate of ≥1% or an AIDS diagnosis rate of ≥1/1000 discharges offer HIV testing routinely to patients aged 15–54.

CDC: Recommendations for HIV testing services for inpatients and outpatients in acute-care hospital settings. MMWR 42(RR-2):1, 1993.

McCarthy BD, et al: Who should be screened for HIV infection?: A cost-effectiveness analysis. Arch Intern Med 153:1107–1116, 1993.

15. Why are HIV-ELISA tests confirmed by Western blot?

For a variety of reasons, the ELISA (enzyme-linked immunosorbent assay) can yield a significant number of false-positive tests for the presence of anti-HIV antibodies. Most laboratories will repeat a positive ELISA, but a repetitively positive result should be confirmed by Western blot to verify that the positive ELISA result is based on true HIV antibodies and not cross-reacting proteins. In populations with a low prevalence of HIV infection, as many as 29 of every 30 positive ELISAs will be false-positives.

Meyer KB, Packer SG: Screening for HIV: Can we afford the false positive rate? N Engl J Med 317:238–241, 1987.

16. How should an "indeterminate" Western blot be followed up?

Assuming that the patient had an initial ELISA test repeatedly positive prior to the indeterminate Western blot, the Western blot should be repeated. If indeterminate again, both the ELISA and Western blot should be repeated in 3 months.

17. What are the diagnostic criteria for AIDS?

The diagnosis depends on the status of the patient's laboratory evidence for or against HIV infection:

1. **For patients *with* laboratory evidence for HIV infection,** a diagnosis of AIDS can be made if the patient has a presumptive or definitive diagnosis of one or more of a list of indicator diseases or a CD4$^+$-lymphocyte count < 200/mm^3.

2. **For patients *without* laboratory evidence for HIV infection,** a diagnosis can be made

if there is no other cause for an underlying immunodeficiency state and the patient has a definitive diagnosis of one or more indicator diseases.

3. **For a patient with laboratory evidence *against* HIV infection,** a diagnosis can be made if the patient has had a definitive diagnosis of *Pneumocystis carinii* pneumonia or has a definitive diagnosis of one or more indicator diseases with a CD4+-lymphocyte count < 400 cells/mm³.

CDC: 1993 Revised classification system for HIV infection and expanded surveillance case definition for AIDS among adolescents and adults. MMWR 41(RR-17):1–19, 1992.

18. What are the AIDS indicator diseases?

Candidiasis of lungs, bronchi, trachea	Lymphoid interstitial pneumonitis
Candidiasis, esophageal	Lymphoma, non-Hodgkin's
Cervical cancer, invasive*	Lymphoma, primary CNS
Coccidioidomycosis, disseminated or extrapulmonary	
Cryptococcosis, extrapulmonary	*Mycobacterium avium,* disseminated or extrapulmonary
Cryptosporidiosis, chronic intestinal	*Mycobacterium kansasii,* disseminated or extrapulmonary
Cytomegalovirus (other than liver, spleen, nodes)	*Mycobacterium* spp., disseminated or extrapulmonary
Cytomegalovirus retinitis	*Mycobacterium tuberculosis,* any site*
Herpes simplex, chronic ulcers or of bronchi, lungs, esophagus	*Pneumocystis carinii* pneumonia (PCP)
Histoplasmosis, disseminated or extrapulmonary	Pneumonia, recurrent bacterial*
HIV encephalopathy	Progressive multifocal leukoencephalopathy
HIV wasting syndrome	*Salmonella* bacteremia, recurrent
Isosporiasis, chronic intestinal	Stronglyloidosis, non-GI
Kaposi's sarcoma	Toxoplasmosis of brain

*Newly added in the 1993 expansion of the AIDS surveillance case definition.

19. What classes of drugs are currently available to treat HIV infection?

From 1987 through late 1995, only one type of drug was available to treat HIV infection, the **nucleoside analog reverse transcriptase inhibitors** (NARTI):

Zidovudine (AZT)	Didanosine (ddI)
Zalcitabine (ddC)	Stavudine (d4T)
Lamivudine (3TC)	

In late 1995 and early 1996, a new class of drugs, the **protease inhibitors,** received FDA approval. These drugs available thus far are:

Saquinavir	Ritonavir	Indinavir

A third class of drugs, the **non-nucleoside reverse transcriptase inhibitors,** is in late clinical trials and one, acvirapine, has been approved.

20. How do the nucleoside analog reverse transcriptase inhibitors (NARTIs) work?

The NARTIs act during the initial infection of a new host cell. They inhibit viral reverse transcriptase during the transcription of viral RNA to host complementary DNA. The NARTIs are analogs that become phosphorylated to a triphosphate form and competitively interfere with transcription, causing DNA chain termination.

21. How do the protease inhibitors work?

In host cells with established infection, following the synthesis of mRNA and then HIV polyproteins, HIV protease must cleave the polyproteins to result in the production of functional proteins. Protease inhibitors act at this stage, preventing cleavage. Viral particles can still be formed and bud from the host cell, but they will be nonfunctional and noninfective.

22. What are the major side effects of the NARTIs?

Zidovudine is associated with hematologic toxicity (mainly anemia and granulocytopenia), nausea, and headache. With chronic use, a myopathy can develop, possibly related to mitochondrial toxicity.

Didanosine causes a peripheral neuropathy and has been associated with pancreatitis, especially in patients with prior pancreatic disease or very advanced-stage HIV infection.

Zalcitabine is associated with the development of peripheral neuropathy as well as oral ulcerations. Stavudine causes a peripheral neuropathy. Lamivudine has not been associated with any major toxicity.

23. Does viral resistance to NARTIs develop?

There is evidence that the HIV can develop decreased sensitivity to almost all of the NARTIs. It many cases, this can become outright resistance. These changes in the viral sensitivities are associated with discrete and specific genetic mutations, which usually occur within 1–6 months of initiating therapy. These changes and mutations have not been demonstrated for stavudine. Clinical correlation with these laboratory findings is, as yet, not known.

Richman DD: Clinical significance of drug resistance in human immunodeficiency virus. Clin Infect Dis 21(suppl 2):S166–S169, 1995.

24. How long does NARTI therapy work?

Long-term studies that have followed patients for 2–3 years or more have tended to show a convergence of the curves of clinical events toward the final months of the studies, implying that the clinical benefit of therapy is about 2–3 years, on average.

25. When should antiretroviral therapy be started?

Since the first anti-HIV medication became available, there has been debate over this question. In patients with advanced disease (AIDs diagnosis or CD4$^+$ count <200/mm^3), antiretroviral therapy has been shown to prolong life. This was seen in the initial antiretroviral trial with zidovudine and now has been demonstrated with the new protease inhibitors. The study of patients in less advanced stages has been hampered by the limited efficacy of the NARTIs. Clinically significant benefit in patients with CD4$^+$ counts of > 500/mm^3 has been difficult to demonstrate, but with the newer prognostic information gained with viral load measurements and the promising strength of combination therapy with NARTIs and protease inhibitors has led authorities to recommend therapy in some of these individuals.

Recommendations for When to Initiate Treatment

STATUS	RECOMMENDATION
Symptomatic HIV disease*	Therapy recommended for all patients
Asymptomatic, CD4+ cell count <0.500×10⁹/L	Therapy recommended[†]
Asymptomatic, CD4+ cell count >0.500×10⁹/L	Therapy recommended for patients with > 30000-50000 HIV RNA copies/mL or rapidly declining CD4+ cell counts
	Therapy should be considered for patients with > 5000-10000 HIV RNA copies/mL

*Symptomatic human immunodeficiency virus (HIV) disease includes symptoms such as recurrent mucosal candidiasis, oral hairy leukoplakia, and chronic and unexplained fever, night sweats, and weight loss.
[†]Some would defer therapy in a subset of patients with stable CD4+ cell counts between 0.350 and 0.500×10⁹/L and plasma HIV RNA levels consistently below 5000-10000 copies/mL.

From Carpenter CCJ, et al: Antiretroviral therapy for HIV infection in 1996: Recommendations of an international panal. JAMA 276:146-154, 1996, with permission.
Ho DD: Time to hit HIV, early and hard. N Engl J Med 333:450–451, 1995.

26. What about combination antiretroviral therapy?

The most recent clinical trial data support the standard use of combination therapy and the relegation of monotherapy to a small subgroup of patients. Didanosine monotherapy remains a regimen that can be considered in patients with less advanced disease. Most of the combinations that have been well studied are zidovudine based. There is litte experience with many of the other possible combinations. The patient groups who may best benefit from any particular combination and the exact combinations to use are unknown at this time.

1. Hammer SM, et al: A trial comparing nucleoside monotherapy with combination therapy in HIV-infected adults with CD4 cell counts from 200 to 500 per cubic millimeter. N Engl J Med 335:1081-1090, 1996.

2. Delta Coordinating Committee: Delta: A randomized double-blind controlled trial comparing combinations of zidovudine plus didanosine or zalcitabine with zidovudine alone in HIV-infected individuals. Lancet 348:283-291, 1996.

27. Does a patient need PCP prophylaxis even though he is on antiretroviral therapy?

Yes. In patients with advanced HIV infection on antiretroviral therapy but not on PCP prophylaxis, approximately half of the opportunistic infections observed are PCP. Therefore, it is recommended that patients also be given PCP prophylaxis once they meet the criteria (see Question 48), regardless of other therapy they may be taking.

28. Can therapy prevent perinatal transmission of HIV infection?

Zidovudine therapy initiated between weeks 14–34 of gestation, continued IV during labor, and administered to the newborn for the first 6 weeks of life was able to decrease the rate of transmission from 25.5% to 8.3%, a 67.5% reduction. Antiretroviral therapy for infected pregnant women is now recommended and has led to greater emphasis on prenatal HIV testing, some states mandating that the test be offered to all pregnant women.

Connor EM, et al: Reduction of maternal-infant transmission of human immunodeficiency virus type 1 with zidovudine treatment. N Engl J Med 331:1173–1180, 1994.

CLINICAL MANIFESTATIONS

29. What is ARC?

ARC, or AIDS-related complex, was a term used to describe patients having symptoms of HIV infection (e.g., oral candidiasis) but not yet diagnosed with an AIDS-defining condition. Lacking a clear-cut or generally accepted definition, this term is no longer in common use.

30. What HIV-related manifestations are seen uniquely in women?

In addition to all the well-known manifestations of HIV infection seen in men, three conditions are specific to women: cervical neoplasia, pelvic inflammatory disease (PID), and vaginal candidiasis. All have their clinical course altered to a more aggressive nature by HIV infection. Invasive cervical cancer was added to the list of AIDS-indicator diseases in the 1993 revision.

Minkoff HL, DeHovitz JA: Care of women infected with the human immunodeficiency virus. JAMA 266:2253–2258, 1991.

31. What is thrush?

Thrush is oropharyngeal pseudomembranous candidiasis, which often presages AIDS. It most often presents as white plaques (pseudomembranes), either scattered small plaques or large sheets, seen on any oral mucosal surface. Candidiasis also may present in an atrophic or erythematous appearance without plaques. Significant oral pain may be present along with altered taste. The diagnosis can be made clinically, with KOH smear, or by culture. A clinician should not confuse thrush with oral hairy leukoplakia, a whitish corrugated growth along the margins of the tongue.

32. How is thrush treated?

Treatment of Oral Thrush

Limited involvement:	Extensive involvement:
Improved oral hygiene with peroxide rinses	Ketoconazole, 200 mg po qd
Nystatin oral suspension	Fluconazole, 50–100 mg po qd
Nystatin vaginal tablets, used oral	
Clotrimazole tablets	

Thrush often indicates significant immune suppression, and if it is found during an initial exam, evaluation should begin for other HIV-related medical interventions, such as PCP prophylaxis.

33. What are some common dermatologic conditions in HIV infection?

Besides Kaposi's sarcoma (KS), there is a multitude of skin findings, including seborrheic dermatitis, psoriasis, and ichthyosis. *Staphylococcus aureus* is the most common bacterial pathogen and typically manifests as folliculitis. Fungal infections such as candidiasis and tinea are common. Rarely, cryptococcosis and histoplasmosis are seen. Viral infections with herpes simplex type 2, varicella zoster, molluscum contagiosum, and condyloma acuminata are common. Rashes due to syphilis must also be considered in these high-risk patients.

Cockerell CJ: Human immunodeficiency virus infection and the skin: A crucial interface. Arch Intern Med 151:1295–1303, 1991.

34. What are the recognized rheumatic conditions known to occur in HIV-positive patients?

- Inflammatory myopathy
- Reiter's syndrome
- Psoriasis
- Sjögren's syndrome
- Vasculitis
- Oligoarticular arthritis

The arthritis does not seem to be responsive to NSAIDs. Also described are painful arthralgias of short duration that often require narcotics for relief. In addition to these clinical syndromes, lab evaluations often reveal low titers of rheumatoid factors, antinuclear antibodies, and anticardiolipin antibodies. Generalized hypergammaglobulinemia is also reported.

Kaye BR: Rheumatologic manifestations of infection with the human immunodeficiency virus (HIV). Ann Intern Med 111:158–167, 1989.

35. Do HIV-infected patients respond to the influenza vaccine?

Administration of the influenza vaccine has been recommended for all persons infected with the HIV, although the antibody response to the vaccine is lower than in non-HIV-infected controls. A two-dose regimen is not superior in efficacy to the traditional single-dose regimen.

Recent studies showing increased HIV viral load and decreased CD4$^+$ counts in study participants receiving influenza vaccine when compared to placebo-injected controls have raised concerns, but no adverse clinical events have been demonstrated. Regardless, since influenza does not seem to have more serious complications in HIV-infected patients, many practitioners have begun to withhold influenza vaccine.

O'Brien WA, et al: HIV-type 1 replication can be increased in peripheral blood of seropositive patients after influenza vaccination. Blood 86:1082–1089, 1995.

36. Do HIV-infected patients respond to the pneumococcal polysaccharide vaccine?

Again, their response is impaired compared to normal controls. The HIV-infected person will mount an adequate antibody response to fewer of the serotypes contained in the 23-valent vaccine, and this response rate decreases with decreasing CD4$^+$ counts. As with influenza vaccination, there appears to be increased HIV viral activity after pneumococcal vaccination, but because morbidity due to pneumococcal disease is clearly and substantially increased in HIV-infected individuals, the risk/benefit ratio supports vaccination.

Rodriguez-Barradas MC, et al: Antibody to capsular polysaccharides of *Streptococcus pneumoniae* after vaccination of HIV-infected subjects with 23-valent pneumococcal vaccine. J Infect Dis 165:553–556, 1992.

36. What is AIDS dementia complex?

Patients with AIDS may develop cognitive, behavioral, and motor dysfunction in the course of their illness. Although multiple opportunistic infections need to be ruled out (cryptococcosis, toxoplasmosis, tuberculosis, etc.), direct CNS infection by HIV seems to cause this complex of signs and symptoms. Early in its course, neuropsychologic testing may be needed to support a clinical suspicion of dementia, but the dementia can progress to a vegetative state. Patients may first complain of concentration difficulties, and family and friends may note personality changes. A thorough neurologic evaluation and investigation into other causes are needed. Zidovudine may be helpful in treating this dementia, probably related to the high drug levels obtainable in the CSF.

McArthur JC, et al: Dementia in AIDS patients: Incidence and risk factors: Multicenter AIDS Cohort Study. Neurology 43:2245–2252, 1993.

37. Do neurologic conditions in AIDS only appear late in the course of the disease?

Not necessarily. Neurologic signs and symptoms may be the earliest manifestations of HIV infection in some patients. The most frequent cause of neurologic abnormality is subacute encephalitis, which may be a part of the initial HIV viral infection in many individuals.

Simpson DM, Tagliati M: Neurologic manifestations of HIV infection. Ann Intern Med 121:769–785, 1994.

38. What is HIV wasting syndrome?

This is an AIDS-defining diagnosis that includes profound weight loss of $> 10\%$ of body weight, with either chronic diarrhea or weakness and fever present for > 30 days. These clinical events should be evaluated for other HIV-related illnesses and, in the absence of other etiologies, a diagnosis of wasting can be made.

Grunfeld C, Feingold KR: Metabolic disturbances and wasting in the acquired immunodeficiency syndrome. N Engl J Med 327:329–337, 1992.

39. How often does HIV infection result in anemia or thrombocytopenia?

Patients with full-blown AIDS are frequently pancytopenic, with anemia occurring in up to 80%, neutropenia in 85%, and thrombocytopenia in 65% of cases. HIV-infected but asymptomatic individuals are much less frequently cytopenic.

Clinically significant thrombocytopenia indistinguishable from that seen in idiopathic thrombocytopenic purpura (ITP) may be a presentation of HIV infection. Typically, there is a normal bone marrow with adequate numbers of megakaryocytes present and behavior much like classic ITP in that patients respond to steroids and splenectomy. It is appropriate to obtain an HIV blood test in most patients presenting with ITP.

Thrombocytopenic patients have improved on zidovudine therapy, although AZT may cause anemia. Of interest is the recent recognition of thrombotic thrombocytopenic purpura (TTP) in association with HIV infection.

Aboulafia DM, Mitsuyasu RT: Hematolic abnormalities in AIDS. Hematol Oncol Clin North Am 5:195–214, 1991.

40. What are the characteristic bone marrow aspirate and biopsy findings in AIDS?

* Decreased cellularity (rarely hypocellular), including dyserythropoiesis
* Increased lymphocytes and plasma cells
* Histiocytic hyperplasia with phagocytosis of red cells, platelets, and WBCs
* Granulomas, marrow fibrosis, serous fat atrophy
* Pure red cell aphasia with giant pronormoblasts (in parvovirus B19 infection)

Also, patients receiving zidovudine often have ineffective hematopoiesis with megaloblastic maturation.

Namiki TS, et al: A comparison of bone marrow findings in patients with acquired immunodeficiency syndrome (AIDS) and AIDS-related conditions. Hematol Oncol 5:99, 1987.

41. What lymphomas are associated with AIDS? How often do they present with extralymphatic presentations?

AIDS is associated with high-grade B-cell lymphomas that arise most often in extralymphatic sites. The histologic types that are seen in 80–90% of patients include small noncleaved cell (resembling Burkitt's) and immunoblastic lymphoma. Extranodal disease is the rule rather than the exception (68–98%). The most frequent extranodal sites are the bone marrow, liver, meninges, lung, soft tissue, primary CNS, rectum, and Waldeyer's tonsillar ring. Additionally, "B" type symptoms are extremely common in this patient group.

Primary CNS lymphomas occur most frequently in patients with a prior AIDS diagnosis and are associated with a median survival of < 3 months. Patients without prior histories of AIDS-related infections (such as PCP) and in good physical condition may respond to standard chemotherapy followed by institution of antiretroviral therapy. Patients who develop systemic lymphoma after other manifestations of AIDS typically do not fare well with chemotherapy. Supportive care only is a reasonable course in these patients.

Levine AM: Acquired immunodeficiency syndrome-related lymphoma. Blood 80:8–20, 1992.

Pneumocystis carinii INFECTION

42. What is PCP?

PCP stands for *Pneumocystis carinii* pneumonia. Prior to routine prophylactic treatments, this infection was the presenting diagnosis in 60% of patients with AIDS and eventually was seen in > 80% of patients with AIDS at some time during their illness. With more active HIV testing and the initiation of effective PCP prophylaxis, the probability of PCP has fallen to < 20%.

43. How does PCP present?

Cough, fever, and dyspnea on exertion are the most common presenting symptoms. The cough is usually nonproductive or productive of only scant, whitish sputum. Patients may also relate a sensation of chest tightness or an inability to take a full, deep inspiration. Other less common complaints include nonspecific weight loss, night sweats, and malaise. Findings on physical examination include fever, tachypnea, persistent cough, and dry rales. Rarely, a patient may endure symptoms at home long enough to present with cyanosis. Laboratory findings include hypoxemia with an elevated A–aO$_2$ gradient. Elevated serum lactate dehydrogenase levels are seen.

Moe AA, Hardy WD: *Pneumocystis carinii* infection in the HIV-seropositive patient. Infect Dis Clin North Am 8:331–364, 1994.

44. How is PCP diagnosed?

By pathologic demonstration of the organism in lung specimens. Several centers have reported success with examination of induced sputum, but most centers rely on bronchoscopy with bronchoalveolar lavage (BAL). Lavage alone has a sensitivity of ~ 95%; thus, transbronchial

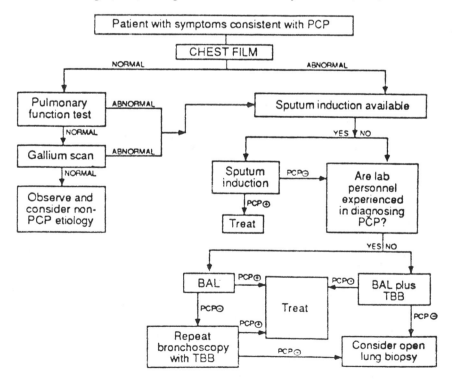

Diagnostic algorithm for PCP. (From Cohen PT, et al (eds): The AIDS Knowledge Base. Waltham, MA, Medical Publishing Group, 1990; with permission.)

biopsy (TBB) is usually withheld except for those cases not diagnosed by BAL. Open lung biopsy is rarely needed.

45. What are the chest x-ray findings in PCP?

Typically seen is a diffuse, bilateral, interstitial infiltrate, often more pronounced in the hilar region (butterfly distribution). Areas of local consolidation are less common, as are cystic and cavitary changes. Normal chest x-rays are also seen, especially in patients presenting early in the illness. Pleural effusion is rare and, if present, should raise the suspicion of another diagnosis.

46. How is PCP treated?

Conventional treatment comes down to a choice among three agents: trimethoprim-sulfamethoxazole (TMP-SMX), pentamidine isethionate, or atovaquone. The first two agents seem to be equally effective in clinical use but differ in routes of administration. Both are available for IV use, but TMP-SMX can also be administered orally, enabling outpatient therapy. The usual daily dose of **TMP-SMX** is 20 mg/kg of TMP and 100 mg/kg of SMX in divided doses, three to four times daily, for 21 days. It appears that a lower dose (15/75 mg/kg) may be equally effective with fewer side effects. Much work is being done to evaluate the role of **inhaled pentamidine** in the acute treatment of PCP, but treatment failures appear too common. Pentamidine is usually given at a dose of 4 mg/kg once a day. The 3-mg/kg once-daily dose may be effective in mild pneumonias.

Atovaquone is an alternative oral therapy for mild to moderate PCP ($PO_2 > 60$ mm Hg, A–a O_2 gradient ≤ 45 mm Hg) in patients who cannot tolerate TMP-SMX. In studies comparing it to TMP-SMX or pentamidine, atovaquone was less toxic and better tolerated. However, it is less effective than TMP-SMX, though equally effective as pentamidine. The dosing regimen with the oral suspension is 750 mg bid, taken with a fatty meal, usually for 21 days.

Dohn MN, et al: Oral atovaquone compared with intravenous pentamidine for *Pneumocystis carinii* pneumonia in patients with AIDS. Ann Intern Med 121:174–180, 1994.

47. What are the expected side effects of treatment of PCP?

Drug-Associated Adverse Effects of TMP/SMX vs Pentamidine

	TMP-SMX	PENTAMIDINE
Fever ($> 37°$ C)	78%	82%
Hypotension	0	27
Nausea, vomiting	25	24
Rash	44	15
Anemia	39	24
Leukopenia	72	47
Thrombocytopenia	3	18
Azotemia	14	64
Alanine aminotransferase	22	15
Alkaline aminotransferase	22	15
Alkaline phosphatase	11	18
Hypoglycemia	0	21
Hypocalcemia	0	3

TMP/SMX is very well tolerated in non-AIDS patients, but it produces side effects in 65–100% of patients with AIDS. Severe rash and neutropenia are often treatment-limiting but reversible with drug cessation.

Progressive renal insufficiency and pancreatitis with dysglycemias are the most serious side effects of pentamidine infusion. Atovaquone is associated with treatment-limiting rash in only 4% of patients and no other adverse reaction in more than 1%.

Sattler FR, et al: TMP-SMX compared with pentamidine for treatment of PCP in AIDS: A prospective, noncrossover study. Ann Intern Med 109:280–287, 1988.

48. Who should receive prophylaxis for PCP?

Indications for PCP Prophylaxis

- Prior episode of PCP (secondary prophylaxis)
- CD4$^+$ count < 200/mm^3 (or CD4$^+$ < 14% of total lymphocytes)
- Earlier initiation warranted for patients with:
  - Oral candidiasis
  - Unexplained fever
  - Rapid fall in CD4$^+$ count

CDC: Recommendations for prophylaxis against *Pneumocystis carinii* pneumonia for adults and adolescents infected with HIV. MMWR 41:1–12, 1992.

49. What are the proper agents and regimens for PCP prophylaxis?

Although many agents are being investigated, TMP-SMX, pentamidine, and dapsone are the three standard agents for prophylactic regimens.

TMP-SMX
- TMP 160 mg/SMX 800 mg daily (one double-strength tablet)
- Side effects similar to but less common than with primary PCP treatment
- Decreasing dose by 50% (one DS tablet 3 ×/wk) may limit side effects while preserving efficacy
- Also provides prophylaxis against CNS toxoplasmosis

Aerosolized pentamidine
- 300 mg once a month via nebulizer.
- Transient taste alterations and coughing or wheezing (can be minimized by pretreatment with inhaled bronchodilators.)
- Evaluate patients for active TB prior to starting therapy

Dapsone (± pyrimethamine)
- 50 mg bid or 100 mg q day
- Provides prophylaxis against toxoplasmosis with addition of pyrimethamine

While TMP-SMX appears virtually 100% effective in those who can tolerate the side effects, dapsone and pentamidine have a 5–10% failure rate per year, with failure meaning that PCP may be mild or atypical. In a very practical, clinically pertinent study comparing these 3 agents, all had similar effectiveness when treatment-limiting toxicities were included.

Bozzette SA, et al: A randomized trial of three antipneumocystis agents in patients with advanced human immunodeficiency virus infection. N Engl J Med 332:693–699, 1995.

50. How does aerosolized pentamidine change the presentation of PCP?

Because this type of prophylaxis is not 100% effective, new episodes of PCP may occur during prophylaxis. These episodes may present with an atypical radiographic appearance, with more upper-lobe infiltrates rather than the traditional diffuse interstitial infiltrates. The yield of BAL for pathologic diagnosis also is decreased.

Jules-Elysee KM, et al: Aerosolized pentamidine: Effect on diagnosis and presentation of *Pneumocystis carinii* pneumonia. Ann Intern Med 112:750–757, 1990.

51. Should PCP patients with respiratory failure be intubated?

Obviously, the answer depends on the patient's previously expressed desires and the clinical setting of respiratory failure. One group of patients has been identified who may benefit from mechanical ventilation. These patients have a shorter duration of symptoms of PCP, a precipitous decline of respiratory status postbronchoscopy, and better arterial oxygenation on admission (PO$_2$ > 60 mm Hg). These patients may have a 1-year survival of up to 80%. To properly advise a critically ill patient about treatment options and outcomes, a practitioner must be aware of these data.

Franklin C, et al: Improving long-term prognosis for survivors of mechanical ventilation in patients with AIDS with PCP and acute respiratory failure. Arch Intern Med 155:91–95, 1995.

52. When should adjunctive steroids be used in therapy for PCP?

- Indicated in patients with $PaO_2 < 70$ mm Hg or $A-aO_2$ gradient > 35 mm Hg on room air
- Corticosteroids begun within 72 hrs of initiating PCP treatment
- Improve clinical outcome and reduce mortality by 50%
- Avoid in presence of coincident pulmonary infection (TB, histoplasmosis) or process (Kaposi's sarcoma)
- Recommended approach: oral prednisone given—
  40 mg twice daily $\times$ 5 days, then
  40 mg once daily $\times$ 5 days, then
  20 mg once daily $\times$ 11 days (total duration 21 days)

Consensus statement on the use of corticosteroids as adjunctive therapy for pneumocystis pneumonia in the acquired immunodeficiency syndrome. N Engl J Med 323:1500–1504, 1990.

Bozzette SA, et al: A controlled trial of early adjunctive treatment with corticosteroids for *Pneumocystis carinii* pneumonia in the acquired immunodeficiency syndrome. New Engl J Med 323:1451–1456, 1990.

53. What is extrapulmonary pneumocystosis?

Pneumocystis infection can involve anatomical sites literally from head (otitis) to foot (vasculitis). The use of nonsystemic (i.e., inhaled) pentamidine therapy for PCP prophylaxis appears to be involved in these cases, although current clinical practice prefers systemic therapy with TMP-SMX or dapsone.

Telzalc EE, et al: Extrapulmonary *Pneumocystis carinii* infections. Rev Infect Dis 12:380–386, 1990.

54. Does the incidence of pneumothorax increase with pentamidine inhalation?

This question arose when patients enrolled in community trials of inhaled pentamidine had several episodes of pneumothorax. It appears that these episodes were related to recurrent episodes of PCP and not to the use of inhalation therapy.

CRYPTOCOCCAL INFECTION

55. How often does *Cryptococcus* cause infection in AIDS?

Depending on which series is examined, *Cryptococcus* may cause 5–10% of AIDS-defining opportunistic infections. Patients also develop cryptococcal infections following a previous AIDS diagnosis, so an overall estimate is between 8–15%. Recent studies have suggested a decreasing incidence of cryptococcosis, possibly related to the more general use of fluconazole for either prophylaxis or treatment for other fungal diseases, such as oral and esophageal candidiasis.

56. How does cryptococcal infection present?

Meningitis is the most common presentation in AIDS. Extraneural disease is frequently seen with meningitis, but is much less common in its absence. Meningismus is present in only 25–30% of patients with meningitis, but fever and headache are seen in 80–90%. Focal neurologic symptoms or signs are seen in a small minority.

Features of Meningeal Cryptococcosis

Symptoms			
Fever	58 (65%)	Altered mentation	25 (28%)
Malaise	68 (76%)	Focal deficits	5 (6%)
Headaches	65 (73%)	Seizures	4 (4%)
Stiff neck	20 (22%)	Cough/dyspnea	28 (31%)
Nausea/vomiting	37 (42%)	Diarrhea	19 (21%)
Photophobia	16 (18%)		
Signs			
Fever	50 (56%)	Altered mentation	15 (17%)
Meningeal signs	24 (27%)	Focal deficits	13 (15%)

Chuck SL, Sande MA: Infections with *Cryptococcus neoformans* in AIDS. N Engl J Med 321:795, 1989.

57. Which patients with cryptococcosis need a lumbar puncture (LP)?

Any and all patients with a culture or a serum antigen titer positive for *Cryptococcus* require an LP, irrespective of which site originally yielded the positive specimen. In any HIV-infected patient having an undiagnosed fever and/or headache in a medically urgent situation, an LP should be considered to examine the possibility of cryptococcal disease. If the situation is less urgent, a serum antigen titer can be obtained.

58. How often should an LP be done?

An LP is performed at the time of diagnosis of cryptococcal infection. If indicative of meningitis and the patient is clinically responding to therapy, a repeat LP should be performed by at least week 2 of therapy to help evaluate the microbial response and to decide on the appropriateness of continued IV or oral therapy. Subsequent LPs should be done as clinically indicated until adequate microbial response is documented. If the clinical response is poor or if the initial opening pressure was elevated, frequent LPs may be needed to relieve increased intracranial pressure and to guide therapy.

59. What cerebrospinal fluid (CSF) findings are seen in cryptococcal meningitis?

CSF Findings in AIDS-Related Cryptococcal Meningitis

	NO. WITH FINDING/NO. TESTED	%
WBC <20 cells/μl	96/128	75%
Glucose >40 mg/dl	87/127	68%
Protein <45 mg/dl	53/127	42%
Positive India ink	92/125	74%
Positive CSF antigen	116/126	92%

The CSF can appear remarkably normal. However you should always perform an India ink test, since this is usually positive and can yield an immediate diagnosis without waiting for other laboratory results.

Chuck SL, Sande MA: Infections with *Cryptococcus neoformans* in the acquired immunodeficiency syndrome. N Engl J Med 321:794–799, 1989.

60. What treatment is recommended for cryptococcosis in AIDS?

Trials comparing amphotericin B with fluconazole for treatment of cryptococcal meningitis have concluded that either therapy is effective. There has been evidence of higher early mortality in patients assigned to fluconazole, and some studies may have used suboptimal doses of both amphotericin B and fluconazole. Due to the concerns of early mortality, most clinicians now recommend an initial 2-week course of amphotericin B at 0.7 mg/kg/day, with or without flucytosine (100 mg/kg/day), followed by fluconazole at 400 mg/day.

Saag MS, et al: Comparison of amphotericin B with fluconazole in the treatment of acute AIDS-associated cryptococcal meningitis. N Engl J Med 326:83–89, 1992.

van der Hort C, et al: Randomized double-blind comparison of amphotericin B plus flucytosine to amphotericin B alone followed by a comparison of fluconazole to itraconazole in the treatment of acute cryptococcal meningitis in patients with AIDS [abstracts I216 and I217]. In Abstracts of the 35th Interscience Conference on Antimicrobial Agents and Chemotherapy, San Francisco, October 1995.

61. Is maintenance anticryptococcal therapy needed?

Cryptococcal infection in AIDS demonstrates a high relapse rate following primary therapy and a high mortality rate during relapse. The standard of care has been to give chronic maintenance or suppressive therapy. Intermittent infusions of amphotericin B as well as oral ketoconazole, itraconazole, or fluconazole have been used, with **fluconazole** (200–400 mg/day) being the agent of choice. All patients should be continued on maintenance therapy for life.

Powderly WG, et al: A controlled trial of fluconazole or amphotericin B to prevent relapse of cryptococcal meningitis in patients with the acquired immunodeficiency syndrome. N Engl J Med 326:793–798, 1992.

62. Are serum cryptococcal antigen levels good indicators of response to therapy?

No. Although the serum antigen test can be very helpful in the diagnosis of cryptococcal infection, it can't be used to judge therapeutic response. In most cases of meningitis, the CSF antigen titer should be determined by repeat lumbar puncture. If after therapy the serum titer does revert to very low titer or negative, an increasing titer in the future should raise concern about a relapse.

63. How is a relapse of cryptococcal infection treated?

Depending upon the patient's previous therapeutic course and compliance with maintenance therapy, relapse should be treated with a reinduction regimen of amphotericin B, followed by fluconazole. Development of resistance has not been demonstrated.

64. What are the poor prognostic indicators in AIDS-related cryptococcosis?

Prognostic Factors Indicating a Poor Response in Cryptococcosis

STUDY	NO. PATIENTS	POOR PROGNOSTIC INDICATORS	
Diamond (1974)	111	India ink-positive	CSF WBC < 20
		High opening pressure	Extra-CNS site of infection
		Low CFS glucose	
Kovacs (1985)	27	No reliable factor identified	Pretreatment CSF antigen
Zugar (1986)	34	India ink-positive	> 1:10,000
		Post-treatment CNS antigen	
		> 1:8	
Chuck (1989)	89	Hyponatremia	Extra-CNS site of infection

In 1974, Diamond and Bennett described multiple prognostic factors in non-AIDS cryptococcal meningitis. Several reports since have attempted to define similar factors in AIDS-related cryptococcosis but for the most part have been unsuccessful.

Cryptococcal disease in patients with AIDS is a less predictable illness than in non-AIDS patients. Often, an adequate response to anticryptococcal therapy is complicated by the development of new adverse clinical events related to the underlying HIV infection.

Diamond RD, Bennett JE: Prognostic factors in cryptococcal meningitis: A study of 111 cases. Ann Intern Med 80:176–181, 1974.

65. Is primary prophylaxis indicated against cryptococcosis?

Some clinicians have adopted primary prophylaxis due to the frequency of other fungal diseases (such as oral and esophageal candidiasis) as well as cryptococcosis. A recent study comparing fluconazole to clotrimazole troches found fluconazole (200 mg/day) to decrease the frequency of cryptococcosis and esophageal candidiasis, especially in persons at highest risk (i.e., $CD4^+$ count < $50/mm^3$). However, no survival benefit was demonstrated, and it was estimated that > 11,000 doses of fluconazole were given to prevent 1 case of invasive fungal disease. Thus, daily fluconazole is not recommended at this time.

Powderly WG, et al: A randomized trial comparing fluconazole with clotrimazole troches for the prevention of fungal infections in patients with advanced human immunodeficiency virus infection. N Engl J Med 332:700–705, 1995.

KAPOSI'S SARCOMA

66. What does Kaposi's sarcoma (KS) look like?

KS in HIV-infected patients is most often seen as **cutaneous** or **oropharyngeal nodules** ranging in size from 0.5–2.0 cm, although multiple nodules may coalesce. These nodules are most often raised and readily palpable, painless and nonpruritic, with no evidence of inflammation or exudate. Rarely, lesions may become friable or verrucous (warty) and weep or bleed with trauma. Their color is usually blue or violet-to-purple, and in darker-skinned patients, they often appear black. These nodules are often multiple when first diagnosed, reflecting the relatively aggressive nature of this malignancy in HIV infection. Any area of the body may be involved, although the palms of the hands are rarely affected despite the more common involvement of the soles of the feet.

67. Does a lesion suspicious for KS need to be biopsied?

In general, yes. If a patient with HIV infection has no previous diagnosis of KS or any opportunistic infection, these suspicious lesions should be uniformly biopsied to establish a diagnosis. In a patient who has had previously diagnosed opportunistic infections and is under regular supervision and care, the need for confirming a clinical diagnosis by biopsy is less clear. However, there are other etiologies for pigmented cutaneous lesions in HIV infection. A patient with previously diagnosed KS does not need new lesions biopsied unless he had been in remission following therapy.

68. Is KS sexually transmitted?

Investigators have demonstrated the presence of genetic material related to human herpesvirus 8 in KS tissue. This raises the possibility of the transmission of an infectious agent related to KS. No causative relationship has been established yet, but this does suggest clues as to why KS is more common in homosexual men than in other HIV risk groups.

Whitby D, et al: Detection of Kaposi's sarcoma associated herpesvirus in peripheral blood of HIV-infected individuals and progression to Kaposi's sarcoma. Lancet 346:799–802, 1995.

69. What treatment is recommended for KS?

There is no single therapeutic approach to KS in patients with AIDS. These patients often have concurrent conditions that should receive priority because, with the exception of pulmonary KS, the disease is rarely threatening to the patient's immediate health—i.e., although AIDS-associated KS is a more aggressive variant of KS, it is relatively benign compared to other AIDS-related processes. In addition, response rates of KS to systemic therapy have not been uniformly high, and myelosuppressive chemotherapy would compromise other life-preserving antimicrobial or antiviral therapies. A general approach to AIDS-associated KS should start with an assessment of the possible course of disease and its effect on the patient's overall condition. The following table can help distinguish between possible indolent disease versus more aggressive KS.

Prognostic Variables in Kaposi's Sarcoma

PREDICTS INDOLENT COURSE	PREDICTS AGGRESSIVE COURSE
Few lesions (< 25)	Many KS lesions (≥ 25)
Low rate of growth	Rapid appearance of new lesions
No visceral KS identified	Intraoral or visceral lesions
No fevers, drenching night sweats, or weight loss	One or more constitutional symptoms
No prior opportunistic infection	One prior or concurrent opportunistic infection
Absolute $CD4^+$ count $> 400/mm^3$	$CD4^+$ count $< 200/mm^3$
Normal ESR	ESR > 40 mm/hr
HIV p24 antigen not detectable	HIV p24 detectable
Normal β_2-microglobulin	β_2-Microglobulin > 5
Normal blood counts	Leukopenia or anemia present

Chaisson RE, Volberding PA: Clinical manifestations of HIV infection. In Mandell GL, et al (eds): Principles and Practice of Infectious Diseases, 4th ed. New York, Churchill Livingstone, 1995, p 1241.

70. What is the life expectancy for a patient with AIDS and KS?

There are no firm numbers with which to answer this question. Since survival statistics were first calculated for patients with AIDS, an AIDS-defining diagnosis of KS (as opposed to another malignancy or opportunistic infection) has carried the best prognosis. This is due to the frequent appearance of KS at a less advanced point in the progressive immunosuppression. The exceptions are patients with pulmonary KS, which is a quickly progressive condition resulting in respiratory failure often within 3–6 months.

71. Is KS always cutaneous?

Sites of Disease and Systemic Signs at Presentation in 49 Patients with Epidemic Kaposi's Sarcoma

Skin lesions		Lymph node involvement	
None	4 (8%)	None	19 (39%)
Generalized	13 (27%)	Generalized	30 (61%)
Locally aggressive	1 (2%)	Splenomegaly	5 (10%)
Visceral involvement		**Systemic signs***	
Bone	1 (2%)	Fever and weight loss	9 (18%)
Hepatomegaly	5 (10%)	Fever only	4 (8%)
Lung	5 (10%)	Weight loss only	1 (2%)
GI tract	22 (45%)	Total with symptoms	14 (29%)

*Unexplained fever > 100°F (orally) and ≥ 10% weight loss.

DeVita, et al (eds): AIDS: Etiology, Diagnosis, Treatment and Prevention, 2nd ed. Philadelphia, J.B. Lippincott, 1988, p 252.

72. Does antiretroviral therapy treat KS?

In general, this therapy does not appear to provide any therapeutic response in KS. However, patients with AIDS-related KS should receive therapy for their HIV infection. This therapy could complicate any myelosuppressive chemotherapy the patient may receive for KS, and care should be taken to recognize the priority of each patient's individual clinical needs.

CYTOMEGALOVIRUS INFECTION

73. What is the cause of blindness experienced by some patients with AIDS?

Chorioretinitis caused by cytomegalovirus (CMV) is a vision-threatening infection experienced by 5–10% of patients with AIDS during the course of their illness. It is an AIDS-defining diagnosis if it occurs as the initial opportunistic infection. Usually, however, this infection appears later in the disease process, after a patient has already been diagnosed with AIDS.

Whitcup SM: Ocular manifestations of AIDS. JAMA 275:142–144, 1996.

74. How is CMV retinitis diagnosed?

Often, a patient presents with nonspecific complaints of blurred vision, decreased visual acuity, or increasing "floaters," but occasionally CMV retinitis may present with a clear visual field cut. Ophthalmologic examination is essential and typically shows large white granular areas with hemorrhage. Diagnosis is based on this characteristic fundoscopic appearance because no tissue is obtained for pathologic examination.

75. What drugs are available to treat CMV retinitis?

Ganciclovir and foscarnet. Usual therapy consists of high-dose "induction" therapy for 2–3 weeks, followed by life-long suppressive therapy. Despite continued therapy, progression of retinitis is seen in most patients. A recent study found that combined ganciclovir and foscarnet therapy for these relapses was superior to either drug alone. The most commonly prescribed doses are:

- Ganciclovir, 5 mg/kg bid × 2 weeks, followed by 10 mg/kg qd
- Foscarnet, 90 mg/kg bid × 2 weeks, followed by 120 mg/kg qd

A ganciclovir-impregnated bead which can be implanted into the vitreous of the involved eye was recently approved by the FDA. This allows for prolonged local therapy.

A third agent, cidofovir, has recently received FDA approval for use in patients who have failed or cannot tolerate the other drugs. Cidofovir is also administered intravenously, but is given only once a week or every other week. It has significant renal toxicity that may significantly limit its use. Despite this toxicity, its efficacy and infrequent dosing make it an attractive alternative.

The SOCA Trial Group: Mortality in patients with the acquired immunodeficiency syndrome treated with either foscarnet or ganciclovir for cytomegalovirus retinitis. N Engl J Med 326:213–220, 1992.

The SOCA Trial Group: Combination foscarnet and ganciclovir therapy vs monotherapy for the treatment of relapsed cytomegalovirus retinitis in patients with AIDS. Arch Ophthalmol 114:23–33, 1996.

76. What are the major toxicities of ganciclovir and foscarnet?

Ganciclovir's most common toxicity is bone marrow suppression, usually seen as neutropenia and/or thrombocytopenia. Almost 40% of treated patients will develop neutrophil counts < 1,000 cells/mm³, and this can become a dose-limiting toxicity. Also seen is CNS toxicity manifested as confusion, headaches, or, rarely, seizures. Nausea, vomiting, and hepatitis may also be seen.

Foscarnet causes progressive renal dysfunction and potential renal failure. Over 25% of recipients have creatinine elevations > 2. Calcium, magnesium, phosphorus, and potassium balances are upset and warrant close monitoring. Seizures can occur, and a fixed drug reaction with penile ulcerations has been described.

77. Should all HIV-infected patients have eye exams?

Because CMV retinitis usually presents later in HIV infection, patients with less-advanced disease do not need an immediate referral to an ophthalmologist. However, there should be a baseline examination performed, with subsequent examinations as clinical symptoms and signs dictate. Patients with CD4⁺-lymphocyte counts chronically below 100/mm³ should be examined regardless of symptoms, with scheduled follow-up 2–3 times per year.

78. How else can CMV infection manifest in HIV infection besides chorioretinitis?

Interstitial pneumonia, colitis, esophagitis, adrenal insufficiency, and encephalitis.

79. Can anti-CMV and antiretroviral therapy be used in combination?

Overlapping toxicity needs to be avoided in these patients with advanced-stage disease. In a more stable patient tolerating therapy with ganciclovir, there is no overwhelming reason not to attempt zidovudine therapy, even though both drugs may exhibit bone marrow toxicity. On the other hand, with an expanded list of therapeutic options, there is no compelling reason to choose a regimen with overlapping toxicity. Close hematologic and chemistry monitoring is imperative.

TUBERCULOSIS AND OTHER MYCOBACTERIOSES

80. What is the relationship between AIDS and tuberculosis (TB)?

Throughout this century, there had been a steady, rapid decline in the morbidity and mortality attributed to TB. However, in the mid-1980s, this decline halted, and in 1986 there occurred the first increase in new TB cases reported since nationwide reporting was initiated in 1953. Several investigators cross-matched statewide public health registers for TB and AIDS cases and found a high number of patients on both lists. Multiple studies now demonstrate the susceptibility of HIV patients to primary TB and the high rate of progression from latent to active TB in those patients with preexisting latent TB and superimposed HIV immunosuppression.

This occurrence is predictable from knowledge of the pathogenesis of each of these separate infections. Control of TB is dependent upon cell-mediated immunity, precisely the most profound deficit seen in HIV infection. The incidence of TB in an HIV-infected population can be expected to mirror that population's previous exposure to *Mycobacterium tuberculosis*. Thus, immigrants, inner-city minorities, and IV drug users, with a high prevalence of both HIV infection and previous TB infection, will develop a high number of active TB cases unless prophylaxis is used.

Shafer RW, Edlin BR: Tuberculosis in patients infected with human immunodeficiency virus: Perspective on the past decade. Clin Infect Dis 22:683–704, 1996.

81. Does TB differ presentation in HIV-infected patients?

TB in HIV-infected patients remains primarily a pulmonary disease, but the incidence of extrapulmonary disease is much higher in the HIV-infected population compared to the general population. Miliary and disseminated TB are more often seen, and "typical" apical or cavitary disease is less common. Although the symptoms of chronic productive cough and hemoptysis are less common, TB in HIV infection remains a progressive, febrile, wasting disease.

The more "typical" TB cases will appear in those HIV-infected patients with a more preserved immune status, whereas the more "atypical" presentations will be in those further along in

HIV-related illness. There appears to be a temporal clustering of TB cases around the time of an AIDS diagnosis.

Jones BE, et al: Relationship of the manifestations of tuberculosis to CD4 cell counts in patients with human immunodeficiency virus infection. Am Rev Respir Dis 148:1292–1297, 1993.

Long R, et al: The chest roentgenogram in pulmonary tuberculosis patients seropositive for human immunodeficiency virus type 1. Chest 99:123–127, 1991.

82. Is TB more contagious in AIDS patients?

Mycobacterium tuberculosis, a communicable pathogen in individuals with normal immunity, represents the rare organism that may be transmitted *from* an HIV-infected individual *to* a noninfected individual. It may be that patients with AIDS are less contagious than non-AIDS patients, but the bottom line is that any patient capable of aerosolizing respiratory droplets containing *M. tuberculosis* is contagious. From the other perspective, patients with AIDS are much more susceptible to TB infection, and care should be taken to minimize any new exposures.

83. What is the treatment of TB in HIV infection?

Thus far, TB appears to be a curable infection in this patient population. The recommended treatment is currently the same for both HIV-infected and non-HIV-infected patients—isoniazid, 300 mg/day, *plus* rifampin, 600 mg/day, *plus* pyrazinamide, 20–30 mg/kg/day, for the first 2 months of therapy. Ethambutol, 25 mg/kg/day, is added initially to protect against the possibility of drug resistance. Tapering down to fewer drugs then depends on sensitivities. Directly observed therapy (DOT) is the standard of care.

American Thoracic Society: Treatment of tuberculosis and tuberculosis infection in adults and children. Am J Respir Crit Care Med 149:1359–1374, 1994.

84. Is a PPD of any use in HIV-infected patients?

The benefits derived from PPD skin testing are dependent on the prevalence of underlying TB infection in the population being screened and the degree of immunosuppression already present. It is currently recommended that all HIV-positive individuals have a PPD placed shortly after the diagnosis of HIV infection. Those persons with a reaction of $\geq$ 5 mm are recommended to receive isoniazid prophylaxis for 12 months, regardless of their age at the time of diagnosis.

Centers for Disease Control: MMWR 38:236–238, 243 250, 1989.

85. What about TB reporting and contact tracing?

TB remains a reportable disease in all states, and cases should be reported. This reporting is wholly independent from reporting HIV infection or cases of AIDS. Many localities have protocols to protect the confidentiality of HIV-infected individuals, so often your report of a TB case may not include HIV status. In areas where these protocols are not present, it is a good idea to add this information, since it assists the local health department in prioritizing its cases.

86. Should TB patients be screened for HIV infection?

Since a larger number of TB cases are now related to HIV infection, and because early diagnosis of HIV infection has many benefits, all TB patients should be asked to consent to HIV testing. In many large cities, the rates on this testing will be as high as 30–40% HIV-positive.

87. What other mycobacterial infections are seen in HIV-infected patients?

Very early in the HIV epidemic, it was noted that a large number of patients had disseminated *Mycobacterium avium* complex (MAC) infection. Autopsy series have demonstrated up to 50% prevalence of this infection at the time of death from AIDS, and clinical studies have shown an annual risk of approx. 20% in AIDS patients.

Multiple other mycobacteria have been found to cause infection in patients with AIDS, but the only one seen in any significant numbers is *M. kansasii.*

Nightingale SD, et al: Incidence of *M. avium-intracellulare* complex bacteremia in human immunodeficiency virus-positive patients. J Infect Dis 165:1082–1085, 1992.

88. How does infection with *Mycobacterium avium* complex (MAC) present?

MAC infection is usually associated with advanced HIV disease, and the patient often has multiple concurrent conditions. Thus, the individual contribution of the MAC infection to the overall condition of the patient can be difficult to ascertain.

Usually seen are systemic symptoms such as fever, night sweats, weight loss, fatigue, and malaise. Laboratory examination may reveal increasing anemia or mild hepatitis. Chronic diarrhea with abdominal pain and/or malabsorption is also seen. The frequency of GI symptoms and pathologic changes suggest this may be the portal of entry.

Diagnosis of MAC infection is made by culture of biopsy specimens or blood. The yield from blood cultures is excellent, and there is often only a short delay while awaiting results. Positive results can be reported in as few as 5–10 days. Specimens from biopsies quickly reveal acid-fast organisms on stains, thus facilitating the diagnosis.

89. Is there a standard therapy for MAC in patients with AIDS?

The development of the new macrolides, clarithromycin and azithromycin, has opened a new door into treatment options for patients with MAC. For the first time, regimens containing these compounds have demonstrated high rates of blood culture sterilization and clinical improvement. The current recommendation is to include one of these agents in addition to at least one second drug—usually ethambutol plus either rifabutin or ciprofloxacin.

CDC: Recommendations on prophylaxis and therapy for disseminated *Mycobacterium avium* complex for adults and adolescents infected with human immunodeficiency virus. MMWR 42(RR-9):14–20, 1993.

90. Is there an effective prophylaxis against MAC?

Three drugs have been approved for prophylaxis against MAC: rifabutin, clarithromycin, and azithromycin. Rifabutin resulted in improved quality of life and decreased the rate of MAC from 18% to 9% in a group of patients with AIDS and a $CD4^+ \leq 200/mm^3$. Clarithromycin also decreased the rate of MAC, from 12.6% to 4.5%, in AIDS patients with a CD4 count $\leq 100/mm^3$. This trial also demonstrated a survival benefit to clarithromycin prophylaxis.

Two concerns arise with these drugs. First, rifabutin could cause cross-resistance to rifampin in a patient with TB who is inadequately evaluated and then treated with this single-drug inadvertently. Second, many MAC breakthroughs on clarithromycin prophylaxis have been shown to be clarithromycin-resistant, thus negating the efficacy of the most active drug used in treatment.

SYPHILIS AND AIDS

91. In which HIV-infected patients should a serologic test for syphilis (STS) be obtained?

Every HIV-infected patient needs an STS as well as a detailed history for all sexually transmitted diseases and past treatments. A growing body of literature suggests the possibility of an accelerated course and unusual progression of syphilis in patients also infected with HIV. With this in mind, and the fact that the routes of transmission for HIV and syphilis are similar, all patients with a positive serology for one should be tested for the other.

Hook EW: Syphilis and HIV infection. J Infect Dis 160:530–534, 1989.

92. What if the STS is positive but the patient gives no history of syphilis?

Due to the concern over altered progression of syphilis in HIV infection, the discrimination between early syphilis, early latent syphilis, and late latent syphilis may be less important, because most practitioners now aggressively treat early infection. A question does arise over the use of lumbar puncture (LP) to evaluate neurosyphilis, as this is not currently recommended in early syphilis but is recommended in late latent (> 1-year duration) syphilis. With no patient history to steer you, it may be best to err on the side of caution and proceed with LP in HIV-infected patients, especially those with any neurologic signs or symptoms or a serum antibody titer >1:32.

An inquiry to the local public health office may provide additional history that the patient has not recalled.

CDC: Recommendations for diagnosing and treating syphilis in HIV-infected patients. MMWR 37:600–608,1988.

93. Which HIV-infected patients with syphilis need a lumbar puncture (LP)?

Although a few authorities would recommend an LP in all of these patients, most would agree that patients with a clear episode of primary or secondary syphilis do *not* need an LP. Examination of the CSF should be done for all HIV-infected patients with syphilis of > 1 year's duration or any clinical signs or symptoms of CNS involvement. Patients with early syphilis whose serologic titers increase or fail to decrease appropriately (4-fold in 6 months) should also undergo an LP to evaluate CNS involvement prior to re-treatment.

94. What is the treatment for neurosyphilis in HIV-infected patients?

It is the same whether or not a patient has HIV infection: aqueous crystalline penicillin G, 2.4 mu IV every 4 hours (12–24 mu/day) for 10–14 days. No non-penicillin-based therapy is considered wholly satisfactory. Patients with remote histories of unclear penicillin allergy may need skin testing.

95. If a chancre is present, is initial therapy changed?

The recommended regimen remains one dose of benzathine penicillin G, 2.4 mu IM, but many authorities would more aggressively treat primary syphilis in patients coinfected with HIV and administer a total of 7.2 mu given as 2.4 mu weekly for 3 consecutive weeks.

Musher DM: How much penicillin cures early syphilis? Ann Intern Med 109:849–851, 1988.

96. How should patients with HIV infection and primary syphilis be followed up?

These patients should have repeat serologic testing at 1, 2, 3, 6, 9, and 12 months. If at any time there is a 4-fold increase in titer, an LP should be done. If by 3 months there has not been a 4-fold decrease in titer, the CSF should be examined.

97. Is HIV-related syphilis reportable to local health authorities?

By all means, yes. The presence of concomitant HIV infection does not change the reporting requirement for syphilis.

98. Should all syphilis patients be tested for HIV?

Again, absolutely. HIV infection may alter the course of syphilis or the response to treatment. Obviously, there are common risk factors for both infections, and in addition, any condition that causes open sores in the genital area can facilitate the transmission of HIV.

TOXOPLASMOSIS

99. What are the most common causes of CNS mass lesions in AIDS?

Cerebral toxoplasmosis and primary CNS lymphoma. Other causes include progressive multifocal leukoencephalopathy (PML), cryptococcoma, tuberculoma, bacterial and fungal abscesses, and metastatic neoplastic disease. The increasing use of TMP-SMX as prophylaxis for PCP may coincidentally be decreasing the proportion of CNS mass lesions attributable to toxoplasmosis.

100. How is the differential diagnosis between CNS toxoplasmosis and lymphoma made?

Most clinicians recommend empirical treatment for toxoplasmosis (pyrimethamine, 100-mg loading dose, then 25 mg/day, and sulfadiazine, 4–6 gm daily in divided doses) and judge clinical response as well as response seen on CT scanning. This response should be rapid (3–5 days) and, if not seen, suggests an etiology other than toxoplasmosis.

101. Are there characteristic CT scan findings in CNS toxoplasmosis?

CT Findings in CNS Toxoplasmosis and Lymphoma

FINDING	TOXOPLASMOSIS	LYMPHOMA
Area involved	Deep gray matter and basal ganglia	White matter, periventricular areas
Mass effect	Yes	Yes
Enhancement	Ring-enhancement	Weakly, not ring-shaped
Number of lesions	Multiple	1–2

102. How long should patients with AIDS be treated for toxoplasmosis?

This is another AIDS-related infection that appears to require lifelong suppressive therapy, much like *Pneumocystis* and *Cryptococcus*. Chronic pyrimethamine and sulfadiazine therapy should be continued indefinitely. Clindamycin is used in sulfa-intolerant patients.

Porter SB, Sande MA: Toxoplasmosis of the central nervous system in the acquired immunodeficiency syndrome. N Engl J Med 327:1643–1648, 1992.

103. Can primary toxoplasmosis prophylaxis be given?

There is gathering evidence that the use of TMP-SMX as prophylaxis against PCP is effective as primary prophylaxis for toxoplasmosis. The same effect is not seen with PCP prophylaxis with dapsone or pentamidine, although the addition of pyrimethamine to dapsone appears effective. In patients with a positive toxoplasma serology, the choice for PCP prophylaxis should be heavily weighted toward TMP-SMX.

Jacobson MA, et al: Primary prophylaxis with pyrimethamine for toxoplasmic encephalitis in patients with advanced human immunodeficiency virus disease: Results of a randomized trial. J Infect Dis 169:384–394, 1994.

BIBLIOGRAPHY

1. Centers for Disease Control: USPHS/IDSA guidelines for the prevention of opportunistic infections in persons infected with human immunodeficiency virus: A summary. MMWR 44(RR-8):1–34, 1995.
2. Cohen PT, et al: The AIDS Knowledge Base, 2nd ed. Waltham, MA, Medical Publishing Group Massachusetts Medical Society, 1994.
3. Harawi SJ, O'Hara CJ: Pathology and Pathophysiology of AIDS and HIV-Related Diseases. St. Louis, Mosby, 1989.
4. Holmes KK, et al: Sexually Transmitted Diseases, 2nd ed. New York, McGraw-Hill, 1990.
5. Makadon HJ, et al: HIV disease in primary care. J Gen Intern Med 6(suppl l):S1–S62, 1991.
6. Mandell GL, Bennett JE, Dolin R: Principles and Practice of Infectious Diseases, 4th ed. New York, Churchill Livingstone, 1995.
7. Sande MA, Volberding PA: The Medical Management of AIDS, 4th ed. Philadelphia, W.B. Saunders, 1995.

14. NEUROLOGY

Loren A. Rolak, M.D., and Anthony P. Weiss, M.D.

*This apoplexy, as I take it, is a kind of lethargy, an't please your lord-
ship; a kind of sleeping in the blood, a whoreson tingling. . . . It hath
it original from much grief, from study and perturbation of the brain.
I have read the cause of his effects in Galen. It is a kind of deafness.*
William Shakespeare (1564–1616)
Description of stroke, Henry IV, Part II

APPROACH TO THE PATIENT

1. What is the initial approach to evaluating patients complaining of neurologic symptoms?
The first step is to localize the lesion to a specific part of the nervous system. Only then should
an etiology be sought, since defining the anatomy usually implies certain causes. Because each
part of the brain, spinal cord, and peripheral nervous system has such specialized functions, lesions in these areas produce specific clinical deficits. Therefore, symptoms can often be localized,
sometimes to the millimeter, to discrete parts of the nervous system.

2. What are the most important regions for anatomic localization?
For clinical purposes, the most important neuroanatomy is limited to a few large regions. The
regions where lesions should be localized are (proceeding from distal to proximal):

1. Muscle	4. Root	7. Cerebellum
2. Neuromuscular junction	5. Spinal cord	8. Subcortical brain
3. Peripheral nerve	6. Brainstem	9. Cortical brain

3. How are symptoms localized to these neuroanatomic regions?
As in all aspects of medicine, the history guides the diagnosis. By asking the proper questions during the history, a clinician can accurately localize most neurologic lesions.
A useful system for diagnosis is to begin distally (with the muscle) and to ask the patient questions about each part of the neurologic anatomy, working backward (proximally) from the muscle, through the neuromuscular junction, peripheral nerve, root, spinal cord, cerebellum, brainstem, subcortex, and ending with the cortex of the brain. By sequentially asking about each of
these areas, you can "examine" the patient thoroughly. Only after the lesion is localized by means
of history-taking should the physical examination begin. If localization of the lesion is still unclear after a careful history, do not begin the physical examination—take a better history!

4. Which clinical features of muscle disease can be elicited by the history?
Muscle disease (myopathy) causes symmetric proximal weakness without sensory loss.
Therefore, questions should elicit these symptoms.
1. **Proximal leg weakness:** Can the patient arise from a chair, get out of a car, get off the toilet, or go up stairs without using his hands?
2. **Proximal arm weakness:** Can the patient lift or carry objects, such as a briefcase, school
books, children, or grocery bags?
3. **Symmetric weakness:** Is the weakness relatively symmetric? Are both sides affected?
(Although most generalized processes are slightly asymmetric, weakness essentially confined to
one limb or one side of the body is unlikely to be a myopathy.)

4. **Sensory loss:** Is there numbness or other loss of normal sensation? (Pain and cramping may occur with some myopathies, but actual sensory loss should not occur with disease that is confined to the muscle.)

5. After a history of muscle disease is elicited, what findings can be expected on physical examination?

The examination should show proximal symmetric weakness without sensory loss. Tone is usually normal or mildly decreased, and reflexes are also normal or mildly decreased. There is seldom significant atrophy unless the process is advanced.

6. Which clinical features of neuromuscular junction disease can be elicited by history?

Neuromuscular junction diseases closely resemble myopathies, causing proximal symmetric weakness without sensory loss. However, the hallmark of disease of the neuromuscular junction is **fatigability:** the weakness worsens with use and recovers with rest. Since strength improves with rest, this fatigability does not usually present as a steady progressive decline throughout the day. Instead, it fluctuates as the muscle first fatigues, then recovers, then fatigues again, then recovers, etc. (Almost *every* medical symptom can be worse at the end of the day. Look for variability or fluctuation as the characteristic of neuromuscular junction fatigability.)

Another feature of neuromuscular junction diseases is that they are usually extremely **proximal.** They often involve muscles of the face resulting in drooping of the eyelids (ptosis), double vision, difficulty in chewing and swallowing, slurred speech, and facial weakness.

7. After a history of neuromuscular junction problems is elicited, what findings can be expected on physical examination?

Examination should show proximal symmetric weakness without sensory loss that results in fatigue. Repetitive testing weakens the muscles, which regain their strength with a minute or so of rest. Similarly, sustained muscular activity (such as upward gaze) leads to fatigability and progressive weakness (such as ptosis). Tone, reflexes, and muscle bulk are all be normal.

8. Which clinical feature of peripheral neuropathies can be elicited by history?

Peripheral neuropathies cause distal, often asymmetric weakness with sensory changes. Atrophy and fasciculations may also appear. Questions should elicit these symptoms:

1. **Distal weakness in the legs:** Does the patient wear out the toes of his shoes or catch his toes and trip, as would be expected with a footdrop?

2. **Distal weakness in the hands:** Does the patient have trouble with his grip, or frequently drop things?

3. **Asymmetric weakness:** Is the process asymmetric? (Some neuropathies are distal, symmetric, stocking-and-glove neuropathies, but most are asymmetric, such as carpal tunnel syndrome or radial nerve palsy.)

4. **Denervation changes:** Has the patient noticed a shrinkage or wasting of the muscle (atrophy) or quivering, twitching muscles (fasciculations)?

5. **Sensory changes:** Is there numbness, tingling, or paresthesia?

9. After a history of peripheral neuropathy is elicited, what findings can be expected on physical examination?

Distal, often asymmetric weakness, with atrophy and fasciculations, and with sensory loss such as decreased pinprick, vibration, and occasionally position sense. Tone is normal or decreased, and reflexes are diminished. Sometimes, there are also trophic changes, such as loss of hair and nails and smooth, shiny skin.

10. Which clinical features of root diseases (radiculopathies) can be elicited by history?

The hallmark of root disease is **pain.** This pain is usually severe, described as sharp, hot, or electric, and commonly radiates down an arm or leg. In addition, radiculopathies usually have similar features to peripheral neuropathies: denervation (weakness, atrophy, fasciculations) with sensory loss. The weakness may be proximal (the most common radiculopathies in the arms involve C5/6 muscles, which are proximal) or distal (the most common radiculopathies in the legs involve L5/S1 muscles, which are distal). The history is therefore the same as for peripheral neuropathies, but with the added element of pain.

11. After a history of radiculopathy is elicited, what findings can be expected on physical examination?

The examination will show weakness in one myotomal group of muscles, such as C5/6 in the arm or L5/S1 in the leg, sometimes with atrophy and fasciculations. Tone is be normal or decreased, and the reflex in those muscles is diminished or absent. There is sensory loss in a dermatomal distribution. Sometimes, maneuvers that stretch the root, such as straight leg raising, will elicit the pain.

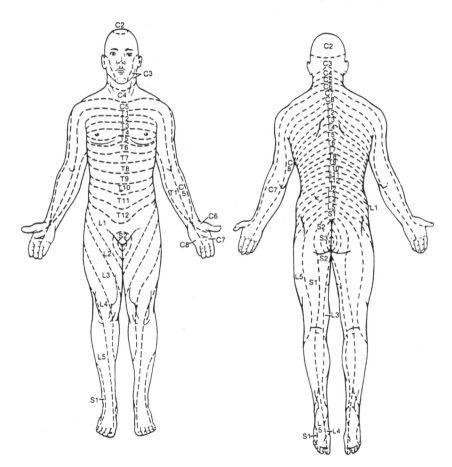

Map of the sensory dermatomes in the anterior and posterior aspects. (From DeJong RN: The Neurologic Examination. Hagerstown, MD, Harper & Row, 1979, with permission.)

12. Spinal cord lesions cause a triad of symptoms. Name these.

1. **A sensory level.** This level, which may occur as a band of sensory change around the thorax or abdomen or as a sharp level below which sensation is lost, is the hallmark of spinal cord disease.

2. **Distal, usually symmetric weakness**

3. **Bowel and bladder changes** (sphincter dysfunction)

13. Which questions should be asked during the history to elicit the symptoms of spinal cord disease?

1. **Distal leg weakness:** Does the patient drag his toes or trip because of the leg weakness? Lesions in the pyramidal tract, also called the corticospinal tract or upper motor neuron, cause weakness that is usually greatest distally and thus can mimic a peripheral neuropathy.

2. **Spasticity:** Are the patient's legs stiff? Pyramidal tract weakness causes spasticity, and many patients report their legs are stiff and that their knees won't bend when they walk.

3. **Sensory level:** Patients sometimes describe this as feeling like a belt or band or "tight swimming trunks" around their waist or abdomen.

4. **Sphincter dysfunction:** Is there retention or incontinence of the bowel or bladder? The bladder is usually much more sensitive to spinal cord injury than the bowel.

14. After a history of spinal cord disease is elicited, what findings can be expected on physical examination?

Examination of a person with spinal cord disease shows distal weakness, usually worse in the legs than the arms, and usually worse in the extensors (dorsiflexors of the feet and extensors of the wrists and fingers) than in the flexors. Tone is increased, reflexes are brisk, and there are often extensor plantar reflexes (positive Babinski signs). Superficial reflexes, such as anal wink, sphincter tone, cremasteric reflex, and abdominal reflexes, are commonly lost. A sensory level can often be found, below which all sensory modalities are diminished.

15. Which clinical features of brainstem disease can be elicited by history?

Cranial nerve abnormalities are the hallmark of brainstem disease. The brainstem is essentially the spinal cord with cranial nerves embedded in it, so symptoms of brainstem disease generally consist of a combination of **long-tract findings** (such as weakness from the pyramidal tract, numbness from the spinothalamic tract, etc.) plus symptoms of cranial nerve impingement. Because the long tracts cross (decussate), the weakness and numbness are not in the distribution of a level, but rather in a hemiparesis or hemianesthesia. Because of the crossing of these long tracts, damage to one side of the brainstem, affecting the cranial nerves on that side, usually results in long tract symptoms that affect the opposite side of the body. These **crossed symptoms** are another hallmark of brainstem disease—e.g., weakness of one side of the face and the opposite side of the body.

16. What are the symptoms of cranial nerve lesions in the brainstem?

Cranial nerve (CN) lesions commonly cause the big "D's":

Diplopia—CN III, IV, VI

Decreased facial sensation—CN V

Decreased facial strength—CN VII

Dizziness—CN VIII

Deafness—CN VIII

Dysarthria and dysphagia—CN IX, X, XII

The history therefore should focus on eliciting these symptoms:

• Is there diplopia, facial weakness or numbness, dizziness, deafness, dysarthria, or dysphagia?

• Are there long-tract findings, such as hemiparesis or hemisensory loss?

• Are the findings crossed or bilateral?

17. After a history of brainstem disease is elicited, what findings can be expected on physical examination?

Examination shows a combination of cranial nerve and long-tract abnormalities.

Checking the **cranial nerves** may reveal ptosis, abnormalities of extraocular movements, diplopia, nystagmus, decreased corneal reflexes, facial weakness or numbness, decreased hearing, dysarthria, paralysis of the palate, decreased gag reflex, or tongue deviation.

Long-tract abnormalities may include in hemiparesis, with a pyramidal pattern of distal weakness with increased reflexes, increased tone, and a positive Babinski sign. Hemisensory loss may include decreased sensation to all modalities.

18. Which clinical features of cerebellar disease can be elicited by history?

The cerebellum is responsible for smoothing out voluntary movements, and impairments produce abnormalities in the rate and rhythm of movements (clumsiness and lack of coordination). Questions should focus on incoordination in the legs and the arms:

1. **Legs:** Does the patient have a staggering, drunken walk? Most laymen use the term "drunken" walk to describe cerebellar disease. (Drinking alcohol does in fact impair the cerebellum, and the characteristic wide-based, ataxic, staggering gait of the intoxicated person is caused by cerebellar dysfunction.)

2. **Arms:** Does the patient have difficulty putting a key in a lock, lighting a cigarette, or performing other target-directed movements? The cerebellar tremor is worse with voluntary, intentional movements that require accurate placement. Fine coordinated movements, such as extending a key and inserting it into the narrow slot of a lock, are perfect examples of difficult tasks for people with cerebellar lesions.

19. After a history of cerebellar disease is elicited, what findings can be expected on physical examination?

Patients with cerebellar disease usually have a staggering gait and difficulty with tandem walking. When they slide a heel down a shin, it wavers unsteadily. In the arms, there is a tremor and wavering when touching the examiner's finger, the patient's own nose, or other targets. Similarly, rapid alternating movements in the limbs are irregular in rate and rhythm

20. How can the history and neurologic exam distinguish between subcortical and cortical brain disease?

Clinically, disease of the brain itself can affect either subcortical or cortical regions. The main features differentiating these are:

1. **Presence of specific cortical deficits:** Does the patient have aphasia (left hemisphere cortex) or visuospatial deficits (right hemisphere cortex)?

2. **Pattern of motor and sensory loss:** If the face and arm are involved, the lesion is cortical; if the face, arm, *and* leg are involved, it is subcortical.

3. **Type of sensory change:** Primary sensations, such as pain, temperature, touch, position, and vibration, are registered in the thalamus (subcortex) and are not much affected by cortical lesions. Deficits seen with cortical damage are secondary sensory changes, such as astereognosis, agraphesthesia, and loss of two-point discrimination. (these are difficult to elicit by history).

4. **Visual field deficits:** Because visual fibers run subcortically (in the optic tract, lateral geniculate, and optic radiations), cortical lesions do not cause field cuts. (Damage to the occipital cortex causes field cuts, but since there are no motor or sensory fibers there, it does not cause any other focal deficits.)

5. **Involuntary movements:** Most movement disorders are thought to arise from subcortical structures, such as the basal ganglia. A history of parkinsonism, chorea, dystonia, or hemiballismus thus suggest a subcortical lesion.

6. **Seizures:** Seizures arise from the paroxysmal discharge of neurons, almost exclusively in the cortex. Subcortical lesions seldom cause seizures.

21. How does the pattern of motor and sensory deficits differ between cortical and subcortical involvement?

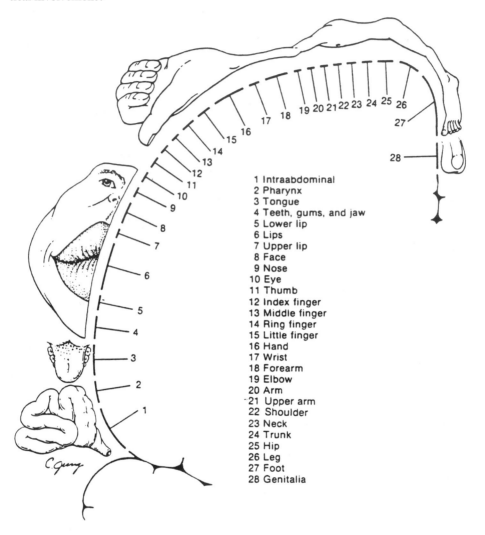

1 Intraabdominal
2 Pharynx
3 Tongue
4 Teeth, gums, and jaw
5 Lower lip
6 Lips
7 Upper lip
8 Face
9 Nose
10 Eye
11 Thumb
12 Index finger
13 Middle finger
14 Ring finger
15 Little finger
16 Hand
17 Wrist
18 Forearm
19 Elbow
20 Arm
21 Upper arm
22 Shoulder
23 Neck
24 Trunk
25 Hip
26 Leg
27 Foot
28 Genitalia

Homunculus showing sensory and motor representation over the cortex. (From Penfield W, Rasmussen T: The Cerebral Cortex. New York, Macmillan, 1950; with permission.)

Motor and sensory neurons corresponding to the various regions of the body are arranged across the cortex in a manner described as a **homunculus.** The parts of the body are draped upside-down over the surface of the outer cortex, with a large face and lips, small neck, a large hand and thumb, and a small trunk, such that a lesion localized to the cortex will result in a deficit in one or more of the anatomic regions. The leg, however, is not over the outside cortex but instead hangs down in the interhemispheric fissure, in the cortex deep between the two brain hemispheres. Most cortical processes, such as a stroke, affect the face and arm but cannot "get to" the leg fibers between the hemispheres, sparing involvement of the leg in these conditions.

Deeper in the brain, in subcortical regions, fibers from the face, arm, and leg lie close together in the pyramidal tract or spinothalamic tract. Even a small lesion in these tracts can affect the face, arm, and leg.

So, if the face and arm are involved, the lesion is cortical. If the face, arm, *and* leg are involved, it is subcortical.

MYOPATHIES

22. What are the most important myopathies?
- Muscular dystrophies: Duchenne's, myotonic, etc.
- Congenital myopathies: Kearns-Sayre, central-core, etc.
- Inflammatory myopathies: polymyositis, dermatomyositis, etc.
- Toxic myopathies: alcohol, zidovudine, clofibrate, steroids, etc.
- Endocrine myopathies: hypothyroidism, hypoadrenalism, etc.
- Infectious myopathies: trichinosis, AIDS, etc.

23. Which of the myopathies are most common on the medical ward?
Polymyositis is the most common. It is an inflammatory, probably autoimmune, disease of the muscles, characterized by the subacute onset of proximal weakness of the arms and legs, often with dysphagia. It may accompany connective tissue disease (such as systemic lupus erythematosus) or vasculitis but usually appears alone. It runs a variable course but can be severe or even fatal.

Dermatomyositis is a distinct clinical entity characterized by similar subacute proximal muscle weakness in association with a rash, often over the face and trunk. Like polymyositis, dermatomyositis may occur alone or in conjunction with other connective tissue diseases. There may also be an increased incidence of concomitant malignancies.

Treatment for polymyositis and dermatomyositis is the same and involves high-dose oral prednisone (at least 1 mg/kg body weight/day) as the mainstay of therapy. Azathioprine or methotrexate may be used in steroid-resistant cases or when complications develop from steroid use. IV immunoglobulin (IVIG), though expensive, may also be safe and effective, especially during acute exacerbations.

Piota PH et al: Myositis: Immunologic contributions to understanding cause, pathogenesis and therapy. Annals Int Med 122:715–724, 1995.

24. Which tests and procedures are used in the diagnostic evaluation of a patient with a myopathy?
The diagnostic evaluation of a myopathy generally entails a triad of tests:
(1) Serum creatine kinase (CK)
(2) Electromyography (EMG)
(3) Muscle biopsy

Muscle destruction usually liberates **CK,** making elevation of this enzyme is a good screening test for muscle disease. (The MM isoenzyme of CK is the most common.) An **EMG** is done by inserting a fine needle electrode into the muscle to record the electrical impulses related to contractions. Myopathies cause low-voltage, short-duration muscle contractions, and this test can thus confirm the presence of myopathy. Finally, a muscle **biopsy** is often needed to define the cause of a myopathy, since most myopathies are clinically similar. The tissue may show inflammation (polymyositis), mitochondrial abnormalities, or other specific diseases.

NEUROMUSCULAR JUNCTION

25. Name the most common neuromuscular junction disease seen on the medical ward?
Myasthenia gravis. MG has a prevalence of 1 case/10,000 population and a bimodal age distribution, occurring in young women in their teens and 20s and old men aged 60 and above. It presents with proximal weakness, especially ptosis and diplopia, with fatigue on use and recovery

with rest. Because MG can involve the respiratory muscles, pulmonary failure is the most feared complication.

26. How is myasthenia gravis treated?

MG is an autoimmune disease in which patients produce antibodies that destroy the acetylcholine receptors on muscle. Acetylcholine is the neurotransmitter that makes muscles contract. Treatment consists of acetylcholinesterase inhibitors, which block the enzymatic break down of acetylcholine, thus allowing for greater concentrations of acetylcholine at the receptor. **Pyridostigmine** (Mestinon) is the drug of choice, but immunosuppressive drugs, including prednisone, azathioprine, and cyclosporine, are often necessary to attack the underlying autoimmune process. Plasmapheresis and IVIG have also been shown to be helpful, usually to provide rapid (but transient) improvement during myasthenic crisis. Finally, all postpubertal patients with MG should undergo surgical thymectomy, due to its strong beneficial effect on disease severity.

Drachman DB: Myasthenia gravis. N Engl J Med 330:1797–1810, 1994.

27. Are some drugs contraindicated for use in patients with neuromuscular junction diseases?

Some drugs can worsen these diseases, including

1. Aminoglycosides
2. Tetracycline antibiotics
3. Corticosteroids (acutely)
4. Thyroid hormone
5. Phenothiazines (i.e., chlorpromazine)
6. Quinidine
7. Lidocaine
8. Propranolol
9. Lithium
10. Dilantin

28. What is the second most common disease causing neuromuscular junction problems?

Lambert-Eaton myasthenic syndrome (LEMS). This LEMS, like MG, is an autoimmune condition, although its target is the presynaptic voltage-gated calcium channel involved in acetylcholine release, not the receptor. It is commonly seen in association with occult carcinoma, especially small cell carcinoma of the lung. LEMS clinically resembles MG because of fluctuating proximal weakness. It is generally treated by therapy for the underlying neoplasm, sometimes accompanied by plasmapheresis and other immune suppressors, especially in cases where no occult cancer can be found. Guanidine may provide symptomatic relief.

Sanders DB: LEMS: Pathogenesis and treatment. Semin Neurol 14(2):111–117, 1994.

29. How do we differentiate myasthenia gravis from Lambert-Eaton myasthenic syndrome?

1. Although MG and LEMS strongly resemble each other clinically, LEMS does not involve the extraocular muscles, so ptosis and diplopia, which are very common with MG, do not occur.

2. By EMG testing, repetitive stimulation of the nerve in MG shows a progressive decline in each muscle contraction, documenting the fatigability with repetitive stimulation. With LEMS, there is a paradoxical increase, rather than decrease, in successive muscle contractions when the nerve is repetitively stimulated. This is due to a progressive increase in the amount of acetylcholine released presynaptically by the stimulated nerve.

30. What triad of tests are useful in the diagnostic evaluation of patients with neuromuscular junction problems?

1. Tensilon test
2. Serum antibody levels
3. Repetitive stimulation on EMG

31. Explain the Tensilon test.

The Tensilon test is performed by administering a small dose of intravenous **edrophonium** (Tensilon), which is a powerful but transient acetylcholinesterase inhibitor. This agent causes a reversal of weakness within 30 seconds to 2 minutes, which lasts approx. 10 minutes before returning to baseline. For example, ptosis of the eyes may transiently resolve after a Tensilon test.

PERIPHERAL NEUROPATHIES

32. Which peripheral neuropathies are seen most common on the medical ward?

Peripheral neuropathies are probably the most frequent neurologic problems seen on a medical ward, unlike myopathies and neuromuscular junction disease which are rare. The most common peripheral neuropathies can be remembered by the mnemonic **DANG THE RAPIST:**

D—Diabetes	R—Remote effects of cancer
A—Alcohol	A—Amyloid
N—Nutritional (vitamin deficiencies, etc.)	P—Porphyria
G—Guillain-Barré	I—Inflammation (collagen vascular disease, etc.)
T—Trauma (carpal tunnel, etc.)	S—Syphilis
H—Hereditary	T—Tumors
E—Environmental (toxins, drugs)	

33. The evaluation of a patient with a peripheral neuropathy usually begins with which study?

An electromyogram and nerve conduction velocity (EMG/NCV) study. This test applies electrical current directly over the nerves and uses an electrode to record the speed with which the nerves conduct the current. It thus documents, extent and degree of slowing and impairment of nerve conduction. The EMG also uses a needle electrode within the muscles to record muscle contractions and thus show denervation of the muscles.

Once a neuropathy has been confirmed, workup for the etiology focuses on the conditions listed in Question 32, requiring evaluation for diabetes, alcoholism, B_{12} deficiency, metabolic abnormalities such as thyroid disease or uremia, familial illnesses, toxic exposure, collagen vascular disease, etc. A spinal tap is often needed to detect inflammatory neuropathies. Only rarely is a nerve biopsy required. The neuropathies usually resolves on treatment of the underlying etiology.

Horowitz SH: Diabetic neuropathy. Clin Orthop 296.78–85, 1993.

34. What is the most common entrapment neuropathy?

Carpal tunnel syndrome, caused by compression of the median nerve at the wrist. Most commonly the result of mechanical overuse, it usually presents with symptoms of pain and tingling in the hand (especially at night), weakness, and/or numbness. Pain in the hand at night is considered carpal tunnel syndrome until proven otherwise. There may be no objective neurologic findings in this condition. As with other peripheral neuropathies, EMG/NCV studies are helpful in making the diagnosis. Treatment is usually surgical, involving open or endoscopic release at the wrist, though conservative measures (such as wrist splinting) may be sufficient for mild cases.

Bracker MS, Ralph LP: The numb arm and hand. Am Fam Physician 31:103–116, 1995.

35. What is the Guillain-Barré syndrome (GBS)?

GBS is an acute inflammatory polyradiculopathy in which there is inflammation of the nerve roots and peripheral nerves. It is presumably autoimmune and often follows viral infections, surgery, pregnancies, and other immune-altering events. It runs a monophasic course, with weakness progressing for several days to weeks, reaching a plateau, and then recovering over a period of several weeks to months. The entire course may take up to 6 months.

Clinically, the diagnosis is confirmed by weakness, often but not always in an ascending pattern (from legs up the trunk to the arms and face). The weakness is hyporeflexive, but there is no significant sensory loss. *Rapidly progressive weakness with absent reflexes and no sensory change is almost always GBS.*

36. Treatment of Guillain-Barré syndrome is based on which of its abnormalities?

Although GBS is presumably autoimmune, no specific antigen or well-defined immune abnormality has been confirmed in this disease. Nevertheless, treatment is directed toward an immunologic cause, consisting of IVIG or plasmapheresis. If done early in the disease, these modalities do seem to shorten the overall course. Because autonomic dysfunction frequently complicates the syndrome and because respiration is often impaired by the weakness, patients usually require management in the intensive care unit. Management thus focuses on the day-to-day concerns of respirators, vital signs, nutrition, and other aspects of critical care.

Van der Mache FGA: The Guillain-Barré syndrome: Plasma exchange or immunoglobulins intravenously. J Neurol Nerosurg Psychiatry 57(suppl):33–34, 1994.

RADICULOPATHIES

37. What is the most common cause of radiculopathies on the medical ward?

Mechanical compression, as from spondylosis or a herniated disc. The common manifestations are neck and low back pain.

38. How should the patient with a radiculopathy be evaluated?

The diagnostic evaluation generally begins with an EMG/NCV to identify specifically which root is involved, and hence which muscles are denervated. The next step is often to image (MRI) the area where the root emerges from the spinal cord, since this is the most common site of disorders causing radiculopathies. If these studies are negative, showing no root compression, then nonmechanical causes such as tumor or infection should be considered.

39. Discuss the treatment for radiculopathies.

For most mechanical radiculopathies, the recommended treatment consists simply of analgesics, such as aspirin or other NSAIDs with avoidance of muscle relaxants and chronic opioid use. There are surprisingly few careful, controlled studies analyzing the value of bedrest, traction, spinal manipulation, or invasive procedures such as acupuncture or trigger point injection. At this time, these methods have no proven benefit in the treatment of radiculopathy.

Bigus S, et al: Acute Low Back Problems in Adults. [Clinical Practice Guideline 14.] Rockville, MD, Agency for Health Care Policy and Research, 1994. [AHCPR publ no. 95–0643.]

40. When is surgery appropriate for a radiculopathy?

One of the most controversial topics arises when radiculopathy due to spondylosis or a herniated nucleus pulposus (slipped disc) requires surgical treatment. Many experts believe that the presence of focal neurologic findings—findings such as weakness, atrophy, or fasciculations in the muscles affected, an absent reflex, or dermatome sensory loss—is a strong indication for surgery. Such hard findings are unlikely to improve spontaneously and may well progress unless pressure on the nerve is relieved.

Much more controversial is surgery for the relief of pain alone, without focal neurologic findings. Even in well-chosen patients with clear lesions and no overlying complications (such as litigation or secondary gain), surgery to alleviate pain is effective in only about half the cases. It is therefore often reserved for patients who have "failed medical management," which is a clinical decision and generally implies persistent, very severe pain after an adequate trial of analgesics.

41. What are the most common causes of back pain?

Only about 20% of back pain is caused by a slipped disc or root compression. There are many other causes, such as arthritis of the facet joints, but most back pain is felt to be musculoskeletal, from strain placed on the tendons, ligaments, and muscles of the back. Many experts feel that this pain is largely mechanical, secondary to the inherent instability of the lordotic spine required for the human upright posture and aggravated by the problems of obesity, lack of exercise, and other precipitating factors in the modern lifestyle. For most such pain, conservative therapy and patience are indicated.

Deyo RA, Rainville J, Kent DL: What can the history and physical tell us about low back pain? JAMA 268:760–765, 1992.

MYELOPATHIES

42. How does spinal cord compression present clinically and what are its most common causes?

Spinal cord compression causes the classic cord syndrome of a sensory level, bowel and bladder changes, and upper motor neuron weakness with spasticity, hyperreflexia, and a positive Babinski sign. Superficial reflexes, such as abdominal reflexes and the anal wink, may be diminished.

The most commonest cause of chronic spinal cord compression is cervical spondylosis. If there is no history of trauma, the acute syndrome is often due to compression by a neoplasm, usually metastatic. Such compression may develop almost instantaneously and may or may not cause back pain.

43. How is spinal cord compression best managed?

The first step is to localize the site of the lesion. Plain x-rays of the spine have a high yield for showing metastatic disease, as evidenced by lytic lesions and erosion of pedicles. Bone scans lack specificity and are generally of low yield. MRI has largely replaced myelography for the definitive documentation of compression.

Surgical intervention is indicated for compression due to cervical spondylosis or mechanical deformation, such as spondylolisthesis. For neoplastic compression, radiation therapy is increasingly favored over surgical decompression, since results are equally good in many studies. Otherwise surgery may be needed for diagnosis as well as treatment. In either case, high-dose IV steroids, such as 100 mg of dexamethasone daily, may provide additional relief.

Byrne TN: Spinal cord compression from epidural metastases. N Engl J Med 327:614–619, 1992.

BRAINSTEM DISEASE

44. A patient presents with a primary complaint of dizziness. What characteristics of the dizziness should be ascertained during evaluation?

When evaluating a patient with dizziness, the first question should be whether this is true vestibular dizziness or "dizziness" because of near-syncope, ataxia, or another etiology. Patients with true vestibular dizziness complain of **vertigo.**

The next step is to determine whether the vertigo is central (due to a brainstem lesion) or peripheral (due to an ear lesion). Although many accompanying signs and symptoms have been promulgated to differentiate central from peripheral vertigo, none has great sensitivity or specificity. The most useful way to diagnose vertigo is by the company it keeps: **brainstem vertigo** is almost always accompanied by other signs of brainstem dysfunction, such as double vision, weakness or numbness of the face, dysarthria, or dysphagia. **Peripheral vertigo** is usually accompanied by tinnitus or hearing loss, but no other neurologic abnormalities.

45. Name the common causes of peripheral vertigo and central vertigo.

Peripheral	Central
Meniere's disease	Stroke
Vestibular neuronitis	Multiple sclerosis
Local trauma	Tumors
Drugs (antibiotics, diuretics)	
Acoustic neuroma	
Benign positional vertigo	

46. Which special procedures are helpful in the diagnostic evaluation of the dizzy patient?

The evaluation depends heavily on the history and physical examination. Audiograms are often useful to determine if there is any disease in the ear. Brainstem auditory evoked potentials can aid evaluation of both the peripheral eighth nerve in the ear and the CNS auditory pathways. Structural lesions, such as acoustic neuromas, are uncommon causes of dizziness, but when strongly suspected, they may be seen using MRI.

47. How is dizziness best treated?

Nonvertigo dizziness (including near-syncope, anxiety, and ataxia) should be treated by addressing the underlying cause. True vertigo can be treated symptomatically, almost regardless of the cause. **Scopolamine** has proved to be the best available treatment in comparative trials against other drugs and placebos. Sympathomimetics, such as ephedrine, also have proved to be helpful. Benzodiazepines and antihistamines are of some value, including meclizine (Antivert) and diazepam.

Ruckenstein MJ: A practical approach to dizziness. Postgrad Med 97:70–81, 1995.

CEREBELLAR DISEASE

48. What is the most common cause of cerebellar disease?

Alcoholism. Alcohol causes an anterior, midline (vernal) atrophy that leads to leg and truncal instability and thus to ataxic gait. Other metabolic causes of cerebellar disease include hypothyroidism and drugs such as 5-fluorouracil and phenytoin. Structural lesions, such as cerebellar infarcts, hemorrhages, and neoplasms (both primary and metastatic), are another cause.

49. What are the main clinical features of cerebellar diseases?

Cerebellar diseases comprise a disturbance of equilibrium, muscle tone, and execution of movement. The following findings can be present: hypotonia, ataxia, dysmetria, dysdiadochokinesia, nystagmus, rebound phenomenon, postural instability, scanning speech, and intention tremor. These findings vay in severity depending on whether the lesion is acute or chronic, bilateral or unilateral, hemispheric or midline. The common findings of cerebellar dysfunction can be remembered by the mnemonic **HANDS Tremor:**

H = Hypotonia (loss of muscle tone)
A = Asynergy (lack of coordination)
N = Nystagmus (ocular oscillation)
D = Dysarthria (speech abnormalities)
S = Station and gait (imbalance, gait ataxia)
Tremor = Tremor (coarse intention tremor)

50. Is there any treatment for cerebellar dysfunction?

Cerebellar tremor, dysmetria, and ataxia are among the most difficult symptoms to mask or treat effectively. Some studies have shown that high doses of isoniazid, 900–1200 mg/day, are superior to placebo for minimizing cerebellar dysfunction. However, the toxic effects on peripheral nerves, requiring pyridoxine supplementation, and on the liver, requiring constant blood monitoring, complicate use of this drug at these high doses. Other medications, such as propranolol, primidone, and trihexyphenidyl, have provided occasional success.

STROKE

51. What is a stroke?

A stroke is focal brain dysfunction due to ischemia. The ischemia may arise from atherosclerotic narrowing of a blood vessel, an embolus, hemorrhage, or other causes.

52. Name the four main kinds of stroke.

Types of Strokes

TYPE	% OF ALL STROKES	ONSET	PRECEDING TIAS (%)	ALTERED MENTAL STATUS (%)	MRI OR CT SCAN	OTHER FEATURES
Thrombotic	40	May be gradual	Up to 50	5	Ischemic infarction	Carotid bruit, stroke during sleep
Embolic	30	Sudden	10	1	Superficial (cortical) infarction	Underlying heart disease, peripheral emboli, or strokes in different vascular territories
Lacunar	20	May be gradual	30	0	Small, deep infarction	Pure motor or pure sensory stroke
Hemorrhagic	10	Sudden	5	25	Hyperdense mass	Nausea and vomiting, decreased mental status

53. What are the clinical features of a thrombotic stroke?

Thrombotic strokes are the most common type and account for approx. 40% of all strokes. They may have a gradual, stuttering, or stepwise onset rather than an abrupt deficit. The cause is generally atherosclerosis affecting large intracranial vessels. The large-vessel involvement explains why these strokes tend to cause considerable neurologic deficit. About one-third to one-half of thrombotic strokes are preceded by transient ischemic attacks (TIAs), which are focal but totally reversible deficits that last from a few minutes to 24 hours.

54. What are the major clinical features of an embolic stroke?

Embolic strokes generally arise from the heart with an underlying cardiac disease, such as atrial arrhythmias, valvular disease, or mural thrombus. They tend to be abrupt in onset, with more rapid resolution, and tend to cause smaller neurologic deficits than a thrombotic stroke. Because the embolus travels in the arterial stream until it reaches a blood vessel of sufficiently small caliber to occlude it, it often travels distally all the way to the cortex. Cortical deficits, such as aphasia, are thus characteristic of embolic strokes.

55. What are the mechanisms of a lacunar stroke?

Lacunar strokes are very small, discrete infarcts, <1 cm^3 in size, occurring deep within the brain or brainstem (*lacune* means little lake or pond). These strokes are due to occlusion of tiny penetrating arterioles that supply the deep brain substance, usually in the region of the basal ganglia, thalamus, and internal capsule, as well as the brainstem. These small strokes cause discrete clinical symptoms, such as a pure motor stroke (hemiparesis without sensory loss) or pure sensory stroke.

56. How do hemorrhagic strokes differ from the other three types?

An intracerebral hemorrhage is classified as a stroke because of its abrupt onset with focal neurologic deficits, but it is due to rupture of a blood vessel with subsequent bleeding and intracerebral mass, rather than to ischemia directly. Intracerebral bleeds have an abrupt onset and are usually accompanied by a significant headache and other signs of increased intracranial pressure, such as nausea, vomiting, and a diminished mental status. These are often devastating events with a poor prognosis. Bleeds tend to occur in the same deep locations as lacunas, i.e., the basal ganglia and brainstem.

57. What are the leading causes of death shortly after a stroke?

The three leading causes of death in the first 30 days after a stroke are not related primarily to the stroke itself or to neurologic deficits.

Leading Causes of Death After a Stroke

| 1. Pneumonia   2. Pulmonary embolus   3. Ischemic heart disease |

58. Discuss the medical management of the patient with acute stroke.

Medical management of the stroke patient should focus on the complications that develop after the stroke. Since the leading cause of death is **pneumonia,** care should be taken that the patient does not aspirate—keep the patient NPO until it is clear that swallowing is not impaired by neurologic damage. Fever should always be presumed to be pneumonia until proven otherwise.

Measures to prevent **pulmonary embolus** should be instituted, including early mobilization, support hose, and low-dose subcutaneous heparin.

Ischemic heart disease commonly causes death, since atherosclerosis affecting the cerebral vasculature probably also involves the coronary arteries. It has not yet been demonstrated that admitting stroke patients to an intensive care unit or that constant cardiac monitoring of such patients actually leads to improved survival or outcome. Nevertheless, cardiac assessment should be individualized.

Unfortunately, there is no current successful therapy for the stroke itself, other than general supportive measures.

59. Do antiplatelet agents have a role in management of cerebrovascular diseases?

Antiplatelet agents, specifically aspirin, have been advocated for the *secondary* prevention of stroke. Patients with TIA or minor stroke are often treated with aspirin, usually one tablet (325 mg) per day, to prevent further episodes of cerebrovascular ischemia.

Despite numerous trials and several meta-analyses, the value of aspirin in cerebrovascular disease has never been proven conclusively. However, because it is likely that aspirin can in fact reduce the risk of stroke and it is a relatively benign therapy for a disease that is otherwise essentially untreatable, it is given routinely.

Dipyridamole has no role in therapy for cerebrovascular disease.

60. Is ticlopidine useful in the prevention of stroke?

Ticlopidine, like aspirin, acts as a platelet inhibitor and similarly decreases the risk of further cerebrovascular ischemia. Unlike aspirin, it does not affect the cyclo-oxygenase pathway and instead acts by interfering with platelet membrane interactions. Its current role is in the prevention of stroke in patients with cerebral ischemia for whom aspirin therapy has failed, has caused intolerable side effects, or is otherwise contraindicated.

61. When is anticoagulation indicated in cerebrovascular disease?

The role of anticoagulation in cerebrovascular disease is very controversial, in part because trials have not been done addressing the most relevant issues. The consensus among neurologists is that anticoagulation is only of benefit, or possible benefit, in two settings:

1. **Stroke in evolution.** Thrombotic stenosis of a large vessel, leading to progressive deficits that slowly worsen over a period of minutes or hours, may be prevented with heparin. Heparin is generally given without a loading bolus, in a dose of ~1000 units/hr by continuous IV drip, to maintain the partial thromboplastin time (PTT) at 1.5 × normal. Some neurologists continue anticoagulation with coumarin for several months, whereas others discontinue anticoagulation once the deficit has stabilized, usually in a few days.

2. **Embolic stroke from the heart.** Following an initial brain embolus from a cardiac source, the risk of subsequent emboli is high, especially within the first few days and weeks, and evidence suggests that immediate anticoagulation dramatically reduces this risk. Although there is a chance that immediate anticoagulation will worsen a stroke by converting the ischemia into hemorrhage, data suggest that this worsening is minimal and more than outweighed by the benefits in preventing further emboli.

Note: Although **recombinant tissue plasminogen activator (rTPA)** is approved for treatment of acute ischemic stroke, data show only modest benefits, with an increased risk of intracranial hemorrhage. The dose is 0.9 mg/kg given over 1 hour; treatment must be initiated within 3 hours of the onset of symptoms and CT of the head must not show any evidence of infarction. There are many contraindications, so thrombolytic therapy is best provided by those skilled in its use.

Barnett HJM, et al: Drugs and surgery in the prevention of ischemic stroke. N Engl J Med 332:238–248, 1995.

62. When is anticoagulation contraindicated in cerebrovascular disease?

Known hypersensitivity to the drugs, bleeding dyscrasias, active bleeding (e.g., from the GI tract or hematuria), massive stroke (defined clinically, based on a clinician's judgment that there has been a major amount of brain tissue infarcted), and very frail health (e.g., elderly, very sick patient).

63. What is the role of carotid endarterectomy in cerebrovascular disease?

For patients with *symptomatic* atherosclerotic stenosis of >70% in the carotid artery, carotid endarterectomy is clearly beneficial, significantly decreasing the risk of ipsilateral stroke. In *asymptomatic* patients with atherosclerotic stenosis of the carotids, its role is less clear. Three large randomized trials done in the early 1990s detected no benefit of endarterectomy in these patients. However, the Asymptomatic Carotid Atherosclerosis Study (ACAS) demonstrated a reduction in cerebral infarction in asymptomatic patients with as little as 60% stenosis, provided perioperative morbidity was kept to a minimum. The benefits were sufficiently modest that not all experts were convinced of the utility of surgery, and considerable individual variation remains among physicians managing such patients. Clearly, any surgical intervention in the treatment of carotid artery stenosis must be used in addition to, not in lieu of, aggressive control of modifiable risk factors.

Executive Committee for ACAS Study: Endarterectomy for asymptomatic carotid artery stenosis. JAMA 273:1421–1428, 1995.

NASCET Collaborators: Beneficial effect of carotid endarterectomy in symptomatic patients with high-grade stenosis. N Engl J Med 325:445–453, 1991.

APHASIA

64. Define aphasia.

Aphasia is an acquired disturbance in language functions (i.e., the ability to manipulate sounds and symbols into concepts, words, and phrases). It must not be confused with dysarthria or slurred speech, which is strictly a problem with the motor control of talking. Aphasics not only have difficulty with talking but also with writing, reading, and all other forms of language production. The most common cause of aphasia in adults is cerebrovascular disease.

65. How do the fluent and nonfluent types of aphasias differ?

1. **Nonfluent aphasias** are generally produced by lesions in the cortex, in the anterior part of the dominant hemisphere around the sylvian fissure, and are often referred to by other expressions such as **Broca's,** motor, expressive, or anterior aphasia. Such patients have difficulty producing language and either cannot speak or do so only in monosyllables and short telegraphic phrases. Naming and repetition are also impaired, but comprehension is relatively preserved.

2. **Fluent aphasias** are due to lesions in the cortex in the posterior part of the dominant hemisphere, around the posterior temporal lobe. Such aphasias—also known as **Wernicke's,** sensory, receptive, or posterior aphasia—result in speech that is fluent and even loquacious, but senseless. These patients can talk but make no sense. They have many neologisms and paraphasic errors, inventing words and sounds as they go along and stringing words together in nongrammatical, meaningless fashions. Such patients usually have impaired naming, repetition, and severely impaired comprehension as well.

Comparison of the Main Types of Aphasia

TYPE	FLUENT	NAMES	REPEATS	COMPREHENDS
Broca's	No	No	No	Yes
Wernicke's	Yes	No	No	No

Damasio AR: Aphasia. N Engl J Med 326:531–539, 1992.

SEIZURES

66. What is an epileptic seizure?

An epileptic seizure is the abnormal discharge of a neuron or group of neurons that leads to excessive electrical activity in the brain, causing disruption of brain function sufficient to produce clinical symptoms such as staring spells or jerking of muscles.

67. What are the main kinds of epileptic seizures?

Generalized seizures	**Partial seizures**
Generalized tonic-clonic (grand mal)	Partial simple (focal)
Generalized absence (petit mal)	Partial complex (psychomotor)

68. Describe the clinical features of partial simple seizures.

Most partial simple seizures encountered in a medical setting consist of the focal jerking or twitching of an arm or leg on one side of the body. This is usually due to a structural lesion in the brain (such as a stroke, abscess, or tumor) that leads to local irritation and an epileptic discharge. If this discharge spreads, the focal seizure also spreads, sometimes involving the other side of the brain and causing twitching or jerking of both arms and legs (generalized tonic-clonic or grand mal seizure). Occasionally, metabolic lesions, especially hyperglycemia and hyperosmolar states, can cause focal lesions and focal partial seizures.

69. What are the clinical features of partial complex seizures?

Partial complex seizures may be preceded by an aura of abnormal smells or tastes, visual sensations, or mental phenomena, such as *deja-vu*. The seizure itself may consist of an episode of staring, lip smacking, and automatic, semipurposeful movements, such as picking at clothes. Often there is no jerking of muscles, no loss of tone, and no falling down. Patients, however, are in a state of significantly altered mental status and often completely unresponsive. After a minute or two the seizure passes, leaving a postictal state of confusion and lethargy.

70. Which group is most likely to develop generalized absence seizures?

Generalized absence seizures, sometimes referred to as petit mal, are seen almost exclusively in **children.** These seizures usually do not have significant aura or postictal state but may consist of just a few seconds of staring and altered mental status. This may be so brief as to escape detection by untrained observers. At other times, children are thought to be daydreaming rather than experiencing a seizure.

71. How do generalized tonic-clonic seizures present?

Generalized tonic-clonic seizures, the so-called grand mal seizures, consist of the sudden onset, often without any preceding aura, of jerking tonic and clonic activity of both arms and both legs, with a generalized increase in muscle tone and loss of consciousness. There may be tongue biting or incontinence. Seizures usually last a minute or two and then resolve, often with a period of postictal lethargy and confusion.

72. How do the identifiable causes of seizures vary by age?

Common Causes of Seizures by Age

NEONATE TO 3 YRS	3–20 YRS	20–60 YRS	>60 YRS
Prenatal injury	Genetic predisposition	Brain tumors	Vascular disease
Perinatal injury	Infections	Trauma	Brain tumors, esp.
Metabolic defects	Trauma	Vascular disease	metastatic tumors
Congenital malformations	Congenital malformations	Infections	Trauma
CNS infections	Metabolic defects		Systemic metabolic
Postnatal-trauma			derangements
			Infections

73. What are the most common causes of seizures seen in the emergency room or on the medical ward?

Anticonvulsant withdrawal. Most patients seen here are known epileptics who have been taking medicine and, for one reason or another, are noncompliant with their drugs. Alcohol withdrawal, drug overdose, and metabolic derangements such as hyponatremia are other common causes. Structural brain disease, including stroke and meningitis, is a less common cause of seizures.

74. How do alcohol withdrawal seizures present?

These seizures generally occur 12–48 hours after cessation or abrupt reduction in the intake of alcohol. These seizures are always generalized tonic-clonic seizures, without locality. They are often single, isolated seizures, but sometimes patients may have two or more over a span of <6 hours. Status epilepticus is rare after alcohol withdrawal but does occasionally occur. Alcohol withdrawal seizures seldom persist and are self-limited.

75. What are the most important principles of seizure management?

Most seizures can be controlled completely, or nearly so, by following a few basic principles:

1. Pick the most appropriate anticonvulsant for the type of seizure the patient is experiencing.

2. Steadily increase the dose of that drug, guided by serum anticonvulsant levels, until seizures are controlled. If drug toxicity develops before the seizures stop, then the drug is not the appropriate one; try a different one. Obviously, increase the new anticonvulsant to therapeutic levels before tapering off the old drug

3. Monotherapy is preferable. Good therapeutic levels of one drug are preferable to subtherapeutic levels of multiple drugs.

76. Which drugs are the most useful anticonvulsants for the different types of seizures?

	PHENY-TOIN	CARBA-MAZEPINE	PHENOBAR-BITAL	ETHO-SUXIMIDE	VAL-PROATE	GABAPENTIN	LAMO-TRIGINE
Partial simple	+	+	+		+	+	
Partial complex	+	+	+			+	+
Generalized absence			+	+			
Generalized tonic-clonic	+	+	+		+		

Adapted from French J: The long-term therapeutic management of epilepsy. Ann Intern Med 120:411–422, 1994.

77. How is status epilepticus treated?

1. Rapid history and physical examination, including airway, breathing, circulation.

2. Start IV and draw blood for CBC, electrolytes, anticonvulsant levels. Administer thiamine and glucose.

3. Infuse phenytoin by slow IV push at 50 mg/min to a dose of ~20 mg/kg (1500 mg). To break a continuous seizure, give diazepam up to 20 mg or lorazepam up to 8 mg.

4. Infuse IV phenobarbital, 100 mg/min up to 600 mg.

5. Institute general anesthesia.

Experts disagree about when to intubate the patient. Some do it in step 2, others wait until step 4. You should always be prepared to immediately intubate any patient in status epilepticus.

Shepherd SM: Management of status epilepticus. Emerg Med Clin North Am 12:941–961, 1994.

MOVEMENT DISORDERS

78. List the four cardinal features of Parkinson's disease.

Cardinal Features of Parkinson's Disease

1. Tremor
2. Rigidity
3. Bradykinesia
4. Postural instability

Parkinson's disease is a gradual, progressive, degenerative disease of the basal ganglia (extrapyramidal) motor system. It is a very common condition, probably affecting 1% of people over age 60. The **tremor** is usually a to-and-fro, pronation-supination, resting tremor that diminishes with voluntary movement. It is coarse and slow and most prominent in the hands and head. Patients have **rigidity,** with a diffuse increase in muscular tone and sometimes a "cog-wheeling" property to their joints when passively moved. **Bradykinesia** refers to slowness of movement. The patients also have a paucity or lack of movement and tend to show minimal axial expression—they often sit quite immobile, almost like statues.

79. What is the differential diagnosis of Parkinson's disease?

A few conditions can cause parkinsonism, a symptom complex that mimics idiopathic Parkinson's disease. The most common causes are the neuroleptic drugs, including phenothiazines (such as chlorpromazine, thioridazine, etc.) and butyrophenones (such as haloperidol). Similar symptoms also can be mimicked by multiple strokes, hydrocephalus, and degenerative conditions such as Alzheimer's disease.

80. How is Parkinson's disease treated?

The best treatment is a combination of L-dopa plus carbidopa (Sinemet). The main cause for the symptoms of Parkinson's disease is a deficiency of dopamine within the pathway running from the substantia nigra to the basal ganglia. Since dopamine cannot be given directly (because it does not cross the blood–brain barrier), it is given as L-dopa. To prevent L-dopa from being decarboxylated and metabolized before it reaches the brain, carbidopa is given in combination.

Other dopamine agonists are sometimes used to supplement Sinemet. The main one is bromocriptine. Anticholinergic agents, which suppress the overactive cholinergic system and bring it into balance with the diminished dopamine system, can alleviate symptoms of Parkinson's disease. The most commonly used agents are trihexyphenidyl and benztropine.

Antioxidants, which may slow the rate of degeneration in the basal ganglia, are probably of some value in slowing the progression of Parkinson's disease. For this reason, MAO inhibitors such as deprenyl are commonly used.

Marsden CD: Parkinson's disease. J Neurol Neurosurg Psychiatry 57:672–681, 1994.

81. What are the other important types of tremors?

Parkinson's disease is a common form of **resting tremor** and can often be recognized by the accompanying rigidity and bradykinesia. Other important types of tremors include:

1. **Essential tremor.** This rapid, fine tremor involving the head and arms especially is pres-

ent at rest but becomes more noticeable with sustained postures or intentional movement. A family history, with an autosomal dominant inheritance, is seen in about half the cases. Treatment may include a β-blocker (propranolol, 80 mg/day) or primidone (starting at 250 mg/day).

2. **Cerebellar tremor.** Damage to the cerebellum disturbs motor control by causing a tremor. This is absent at rest and only appears with intentional or voluntary movements. It is a slow, coarse, dyssynergic tremor. Other evidence of cerebellar dysfunction may be present. Pharmacologic treatment is generally unsatisfactory.

Sandroni P, Young RR: Tremor: Classification, diagnosis and Management. Am Fam Physician 50:1505–1512, 1994.

82. What are dystonias?

Dystonias, as the name suggests, are disorders of muscle tone which result in involuntary, sustained muscle contractions. These can lead to abnormal posturing or unique repetitive movements. Examples include spasmodic torticollis, blepharospasm, and oromandibular dystonia.

83. How is botulinum toxin used in the treatment of dystonias?

Botulinum toxin type A (Botox), one of the most potent toxins found in the environment, has become the treatment of choice for focal dystonias such as blepharospasm and torticollis. Carefully localized intramuscular injections act to block the release of acetylcholine at the presynaptic membrane of the neuromuscular junction, thereby decreasing excessive muscle activity.

Treatment has been quite successful, with improvement noted in 70–90% of patients. The effects can last up to 4 months. Botulinum toxin has proven to be quite safe if administered properly, with temporary localized weakness as the only major side effect.

Hughes AJ: Botulinum toxin in clinical practice. Drugs 48:888–893, 1994.

HEADACHE

84. What are the key principles in evaluating headache?

1. The brain is anesthetic. This means that most causes of head pain do not arise from the brain itself but rather from surrounding structures, such as blood vessels, periosteum etc. Since most headaches are not caused by brain disease, most are benign.

2. The more severe the headache, the more benign the disease. The exception to this is intracranial hemorrhage, but in general, most severe headaches are due to self-limited causes.

3. Eye problems and sinus disease seldom cause headaches. Patients tend to blame their headaches on eye strain or sinusitis, but in fact these are rare etiologies.

85. What are the common types of headache?

1. Common migraine (without aura)
2. Classic migraine (with aura)
3. Tension headaches

Other less common or rare types of headaches include cluster headaches and headaches from brain tumor, meningeal irritation, and temporal arteritis.

86. Which serious diseases capable of causing permanent neurologic dysfunction can present as headaches?

Most processes causing headache are benign, but some are serious, as follows:

Serious Diseases That May Present as a Headache

1. Primary brain tumor	7. Meningitis
2. Metastatic brain tumor	8. Temporal arteritis
3. Abscess	9. Hypertension
4. Subdural hematoma	10. Hydrocephalus
5. Intracerebral hemorrhage	11. Glaucoma
6. Subarachnoid hemorrhage	

87. How can you tell if your headache is due to a brain tumor?

Brain tumors generally cause a mild-to-moderate headache, seldom severe, that is rather non-specific in its symptoms. It is dull, chronic, and throughout the whole head. Often, it is not localized to the region of the tumor. The headache is usually worse with maneuvers that cause the tumor to shift around, such as changes in position (e.g., getting out of bed, bending over). Valsalva maneuvers, which increase intracranial pressure, also worsen the headache. Most brain tumors produce abnormal findings on physical examination, such as altered mental status, papilledema, or focal weakness or numbness. A headache with a normal neurologic examination is unlikely to be a brain tumor.

88. What clinical features are seen with increased intracranial pressure (ICP)?

Because the brain is completely surrounded by the hard bony skull, any increase in ICP can impair brain function. The most sensitive indicator of increased ICP is an altered mental status, and it is usually the first symptom to change as the pressure rises. With increased pressure, the brain can herniate downward through the foramen magnum, compressing and destroying the brainstem. Herniation can be recognized by the development of brainstem signs as the top of the brainstem (midbrain) becomes impaired. In addition to altered mental status, these signs include dilatation of one or both pupils ("blown pupil"), hyperventilation, and focal neurologic signs such as hemiparesis. Herniation can progress to coma and death.

89. How can intracranial pressure be lowered?

Lowering ICP requires reduction of the intracranial contents to make room for the mass lesion and increased pressure. The intracranial contents consist essentially of the brain, cerebrospinal fluid (CSF) filling the ventricles, and blood within the blood vessels.

1. **Lowering blood pressure** lowers the ICP and can be accomplished with a diuretic such as furosemide. Osmotic diuresis is particularly effective, and therefore mannitol is the mainstay of therapy. It is given IV in a dose of 100 mg, followed, if necessary, by 50 mg boluses every 2 hours.

2. **Incubation and hyperventilation** cause vasospasm that reduces the blood volume intracranially. This temporarily lowers ICP, but because of compensatory re-equilibration, it provides only a few hours of relief.

3. **Steroids** can reduce swelling secondary to vasogenic edema, such as occurs with neoplasms, but they are not useful for edema that is cytotoxic, such as develops after a stroke or intracerebral hemorrhage. They may take hours or days to work and have little value acutely.

4. **Shuinting** can be used in emergency situations to remove CSF and so lower ICP.

90. How do subarachnoid and intracerebral hemorrhage differ in clinical presentation?

Intracranial hemorrhage causes the abrupt onset of an extremely severe headache. Patients report that it is "the worst headache in my life." The bleeding may result from the rupture of a vessel outside the brain (subarachnoid hemorrhage) or inside the brain (intracerebral hematoma).

Subarachnoid hemorrhage is usually due to the rupture of a small intracranial aneurysm, called a berry aneurysm, often located on the anterior communicating artery, middle cerebral artery, or their branches. Approximately half of the patients die at the time of the bleed. The remainder usually present to an emergency room with an altered mental status but may not have significant focal neurologic findings.

Intracerebral hemorrhage also causes collapse, coma, and death in a high percentage of patients, but since it occurs within the parenchyma of the brain, there are almost always focal neurologic findings, such as hemiparesis. Most patients also have altered mental status. It is strongly associated with hypertension.

91. What are the clinical features of headache due to meningitis?

The headache of meningitis, as in other severe illnesses, is often mild-to-moderate rather than extremely intense. It is a diffuse pain throughout the head, sometimes accompanied by photophobia, and shows signs of irritation of the brain and meninges, such as a stiff neck.

Meningitis is unlikely to be overlooked in the differential diagnosis of headache because of the accompanying signs of fever, elevated WBC count, and other evidence of infection. It usually presents as an infectious, toxic process rather than as a headache.

92. What is temporal arteritis?

Temporal arteritis is the confusing term used to describe a **giant cell arteritis** which may present as a headache. It is confusing because the process is not confined to the temporal arteries, but rather is a systemic illness with generalized symptoms such as fevers, myalgias, arthralgias (polymyalgia rheumatica), anemia, and elevated liver function tests. The headache is a mild-to-moderate diffuse pain, not necessarily confined to the temples or frontal region of the head. The disease should be suspected in elderly people, over age 55, who develop new headaches. The ESR is usually very elevated, >100 mm/min, and is a good screening test. The confirmatory test is a temporal artery biopsy showing granulomatous arteritis.

93. How do you treat temporal arteritis?

High-dose steroids for a period of 1–2 years are often required, sometimes in doses of 60 mg/day of prednisone equivalent or more. This is effective in controlling most symptoms of temporal arteritis, including the most tragic symptom, which is blindness from vasculitic involvement of the ophthalmic blood supply. Approximately 15% of these patients, if left untreated, develop significant visual loss.

MIGRAINE AND TENSION HEADACHE

94. At what age do migraine headaches have their onset?

Migraines typically begin in the teenage years, sometimes even in childhood, and diminish in both frequency and intensity of attacks in later adulthood. About half of all patients with migraine have a family history of the problem.

95. How frequently do migraine headaches occur?

Migraine headaches are paroxysmal, intermittent headaches occurring on an average of once a month and lasting from 4–12 hours or more. The frequency is highly variable, with some patients reporting 2–4 attacks a month and some 3–4 a year.

96. What are the common symptoms of migraines?

1. About one-third of patients have hemicranial pain, but in two-thirds the headache is diffuse over the entire head.

2. Some patients have a preceding aura for 20–40 minutes before the headache. This often consists of visual changes, such as flashing lights.

3. Gastrointestinal disturbances are very common, including nausea, vomiting, and anorexia. If you can eat during your headache, it is probably not migraine!

4. Photophobia and phonophobia

5. Mood changes

6. Visual or sensory loss

97. What triggers migraine headaches?

Many patients have triggering factors that set off their headaches. Hormonal triggers are common, and many women have headaches at the time of menstruation or ovulation. Alcohol, emotional stress, and some foods such as chocolate can also trigger headaches.

Some Precipitating Factors in Migraine Headaches

1. Head trauma	5. Diet: chocolate, alcohol, MSG
2. Psychological stress	6. Hormonal changes
3. Sleep	7. Physical exertion
4. Changes in weather (barometric pressure)	

98. Is the cause of migraine headaches known?

No. Probably low **serotonin** levels in the brain trigger brainstem neurons to fire, which alters cerebral blood flow. The neurologic deficits and the head pain result from low brain serotonin levels, aggravated by concomitant vascular changes.

99. What is the best treatment for a migraine headache?

For symptomatic relief from mild to moderate migraines, simple analgesics or NSAIDs such as aspirin or naproxen may be sufficient. For more severe attacks, the newer preparations of ergotamine or sumatriptan (Imitrex) are effective.

Sumatriptan, a 5-hydroxytryptamine receptor agonist, is the most effective antimigraine agent currently available, but patients should be warned of the flushing, sweating, and chest tightness that can occur within seconds after injection. These effects are transient and benign. The oral preparation, in doses of 25–50 mg, also provides good relief.

100. Which agents are useful as prophylactic therapies?

For patients having very frequent headaches (2–3/month or more) or for the occasional patient whose headache is complicated by persistent neurologic deficits, prophylactic treatment may be indicated. A variety of drugs from different classes are helpful:

1. **Amitriptyline,** a tricyclic compound. Doses of 100 mg/day or more may be necessary. Most other tricyclics are not effective.

2. **Propranolol,** a β-adrenergic blocking agent. Again, doses of 100 mg/day or more may be needed. Most other β-adrenergic blockers are not effective.

3. **Calcium channel blockers.** Both nifedipine and verapamil are useful.

Welch KMA: Drug therapy of migraine. N Engl J Med 329:1476–1483, 1993.

101. What are the clinical features of tension headaches?

Tension headaches are diffuse headaches, often described as a band around the head, usually bifrontal but sometimes occipital. Patients with chronic, persistent tension headaches report that the pain is very severe (though it seldom seems so to the physician). Unlike migraine, these headaches are usually not paroxysmal but are constant and chronic. Like migraine, they are more common in women and generally begin early in life. About half of the patients have a family history. Usually, there are no associated neurologic symptoms (such as visual changes) or nausea and vomiting.

Tension and migraine headaches commonly coexist in the same patient.

102. What causes tension headaches?

The cause is not known. There is no convincing evidence that they are due to psychological factors or emotional stress, nor are there good data showing they are related to muscle contraction.

103. How should tension headaches be treated?

Amitriptyline, up to 75–150 mg/day, works independently of its antidepressant effects. NSAIDs are useful for common headaches but are seldom successful in chronic persistent tension headache. Muscle relaxants also are not effective (not surprising, since muscle contraction is not the cause of the headache).

DEMENTIA

104. What is dementia?

Dementia is a progressive decline in cognitive and intellectual functions in the presence of a clear sensorium. Dementia implies that the person has lost intellectual function from a baseline state—i.e., he or she was not born mentally retarded (this is an acquired process) and is not delirious, lethargic, or otherwise suffering from an impaired level of consciousness.

105. What causes dementia?

Etiologies of Dementia

Senile dementia of Alzheimer's type	50–60%
Multi-infarct dementia (MID)	10–20%
Combination Alzheimer's and MID	10–20%
Other disorders	5–10%
Reversible or partially reversible	20–30%

Other causes of dementia include neurosyphilis, hypothyroidism, HIV infection, neoplasm, subdural hematoma, and head trauma. The old belief that generalized atherosclerosis and global reduction in blood flow can cause dementia has proven correct in only rare cases. Cerebrovascular disease essentially does not cause dementia except by actual destruction (infarction) of brain tissue, as in MID.

Winograd CH, et al: Physician management of the demented patient. J Am Geriatr Soc 34:295–308, 1986.

106. What is the diagnostic approach to the patient with dementia?

Most dementias, such as Alzheimer's disease, have no effective treatment, so the evaluation of any patient presenting with dementia generally focuses on finding the treatable causes, even though these are uncommon.

Reversible Causes of Dementia

D—Drugs
E—Emotional disorders (pseudodementia or depression)
M—Metabolic and endocrine disorders (hepatic encephaolpthy, hypothyroidism, chronic renal failure)
E—Eye and ear dysfunction
N—Nutritional deficiencies, normal pressure hydrocephalus (NPH)
T—Tumor, trauma (including chronic subdural hematoma)
I—Infections (neurosyphilis, chronic meningitis)
A—Alcohol, arteriosclerotic complications

Screening for Reversible Dementias, in Addition to History and Physical Examination

Thyroid function tests	Vitamin B_{12} level
Serum chemistries (including CA^{2+})	Head CT or MRI
Examination of CSF for possible NPH	Syphilis serology
or if RPR positive or if cranial nerve abnor-	CBC
malities are present (consistent with meningitis)	Serum folate level

A workup includes CT scan or MRI to image the brain, an EEG to show metabolic encephalopathies, (diffuse slowing) or some specific dementias (e.g., periodic sharp waves seen in Creutzfeldt-Jakob disease), and sometimes lumbar puncture to rule out neurosyphilis, cryptococcal meningitis, or other chronic infections. Blood studies detect most other causes of dementia, such as hypothyroidism, B_{12} deficiency, and vasculitis.

Morris JC: Differential diagnosis of Alzheimer's Disease. Clin Geriatr Med 10(2):257–276, 1994.

107. What is Alzheimer's disease?

Alzheimer's disease is a degenerative dementing process of unknown etiology. Most elderly patients who were once termed "senile" probably had Alzheimer's disease, which is now felt to be a specific, distinct disease entity rather than the mere loss of intellectual function with normal aging.

Pathologically, Alzheimer's disease is characterized by degenerative changes in the brain, especially senile plaques, neurofibrillary tangles, and granulovacuolar degeneration. These degenerative changes are seen in great concentration in the hippocampus.

108. How is Alzheimer's disease diagnosed?

There is no biological marker or specific test for Alzheimer's disease, so the clinical diagnosis is largely one of exclusion. The criteria for the diagnosis of Alzheimer's disease, short of a brain biopsy, are summarized below:

Clinical Diagnosis of Alzheimer's Disease

1. Proof of dementia by neuropsychologic testing
2. Deficits in 2 or more areas of cognition (i.e., not just memory loss)
3. Progressive worsening
4. No disturbance of consciousness
5. Onset between ages 40–90 (usually after age 65)
6. Absence of other causes of dementia

109. Is there any treatment for Alzheimer's disease?

Tacrine recently became the first drug accepted for use in the treatment of Alzheimer's disease. While it does not seem to alter the course of the underlying disease, tacrine was shown to slow the rate of cognitive decline when compared with placebo in multiple clinical trials. Tacrine therapy carries with it a risk of hepatotoxicity, with significant (albeit temporary) elevations of serum enzymes in half of patients receiving the drug.

Davis KL, Powchik P: Tacrine. Lancet 345:625–630, 1995.

MULTIPLE SCLEROSIS

110. What is multiple sclerosis (MS)?

MS is the most common disabling neurologic disease of young people under age 40, affecting approx. 250,000 Americans. It is probably an autoimmune disease, characterized by relapsing and remitting episodes of inflammation in the brain and spinal cord. This inflammation destroys the myelin, which is the insulating sheath around nerve cells, and hence destroys the ability of the nerves to conduct electrical impulses (action potentials).

111. What are the clinical symptoms of MS?

Clinically, MS may affect almost any part of the brain or spinal cord. Generally, symptoms come on fairly abruptly, over a period of hours to days, persist for several weeks, and then resolve over a period of several more weeks, often returning completely to normal. On average, patients have one attack per year, although about 20% of patients have a chronic progressive course with steady worsening deficit, without abrupt attacks.

The highly variable presentation of MS reflects the fact that it may involve the optic nerves, spinal cord, pyramidal tracts, spinothalamic tracts, brainstem, or cerebellum. Common symptoms include:

Most Common Symptoms of Multiple Sclerosis

Focal weakness	45%	Cerebellar ataxia	30%
Optic neuritis	40%	Diplopia and nystagmus	25%
Focal numbness	35%	Bowel and bladder changes	20%

112. How is the diagnosis of MS made?

Schumacher Criteria for Definite Multiple Sclerosis

1. Two separate CNS lesions	4. Objective deficits on examination
2. Two separate attacks of symptoms	5. Age 10–50 years (usually 20–40)
3. Symptoms must be consistent with a white matter (myelin) lesion	6. No other disease to explain symptoms

The diagnosis of MS is often difficult given the great variability in signs and symptoms. Generally, young people who have had two separate lesions in the CNS at two separate times have a strong likelihood of having MS.

113. Does laboratory testing or imaging have any role in diagnosing MS?

Although the Schumacher criteria are quite accurate, it is not possible to use them to diagnose MS when the first symptom appears. A definitive diagnosis requires two separate symptoms. For this reason, patients suspected of having MS often undergo further testing to provide some laboratory confirmation of the diagnosis.

- **MRI** of the head is very sensitive for showing the white matter lesions of MS, but not very specific.
- Spinal fluid usually shows immunologic abnormalities, specifically the presence of multiple polyclonal concentrations of IgG.
- Evoked potentials is a technique in which visual, auditory, or electrical stimulation is flashed to the brain, whose reactions are recorded using electrodes, similar to an EEG. A delay in the impulses evoked by the stimuli often indicates an underlying lesion in patients with MS.

114. How are the symptoms of MS best managed?

Because the cause of MS is not known, there is no cure. Steroids often help alleviate attacks by reducing inflammation. However, they do not appear to alter the natural history of the disease.

Symptomatic management consists of medications to improve spasticity (such as baclofen), management of the neurogenic bladder, and braces or other aids to ambulation.

115. Can any treatments alter the natural course of MS?

While a cure for MS remains elusive, two novel therapies may actually alter the natural course of MS. Both β-**Interferon** and **copolymer-1** decrease the number of yearly relapses in patients with MS, as demonstrated in large clinical trials. The drugs seem equally effective, cutting attacks by approx. one-third. Both medications are given subcutaneously. Major side effects of β-interferon include flu-like symptoms, depression, and leukopenia. Copolymer-1 has relatively few side effects, mild injection site inflammation being the only one of note.

Despite their apparent benefit in decreasing relapses of MS, neither drug has been shown to affect patients with chronic progressive MS, nor to clearly prevent disability.

Johnson KP, et al: Copolymer-1 reduces relapse rate and improves disability in relapsing-remitting MS. Neurology 95:1268–1275, 1995.

The IFNB MS Study Group: IFNB-1b in the treatment of MS. Neurology 95:1277–1285, 1995.

116. How long do patients survive after the onset of MS?

Most patients live 40 years or longer. MS may be disabling but is seldom fatal.

COMA

117. What are the most common causes of coma?

1. Drugs (including alcohol, illicit drugs, accidental or intentional overdose, etc.)
2. Hypoxia
3. Hypoglycemia
4. Other metabolic derangements (sepsis, uremia, hepatic failure, etc.)
5. Structural brain disease (stroke, intracranial hemorrhage, etc.)

Most etiologies of coma are medical problems, not primary neurologic diseases.

118. What is the approach to the patient in coma?

1. ABCs—protect the airway, breathing, and circulation.
2. Draw blood to check for metabolic derangements, infection, and drugs.
3. Infuse glucose, thiamine, and naloxone.

4. History and physical exam for clues to the cause of coma. Focus on pupils and extraocular movements for evidence of brainstem dysfunction.

5. Definitive diagnosis (and therapy) may require CT scanning, lumbar puncture, EEG, and other studies depending on the situation.

119. What is the prognosis of coma?

Almost 70% of patients admitted to a hospital in coma die. Brainstem abnormalities—absent extraocular movements, gag reflex, or spontaneous respirations, or unreactive pupils—carry an especially grim prognosis.

Hamel MB, et al: Identification of comatose patients at high risk for death or severe disability. JAMA 273:1842–1848, 1995.

OTHER MEDICAL CONDITIONS

120. How does alcohol affect the nervous system?

Alcohol can affect virtually any part of the nervous system:

- Alcoholic myopathy—occurs in heavy drinkers in a fashion analogous to alcoholic cardiomyopathy.
- Acute rhabdomyolysis—rare, associated with heavy alcohol consumption.
- Peripheral neuropathy—usually a distal, symmetric, stocking-and-glove sensory and motor polyneuropathy.
- Nerve compression—increased susceptibility in alcoholics (e.g., "Saturday night" palsy)
- Fulminant necrotic myelopathy—rare, associated with heavy alcoholic intake.
- Wernicke's encephalopathy—due to thiamine deficiency secondary to alcoholism
- Cerebellar ataxia—alcohol leads to degeneration of the anterior (dermis) region of the cerebellum, causing a very ataxic gait.
- Alcoholic dementia—amnesia (Korsakoff's syndrome) and generalized dementia.

Diamond I, Messing RO: Neurologic effects of alcoholism. West J Med 161:279–287, 1994.

121. What triad of findings is seen in Wiernicke's encephalopathy?

Alcohol can affect the brainstem in the classic Wernicke's encephalopathy, which causes a triad of:

(1) Nystagmus with extraocular abnormalities

(2) Cerebellar ataxia

(3) Confusion

Wernicke's is really due to a thiamine deficiency rather than to alcohol ingestion itself. The brainstem signs reverse readily with parenteral thiamine infusion, but the confusion resolves more slowly.

122. Does HIV affect the nervous system?

HIV can cause widespread damage in the nervous system, probably entering through macrophages that cross the blood-brain barrier. Approx. 10% of all AIDS patients present initially with neurologic symptoms, and up to 50% develop neurologic complications at some point during their illness.

- Inflammatory myopathy—similar to polymyositis, with symptoms of slowly progressive proximal weakness. Zidovudine may also cause a similar reversible myopathy.
- Peripheral neuropathy—distal symmetric (glove and stocking) pattern, with distal burning and other dysesthesias, seen in approx. 30% of patients.
- Acute inflammatory demyelinating polyneuropathy—like Guillain-Barré syndrome but with CSF pleocytosis.
- AIDS myelopathy—vacuolar degeneration resembling B_{12} deficiency, a chronic progressive spinal cord syndrome.
- HIV encephalopathy—progressive dementia manifested by apathy, personality change, and/or loss of higher cognitive functions.
- Aseptic meningitis—due to HIV itself

Newton HB: Common neurologic complications of HIV-1 infection and AIDS. Am Fam Physician 51:387–398, 1995.

123. What two conditions should be suspected when a CT scan reveals CNS mass lesions in a patient with AIDS?

Cerebral toxoplasmosis and primary CNS lymphoma.

124. What are the effects of diabetes mellitus (DM) on the peripheral nervous system?

The primary effect of DM on the nervous system is on the peripheral nerves. The most frequent problem is a distal, symmetric, stocking-and-glove sensory and motor **polyneuropathy.** This usually begins in the feet, generally with numbness, and then ascends to the hands. Often, there are burning, painful paresthesias. In severe cases, proprioceptive loss may be sufficiently significant to cause Charcot joints. A motor neuropathy frequently accompanies the sensory changes.

Mononeuropathy can occur because the small vessel disease that accompanies DM frequently leads to infarction of nerves by occlusion of the vasa nervorum. Femoral neuropathies and cranial nerve palsies are particularly common. Another type of neuropathy is thoracoabdominal neuropathy, in which a thoracic root is damaged, again possibly by infarction, leading to severe chest or abdominal pain that is often mistaken for a visceral crisis.

Finally, the autonomic peripheral nervous system may be affected, leading to impotence, bowel and bladder dysfunction, gastroparesis, orthostatic hypotension, or arrhythmias.

125. In what ways does diabetes affect the CNS?

Involvement of the CNS by diabetes is more indirect than its effects on the peripheral nerves. Because diabetes is a risk factor for **atherosclerosis,** there is an increased incidence of stroke. **Hypoglycemia** from overmedication can lead to focal neurologic findings, such as hemiparesis or aphasia, or, if severe, altered mental status including coma. **Hyperglycemia,** from diabetic ketoacidosis or from nonketotic hyperosmolar states, also causes altered mental status, sometimes accompanied by seizures.

126. How does renal failure affect the nervous system?

1. Uremia is one of the most common metabolic abnormalities affecting the nervous system, especially the peripheral nerves, where there is a stocking and-glove distal, symmetric, **sensorimotor neuropathy.**

2. Patients with renal failure are prone to **metabolic encephalopathies** causing confusion, lethargy, and even coma. This may be aggravated by fluid and electrolyte shifts during dialysis.

3. Because of the anticoagulation necessary for dialysis, there is an increased incidence of **intracerebral hemorrhage,** such as subdural hematomas.

4. A special type of mental status change is the syndrome of **dialysis encephalopathy,** which is a progressive deterioration in mental status, with hyperreflexia and dysarthria, usually accompanied by myoclonus and seizures. This syndrome is often irreversible and progressive until death.

Fraser CL, Arieff Al: Nervous system complications in uremia. Ann Intern Med 109:143–153, 1988.

127. How does metastatic cancer present in the nervous system?

Cancer affects the nervous system primarily by direct invasion. Metastases to the brain occur in 10–30% of patients with primary neoplasms, most commonly in lung and colon cancer in males and breast cancer in females. Metastatic cancer usually presents as a focal neurologic deficit, such as hemiparesis, but may also cause seizures. As the tumor enlarges, it produces increased ICP, leading to headache, altered mental status, and ultimately herniation and death.

Cancer may metastasize or spread locally to the spinal cord, leading to acute spinal cord compression. Usually, this is accompanied by back pain from vertebral body destruction. The onset of symptoms may be sudden with paraparesis, a sensory level, and bowel and bladder disturbances.

128. What other effects of cancer may be seen?

Carcinomatous meningitis is most common in lymphomas and leukemias, but can be seen with solid tumors as well. Usually this presents as altered mental status, sometimes with fever, and sometimes with focal neurologic deficits as the cancer invades cranial nerves and roots as they emerge from the CNS.

Involvement of the peripheral nervous system by direct extension is sometimes seen, such as when a Pancoast tumor invades the brachial plexus. Peripheral neuropathies are uncommon.

Paraneoplastic syndromes, or remote effects of cancer, are quite rare. They may include myopathy (polymyositis), neuromuscular junction deficit (Lambert-Eaton myasthenic syndrome), and a peripheral neuropathy, predominantly sensory.

There is also a condition of diffuse cerebellar ataxia, likely caused by circulating immunologic proteins or antibodies which cross-react with neurologic tissues.

BIBLIOGRAPHY

1. Adams RD, Victor M: Principles of Neurology, 6th ed. New York, McGraw-Hill, 1997.
2. Aminoff M: Neurology and General Medicine, 2nd ed. New York, Churchill-Livingstone, 1995.
3. Asbury AK, Thomas PK: Peripheral Nerve Disorders, 2nd ed. New York, Butterworth-Heinemann, 1995.
4. Caplan LR: Stroke: A Clinical Approach. New York, Butterworth-Heinemann, 1993.
5. Feldmann E: Current Diagnosis in Neurology. St. Louis, Mosby, 1994.
6. Johnson RT, Griffin JW: Current Therapy in Neurologic Disease, 5th ed. St. Louis, Mosby, 1997.
7. Matthews WB (ed): McAlpine's Multiple Sclerosis, 2nd ed. New York, Churchill Livingstone, 1991.
8. Plum F, Posner JB: The Diagnosis of Stupor and Coma, 3rd ed. Philadelphia, F.A. Davis, 1982.
9. Rolak LA: Neurology Secrets. Philadelphia, Hanley & Belfus, 1993.
10. Wyllie E: The Treatment of Epilepsy: Principles and Practice. Philadelphia, Lea & Febiger, 1993.

15. MEDICAL CONSULTATION

Carol M. Ashton, M.D., M.P.H., and Nelda P. Wray, M.D., M.P.H.

Physicians who meet in consultation must never quarrel or jeer at one another.

Hippocrates
Precepts VIII

Whenever he (Thomas Jefferson) saw three physicians together, he looked up to discover whether there was not a turkey buzzard in the neighborhood.

Quoted by Dr. Everett, private secretary to James Monroe

GENERAL PERIOPERATIVE EVALUATION AND CARE

1. What hemodynamic changes occur with spinal anesthesia?

Spinal anesthesia, the injection of local anesthetic into the subarachnoid space, blocks transmission of the impulses from the sympathetic nervous system as well as those mediating motor and sensory functions. The sympathetic nervous system controls the caliber of the blood vessels. At basal levels of sympathetic tone, the vessels are maintained at about half their maximum diameter. Sympathetic stimulation causes vasoconstriction, whereas sympathetic enervation, as in spinal anesthesia, causes vasodilatation. The vasodilatation causes a drop in systemic vascular resistance and consequent pooling of blood in the lower extremities. Arterial blood pressure usually decreases with administration of spinal anesthesia, and the drop is more severe in patients who are volume-depleted prior to the anesthetic. Patients with hypertension (whether controlled or not) also have a tendency to have exaggerated hypotensive responses to spinal anesthesia.

2. What are the four most common causes of hypertension in recovery room patients?

Pain, a full bladder, hypothermia with shivering and vasoconstriction, and hypercarbia. Resolving these problems almost always reduces the arterial pressure without the need for specific antihypertensive therapy.

3. Describe the correct approach to evaluating hypertension in the recovery room.

The first task is to verify the accuracy of the blood pressure (BP) measurement, and the second is to assess the immediacy and severity of the situation. This is done by ascertaining whether the elevated BP is causing or worsening acute organ dysfunction. A useful approach is to categorize the situation as:

1. **Hypertensive emergency**—BP should be lowered within the hour
2. **Hypertensive urgency**—BP should be controlled within 24 hours
3. **Simple hypertension**—there is no immediacy to lowering BP.

A hypertensive emergency is defined by markedly elevated BP and cerebral dysfunction (malignant hypertension or encephalopathy) or an acute intracranial event, myocardial ischemia, aortic dissection, acute pulmonary edema, pheochromocytoma crisis, or postoperative bleeding. Hypertensive urgencies include markedly elevated BP in conjunction with retinal hemorrhages and exudates (but no papilledema), congestive heart failure, stable angina, transient ischemic attacks, and renal insufficiency. In simple hypertension, the BP may be quite elevated but there is no acute or worsening chronic organ dysfunction.

Reeler JB, Magarian GJ: Hypertensive emergencies and urgencies: Definition, recognition, and management. J Gen Intern Med 3:64–74, 1988.

4. Intraoperative hemodynamic monitoring using a pulmonary artery catheter is often contemplated in the high-risk surgical patient. What are the potential benefits of such monitoring?

The hemodynamic parameters directly measurable using a pulmonary artery catheter include pulmonary artery systolic, diastolic, and wedge pressures, as well as right atrial or central venous pressure. The mixed venous oxygen content, a measure of the adequacy of peripheral perfusion and tissue oxygenation, can be measured from blood obtained via the catheter. Indirect measurement of cardiac output can be performed, and several other parameters such as systemic vascular resistance can be calculated.

By far, the most clinically relevant use of the pulmonary artery catheter in the perioperative period is the management of intravascular volume. The pulmonary capillary wedge pressure (PCWP) (and also pulmonary artery diastolic pressure) is an indicator of left ventricular (LV) filling pressure (preload); it should be interpreted and manipulated in light of simultaneous measures of cardiac output. Intraoperative hemodynamic monitoring using a pulmonary artery catheter has not yet been proven to reduce perioperative complications in patients undergoing noncardiac surgery. The pulmonary artery catheter is probably a more important tool in the early postoperative period than the intraoperative period.

Sola JE, Bender JS: Use of the pulmonary artery catheter to reduce operative complications. Surg Clin North Am 73:253–263, 1993.

5. What are the risks of hemodynamic monitoring via a pulmonary artery catheter?

Complications associated with catheter insertion include pneumothorax, accidental arterial puncture, and ventricular ectopy and dysrhythmias. Dysrhythmias are a common occurrence but, in most cases, are self-limited or at least nonfatal. However, insertion of a catheter through the right heart in the patient with a left bundle branch block may interrupt right bundle branch conduction, leading to complete AV block.

Complications that occur while the catheter is in place include pulmonary infarction and perforation or rupture of the pulmonary artery. The latter is a rare complication but almost always fatal. Catheter-related sepsis and venous thrombosis are complications usually associated with longer-term (days rather than hours) catheterization.

Matthay MA, Chatterjee K: Bedside catheterization of the pulmonary artery: Risks compared with benefits. Ann Intern Med 109:826–834, 1988.

6. What are the general principles governing the use of perioperative antibiotics for prophylaxis of infection in "clean" surgical procedures?

Clean procedures are those that do not cross a mucous membrane or involve a break in surgical technique. Generally, prophylactic antibiotics are not given for clean procedures unless the operation involves the insertion of some prosthetic material, such as a cardiac valve or artificial joint. In those cases, the drastic consequences of an infection make the use of antibiotics worthwhile, even though the risk is very low. Evidence suggests that prophylactic antibiotics may be cost-effective in some clean procedures not involving prostheses.

Clean-contaminated procedures are those that cross a mucous membrane such as the urinary tract but do not involve a break in surgical technique. Prophylactic antibiotics reduce endogenous flora and are effective in reducing the rate of postoperative infections. **Contaminated procedures**—those involving traumatic wounds, spillage of GI tract contents, or breaks in surgical technique—have a higher rate of infection, and antibiotics are effective in reducing subsequent infection. The timing of perioperative antibiotics is an important factor in their efficacy.

7. When should preoperative antibiotics be initiated in "dirty" surgical procedures?

Dirty cases, those involving pus or old traumatic wounds, have the highest rate of surgical infection, and antibiotics are always indicated. Because the goal is to attain antimicrobial levels in the tissues by the time bacteria are likely to seed the wound or bloodstream, antibiotics should be given not more than 2 hours before the procedure. Often they are administered with the preoperative sedatives. In general, the duration of therapy need not be longer than 24 hours, and in many cases one preoperative dose will do.

Classen DC, et al: The timing of prophylactic administration of antibiotics and the risk of surgical wound infection. N Engl J Med 325:281–286, 1992.

8. Discuss the pros and cons of substituting spinal anesthesia for general endotracheal anesthesia in patients with lung disease.

Pros: Endotracheal intubation breaches the mechanical barriers to lower respiratory tract infection, which is of special concern in the patient with chronic lung disease, whose defenses are already impaired and in whom respiratory infection carries a high mortality. Intubation is also associated with increased bronchial secretions, which may be difficult for the chronic lung patient to clear, and may cause bronchospasm in the patient with reactive airways. However, these risks are more than balanced by the fact that intubation and mechanical ventilation allow a measure of control over alveolar ventilation and gas exchange that is not possible in the nonintubated patient.

Cons: Spinal anesthesia may cause serious respiratory compromise in the chronic lung patient, depending on the level of the spinal cord to which anesthesia extends. Expiration is a passive process during quiet breathing in normal persons, but in patients with obstructive lung disease, expiration is an active process, requiring muscular effort. The most important expiratory muscles are those of the abdominal wall (rectus, internal and external oblique, and transverse) and the internal intercostal. These are innervated by the thoracic nerves (T1–L1). The most important muscle of inspiration is the diaphragm. Because this muscle is innervated by the phrenic nerve (C3,4,5), it is very unusual for the diaphragm to be paralyzed by spinal anesthesia. However, during abdominal surgery retractors and packs may interfere with diaphragmatic excursion and compromise the patient with limited respiratory reserve.

9. What are the metabolic-hormonal responses to major surgery?

The most important metabolic-hormonal response to surgery is the **stress response.** Although anesthesia prevents conscious perception of bodily injury, the body responds to major surgery as it does to any other noxious stimulus, with an outpouring of catecholamines and cortisol. In addition to their multiple hemodynamic effects, the catecholamines epinephrine and norepinephrine stimulate the pituitary gland to produce ACTH. ACTH stimulates the adrenal gland to secrete glucocorticoids (e.g., cortisol) and mineralocorticoids (e.g., aldosterone). Glucocorticoids promote gluconeogenesis by a variety of mechanisms, most of which are catabolic. Postoperative hyperglycemia, seen even in nondiabetics, often results. Aldosterone acts on renal tubular cells to increase the conservation of sodium (potassium is excreted in exchange). The net effect is to increase the extracellular fluid volume, and ultimately, intravascular volume. Surgical trauma and postoperative pain also may increase the secretion of antidiuretic hormone (ADH) (arginine vasopressin), which decreases free-water excretion by the kidneys.

These mechanisms are all devoted to protecting the organism, but at times they overshoot. Starvation, water deprivation, pain, infection, hemorrhage, and drugs often exaggerate their effects. It has been demonstrated that epidural anesthesia is associated with a muted neural-hormonal-metabolic stress response compared with general anesthesia.

10. Shifts in blood pressure are most common at what times during the intraoperative course of the patient undergoing general endotracheal anesthesia?

Induction of anesthesia is almost always accompanied by a drop in the mean arterial BP. The drop can be quite marked in hypertensives (whether or not they are well-controlled preoperatively) and in patients with volume depletion. Laryngoscopy and tracheal intubation are often associated with tachycardia and hypertension. BP usually levels out during the procedure.

11. In the patient on long-term antianginal or antihypertensive therapy, how should the medications be handled perioperatively?

Antihypertensive and antianginal agents should be continued up until the day of surgery. On the morning of surgery, they should be administered with a sip of water. The patient should resume a normal schedule as soon as possible postoperatively.

One occasional exception to this practice is the patient on chronic diuretic therapy for hypertension. Rarely, such a patient is truly volume-depleted as a result of this therapy. Volume status can be assessed by determining whether postural changes occur in the BP and heart rate. If the patient is volume-depleted, diuretics should be withheld and the intravascular volume restored prior to surgery.

12. In which surgical populations is it *not* cost-effective to obtain a preoperative screening ECG? A screening chest radiograph? Screening coagulation studies?

A "screening" test is a test performed on a person who has no clinical evidence of the disease in question. Because of sensitivity and specificity issues, not all tests are good screening tests. Furthermore, screening is justifiable only for certain diseases.

Routine preoperative screening ECGs, chest radiographs, and coagulation studies have been shown to be *not* cost-effective because the prevalence of clinically silent but perioperatively important heart, lung, and coagulation disorders is low in asymptomatic patients. In situations in which the prevalence of these conditions is higher, or there is some indication from history or examination that disease may be present, preoperative tests may be justified. Some believe that all patients over age 45 should have an ECG and chest radiograph before elective surgery. Others obtain those tests only in patients suspected of having heart or lung disease.

It is a common practice to obtain routine preoperative screening coagulation studies, but no studies have shown this to be cost-effective or beneficial. It is recommended that coagulation studies for elective surgery be reserved for patients with a personal or family history of coagulopathy or liver disease. In some patients, preoperative testing can be reduced by using the results of previous tests, provided results were normal and no indication for retesting is present.

MacPherson DS, Snow R, Lofgren RP: Preoperative screening: value of previous tests. Ann Intern Med 113:969–973, 1990.

13. When should total parenteral nutrition (TPN) be used in surgical patients?

The hypermetabolic, catabolic state induced by major surgery is compounded by a state of relative starvation in the perioperative period. Though this presents little problem to the well-nourished individual, the incidence of postoperative complications is highly correlated with the severity of malnutrition in less robust patients.

Because of its significant risks and costs, TPN should not be used indiscriminately in surgical patients. Three groups of high-risk patients almost always benefit from perioperative parenteral nutrition:

(1) Severely malnourished patients undergoing major intrathoracic or intra-abdominal surgery

(2) Moderately malnourished or previously well-nourished patients having procedures that result in prolonged (>1 wk) periods of inadequate intake (e.g., pancreaticoduodenectomy)

(3) Previously well-nourished patients who develop postoperative complications likely to result in a prolonged period of inadequate oral intake.

American College of Physicians: Perioperative parenteral nutrition. Ann Intern Med 107:252–253, 1987.

14. Induction, maintenance, and reversal are the three phases of general anesthesia. What is induction and what are some of the problems that may occur at induction?

Induction of anesthesia consists of administering medication to the conscious, perceiving patient in order to produce a state of unconsciousness and lack of perception. Though inhalational agents can be used to induce anesthesia, in current practice induction is usually accomplished by the intravenous (IV) route. Though it is advisable to intubate some patients before induction of anesthesia, endotracheal intubation is usually carried out immediately after induction. Problems that may occur include retching, vomiting, aspiration, cough, laryngospasm, hypotension, and cardiac dysrhythmias.

15. What is regional anesthesia?

Any anesthesia that is not general is regional. This includes spinal anesthesia (injection of anesthetic into the subarachnoid space), epidural anesthesia, peridural and caudal nerve blocks, regional nerve blocks (e.g., brachial plexus block), and local anesthesia. In many cases there are significant advantages to using regional anesthesia instead of general. However, regional anesthesia demands more technical skill from the anesthetist, modified behavior in the operating room by all members of the surgical team, and considerable psychologic support of the patient during the operation.

SURGERY AND HEART DISEASE

16. What are the components of Goldman's cardiac risk index? How do the levels of risk as determined by the index correlate with the likelihood of cardiac complications?

Goldman found that nine factors affect the likelihood of a cardiac complication with noncardiac surgery:

Computation of Cardiac Risk Index

FACTOR	POINTS
1. Age >70 yrs	5
2. Myocardial infarction (MI) in prior 6 mos	10
3. S_3 gallop	11
4. Important valvular aortic stenosis	3
5. Cardiac rhythm other than sinus, or PACs on last preoperative ECG	7
6. >5 PVCs/minute documented at any time prior to operation	7
7. Poor general medical status (PaO_2 < 60 or $PaCO_2$ > 50 mm Hg, K^+ < 3.0 or HCO_3^- < 20 meq/1, BUN >50 or Cr >3.0 mg/dl, abnormal AST, signs of chronic liver disease, or patient bedridden from noncardiac causes)	3
8. Intraperitoneal, intrathoracic, or aortic operation	3
9. Emergency operation	4
Total possible	53 points

PAC = premature atrial contraction; PVC = premature ventricular contraction.

The risk of a life-threatening cardiac complication (MI, pulmonary edema, or ventricular tachycardia) increased with the number of points:

<5 points = Negligible risk

6–12 points = 5% risk

13–25 points = 11% risk

≥26 points = 22% risk

This index is now 20 years old, however, and the predictive accuracy of scores in present-day practice is unknown. The best use of the index is as a list of factors to look for during the preoperative evaluation. If possible, it is advisable to delay the surgical procedure to correct whatever modifiable problems the patient has.

Goldman L, et al: Multifactorial index of cardiac risk in noncardiac surgical procedures. N Engl J Med 297:845–850, 1977.

17. What are the important issues relating to the perioperative care of the patient with a permanent cardiac pacemaker?

Two issues must be addressed: the cardiac status of the patient, including an assessment of adequacy of pacemaker function, and safety in the operating room. In general, the adequately functioning pacemaker (1) senses the patient's own intracardiac signals and (2) delivers an electric stimulus to depolarize the myocardium at a time when it is excitable and at an appropriate rate. Pacemaker function should be assessed sometime during the month before elective surgery at the patient's usual source of pacemaker care.

In the OR, electromagnetic interference (usually from the electrocautery) may cause the demand pacemaker to fail to pace. This problem can be solved by converting the pacemaker from a demand mode to a fixed-rate mode by placing a high-powered magnet over the generator. The possibility of electromagnetic interference can be minimized by placing the ground plate as far from the generator as possible and by using the electrocautery in short bursts. In the patient with a temporary pacemaker, the pacemaker leads provide a direct pathway by which extraneous external electrical impulses can go directly to the heart. The contact points between the leads and the generator should be covered with a surgical glove, and gloves should be worn when handling the unit.

18. What common postoperative dysrhythmia typically presents with a heart rate of 150?

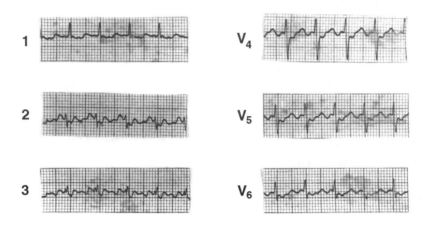

Atrial flutter, a supraventricular tachycardia, is one of the most common dysrhythmias observed in the postoperative period. It may occur in persons with or without heart disease. In atrial flutter, the atrial rate is about 300 bpm. Atrial flutter with a 2:1 conduction ratio should be suspected in the patient with a supraventricular dysrhythmia who has a heart rate of 150 bpm.

19. Hemodynamically, why do general anesthesia and surgery carry a higher risk for perioperative cardiac complications in the patient who has asymptomatic but significant aortic stenosis (AS)?

The stenotic aortic valve presents a fixed obstruction to the outflow of blood from the left ventricle (LV). In other words, the stenotic orifice limits the maximum cardiac output (CO) that can be achieved. In early AS, CO is maintained and the pressure gradient across the stenotic valve during systole increases with increased flow (i.e., increased CO). As the valve orifice decreases in diameter, the LV hypertrophies in response to the chronic pressure overload. As outflow obstruction worsens, though CO is normal at rest, there is an inability to increase it appropriately with exercise.

In normal individuals, when tissue demands for oxygen go up (such as with exercise), CO is increased by three mechanisms: (1) arterial dilatation with a drop in LV afterload; (2) enhanced myocardial contractility; and (3) a drop in venous capacitance with increased return to the heart and thus increased preload. In patients with moderately severe AS, arterial dilatation has little effect on improving CO, because the stenotic valve remains the major obstruction to outflow. Because such patients do not have an appropriate response to peripheral dilatation, they are prone to have hypotension with exercise or any other situation in which peripheral dilatation is induced (e.g., anesthesia). Furthermore, because of LV hypertrophy these patients have stiff ventricles, such that for any given intracavitary volume the pressure is higher than normal. When cardiac return is increased in an effort to augment CO, there is the potential for rapid rises in filling pressures and resultant pulmonary edema.

As would be expected in this pathophysiologic state, at the time of surgery, persons with AS are at risk for hypotension, pulmonary edema, and MI. Ischemia can develop in the patient with AS for several reasons. First, atherosclerotic coronary disease frequently coexists with AS. In addition, the pathophysiologic features of AS also affect myocardial O_2 balance unfavorably. Myocardial hypertrophy is associated with an increase in myocardial O_2 demand, and decreases in aortic pressure, especially during diastole, lead to decreases in myocardial O_2 delivery.

20. What is the risk of reinfarction with noncardiac surgery after myocardial infarction (MI)?

In general, the more recent the MI, the higher the chance of reinfarction with noncardiac surgery. In the 1970s, it was shown that patients operated on within 3 months of an MI had a reinfarction rate as high as 25%. The rate stabilized at 3–5% after 6 months. In more recent studies, reinfarction rates appear to be lower. At some centers, it is now the practice to defer elective surgery for 3 rather than 6 months after acute MI. The safety of this approach has not been formally evaluated.

Steen PA, et al: Myocardial reinfarction after anesthesia and surgery. JAMA 239:2566–2570, 1978.

21. How is it possible to determine whether myocardial ischemia is occurring intraoperatively?

Continuous ECG monitoring of ST-T wave morphology in lead V_5 (one of the "exercise" leads) is the easiest and most reliable way to check for ischemia intraoperatively. Intraoperative transesophageal echocardiography detects transient wall motion abnormalities in the patient having an episode of ischemia. Another possible way is to use changes in pulmonary capillary wedge pressure (PCWP) obtained via the pulmonary artery catheter. During ischemia, the diastolic stiffness of the LV increases, leading to an increase in PCWP. This last technique has very little real clinical utility because of the many factors that interfere with the interpretation of the PCWP in the operating room: operative position, blood loss, and fluid and drug administration.

22. What are the risk factors for perioperative MI with noncardiac surgery?

In theory, anything that increases myocardial O_2 demand or decreases O_2 supply to the myocardium such that irreversible cell injury occurs is a risk factor for perioperative MI. In practice, however, because of the remarkable range of the autoregulation of perfusion across the coronary bed in the person with normal coronaries and myocardium, the most important risk factor is some sort of heart disease, such as stenotic coronary arteries, hypertrophied muscle, or dilated chambers. These conditions make the heart less able to compensate for the perturbations of myocardial O_2 demand and supply that may occur with anesthesia and surgery. In other words, they abbreviate cardiac reserve.

The occurrence of sustained hypotension intraoperatively seems to be the most important extraneous risk factor. Sustained intraoperative hypertension does not seem to be as important.

Ashton CM: Perioperative myocardial infarction with noncardiac surgery. Am J Med Sci 308:41–48, 1994.

23. How do you make the diagnosis of MI in the postoperative patient?

Just as in other settings, the diagnosis rests on the triad of typical symptoms, a typical pattern of change in cardiac enzymes, and ECG changes. However, the postoperative patient presents some diagnostic challenges. Up to half of these patients may never have the chest pain typical of MI. Instead, they present with unexplained hypotension, dysrhythmias, pulmonary congestion, mental status changes, and restlessness. Though the symptoms are atypical for MI, the truly asymptomatic perioperative MI is an uncommon occurrence.

Secondly, of all the so-called cardiac enzymes, only the MB fraction of creatine kinase (CK) is not elevated by the muscle trauma associated with anesthesia and surgery. So, although the total CK may be "falsely" elevated in the postoperative patient, CK-MB retains its excellent sensitivity and specificity for acute MI.

ECG changes are very common in the postoperative setting, so the ECG by itself is of little utility in diagnosing infarction. Up to 20% of postoperative patients will have new ECG abnormalities, usually minor changes such as T-wave inversion or flattening. In any setting, Q waves pathognomonic for infarction develop in only 60% of patients with documented MIs.

24. What are the principles of evaluation and management of the patient with congestive heart failure (CHF) who must undergo noncardiac surgery?

In the patient with CHF, whether from systolic impairment or diastolic dysfunction, determining the state of compensation for CHF is the most important component of the preoperative evaluation, even more important than knowing the ejection fraction. The ejection fraction tells nothing about the state of compensation, and no consistent relationship has been found between ejection fraction and exercise tolerance as determined on a treadmill. Dyspnea on exertion is the earliest and most reliable symptom of CHF. Recent declines in exercise tolerance, increasing fatigue, orthopnea, and paroxysmal nocturnal dyspnea are the symptoms of decompensation. The signs of decompensation are weight increase, jugular venous distention, S_3 gallop, hepatomegaly, and edema. It is important to have the patient as well compensated as possible before surgery. CHF seems to be an independent risk factor for perioperative cardiac complications. Monitoring right atrial or pulmonary wedge pressure intraoperatively and, even more importantly, postoperatively can help in the management of intravascular volume.

25. How commonly do patients with atherosclerotic peripheral vascular disease and no symptoms or signs of coronary artery disease (CAD) actually have silent, significant (≥70% stenosis of at least one vessel) CAD?

Concomitant coronary atherosclerosis is frequently observed in patients who have atherosclerotic disease in other circulations, such as the cerebral vessels and aorta, and are scheduled to undergo vascular procedures. Usually the CAD is obvious: the patient has a history of MI, angina, or both. But a significant number (about 30%) of patients with peripheral vascular disease who have no historical, clinical, or ECG evidence of CAD will be found to have significant stenosis if coronary angiography is done. This is not to say that all patients should undergo coronary angiography in preparation for vascular surgery. If the goal is to reduce the likelihood that the vascular procedure may precipitate an MI, then the risk of mortality and morbidity from the coronary angiography and subsequent coronary revascularization must be *less than* the chance the patient will have a fatal perioperative MI with the peripheral vascular procedure. This is certainly not the case for most patients.

SURGERY AND LUNG DISEASE

26. What changes in respiration occur postoperatively with upper abdominal surgery?

Vital capacity (VC) is reduced in the early postoperative period after upper abdominal surgery. (VC includes three lung volumes: inspiratory reserve volume, tidal volume, and expiratory reserve volume.) Though pain is an important factor, the reduction in VC is attributable to diaphragmatic dysfunction and not simply to pain.

Respirations are shallower and faster, and sighs occur less frequently. When respiration at lower-than-normal lung volumes persists, airways at the lung bases are compressed, leading to collapse and atelectasis. Atelectasis causes ventilation/perfusion imbalance, and hypoxemia results. Preoperative and postoperative breathing exercises can minimize the probability of postoperative atelectasis.

27. What are the most common causes of postoperative respiratory failure?

Respiratory failure is defined as a decline in the ventilatory performance accompanied by an arterial PO_2 < 50 mm Hg and/or PCO_2 > 50 mm Hg. Simply stated, respiratory failure means that the lung is not performing its gas exchange function adequately.

By far the commonest causes of postoperative respiratory failure are **atelectasis** due to secretion retention and **nosocomial pneumonia.** Aspiration pneumonia (true infection) due to aspiration of oropharyngeal secretions is observed more commonly than pneumonitis due to aspiration of gastric contents (infection is not invariable in this setting). The adult respiratory distress syndrome (ARDS), a noncardiogenic pulmonary edema, frequently occurs in the setting of massive aspiration of gastric contents. However, the overall incidence of postoperative ARDS seems to be decreasing. Other infrequent pulmonary complications associated with respiratory failure include massive pulmonary thromboembolism and fat embolism.

28. Describe the symptoms and signs of pulmonary embolism (PE) in the postoperative patient.

Depending on the size of the embolus and the cardiopulmonary reserve of the patient, the clinical signs and symptoms of PE can be dramatic or subtle, ranging from cardiac arrest to mild dyspnea. Dyspnea is the most common symptom and, together with pleuritic pain, occurs in over half of patients. Cough may or may not be present. Hemoptysis is observed in fewer than a third of patients. Syncope occurs infrequently, but PE should be in the differential diagnosis when a patient suffers a syncopal attack on his or her first postoperative ambulation. Tachypnea is observed in most patients, but rales, tachycardia, an increased P_2 on cardiac auscultation, fever, and clinical signs of phlebitis are observed in fewer than half of the patients.

The diagnostic triad of hemoptysis, pleuritic pain, and dyspnea is seen in <20% of patients, even when massive embolus is present.

29. What are the classic ECG findings in the patient with acute PE? What are the classic arterial blood gas (ABG) findings?

One or more of the "classic" ECG findings of acute cor pulmonale—$S_1Q_3T_3$, right bundle branch block (RBBB), P pulmonale, or right axis deviation (RAD)—are observed in <25% of patients. Over 10% of patients have unchanged ECGs. ECG changes are observed more commonly in patients with preexisting cardiopulmonary disease and in patients with massive emboli. In most patients with PE, the ECG shows only sinus tachycardia and/or ST-segment and T-wave abnormalities.

In most patients with clinically detectable PE, the arterial PO_2 is <90 mm Hg, and a mild respiratory alkalosis is usually seen. ABGs cannot be relied upon to rule in or rule out the diagnosis of PE, but they are useful in determining the adequacy of the patient's ventilation.

30. Which test of pulmonary function is the best predictor of postoperative morbidity in the patient with lung disease?

An elevated $PaCO_2$. Patients who have chronic hypercapnea are at high risk for perioperative morbidity and mortality from all causes. Most practitioners believe that there is no place for elective surgery in patients who have chronic hypercapnea.

31. What is atelectasis? What effect does it have on gas exchange?

Atelectasis is alveolar collapse. Microatelectasis (*micro* because it is not radiographically apparent) is a prominent feature of ARDS, whereby defects in the pulmonary surfactant system lead to alveolar instability and collapse. With endobronchial obstruction, radiographically apparent subsegmental, segmental, or lobar atelectasis occurs. Atelectasis is associated with intrapulmonic shunting—i.e., the blood courses past poorly ventilated alveoli, with resulting "venous admixture" and arterial hypoxemia.

32. How frequently does aspiration of gastric contents occur with tracheal incubation in the operating room? What are its consequences?

The true incidence is unknown, but aspiration of small amounts of gastric contents may be quite common, occurring in as many as 1 in 4 patients. Most times, this has no clinically evident consequences. Aspiration of large amounts of gastric contents is uncommon and is immediately apparent to the anesthesiologist. The risk is greatest in nonfasting parturients and patients undergoing emergency operations. Patients with intestinal obstruction or esophageal disorders are also at risk.

Sequelae depend on the amount and type of aspirate. Aspiration of large amounts of acid gastric contents (pH < 2.5) causes a chemical burn of the lung, pneumonitis, which results in immediate, intense bronchoconstriction and eventual respiratory distress and insufficiency. Radiographic "white out" of the lungs occurs, and the full-blown ARDS develops. The consequences of aspiration of nonacid gastric contents (pH > 2.5) depend on whether bacteria and/or particulate matter is present in the aspirate. Aspiration of bacteria-containing material leads to infection, i.e., aspiration pneumonia. Aspiration of food particles causes obstruction of airways.

Warner MA, Warner ME, Weber JG: Clinical significance of pulmonary aspiration during the perioperative period. Anesthesiology 78:56–62, 1993.

33. What are the principles of managing the cigarette smoker who must undergo nonpulmonary surgery?

It is important to note that while most smokers do not have chronic obstructive lung disease (COPD), almost all smokers *do* have chronic bronchitis. Chronic bronchitis, a clinical diagnosis, is present if a productive cough has been present for 3 months of the year for 2 consecutive years. The excessive mucus production in smokers/chronic bronchitics is what leads to an increased incidence of postoperative pulmonary complications. Secretion retention and mucus plugging of airways in the postoperative period are associated with microatelectasis or radiographically apparent atelectasis. Atelectasis leads to gas-exchange abnormalities.

There is evidence to suggest that smokers who can stop smoking for at least 8 weeks before surgery have a reduced likelihood of postoperative complications. This is probably because the tracheobronchial mucosa can repair itself in that time period and mucus production returns toward normal. Smokers who have a productive cough may benefit from a preoperative pulmonary toilet program, and, in general, the greater the amount of secretions, the more vigorous the program should be. The presence of a productive cough can be best ascertained at the bedside by asking the patient to cough and listening to how much "rattle" is present. Simply asking the patient about productive cough is much less reliable, since most smokers fail to notice their own cough.

34. What are the principles of management for the asthmatic who must undergo nonpulmonary surgery?

The two major principles of managing the asthmatic are **control of bronchospasm** and **control of secretions**. Tracheal intubation can exacerbate bronchospasm and is also associated with increased sputum production. This can be minimized by ensuring that bronchospasm is under optimal control before the patient goes to the operating room. Inhaled bronchodilators should be administered on a regular schedule, and if the patient is receiving theophylline, the serum level should be kept in the therapeutic range. Secretions can be managed by a pulmonary toilet program perioperatively. Such a program includes incentive spirometry in addition to inhaled bronchodilators. Steroid-dependent asthmatics, in whom adrenal function is often suppressed, should receive IV corticosteroids in the perioperative period to cover them for the stress of anesthesia and surgery.

35. What are the principles of management for the patient with severe COPD who must undergo nonpulmonary surgery?

Postoperative pulmonary complications are most likely with upper abdominal surgery and occur much less commonly with peripheral procedures such as hip replacement. Nevertheless, the principles of management remain the same: control of secretions with a program of pulmonary toilet (aerosol bronchodilators, chest physiotherapy, coughing and deep breathing exercises, early ambulation); substitution of non-narcotic analgesics to avoid the suppression of respiratory drive and coughing associated with narcotic analgesics and sedatives; and monitoring of gas exchange status with arterial blood gas measurements. In addition, postanesthesia extubation of patients with severe COPD should be postponed until the patient is fully awake and able to cough vigorously.

36. Of what benefit are preoperative basic pulmonary function tests (PFTs)?

PFTs—spirometry and lung volume measurement—are an essential part of the workup of the patient who is facing pneumonectomy, lobectomy, or segmentectomy. In that setting, preoperative PFTs can help the clinician estimate the amount of respiratory function the patient will have after lung resection.

In nonthoracic surgery, however, the place of preoperative PFTs is much less clear. For preoperative PFTs to be of benefit, two conditions must apply:

- PFTs must provide relevant diagnostic information over and above that which is available from the history and physical examination.
- PFTs must be able to predict more accurately than the clinician which patients are at risk for postoperative pulmonary complications.

Neither of these conditions has been satisfied. Basic PFTs can diagnose only two conditions: obstructive lung disease and restrictive lung disease. These diagnoses can almost always be made and their severity estimated on clinical grounds, without the need for PFTs.

Postoperative pulmonary complications occur most commonly with upper abdominal surgery, and the more severe the respiratory impairment, the more likely it is that complications will occur. The degree of respiratory impairment and the likelihood of postoperative pulmonary complications can be quite accurately assessed by questioning the patient about exercise tolerance (or observing it during a walk around the ward), estimating the amount of tracheobronchial secretions the patient produces, and checking the arterial blood gases. These maneuvers cost quite a bit less than PFTs. The chance of postoperative pulmonary complications can be minimized by a pulmonary toilet program, which is safe, noninvasive, and inexpensive.

Lawrence VA, et at: Preoperative spirometry before abdominal operations: A critical appraisal of its predictive value. Arch Intern Med 149:280–285, 1989.

37. What is the "lesion" in postoperative adult respiratory distress syndrome (ARDS)?

ARDS is a type of pulmonary edema. Pulmonary edema is of two types: **cardiogenic,** in which alteration of Starling forces is responsible for increases in water content of the interstitium and alveoli; and **noncardiogenic,** in which the Starling forces are not deranged, but interstitial and alveolar water accumulates because of an increase in capillary permeability. The "lesion" in ARDS is an **injured pulmonary capillary epithelium.** (The Starling forces include the hydrostatic pressure inside the capillary, hydrostatic forces in the interstitium, oncotic pressure inside the capillary, and oncotic pressure in the interstitium.)

It is impossible to distinguish noncardiogenic pulmonary edema (ARDS) from cardiogenic pulmonary edema on the basis of the clinical presentation and radiographic findings. The two conditions can be differentiated by measurement of the pulmonary capillary wedge pressure (PCWP), which reflects LV filling pressures and is normally 6–12 mm Hg. The PCWP is elevated in cardiogenic pulmonary edema, reflecting the elevated LV filling pressures. It is normal in ARDS, because LV filling pressures are normal since the defect is at the alveolocapillary membrane.

38. Who is at special risk for postoperative ARDS?

Factors that seem to predispose the postoperative patient (as well as nonoperative patients) to ARDS include massive aspiration of gastric contents, sepsis, massive transfusion of blood products, fat embolism, and disseminated intravascular coagulation (DIC). Patients with more than one of these factors are at greatest risk.

39. How does fat embolism present clinically?

The fat embolism syndrome is a constellation of findings that includes mental status changes, respiratory and sometimes renal insufficiency, and a petechial rash. The syndrome is most commonly observed after fractures of long bones, but occasionally occurs after total hip arthroplasty. Although its delayed appearance lessens its diagnostic usefulness, the petechial rash is very specific for the syndrome. It develops only on the upper torso and in the absence of thrombocytopenia. The mortality rate of fat embolism may be as high as 20%, with respiratory failure accounting for most deaths. There is some evidence that corticosteroids may favorably alter the course. An index has been developed that, when used in the appropriate clinical setting, may lead to earlier diagnosis.

*Fat Embolism Index**

FACTOR	SCORE
Petechiae	5
Diffuse alveolar infiltrates	4
PaO_2 < 70 mm Hg	3
Confusion	1
Fever ≥ 100.4°F	1
Heart rate >120 bpm	1
Respiratory rate >30/min	1

*A minimum of 5 points must be present for the diagnosis to be considered highly probable. (Schonfeld SA, et al: Fat embolism prophylaxis with corticosteroids. Ann Intern Med 99:438–443, 1983.)

SURGERY AND KIDNEY DISEASE

40. What are the most common causes of postoperative renal insufficiency?

Most cases are due to prerenal causes. Renal parenchymal insults resulting in acute renal failure occur next in frequency. The most common insults are prolonged cross-clamping of the aorta at the time of vascular procedures, leading to renal ischemia, and nephrotoxic agents. Though contrast agents and aminoglycoside antibiotics are the most frequent nephrotoxins, NSAIDs also can cause acute renal failure. Postrenal causes of postoperative azotemia are least frequent and include urinary retention from prostatic hypertrophy or a kinked indwelling bladder catheter.

41. How can the incidence of contrast-related nephropathy be minimized in the patient with peripheral vascular disease who must undergo preoperative angiography?

Patients who are at highest risk for the development of dye-induced nephropathy are those who have preexisting renal insufficiency regardless of the cause. Volume depletion at the time of the study is an important additive risk factor. Also, the risk increases with the amount of dye injected. A two-pronged approach should be used:

1. The patient must be adequately hydrated before the procedure.

2. The amount of dye injected should be kept to the minimum. Normal or half-normal saline should be infused before, during, and after the procedure. Some nephrologists also prescribe a 20% solution of mannitol IV for prophylaxis. If two contrast procedures are necessary, the serum creatinine should be allowed to return to baseline before the second procedure. The evidence that low-osmolality radiocontrast agents are associated with a lower incidence of contrast nephropathy is suggestive but not compelling.

42. How should you determine the cause of new-onset renal insufficiency in the postoperative patient?

In the postoperative patient, as in other settings, it is useful to classify new-onset renal insufficiency as prerenal, renal, or postrenal. **Prerenal azotemia** results from decreased renal perfusion. Its causes include intravascular volume depletion due to hemorrhage, GI losses (as with nasogastric suction or ileostomy), or third-spacing of fluids (as with peritonitis); decreased cardiac function due to pump failure, valvular abnormalities, dysrhythmias, or pericardial tamponade; excessive peripheral vasodilatation as seen in sepsis or with afterload-reducing agents; and obstruction of blood flow through renal arteries or veins.

To evaluate for the presence of prerenal causes, a careful history and physical examination should be performed, with special reference to the cardiovascular system. In prerenal azotemia, the BUN:creatinine ratio approaches 20:1 rather than its normal 10:1. Urinary sodium measures also are extremely helpful. Because the kidney has only one stereotypical response to what it perceives as a threat to intravascular volume, i.e., conservation of sodium (and hence water), in prerenal azotemia the urinary sodium is very low, <10 meq/l.

Obstruction to urine flow causes **postrenal azotemia.** In the workup of postoperative renal insufficiency, obstruction at or below the bladder neck should be ruled out by the insertion of a catheter. For obstruction above the bladder to cause renal failure, it must be bilateral. Inadvertent ligation of the ureters during abdominopelvic surgery occasionally occurs. The presence of hydronephrosis/hydroureter can be ascertained by renal ultrasonography.

Renal parenchymal causes of postoperative azotemia include ischemia, as can occur with abdominal aortic aneurysm surgeries, and exposure to nephrotoxins, such as contrast agents and aminoglycosides. The diagnosis is suggested by a BUN:creatinine ratio of >20:1 and a urine sodium of >10 meq/l. The urine sodium is elevated because the injured parenchyma is unable to conserve sodium.

43. Who is at special risk for postoperative renal insufficiency?

> **Prerenal azotemia**—patients with cardiac disease
> **Renal azotemia**—elderly patients (GFR falls progressively with aging), diabetics, hypertensives, and patients with preexisting renal insufficiency
> **Postrenal azotemia**—patients with structural abnormalities of the lower urinary tract, i.e., prostatic hypertrophy or urethral stricture

44. How should you manage the patient with chronic renal failure in the perioperative period?

Preoperatively, a thorough history, physical examination, and laboratory evaluation should be performed to quantitate the degree of renal dysfunction present. A convenient way to classify renal dysfunction is:

> Stage 1: decreased renal reserve
> Stage 2: renal insufficiency
> Stage 3: moderate renal failure
> Stage 4: severe renal failure

Patients in stage 1 are completely asymptomatic but have a GFR of only 50–60% of normal. BUN is <20 mg/dl, and serum creatinine is <2 mg/dl. Elderly patients fall into this stage because of age-related decrements in GFR. In the elderly, BUN and creatinine may be normal in the face of the decline in GFR, because muscle mass is lost with aging. Patients in stage 1 are at increased risk for postoperative renal failure from nephrotoxins.

Stages 2–4 are characterized by progressive azotemia accompanied by symptoms and signs of uremia. These patients are unable to excrete volume and salt loads and are at risk for volume overload manifested by pulmonary edema and peripheral edema. In these patients, during the perioperative period, scrupulous attention must be given to intake and output. A pulmonary artery catheter, which allows measurement of intravascular volume and pulmonary wedge pressure, is very helpful in managing these patients postoperatively.

45. What effect do anesthesia and surgery have on antidiuretic hormone (ADH)? What clinical significance does that effect have?

Anesthesia and surgery seem to provide "nonosmotic" stimuli for the release of ADH from the posterior pituitary. ADH has a central role in water excretion by the kidney by increasing the permeability of the collecting tubules to water. Without ADH, the collecting tubules are not permeable to water, and large volumes of water are excreted in urine. In the presence of ADH, water flows down its concentration gradient from the lumen into the interstitium, and a concentrated urine is excreted. Serum sodium drops. Hyperosmolality is the most potent stimulus for ADH release, though volume depletion is also a potent stimulus.

Depending on the severity of the hyponatremia (and the consequent serum hypo-osmolality) and the rapidity with which it develops, postoperative hyponatremia may cause brain swelling and significant neurologic impairment. The careless administration of high volumes of hypotonic fluids to the postoperative patient can have disastrous consequences.

46. What is the correct diagnostic approach to the patient with postoperative hyponatremia (i.e., serum Na$^+$ of 127 meq/l)?

The plasma concentration of sodium, the primary determinant of serum osmolality, is maintained within a narrow normal range by means of a balance of water intake, regulated by the thirst mechanism, and water excretion by the kidney. The normal kidney can excrete up to 10 liters of water per day. Consequently, hyponatremia is only rarely caused by excessive water intake. The most common cause of hyponatremia is a defect in the renal excretion of water.

The following is a time-honored approach to the hyponatremic patient. The first step is to assess the patient's volume status by performing a physical examination. Three possibilities exist, each with its own differential:

1. The **volume-depleted patient** is salt-and water-depleted, with the salt deficit exceeding the water deficit. These deficits result from either renal losses (e.g., diuretic excess) or extrarenal losses (e.g., GI losses).

2. The **edematous patient** has an excess of total body water and salt, with the water excess greater than the salt excess. The excesses result from the kidney's retention of salt and water in conditions such as cardiac failure and cirrhosis, where it perceives a decrease in the "effective arterial blood volume." Salt and water excess is also seen in nephrosis and advanced renal failure, though the inciting causes are different.

3. The hyponatremic patient who appears to be **euvolemic** is usually modestly volume-expanded and has an excess of total body water, though this is not detectable on examination. The most likely explanation for "euvolemic" hyponatremia is prolonged release of ADH in the face of persistent water intake. Postoperative pain is one stimulus for ADH release.

Measurement of the urinary sodium concentration is a useful adjunct in distinguishing among the diagnostic possibilities in these three categories.

Hyponatremia is very common in postoperative patients. Usually it results from a combination of hypotonic fluid administration and release of ADH. It should be kept in mind that hyperglycemia can cause a "factitious" hyponatremia (called factitious because though sodium is low, plasma osmolality is normal or high). This is an important consideration in the postoperative diabetic with hyponatremia.

Berl T, Schrier RW: Disorders of water metabolism. In Schrier RW (ed): Renal and Electrolyte Disorders, 4th ed. Boston, Little, Brown, 1992, pp 50–67.

SURGERY AND DIABETES AND OTHER ENDOCRINE DISEASES

47. What hormonal changes does the patient with insulin-dependent (type I) diabetes mellitus (IDDM) experience with major surgery?

Just as with the nondiabetic, the diabetic experiences a catabolic state that results from perioperative starvation and the physiologic stress of anesthesia and surgery. However, insulin plays a major role in muting some of the catabolic processes, and the patient with IDDM may develop severe diabetic ketoacidosis postoperatively.

Starvation is associated with a drop in plasma glucose and insulin. Lipid metabolites rise as the body switches to alternative fuels. In nondiabetics, basal insulin secretion serves to place a brake on catabolism, but in the IDDM patient, lipolysis is uncontrolled. Added to the effects of starvation are the catabolic effects of the "stress response." Surgery causes an outpouring of catecholamines, which in addition to various hemodynamic effects act on the pituitary. ACTH from the pituitary causes release of glucocorticoids from the adrenals. Glucagon and growth hormone are also secreted. By their various pathways, these catabolic hormones lead to gluconeogenesis. In the IDDM patient, severe hyperglycemia develops; lipid mobilization persists unchecked by insulin; and fatty acid and ketone body concentrations rise, causing diabetic ketoacidosis.

It should be clear that insulin administration to type 1 diabetics is the cornerstone of keeping perioperative catabolic processes under control.

48. How should the oral hypoglycemic agents be handled in the type II diabetic in the perioperative period?

In contrast to type I diabetics, who suffer from insulin deficiency, type II diabetics have three abnormalities contributing to their hyperglycemia:

1. Impaired insulin secretion from pancreatic beta cells.
2. Insulin resistance in peripheral tissues.
3. Increased production of glucose by the liver.

Sulfonylureas are the most commonly used oral hypoglycemics. Though the precise intra-cellular events are still unknown, sulfonylureas act on the pancreatic beta cell to increase insulin secretion. The duration of action of these agents is very important in the perioperative patient. The longest-acting drugs are chlorpropamide (duration of action up to 72 hours) and glyburide (up to 24 hours). Hypoglycemia resulting from sulfonylureas is likely to be prolonged, and its signs and symptoms may be inapparent in the perioperative patient.

Sulfonylureas should be stopped before major surgery, with the timing of discontinuation based on the duration of action of the particular drug. Insulin can be used in the perioperative pe-riod. With minor surgery in otherwise healthy patients, who will almost certainly be eating regu-lar meals the day of surgery, the drug need not be interrupted. Frequent measurement of the blood sugar is essential in management, and it should be kept in mind that inaccuracy of glucose mon-itoring using fingerstick test strips is greatest at low levels of blood glucose.

49. What are the adverse consequences of hyperglycemia (serum glucose > 300 mg/dl) in the postoperative diabetic?

Despite the difficulty of proving the assertion, most believe that **wound healing** is impaired in the poorly controlled diabetic. A second adverse consequence may be a predisposition to **in-fection.** Although the clinical ramifications are not yet known, several defects in host defense mechanisms have been shown to be present in poorly controlled diabetics. These include impaired leukocyte chemotaxis, decreased intracellular bactericidal activity, and an impaired cell-mediated immune response.

A third, often forgotten adverse effect is the **osmotic diuresis** hyperglycemia induces. In the renal tubule, the T_m (maximum tubular transport capacity) for glucose is about 375 mg/min. Once the filtercd load of glucose exceeds the T_m, no more glucose can be reabsorbed, and glucose ap-pears in the urine. The osmotic presence of glucose in the renal tubular fluid retards water and salt reabsorption. In the postoperative patient (as in other settings), this may lead to volume depletion and prerenal azotemia.

50. What is the approach to managing the insulin regimen in the type I diabetic undergo-ing major surgery?

One approach to perioperative management is the **partial-dose approach,** in which the pa-tient is given one-half or two-thirds of his or her usual intermediate-acting insulin on the morn-ing of surgery. Insulin can be administered postoperatively using a sliding scale approach. Alter-natively, a **continuous low-dose infusion** of insulin can be used perioperatively. Several different treatment protocols for continuous infusions have been proposed.

Schiff RL, Emanuele MA: The surgical patient with diabetes mellitus: Guidelines for management. J Gen Intern Med 10:154–61, 1995.

51. Occasionally, a hyperosmolar, hyperglycemic state (HHS) develops in the postoperative period in the previously undiagnosed type II diabetic. What are the symptoms, signs, and management of this syndrome?

The HHS represents an acute decompensation of diabetes mellitus. The syndrome is marked by severe hyperglycemia (levels as high as 2,400 mg/dl have been observed), a serum osmolar-ity > 325 mOsm/l, and little or no acidosis. The prodrome, which may last from days to weeks, consists of polyuria, polydipsia, progressive volume depletion as a result of a relentless osmotic diuresis, and mental status changes that progress from lethargy to coma. Occasionally HHS is pre-cipitated by the stress response associated with major surgery. Treatment is directed first at re-placement of fluid and electrolyte losses. Fluid losses with HHS may be as much as 20% of body weight. Insulin requirements are much less than with diabetic ketoacidosis. Mortality, which is still quite high, generally results from thrombotic phenomena.

52. What are the symptoms and signs of postoperative adrenal insufficiency?

Adrenal insufficiency occurring in the perioperative period is rare, and although it is an em-inently treatable condition, clinicians often omit it from the differential diagnosis of intra- or post-operative deterioration.

Surgery is a physiologically stressful situation that may unmask chronic adrenal insufficiency. The first sign may be persistent intraoperative hypotension. Postoperatively, the patient may be febrile to 103°F, with nausea, vomiting, and severe abdominal pain, findings which are often misdiagnosed as an intra-abdominal catastrophe. Hypotension and shock can develop. Whenever the diagnosis is entertained, a serum cortisol level should be drawn, and without waiting for the result, corticosteroids should be administered.

It is the patient with chronic adrenal insufficiency who is at risk for an adrenal crisis precipitated by surgery. The symptoms and signs of chronic adrenal insufficiency are asthenia, fatigue, muscle weakness, postural hypotension, nausea, vomiting, anorexia, weight loss, abdominal pain, hyperkalemia, hyponatremia, anemia, and eosinophilia. Hyperpigmentation may or may not be present. Though very helpful if elicited as part of the preoperative evaluation, these findings seen in the postoperative patient are difficult to interpret because they can be attributed to iatrogenic causes, such as anesthesia, surgery, and fluid and electrolyte administration.

53. What problems might occur in the perioperative period in the patient with undiagnosed hyperthyroidism undergoing major surgery?

Thyroid hormone has important effects on many organ systems, but in the perioperative patient, its effects on heart and lungs are of greatest importance. Thyroid hormone has direct effects on the cardiovascular system that resemble, but are distinct from, the effects of **catecholamines.** These effects include an increase in myocardial contractility, an increase in heart rate, and a decrease in peripheral vascular resistance. Stroke volume and cardiac output are increased. High output cardiac failure and consequent pulmonary vascular congestion may occur. The "stress response" evoked by surgery and general anesthesia involves an outpouring of catecholamines, with the hemodynamic effects of the catecholamines being additive to the sympathomimetic effects of excess thyroid hormone. Because of the increase in myocardial O_2 requirements, angina pectoris may occur. Cardiac failure may be precipitated or worsened.

Excess thyroid hormone is associated with **increased ventilatory demands** (because of increased O_2 demand and increased production of CO_2) and with weakness of the respiratory muscles. This may be a lethal combination in the postoperative patient whose respirations may be further depressed by anesthesia and analgesia, and whose ventilatory capacity is reduced by upper abdominal surgery.

Finally, surgery is known to be one of the precipitating causes of **thyrotoxic crisis.** This condition occurs intraoperatively or later on the day of operation and presents with fever, diaphoresis, tachycardia (and frequently other dysrhythmias), and sometimes hypotension. Thyrotoxic crisis can be mistaken for malignant hyperthermia, sepsis, or delirium tremens in the surgical patient.

54. How is the patient on chronic corticosteroid therapy managed during the perioperative period?

Atrophy of the adrenal glands can be induced by exogenous corticosteroids in a matter of weeks. The glands atrophy because the exogenous hormone suppresses pituitary secretion of ACTH. ACTH is trophic for the adrenals—i.e., it is necessary for normal structure and function.

In the preoperative patient on chronic corticosteroids, it is possible to determine whether the hypothalamic-pituitary-adrenal axis is suppressed and, if it is, to administer extra corticosteroids to cover the stress of surgery. However, most clinicians simply assume the axis is suppressed and treat accordingly. A variety of corticosteroid preparations are available, and they differ in potency. Dosing and administration schedules are largely empiric. For minor surgery, hydrocortisone, 100 mg (or its equivalent), should be administered parenterally every 6 hours during the day of surgery. Dosing can begin when the premedication is given. (Some recommend beginning the evening before surgery.) The regular dose and schedule can resume the day after surgery. For major surgery, every-6-hour dosing can begin when the premedication is given and continue for 2 or 3 days postoperatively. If complications occur, this may need to be extended. There is no need to taper the dose to return to usual maintenance doses.

SURGERY IN THE ELDERLY

55. Delirium is a fairly common postoperative problem in the elderly. How is it diagnosed? What causes it?

The key diagnostic points are:

1. Delirium affects the main aspects of cognition—thinking, perception, memory.

2. Delirium is frequently accompanied by frightening visual (and sometimes auditory) hallucinations.

3. An attention disorder is present, and the level of alertness waxes and wanes throughout the day.

4. The sleep-wake cycle is disturbed, with symptoms typically worse at night.

Delirium is an organic disease. It is a medical emergency, and its cause should be sought immediately. Up to 20% of elderly patients develop postoperative delirium, and the incidence may be higher in patients with Parkinson's disease. Drugs, especially anticholinergics, are the commonest cause of delirium.

However, in the elderly, delirium is often the presenting finding in acute MI, pneumonia and other infections, and electrolyte abnormalities. Thus, "postoperative" delirium should be considered a diagnosis of exclusion and made only after these other considerations have been ruled out.

Lipowski Z: geriatrics: Delirium in the elderly patient. N Engl J Med 320:578–582, 1989.

56. How frequently does postoperative delirium occur? Who is at risk, and how do you treat it?

The precise incidence is uncertain, but by patients' self-report, it is surprisingly high. Six of 10 patients report that they experience cognitive problems in the early postoperative period. Risk factors include age >70, alcohol abuse, poor baseline cognitive status, poor functional status, abnormal preoperative sodium, potassium, or glucose, noncardiac thoracic surgery, and aortic aneurysm surgery. Anesthesia type does not seem to be a strong predictor. Haloperidol in low doses (0.5 mg twice a day) usually provides good sedation without severe side effects.

However, vigilant supportive nursing and medical care are essential in preventing complications and keeping the period of delirium as brief as possible. Nutritional, fluid, and electrolyte needs must be addressed, and any signs of infection must be investigated promptly. A brightly lit room with a clock and calendar is helpful. Sensory stimuli should be limited. The presence of family members is often calming to the patient.

Marcantonio ER, Goldman L, Mangione CM, et al: A clinical prediction rule for delirium after noncardiac surgery. JAMA 271:134–139, 1994.

57. In the healthy elderly, what age-related changes increase the risk of postoperative morbidity due to fluid and electrolyte abnormalities and drug toxicity?

1. Changes in body composition, with loss of lean muscle mass and increase in adipose tissue, such that total body water is decreased

2. Decrease in glomerular filtration rate (GFR)

3. Decrease in kidney's ability to conserve water

4. Decrease in kidney's ability to conserve sodium

5. Decrease in perception of thirst

These five factors work together to increase the risk of serious volume depletion, which is likely to be hypertonic in situations where the patient's access to free water is impeded, as in the postoperative period. Changes in body composition change the volume of distribution of drugs. This factor, together with the decline in the kidney's ability to metabolize and excrete certain drugs, increases the risk of drug toxicity.

58. Why would an elderly patient be more likely than a young patient to experience a delay in "waking up" in the recovery room after general anesthesia?

Unrecognized hypothermia in the recovery room can occasionally be the cause of delayed awakening from general anesthesia. Age-related changes in the autonomic nervous system impair the ability to generate and conserve heat. However, by far the most common cause of delayed awakening in the elderly is **delayed metabolism and excretion** of drugs used in anesthesia.

Opiates, which can be used as primary or supplementary anesthetics, probably account for most cases of delayed awakening in the elderly. Older people are much more sensitive than younger people to the anesthetic and respiratory depressant effects of opiates. Their increased sensitivity is related to greater plasma drug concentrations, which may be due to age-related changes in the drug's volume of distribution and clearance. In older people slow to react in the recovery room, CO_2 narcosis resulting from opiate-related respiratory depression should be ruled out by measuring the arterial PCO_2.

MISCELLANEOUS PERIOPERATIVE ISSUES

59. How do you manage the anticoagulants in a patient who has a prosthetic aortic valve and must undergo transurethral prostate resection?

In the anticoagulated patient facing surgery, the task is to balance the risk of bleeding with the risk of thrombosis. It takes 3–5 days for the coagulation cascade to normalize after warfarin is stopped. Many recommend that patients with prosthetic heart valves be admitted 3 days before the planned surgery. At that time, the warfarin should be stopped and the patient should be anti-coagulated with heparin. Heparin should be stopped 6 hours before the operation. Warfarin should be restarted as soon as the patient can tolerate oral intake, and the prothrombin time will be prolonged within 3 days. The risk of thromboembolism during the period the patient is not anticoagulated seems greatest in patients with a prosthetic valve in the mitral position. In these patients, heparin should be restarted 6–12 hours postoperatively and continued until warfarin has prolonged the prothrombin time.

White RH, et al: Temporary discontinuation of warfarin therapy: Changes in the international normalized ratio. Ann Intern Med 122:40–42, 1995.

60. Is prophylaxis against infective endocarditis necessary in the patient with mitral valve prolapse (MVP)?

MVP is a common valve abnormality estimated to be present in up to 10% of people. When associated regurgitation is present, MVP is considered to place the patient at an intermediate risk for infective endocarditis; when it is not, the risk is negligible.

Clinical practice varies, with some physicians prescribing prophylactic antibiotics in all patients with MVP, others using prophylaxis only in MVP patients who have associated mitral insufficiency, and still others who believe prophylaxis is simply not necessary in patients with MVP.

61. What are the three general principles of prophylaxis against infective endocarditis?

1. Certain types of congenital or acquired structural cardiac lesions place patients at risk for infective endocarditis.

2. Surgery/invasive procedures that traverse a mucous membrane (oral, GU, and GI) are more commonly associated with transient bacteremia than incisions across a sterile field.

3. The presence of circulating antibiotics with appropriate antimicrobial activity during the time of bacteremia reduces the incidence of bacterial seeding and infection of cardiac structures.

Durack DT: Prevention of infective endocarditis. N Engl J Med 332:38–44, 1995.

62. What is the risk of transmission of hepatitis C virus (HCV) from a blood transfusion? Of HIV transmission?

Current blood-banking protocols have reduced the risk for transmission of HCV dramatically, to about 3 cases/10,000 transfusions. The risk for transmission of the HIV is 1 case/40,000–225,000 transfusions.

Rutherford CJ, Kaplan HS: Autologous blood donation—Can we bank on it? N Engl J Med 332:740–742, 1995.

63. How can you minimize the possibility of the infective and noninfective complications of blood transfusion in a patient who will need perioperative transfusions?

Advances in the ability to test for blood-borne infections, such as HIV and hepatitis B and C viruses, in blood-banking practices have reduced the risk for infective complications of allogeneic transfusion (blood from volunteer donors) to extremely low levels. The banking and handling of autologous blood (blood from the person who is to receive the blood) are associated with higher costs than those for allogeneic blood. Consequently, autologous blood banking is no longer a cost-effective way to reduce the risk for transmission of blood-borne infections. Nevertheless, the use of autologous blood increases patients' peace of mind and, in addition, reduces the risk for non-infective transfusion-associated complications that cause significant morbidity, such as febrile, allergic, and delayed hemolytic reactions.

Intraoperatve hemodilution is a simple and inexpensive form of autologous blood donation that is coming into wider use. In this approach, one or two units of blood are withdrawn immediately before surgery and replaced with crystalloid. The withdrawn blood is held in the operating room at room temperature and is reinfused at the end of the procedure.

Rutherford CJ, Kaplan HS: Autologous blood donation—Can we bank on it? N Engl J Med 332:740–742, 1995.

64. What is malignant hyperthermia?

Malignant hyperthermia is an extremely rare complication of anesthesia with halogenated inhalational agents or the neuromuscular blocking agent succinylcholine. Its incidence is estimated to be 1 in 50,000–100,000 anesthetic episodes.

Many genetic, environmental, and pathophysiologic features of the syndrome are incompletely understood. It is believed to be due to a defect in muscle whereby calcium is handled abnormally by the sarcoplasmic reticulum. An increase in the sarcoplasmic calcium concentration precipitates a generalized hypermetabolic state in muscle. The syndrome is usually heralded by a rise in body temperature, which can reach 108°F. Tachycardia is often the first sign noted by the anesthesiologist. Muscle rigidity is a late finding.

65. How is malignant hyperthermia managed?

As soon as malignant hyperthermia is suspected, the operative procedure should be terminated, and respiratory support, circulatory support, body-cooling measures, and fluid and electrolyte therapy should be instituted. Dantrolene sodium, available in all operating suites, is specific therapy.

66. How commonly does deep venous thrombosis (DVT) occur with repair of hip fracture and transurethral prostate resection?

Although the incidence of clinically evident postoperative pulmonary embolism is low, DVT is a common occurrence in postoperative patients. Over 40% of patients undergoing hip fracture repair develop DVT postoperatively. In 30% of patients, the thrombus is in the proximal veins, which is thought to carry a higher risk of embolization than distal DVT. With transurethral prostate resection, the incidence is lower, about 10%.

67. What prophylaxis against perioperative thromboembolic disease has been found to be successful (without causing significant bleeding) in general, urologic, orthopedic, and gynecologic surgery?

Though many of the clinical trials of measures to prevent postoperative venous thromboembolism were too small to detect protective effects, an analysis of the compiled results from multiple studies has provided strong evidence that **low-dose heparin,** given perioperatively, confers significant protection against venous thromboembolism without causing significant bleeding. The heparin regimen is 5000 units administered subcutaneously every 8 or 12 hours, beginning before surgery and continuing until the patient is fully ambulatory. Other measures that confer some protection against postoperative thromboembolic disease (at least in some surgical groups) are dextran infusion and mechanical lower limb compression devices.

Some practitioners are unwilling to begin pharmacologic prophylaxis against thromboembolic disease preoperatively because of fears of operative bleeding complications. It appears that pharmacologic and nonpharmacologic methods of prophylaxis retain much of their efficacy even when started postoperatively.

Kearon C, Hirsh J: Starting prophylaxis for venous thromboembolism postoperatively. Arch Intern Med 155:366–372, 1995.

68. Occasionally, a patient abruptly develops hypertension, tachycardia, diaphoresis, disorientation, hallucinations, and tremor in the postoperative period. What is the most likely diagnosis?

The most likely diagnosis is **delirium tremens** (DTs), the most serious of the alcohol withdrawal syndromes. Alcoholism is underdiagnosed in general hospitals in the U.S., with its prevalence in adults admitted for general medical problems estimated to be as high as 30%. The abstinence from alcohol necessitated by hospitalization, anesthesia, and surgery can precipitate DTs, and its development can be quite surprising to the clinician who was unaware of the patient's alcoholism. The syndrome carries a mortality rate of 10–15% and is associated with marked autonomic hyperactivity manifested by fever, tachycardia, hypertension, diaphoresis, and tremor. The patient is profoundly disoriented and difficult to control. There are massive fluid and electrolyte losses. Treatment is supportive, and benzodiazepines are used for sedation.

PSYCHIATRIC DISORDERS

69. What is somatization disorder?

According to the *DSM-IV*, it is a psychiatric condition characterized by multiple, recurrent physical complaints for which no organic basis can be found. The disorder begins before age 30 and is more common in females. Common physical complaints include vomiting, pain in the extremities, shortness of breath, amnesia, pain in sexual organs or rectum, and dysmenorrhea.

The patient makes frequent visits to physicians because of the physical symptoms, often seeing several physicians concomitantly. Patients undergo extensive, repetitive diagnostic workups for their symptoms, take many prescription drugs, and often undergo surgical procedures. None of these interventions reveals an organic basis for the symptoms. There is no known effective therapy for somatization disorder.

70. How should the internist approach the patient with somatization disorder?

Because the cycle in somatization disorder (or any somatoform disorder) often is "physical complaint → unrevealing workup → empiric therapy," the danger of iatrogenic disease is very real. The physician who can establish a long-lasting relationship with a patient who has somatization disorder is occasionally able to break the cycle. To be successful, the physician must have confidence in his or her history-taking and physical examination ability and must be able to exercise diagnostic and therapeutic restraint. Care of the somaticizing patient is extremely difficult in public hospital or clinic settings, because a new physician may see the patient at each visit.

71. Is the patient with a schizophrenic disorder competent to make decisions about his medical care?

The three elements of informed decision-making (consent or refusal) are:

1. The physician must disclose an adequate amount of information about the risks, benefits, and alternatives of the proposed medical intervention.

2. The patient must understand the information provided (i.e., be able to receive, retain, retrieve, and rationally manipulate information).

3. The patient must be able to make a voluntary decision, free from internal and external compulsions.

The natural history of schizophrenia varies. Apparently, 20% of patients recover completely, usually after one episode. Obviously, such patients are competent to make informed decisions about their medical therapy, except during the active phase of their illness. Another 40% have a waxing and waning course marked by remissions and exacerbations. These patients generally become more impaired with each cycle, and competence may be permanently impaired. The remaining 40% of patients have persistent symptoms and signs of schizophrenia, and they may or may not be capable of making informed decisions.

In the individual, the severity of the symptoms and signs of schizophrenia fluctuate markedly over time. During the active phase, significant disturbances exist in several areas that almost certainly affect an individual's ability to make informed choices for his or her care, including language and communication, thought content, perception, affect, sense of self, volition, and relationship to the environment. With schizophrenics who are not in the active phase of illness, competence to make choices regarding personal medical care must be assessed on a case-by-case, and within the same patient, on an encounter-by-encounter basis. Competence evaluations should be motivated by respect for the patient's autonomy.

72. What is a personality disorder? How might it interfere in the relationship between patient and physician?

Personality disorders are very common in medical as well as psychiatric practice. A personality disorder is present when the patient's patterns of relating to, experiencing, and thinking about him or herself, others, and the environment cause internal distress or interfere with the person's social and occupational performance. There are various types of personality disorders, and the manner in which these types would hinder the relationship between internist and patient is fairly predictable. For example, the treatment of the patient with a paranoid personality disorder might be hampered by the patient's suspiciousness about the physician's diagnostic and therapeutic intent. The physician treating the patient with a histrionic personality disorder for a medical problem may have to deal with seductive behavior on the part of the patient. Another problem with this type of patient is that physical complaints are related to the physician in an excessively dramatic way, which can interfere with the physician's ability to assess the severity of the medical illness.

73. How do you differentiate between delirium and dementia?

In both, there is impairment of the three main aspects of cognition: thinking, perception, and memory. However, in dementia, the cognitive impairment develops insidiously and is enduring, whereas in delirium, the impairment has an abrupt onset and is short-lived.

Differentiation of Delirium and Dementia

CHARACTERISTIC	DELIRIUM	DEMENTIA
Onset	Sudden	Insidious
Course over 24 hrs	Fluctuating, worse at night	Stable
Consciousness	Reduced	Clear
Attention	Disordered	Normal except in severe cases
Cognition	Disordered	Disordered
Hallucinations	Visual or auditory	Often absent
Delusions	Poorly systematized	Often absent
Orientation	Usually impaired	Often impaired
Psychomotor activity	Variable	Often normal
Speech	Often incoherent	Difficulty in word-finding, perseveration
Involuntary movements	Asterixis/coarse tremor	Often absent
Physical illness or drug toxicity	One or both present	Often absent

Adapted from Lipowski ZJ: Delirium in the elderly patient. N Engl J Med 320:578–582, 1989.

74. Discuss the appropriate approach to the delirious patient.

Delirium is a medical, not a psychiatric, emergency. After the diagnosis has been made and the patient's immediate safety ensured, the possible causes of delirium should be investigated. In the elderly, delirium is often the herald of serious systemic disease; therefore, the first group of diagnostic possibilities to be explored includes acute MI, pneumonia and other infections, hyper- or hypoglycemia, azotemia, acid-base disorders, and fluid and electrolyte disturbances. The second group of possibilities consists of drug toxicities, including alcohol withdrawal. Almost any drug can cause changes in mental status, even when ingested in "therapeutic" doses.

75. What are the somatic signs of depression?

Though nonspecific somatic complaints such as fatigue, headache, and GI disorders can accompany depression, by far the most common somatic signs involve sleeping, eating, and sexual function. Sleep disturbances include difficulty in falling asleep and early morning awakening, with the patient sometimes awakening 2 or 3 hours before his or her habitual rising time. On the other hand, hypersomnia occasionally occurs. Often, the patient complains that food has lost its taste. Loss of appetite and weight occur more commonly than increases in appetite and weight. Libido may be completely lost.

MEDICAL CARE OF THE PSYCHIATRIC PATIENT

76. What is a rational approach to the treatment of chronic hypertension in the patient with depression?

Depression has been reported to occur with (or be exacerbated by) many antihypertensive agents. However, depression is also reported by patients in the placebo arms of clinical trials almost as commonly as in patients on active therapy, and so the clinician should be wary of changing medication without substantial indications that the symptom is a side effect of drugs.

Evidence has suggested that ACE inhibitors may be a very good choice in the patient with depression. A study comparing the effect of captopril, propranolol, and methyldopa on patient-perceived quality of life found that captopril was associated with an improved performance on the quality-of-life scale. Captopril has also been reported to produce mood elevation in depressed patients. Even within the class of ACE inhibitors, different agents may have different effects on mood and quality of life. For example, in one study, captopril and enalapril were equivalent in terms of safety and efficacy in hypertensive men, but captopril had more favorable effects on quality of life, general health, health status, sleep, and emotional control. Selection of antihypertensive agents must be individualized based on the patient's age, race, coexisting conditions, and concurrent medications.

Testa MA, et al. Quality of life and antihypertensive therapy in men: A comparison of captopril with enalapril. N Engl J Med 328:907–913, 1993.

77. What is a rational approach to the treatment of chronic hypertension in the patient with psychosis or a major affective disorder?

There are four basic points to remember when treating such a hypertensive patient:

1. Because of severe agitation and autonomic overactivity, blood pressure will be elevated during a period of acute decompensation. Overzealous use of antihypertensives during this time can be disastrous.

2. Avoid selecting for chronic use agents known to cause rebound hypertension when abruptly discontinued (such as clonidine). Transdermal delivery of antihypertensive medication by means of a skin patch may help in avoiding such a situation in patients with particularly unpredictable behavior.

3. Diuretics should be used as antihypertensives with great caution in patients receiving lithium, and serum lithium levels should be monitored frequently during therapy.

4. Patients are more likely to comply with simple once-a-day regimens.

78. How does the acute ingestion of cocaine affect the cardiovascular system?

Cocaine blocks the presynaptic re-uptake of norepinephrine. Thus, acute ingestion has predictable cardiovascular manifestations consistent with sympathetic nervous system overactivity, including vasoconstriction, an acute rise in arterial pressure, tachycardia, and a predisposition to ventricular dysrhythmias. Acute MI occasionally occurs secondary to cocaine ingestion. The increases in heart rate and blood pressure increase myocardial O_2 demand. Though persons with coronary artery disease are at greatest risk for cocaine-induced MI, MI after cocaine use has also been found to occur in persons with normal coronary arteries. Cocaine ingestion predisposes to such cardiac arrhythmias as sinus tachycardia, ventricular ectopy, ventricular tachycardia and fibrillation, and asystole.

Hollander JE: The management of cocaine-associated myocardial ischemia. N Engl J Med 333:1267–1272, 1995.

79. What should be included in the medical evaluation of the elderly depressed patient scheduled to begin a course of electroconvulsive therapy (ECT)?

ECT is often more effective than drugs in the treatment of depression. It acts more quickly than drugs, an important consideration when there is a significant risk of suicide. ECT may be of particular value in the depressed elderly because age-related changes, coexisting disease, and the need for concomitant medications often lead to intolerable side effects with antidepressant drugs.

In contrast to the manner in which ECT was provided in the past, in current practice ECT is delivered under controlled conditions, and the patient's cardiovascular and ventilatory status are carefully monitored. The patient receives a short-acting general anesthetic for comfort and a neuromuscular blocking agent to attenuate the seizure. Supplemental oxygen is administered to prevent the development of hypoxia during the seizure, and anticholinergics are given to control secretions and lessen the bradycardia that occurs when the seizure begins.

The most common complications of ECT are cardiac dysrhythmias and exaggerated hypertensive responses. Very rarely, MI occurs. Dysrhythmias are quite common. The pretreatment evaluation should be directed at assessing the presence and control of hypertension, the presence and state of compensation of congestive heart failure, the presence and severity of angina, and the history of cardiac dysrhythmias. A careful history, physical examination, and ECG are usually the only diagnostic workup indicated.

MEDICAL DISEASE DUE TO PSYCHIATRIC DRUGS

80. Name the four categories of drugs used to treat psychiatric conditions. List the most common, medically important side effects of each group.

Major Classes of Psychiatric Drugs and Their Side Effects

Antipsychotics	Dry mouth
Phenothiazines	Urinary retention
Thioxanthines	Constipation
Butyrophenones	Orthostatic hypotension
Miscellaneous compounds	
Mood stabilizers	Polyuria/polydipsia
Lithium	Nephrogenic diabetes insipidus
Antidepressants	Dry mouth
Tricyclics	Urinary retention
Monamine oxidase inhibitors	Delirium
Tetracyclics	Tachycardia
Others (e.g., fluoxetine, trazodone)	Orthostatic hypotension
Sedative-hypnotics	Drowsiness
Benzodiazepines	Diminished motor skills (incl. falls in elderly)
Barbiturates	Delirium (esp. in elderly)
Miscellaneous compounds	

81. How does lithium affect salt- and water-handling by the kidney?

When first administered, lithium can cause a brief (1–2 day), transient natriuresis that is usually of no clinical significance. Though there are many similarities in the way the kidney handles lithium and sodium, by far the most important effect of lithium is on the handling of water.

Antidiuretic hormone (ADH), a hormone secreted by the posterior pituitary, makes the normally water-impermeable collecting tubules in the kidney permeable to water. In the absence of ADH, or with reduced tubular responsiveness to ADH, water is not reabsorbed in the tubules, and large amounts of water are excreted in the urine. ADH levels in patients receiving lithium are normal or elevated in the face of impaired free-water conservation. This indicates that lithium interferes with the action of ADH on renal tubular epithelium. The urinary concentrating deficit is usually reversible when lithium is stopped.

82. What are the signs of lithium toxicity?

Early signs of lithium toxicity can be quite subtle. Unrecognized, toxicity gradually worsens over several days to weeks.

Serum levels <1.5 mmol/l—fine intention tremor, lethargy, weakness, difficulties with concentration and memory

Serum levels >1.5 mmol/1—coarse resting tremor, muscle fasciculations, increased muscle tone, hyperreflexia, confusion, visual disturbances, ataxia, dysarthria, extrapyramidal signs

Serum levels >3 mmol/1—seizures, coma, flaccid paralysis, death

Dialysis is indicated when levels are above 3 and may be indicated with lower levels, depending on the clinical state. Elderly people can develop lithium toxicity when serum levels are in the so-called therapeutic range.

83. What are extrapyramidal side effects? How are they treated?

Extrapyramidal side-effects (EPS) can be classified into four syndromes, three of which are early and one which is late. The early syndromes consist of a **parkinsonian complex** indistinguishable from Parkinson's disease; **akathisia,** in which the patient is in constant motion; and **acute dystonia,** which can range from grimacing to oculogyric crisis. **Tardive dyskinesia,** the late syndrome, consists of a syndrome of involuntary movements such as buccolingual masticatory movements, choreoathetoid movements of the limbs, and facial tics, which develops after months to years of neuroleptic medication usage.

All three of the early syndromes are reversible if the drug is stopped or the dose reduced (although tardive dyskinesia may be persistent). The danger is that the EPS syndromes may be misinterpreted as signs of worsening psychiatric disease rather than drug toxicity, with a consequent increase of the dose. Anticholinergics such as benztropine or diphenhydramine relieve the early EPS syndromes promptly.

84. What salt and water changes would occur if a patient on long-term lithium therapy developed gastric outlet obstruction and persistent vomiting, but still took his lithium?

The kidney handles lithium much the same way it handles sodium, and this has important implications for patients taking lithium who, for whatever reason, experience changes in intravascular volume while on the drug. Like sodium, about 75% of filtered lithium is absorbed in the proximal tubule. Thus, in states of volume depletion, such as in the patient described, the kidney conserves sodium (to protect the intravascular volume), and it also "conserves" lithium. Lithium levels rise and toxicity develops. Conversely, in volume-expanded states, where the kidney is excreting salt, the kidney also is excreting lithium, and doses may need to be increased to maintain therapeutic serum levels.

85. What is "steroid psychosis"?

Corticosteroid use is frequently associated with changes in mood (euphoria, dysphoria, or emotional lability), sleep pattern (insomnia, weird dreams, nightmares), and appetite (usually increased). Corticosteroids also can have important effects on behavior and thought processes, inducing frank psychosis in persons without a prior history of psychiatric disturbance or causing a decompensation in the known psychotic.

86. Chlorpromazine can occasionally cause liver problems. What are the clinical, laboratory, and histologic findings with chlorpromazine-induced liver problems?

Chlorpromazine caused a therapeutic revolution in psychiatry when it was introduced in the early 1950s, and continues to be used quite often. The liver problem that chlorpromazine causes is **cholestatic jaundice.** This occurs in 1–2% of patients, but the incidence may have decreased in the last decade. Previously this problem was thought to be related to hypersensitivity, but evidence now indicates that chlorpromazine is toxic to the liver and that subclinical cholestasis occurs in most patients receiving the drug. It is not known why some patients develop overt cholestasis.

Laboratory findings consistent with biliary obstruction are observed, but fever and right upper quadrant tenderness are minimal. Jaundice becomes apparent during the second through fourth week of therapy. Pathologically, the liver shows bile plugs, portal inflammation, and hepatocellular necrosis. The treatment is discontinuation of the drug. Weeks may elapse before laboratory evidence of cholestasis resolves.

87. What commonly used psychotropic agents cause orthostatic hypotension?

Orthostatic hypotension is a common occurrence with some of the antipsychotics, particularly chlorpromazine, and the tricyclic antidepressants. Tricyclics are widely used in the elderly, because the prevalence of depression in that age group. Many elderly have age-related degenerative changes in the autonomic nervous system and/or are taking other medications, such as diuretics or antihypertensives, that exacerbate the postural drop in blood pressure (BP) caused by tricyclics. Postural BP changes can cause syncope or near-syncope, with consequent injury from falls. The propensity to cause orthostasis seems to vary somewhat among agents based on affinity for the α-adrenergic receptor. Lower-affinity agents should, at least in theory, produce fewer postural BP changes. From highest affinity to lowest, the rank is doxepin > amitriptyline > nortriptyline and imipramine > protriptyline > desipramine.

88. Discuss the cardiovascular effects seen with therapeutic doses of tricyclic antidepressants (TCAs).

TCAs are commonly associated with orthostatic hypotension, changes in the ECG, and, anecdotally, development of high-grade heart block in patients with preexisting intraventricular conduction abnormalities. Heart rate increases in some patients. Some of the tricyclics (imipramine) actually seem to decrease ventricular ectopy, and atrial or ventricular ectopy should not automatically preclude the careful use of TCAs. Early animal studies suggested that TCAs decrease myocardial contractility, and for a long time these agents were avoided in patients with myocardial dysfunction, but a 1982 study indicated that LV function in patients with chronic heart disease is not adversely affected by therapeutic doses of imipramine or doxepin.

Veith RC, et al: Cardiovascular effects of tricyclic antidepressants in depressed patients with heart disease. N Engl J Med 306:954, 1982.

89. What changes can lithium produce in the ECG? Tricyclics? Chlorpromazine?

About 20% of patients taking lithium exhibit flattening of the T wave. Occasionally, ST-segment depression is found, especially in patients with supratherapeutic levels.

The TCAs produce minor ST-segment changes, but their effect on intramyocardial conduction seems to be more important. In fact, in patients taking TCA overdoses, the duration of the QRS complex is a good predictor (even better than serum drug levels) of the likelihood that seizures or ventricular arrhythmias will occur. In patients taking therapeutic amounts of TCAs, some prolongation of the PR interval, QRS complex, and QT interval may be observed. In patients with preexisting conduction disorders, tricyclics can provoke heart block.

The most common ECG changes observed in patients taking chlorpromazine (and other phenothiazines) consist of T-wave flattening or inversion. ST-segment depression and prolongation of the PR interval and QRS complex are less commonly seen.

90. What is neuroleptic malignant syndrome (NMS)? How often does it occur?

NMS is a rare complication associated with use of antipsychotic agents. The precise incidence is unknown but is estimated at <0.5% of patients receiving antipsychotics. A significant proportion of patients who develop NMS have taken antipsychotics in the past without incident.

The diagnosis is made clinically. The constellation of signs and symptoms includes delirium, fever (as high as 105°F), tachycardia, BP instability, diaphoresis, and muscle rigidity. The complex develops over 24–72 hours and seems to be occasionally precipitated by, or at least associated with, volume depletion, physical exhaustion, and use of lithium along with the antipsychotic. The pathophysiology of NMS is unknown. Treatment is supportive. Antipsychotics must be stopped when the diagnosis is suspected; continued administration is lethal. The mortality rate is as high as 30%.

Rosebush P, Stewart T: A prospective analysis of 24 episodes of neuroleptic malignant syndrome. Am J Psychiatry 146:717–725, 1989.

BIBLIOGRAPHY

1. Goldmann DR, et al (eds): Perioperative Medicine: The Medical Care of the Surgical Patient, 2nd ed. New York, McGraw-Hill, 1994.
2. Kammerer WS, Gross RJ (eds): Medical Consultation: Role of the Internist on Surgical, Obstetric, and Psychiatric Services, 2nd ed. Baltimore, Williams & Wilkins, 1990.
3. Lubin MF, et al (eds): Medical Management of the Surgical Patient, 3rd ed. Boston, Butterworth, 1995.

16. AMBULATORY CARE

Mary P. Harward, M.D.

Here, at whatever hour you come, you will find light and help and human kindness.

Albert Schweitzer (1875–1965)

The sooner patients can be removed from the depressing influence of general hospital life the more rapid their convalescence.

Charles H. Mayo (1865–1939)
The Lancet, 1916

1. What are the most common reasons that patients are seen in ambulatory care clinics?

Common Reasons for Ambulatory Visits to Office-based Internists

REASONS NAMED BY PATIENTS	REASONS NAMED BY PHYSICIANS
General medical examination	Essential hypertension
Hypertension	Diabetes mellitus
Progress visit, no other symptoms	Chronic ischemic heart disease
Chest pain and related symptoms	Acute upper respiratory infection
Cough	General medical examination
Blood pressure test	Osteoarthritis and allied diseases
Diabetes mellitus	General symptoms
Symptoms referable to throat	Chronic airway obstruction
Abdominal pain, cramps, spasms	Asthma
Headache, pain in head	Bronchitis
Upper respiratory infection, (head cold, coryza)	Neurotic disorders
Back symptoms	Angina pectoris
Vertigo, dizziness	Chronic sinusitis
Shortness of breath	Acute pharyngitis
Tiredness, exhaustion	Cardiac dysrhythmia
Leg symptoms	Misc. (diagnosis missing or illegible)
Shoulder symptoms	Other disorders of soft tissue
Neck symptoms	Other respiratory symptoms
Ischemic heart disease	Congestive heart failure
	Peripheral enthesopathies

*National Ambulatory Medical Care Survey.

(Barker LR: Curriculum for ambulatory care training in medical residency: Rationale, attitudes and generic proficiencies. J Gen Intern Med 5(suppl 1):S3–S14, 1990.

2. How should you initially evaluate a 45-year-old black man whose blood pressure (BP), measured on several occasions, has been between 140/95 and 155/105 mm Hg?

The initial evaluation of a recently identified and confirmed hypertensive patient must uncover treatable causes of secondary hypertension. Extensive evaluations are not useful, though, if the treatment will not change. Also, baseline evaluation of any systemic effects of hypertension is useful in evaluating future therapies.

The history and physical evaluation, when thoroughly done, and limited diagnostic tests will suggest the presence of most secondary causes, assess organ function, identify other risk factors for heart disease, and establish baseline for monitoring of future effects of hypertension or medication side effects. In general, secondary hypertension causes are more likely in patients whose hypertension begins during adolescence or over age 50 or have hypertension resistant to therapy.

447

Diagnostic Evaluation of the Newly Diagnosed Hypertensive Patient (to Identify Secondary Causes and End-organ Effect and Establish Baseline)

DIAGNOSTIC TEST	SECONDARY CAUSE OR END-ORGAN EFFECT	SIDE EFFECT
Urinalysis	Renal parenchymal disease	Proteinuria
BUN, creatinine	Renal parenchymal disease	Dehydration, renal insufficiency/failure
Glucose	Diabetes mellitus	Hyperglycemia
Calcium	Hyperparathyroidism	Hypercalcemia
Potassium	Hyperaldosteronism	Hypokalemia
Uric acid	NA	Hyperuricemia
Total cholesterol and HDL	Additional risk factor for heart disease	Hypercholesterolemia
ECG	Presence of LV hypertrophy	Conduction disturbance

3. What findings on history and physical examination suggest the presence of secondary hypertension?

Finding	*Implication*
Positive CAGE questionnaire*	Alcoholism
History of drug use	Stimulant use
Obesity, facial hair, striae	Cushing's syndrome
Anxiety, tremor, tachycardia	Pheochromocytoma, hyperthyroidism
Goiter, exophthalmos	Hyperthyroidism
Pallor, diaphoresis	Pheochromocytoma
Muscle cramps, weakness	Hyperaldosteronism
Hypersomnolence, snoring, obesity	Sleep apnea
Diminished femoral pulses, heart murmur, bruit best heard over back	Aortic coarctation
Periumbilical bruit	Renovascular disease
Fatigue, confusion, constipation	Hyperparathyroidism

*For CAGE, see Question 84.

4. How often should you screen for hypertension in normotensive adults?
Normotensive adults (diastolic BP < 85 mm Hg and systolic BP < 140 mm Hg) should have their BP measured at least every 2 years. Adults with diastolic BPs between 85–89 mm Hg should be screened annually.

5. Name some of the nonpharmacologic treatments for hypertension.
- Weight loss
- Smoking cessation
- No-added salt diet
- Regular exercise
- Decreased alcohol intake
- Biofeedback/relaxation techniques
- Stress reduction

6. How would you manage an asymptomatic hypertensive patient with a BP of 170/119 who stopped his medication 1 week ago?
If the patient has no signs or symptoms of a hypertensive emergency, slowly lowering the BP over a 24 hour period by restarting the prescribed maintenance dose of the patient's antihypertensive medications and maintaining close outpatient follow-up will be sufficient.

7. What test(s) should be ordered to screen for hyperlipidemia?
A nonfasting serum cholesterol and high-density lipoprotein (HDL) cholesterol should be measured. Lipoprotein analysis (fasting levels of total cholesterol, total triglyceride, and HDL-cholesterol) and calculation of the low-density lipoprotein (LDL) cholesterol should be done for all patients with screening total cholesterol ≥ 240 mg/dl or HDL of 35 mg/dl. If a patient has a total cholesterol between 200–239 mg/dL, an HDL of 35 mg/dl and two or more risk factors for coronary artery disease, a lipoprotein analysis should also be done. The LDL is calculated as follows:

$$LDL = \text{total cholesterol} - HDL - (\text{triglycerides}/5)$$

Second report of the National Cholesterol Education Program Expert Panel on Detection, Evaluation, and Treatment of High Blood Cholesterol in Adults. Washington, DC, National Institutes of Health, 1993.

8. What advice about sexual activity would you give a patient recovering from an uncomplicated MI?

Sexual intercourse requires about 3–5 METs of exertion. (One MET is the amount of energy expended at rest.) Most patients recovering from an uncomplicated MI can tolerate this without difficulty. It may be more strenuous for a man to support his weight on his arms in a superior position, and, therefore, other positions for intercourse should be considered.

9. Describe the physical findings of an innocent murmur and the murmur of mitral valve prolapse.

Physical Findings in Innocent and Mitral Valve Prolapse (MVP) Murmurs

FINDING	INNOCENT	MVP
Location	Base	Apex (left lateral decubitus position)
Intensity	< 3/6	≥ 3/6
Timing	Early systole	Late systole
Response to maneuvers	Decreases with standing and Valsalva	Begins earlier in systole with standing and Valsalva
Associated signs	Normal S_2	Midsystolic click

10. What are your recommendations for prophylactic antibiotics to a patient with mitral valve prolapse scheduled for an elective dental procedure? To a patient with a prosthetic aortic valve?

Antibiotic prophylaxis against endocarditis is recommended for patients with congenital heart disease (except uncomplicated secundum atrial septal defect), rheumatic or acquired valvular disease, hypertrophic cardiomyopathy, MVP with mitral insufficiency, prosthetic heart valves, or a history of previous endocarditis who are undergoing procedures that will likely lead to bacteremia with pathogenic organisms. Viridans streptococci are the most common cause of endocarditis after dental or upper respiratory procedures; enterococci are the most common cause of endocarditis after GI or GU procedures.

Prophlactic Antibiotics for Adults Undergoing Invasive Procedures

PROCEDURE	ORAL REGIMEN	PARENTERAL REGIMEN
Upper respiratory or dental	Amoxicillin, 3 gm po 2 hr before, then 1.5 gm 6 hr after initial dose; *OR* Erythromycin ethylsuccinate, 800 mg po, or erythromycin stearate, 1 gm po 2 hr before, then half-dose 6 hr after initial; *OR* Clindamycin, 300 mg po, 1 hr before, then 150 mg 6 after	Ampicillin, 2 gm IV or IM 30 min before, then ampicillin 1 g IV or IM or amoxicillin 1.5 gm po 6 hrs later; *OR* Clindamycin, 300 mg IV 30 min before, then 150 mg IV or IM 6 hr after
GI or GU	Amoxicillin, 3 gm po 1 hr before, then 1.5 gm po 6 hr later	Ampicillin, 2 gm IM or IV, plus gentamicin, 1.5 mg/kg IM or IV, 30 min before; then repeat parenteral dose or amoxicillin, 1.5 gm po 6 hr after *OR* Vancomycin, 1 gm IV infused over 1 hr starting 1 hr before procedure, plus gentamicin, 1.5 mg/kg IM or IV 1 hr before, then may repeat 8 hr later

Adapted from Karchmer AW, et al: Infectious endocarditis. In Dale DC, Federman DD (eds): Scientific American Medicine. New York, Scientific American Inc., 1995, 7:XVIII:14.

11. How do you evaluate an asymptomatic patient with new-onset atrial fibrillation?

The evaluation should specifically look for the causes of atrial fibrillation and evidence of cardiac dysfunction.

Evaluation for the Causes of Atrial Fibrillation

CAUSE	HISTORY	PHYSICAL EXAM	LABORATORY
Alcohol use	Daily use, binging	Jaundice, spider angiomata, palmar erythema, hepatomegaly	Liver function tests
Medications	Digoxin	—	Digoxin level, ECG
Drug use	Stimulant use	—	Toxin screen
Congestive heart failure	Dyspnea on exertion, paroxysmal nocturnal dyspnea, peripheral edema, nocturia	Jugular venous distension, rales, edema, S_3	Chest x-ray
Pulmonary embolism	Chest pain, dyspnea, calf pain, predisposing factors (recent surgery, immobilization)	Calf swelling, pleural rub	ABG, chest x-ray, consider V/Q
Myocardial infarction	Chest pain	S_4	ECG, cardiac enzymes
Cerebrovascular accident	Paresis, paralysis, aphasia, visual loss, numbness	Muscle weakness, sensory loss, dysarthria, reflex changes	Head CT scan or MRI
Mitral valve disease	Rheumatic fever or valvular disease	Heart murmur	Echocardiogram
Organic heart disease	Hypertension or heart disease	S_3, S_4, elevated BP	Chest x-ray, ECG, echocardiogram
Hyperthyroidism	Weight loss, depression	Goiter	Thyroid function tests
Wolff-Parkinson-White syndrome	Palpitations	—	ECG
Sick sinus syndrome	Syncope	—	Holter or event monitor

ABG = arterial blood gas; V/Q = ventilation/perfusion scan.

12. What are the LEOPARD and LAMB syndromes?

These acronyms refer to constellations of findings, but both are characterized as hyperpigmentation disorders because of the presence of lentigines.

L—Lentigines (hundreds covering the body, developing in childhood)
E—ECG abnormalities, primarily conduction disorders
O—Ocular hypertelorism
P—Pulmonary stenosis and subaortic valvular stenosis
A—Abnormal genitalia
R—Retardation of growth
D—Deafness

L—Lentigines
A—Atrial myxomas
M—Mucocutaneous myxomas
B—Blue nevi

13. What should be the therapeutic plan for an adolescent with a moderate case of acne vulgaris?

1. Avoid oily cosmetics.
2. Use mild cleansing soap.
3. Use topical 2.5% benzoyl peroxide gel once or twice daily to cause slight erythema and scaling. If this does not improve the acne, increase the concentration up to 10% benzoyl peroxide or add topical clindamycin daily.

4. If pustules are present, apply topical clindamycin daily.

5. Use oral tetracycline (500 mg bid) for 6 weeks for severe cases. Stop the antibiotics periodically to assess continued need. Chronic antibiotic use may cause vaginitis in women.

6. Refer to a dermatologist if intralesional steroids or 13-cis-retinoic acid is needed.

7. Avoid oral contraceptives for women containing norgestrel or norethidrone.

14. What is hidradenitis suppurativa?

Hidradenitis suppurativa is an infection of the apocrine sweat glands that leads to chronic inflammation and scarring. It occurs in the axilla, groin, and buttocks and under women's breasts. Antibiotic therapy (erythromycin or dicloxacillin) can be useful, but sometimes surgical excision is required.

15. What are the typical locations and appearance of psoriasis?

Psoriasis typically occurs on the extensor surfaces (elbows and knees), waistline, umbilicus, external genitalia, and gluteal fold. The typical lesions are elevated, reddish-brown plaques and papules with silvery scale. Bleeding points occur where the scale is removed (Auspitz's sign). In addition, the nails may be pitted. Some patients have arthritic involvement of the distal interphalangeal (DIP) joints.

16. Name some causes of alopecia.

NONSCARRING	SCARRING
(Permanent hair follicles not permanently lost or damaged)	(Permanent loss of hair follicles)
Male-pattern baldness	Discoid lupus erythematous
Stress, childbirth, general anesthesia, weight loss	Tinea capitis
Malnutrition	Pemphigoid
Medications	Lichen planus
Androgens, anticoagulants, anticonvulsants, corticosteroids, lipid-lowering agents, chemotherapy	
Alopecia areata	

17. Describe the characteristic appearance of tinea versicolor. How do you treat it?

Tinea versicolor, caused by infection with the fungus *Malassezia furfur,* has various colors (red, pink, brown) and is usually macular with slight scaling. The involved areas of skin do not tan well, and the infection becomes particularly obvious in the summer, when the involved areas are hypopigmented. The lesions fluoresce orange and gold under Wood's light.

It should be treated with 2.5% selenium sulfide suspension applied to the entire body at bedtime and rinsed the following morning. Recurrences are common. Topical antifungal agents (clotrimazole, miconazole) can be used for small areas. Systemic antifungal agents (ketoconazole) can be used in severe cases.

18. How does *Candida albicans* look on a potassium hydroxide (KOH) preparation? How about tinea cruris?

Candida has pseudohyphae and budding spores. Tinea cruris has septate hyphae and spores with the appearance of "spaghetti and meatballs."

19. What is the proper technique for a KOH preparation of a skin lesion?

Moisten the involved skin with water and scrape with a sterile number 10 or 15 scalpel. Place the scrapings on a glass slide and add 1–2 drops of 20% KOH and 40% dimethyl sulfoxide (DMSO). Cover the preparation with a coverslip. Examine the slide under the 10× and 40× objectives.

20. Describe the routine follow-up for a patient with diabetes mellitus.

Diabetics should be seen at least semiannually if their glycemic control is stable. If their regimen requires a change, more frequent visits are needed. Individualized goals for glycemic control should be established with the patient. At the visit, obtain historical information regarding the frequency, cause, and severity of hypoglycemic or hyperglycemic episodes; home glucose monitoring records; current medications; other illnesses; lifestyle changes; life stressors; and patient difficulty with compliance with treatment recommendations. Weight and blood pressure, optic fundi, and any symptom-directed organ system should be thoroughly examined. A foot examination is especially important and should include inspection for trauma, callouses, and nail skin conditions; palpation of pedal pulses; and sensory exam. Annual ophthalmologic exams are necessary.

Regular lab tests include glycohemoglobin (Hgb A1C) at least quarterly or as often as needed to establish control. Fasting glucose may provide additional information. Lipid profiles (including fasting total cholesterol, triglycerides, and HDL) should be tested at least annually if abnormal or every 5 years if normal. Additional monitoring may be needed if therapeutic changes are made. An annual urinalysis is recommended, as is a timed urine collection for detection of microalbumin. Diabetics require pneumococcal vaccine (once), influenza vaccine (annually), and tetanus/diphtheria toxoid (every 10 years).

American Diabetes Association: Standards of medical care for patients with diabetes mellitus. Diabetes Care 17:616, 1994.

21. Name the two most frequent causes of mild, asymptomatic hypercalcemia in the ambulatory population.

Thiazide drugs and hyperparathyroidism.

22. What are some of the adverse consequences of obesity?

Obese patients are more likely to have hypertension, diabetes mellitus, and coronary artery disease than patients who are not overweight. Obesity can complicate chronic obstructive pulmonary disease (COPD) and osteoarthritis. Obese patients will have difficulty following a regular exercise program. They may have a depressed mood and poor self-esteem.

23. What should be included in a treatment regimen for a patient with chronic, idiopathic constipation?

1. Regular bowel habits with attempted bowel movements at the same time each day (15–20 minutes after breakfast when the gastrocolic reflex is the strongest).

2. High-fiber diet, including beans (navy, lima, kidney), baked potato with skin, broccoli, peas, corn, apple with peel, oranges, peaches, raspberries, wheat bread, bran cereals.

3. Adequate fluid intake (at least eight 8-oz glasses of water each day).

4. Bulk laxative (psyllium), if needed.

5. Daily exercise.

24. Give causes of chronic constipation.

Causes of Chronic Constipation

Medications	Calcium channel blockers, antihistamines, opiates, iron, antidepressants, aluminum and calcium antacids, and laxatives (if abused)
Endocrine/metabolic	Hypothyroidism, diabetes mellitus, hyperparathyroidism, hypokalemia
Mechanical obstruction	Tumors, strictures
Neurogenic	Spinal cord disease, multiple sclerosis, scleroderma
Rectal disease	Hemorrhoids, anal fissure
Psychological	Major depression, personality disorder
GI disease	Irritable bowel syndrome, diverticular disease
Physical inactivity	Television

25. Describe the office evaluation of a patient having acute diarrhea for < 24 hours.

Most causes of acute diarrhea are infectious, and many are self-limited. The history and physical examination will help guide further evaluation. In the history, inquire about recent travel; food ingestion (particularly raw meats and poultry and custards); exposure to animals or people with similar symptoms; frequency, volume, and appearance of stool; associated symptoms (including fever, abdominal pain, tenesmus, blood in the stool, and skin rash); and current medications. During the physical examination, check the temperature, abdomen, and rectum (including a test for fecal occult blood). The examination should include a check for the presence of orthostatic changes in the BP and pulse and a skin rash.

A patient with few associated symptoms needs no further evaluation unless the diarrhea does not resolve within a week. In a patient with severe systemic symptoms or bloody diarrhea, a search for and treatment of specific pathogens is needed and can best be accomplished by flexible sigmoidoscopy. In addition to directly visualizing the mucosa, samples can be obtained for fecal leukocytes and cultures.

26. Describe the office evaluation of a patient having diarrhea persisting for 2–3 weeks.

Fecal blood and leukocytes should be rechecked and cultures repeated, with a specific request for ova and parasite examination. Sometimes, as many as three specimens are needed for identification of the pathogen. The diagnostic yield can be increased if the examination is done on a fresh stool specimen.

Complete blood count, serum electrolytes, calcium, glucose, liver function tests, and amylase may indicate a systemic illness. Sigmoidoscopy is indicated. In certain patients with evidence of malabsorption such as weight loss, a Sudan stain for fat followed by quantitative 72-hour fecal fat collection will be useful. If no etiology is determined, additional evaluations are needed.

27. What are the symptoms of irritable bowel syndrome (IBS)? How do you treat it?

Because it is the most common GI disease seen in clinical practice, most physicians are all too familiar with IBS. However, its management can be frustrating.

Patients with IBS often complain of diarrhea alternating with constipation for months to years. The stools may contain excessive mucous, but no blood. Frequently audible bowel sounds, left lower quadrant or generalized abdominal pain, and urgency to defecate accompany the diarrhea or constipation. Patients may even describe left arm shoulder pain with the splenic-flexure syndrome. Associated symptoms include anxiety, depression, and signs of vasomotor instability such as palpitations, hyperventilation, sweating, and headaches.

The treatment of IBS includes acknowledgment of the symptoms, identification of and counseling for any underlying psychiatric stress or illness, education about the benign nature of the disorder, and therapy for chronic constipation or diarrhea (increased dietary fiber). Increased physical activity is also beneficial. Short-term limited use of anticholinergic medications is useful in a few patients but should not be the sole therapy.

28. How do you manage an anal fissure?

The patient having an anal fissure usually complains of severe pain with defecation, sometimes associated with bleeding. Most fissures are located in the midline and are visible. Conservative management with warm baths, stool softeners, and bulk laxatives improves the ease of defecation. Drugs that cause constipation should be avoided. If this therapy fails, the patient should be referred for consideration of surgical repair.

29. What is proctalgia fugax?

A fleeting, deep pain in the rectum, probably caused by muscle spasm.

30. Which tests are most useful in determining if an acute hepatitis is viral in etiology?

If one suspects viral hepatitis based on history, physical examination, and elevated liver transaminases, a hepatitis B surface antigen (HBsAg) should be ordered first. If this is negative, an IgM hepatitis B core antibody-IgM (anti-HBc) will pick up additional cases of acute hepatitis B that are antigen-negative. Hepatitis A can be detected through hepatitis A antibody-IgM (IgM anti-HAV). Hepatitis C antibody can be detected through commercially available assays using enzyme-linked immunosorbent assays (ELISA) or polymerase chain reaction (PCR) methods.

31. How do you diagnose cervicitis due to *Chlamydia?*

Chlamydiosis is diagnosed by a variety of immunologic techniques that utilize direct immunofluorescence techniques, ELISA, or PCR. Chlamydial cervicitis is suspected in a sexually active woman when a mucopurulent discharge with cervical erythema, ulceration, and friability (easy bleeding) are seen during speculum examination of the vagina. Chlamydia infections may also be asymptomatic.

32. How should you evaluate a 20-year-old sexually active woman who complains of acute dysuria?

The multiple causes of dysuria include urethritis, cystitis, vaginitis, and cervicitis. A history of sexual activity (particularly with a new partner) may point toward a vaginitis or cervicitis. The history should focus on the presence of hematuria, vaginal discharge, flank pain, fever, and chills. The physical examination should be include temperature, pulse, BP (with orthostatic changes, if symptoms are severe), and bimanual pelvic examination. Any vaginal discharge should be examined microscopically. Appropriate testing for *Neisseria gonorrhoea* and *Chlamydia* should be done if a mucopurulent cervicitis is present. If the history and physical examination suggest acute uncomplicated cystitis, the patient may be empirically treated with trimethoprim-sulfamethoxazole or a fluoroquinolone without urine testing. If she remains symptomatic after 3–7 days of treatment, a urinalysis and urine culture should be done.

33. What are some causes of abnormal vaginal bleeding in a premenopausal woman?

Causes of Premenopausal Abnormal Vaginal Bleeding

Dysfunctional uterine bleeding	Idiopathic, Stein-Leventhal syndrome
Pregnancy	Threatened or complete abortion, ectopic pregnancy
Medical conditions	Thrombocytopenia, hypothyroidism, bleeding diathesis
Medications	Anticoagulants, oral contraceptives
Anatomic causes	
Perineal	Bladder pathology, hemorrhoids
Vulvar	Infection, laceration, tumor
Vaginal	Infection, laceration, tumor, foreign body
Cervical	Infection, erosion, polyp, carcinoma
Uterine	Infection, polyp, leiomyomata, carcinoma, intrauterine device
Ovarian	Infection

34. How do you manage a woman with postmenopausal vaginal bleeding?

The woman should be referred to a gynecologist for consideration of a dilatation and currettage (D&C) of the uterus to detect endometrial carcinoma.

35. Describe the characteristic vaginal discharges caused by *Candida albicans, Neisseria gonorrhoeae, Gardnerella vaginalis,* and *Trichomonas vaginalis.*

Causative Organisms and Characteristics of Vaginal Discharges

ORGANISM	DISCHARGE CHARACTERISTICS
C. albicans	Thick, white, curdlike, adherent to vaginal wall with erythema or perineal satellite lesions
N. gonorrhoeae	Mucopurulent with cervicitis
G. vaginalis	Foul-smelling ("fishy" odor with KOH), thin, scanty, nonpruritic, adherent to vaginal wall
T. vaginalis	Copious, yellow-green, frothy

36. What are clue cells?

Clue cells are seen in the discharge of vaginal infections caused by *Gardnerella vaginalis.* Microscopically, they appear on a wet mount of vaginal secretions as epithelial cells covered with coccobacilli or curved rods.

37. What advice should you give a woman taking combination oral contraceptives who missed a pill?

She should take the missed pill as soon as she is aware of the missed dose, then continue the remainder of her pills as scheduled. After a missed pill, it is prudent to use additional barrier contraception until the next menses to prevent pregnancy.

38. What are the absolute contraindications to oral contraceptive use?

Pregnancy

Hepatic adenomas

Estrogen-dependent neoplasms

Cardiovascular disease

Severely impaired liver function

Breast carcinoma

Thromboembolic disease

39. How would you evaluate a new breast nodule discovered during a routine physical examination of a woman?

The nodule's characteristics (size, firmness, mobility) are not predictive of the likelihood of malignancy. If multiple, cystic nodules are present and the woman is premenopausal, she should be followed through several menses for any changes in the nodule. Any solitary nodule requires referral for biopsy. A mammogram may be useful for localization of the nodule, but a normal mammogram should not preclude the need for biopsy of a solitary nodule.

40. Is there a proven, validated drug therapy for premenstrual syndrome (PMS)?

Although many agents have been used in the management of PMS (including antidepressants, bromocriptine, danazol, evening primrose oil, spironolactone, progesterone, and prostaglandin synthetase inhibitors), there is as yet no scientifically proven therapy. The selective serotonin-reuptake-inhibiting antidepressants may hold some promise for future use.

41. What are some pharmacologic therapies for osteoporosis?

Adequate calcium intake is a necessary treatment for osteoporosis, either through the diet or as nutritional supplement. Two Tums 3 times a day are sufficient. In addition, estrogen, bisphosphonates (etidronate, pamidronate, alendronate), salmon calcitonin (now available as nasal spray), and slow-release sodium fluoride can be useful in combination with calcium.

New drugs for osteoporosis. Med Let 38:1, 1996.

42. What are the clinical symptoms of influenza?

Influenza typically presents with the sudden onset of high fever, malaise, myalgia, coryza, headache, and sore throat. There may be GI symptoms (nausea, vomiting, diarrhea). With complications, symptoms of pneumonia, encephalitis, hepatitis, pancreatitis, or myositis may develop.

43. How do you differentiate influenza from other acute respiratory illnesses?

It is difficult to distinguish influenza on clinical grounds alone. Although a patient presenting with characteristic symptoms during an outbreak of influenza in the winter months most probably has the disease, laboratory diagnosis is the only way to be certain and can be made during acute illness from sputum samples, a throat swab, or nasopharyngeal washes.

Streptococcal pharyngitis and early bacterial pneumonia can resemble influenza. Unlike influenza, bacterial pneumonia is generally not self-limited. Streptococcal pharyngitis can be identified through commercially available rapid antigen detection kits or throat culture.

44. Who should receive the influenza vaccine?

Vaccination with inactivated, trivalent influenza virus vaccine is recommended annually for the following groups:

1. Individuals at increased risk for the complications of influenza virus infection (including death, influenza pneumonia, and secondary bacterial pneumonia):

    a. Adults and children with chronic pulmonary or cardiovascular illnesses (including asthma)

    b. Residents of nursing homes or other chronic care facilities with any chronic medical condition

    c. Adults 65 years of age and older

    d. Adults or children with chronic medical conditions requiring regular medical follow-up or hospitalization during the preceding year (including diabetes mellitus, renal dysfunction, hemoglobinopathies, or immunosuppression)

    e. Children and teenagers (aged 6 months to 18 years) who are receiving long-term aspirin therapy and are therefore at increased risk for developing Reye's syndrome after an influenza infection

2. Individuals capable of transmitting influenza to high-risk persons:

    a. Physicians, nurses, students, and other personnel in both inpatient and outpatient settings who have extensive contact with high-risk patients in all age groups

    b. Providers of home care to high-risk patients

    c. Household members (including children) of high-risk persons

3. Other groups:

    a. Anyone, especially those providing essential services, who wishes to reduce his or her chance of acquiring influenza infection

    b. All HIV-infected persons

    c. Persons embarking on foreign travel during their destination's influenza season

ACP Task Force on Adult Immunization: Guide for Adult Immunization, 3rd ed. Philadelphia, American College of Physicians, 1994.

45. When is amantadine or rimantadine indicated in influenza management?

Amantadine and rimantadine may be used for prophylaxis and treatment of influenza A but are not effective against influenza B. Prophylactic use is indicated during influenza epidemics for high-risk patients who have not been immunized or have contraindications to vaccination. Both agents are given at dosages of 200 mg/day and should be continued throughout the epidemic. If a person is immunized during an outbreak, amantadine or rimantadine should be continued for 2 weeks after immunization, at which time adequate antibody should have developed.

If used for influenza A treatment, amantadine or rimantadine must be started within 48 hours of the onset of symptoms. Rimantadine causes fewer side effects. The usual dosage is 200 mg/day of each but should be reduced to 100 mg/day for elderly patients or those with an renal insufficiency.

46. When are combined tetanus/diphtheria toxoid (Td) and tetanus immune globulin (TIG) indicated in wound management?

If a patient does not have a definite history of receipt of at least 3 previous doses of Td, TIG should be given also if the wound is contaminated with dirt, feces, or saliva or results from puncture or sharp object penetration, frostbite, or burn.

47. What organisms commonly cause nongonoccal urethritis in men?

Chlamydia trachomatis and *Ureaplasma urealyticum.*

48. What organisms commonly cause epididymitis?

Chlamydia trachomatis, Neisseria gonorrohoeae, and Gram-negative rods. Rarely, mumps can cause epididymitis, as can fungal and tubercular infections. Appropriate antimicrobial therapy will be guided by cultures.

49. How do you differentiate acute epididymitis from testicular torsion?

Differentiation of Epididymitis and Torsion

	EPIDIDYMITIS	TORSION
Age	Older	Prepubertal
Pyuria	+	−
Bacteriuria	+	−
Urethritis symptoms	+	−
Physical exam	Palpable epididymis	Firm, tender mass

50. What are the symptoms of atypical pneumonia? What are its causes?

The cough of atypical pneumonia is usually dry. A prodrome of headache and myalgias is frequently found. The chest radiograph has a diffuse infiltrate and typically "looks worse" than the patient. Common causes of the atypical pneumonia syndrome include *Mycoplasma pneumoniae,* viruses (influenza A and B, adenovirus, respiratory syncytial, and parainfluenza), *Chlamydia psittaci* (psittacosis), *Chlamydia pneumoniae* (TWAR strain), rickettsia (Q fever), fungi (histoplasmosis, coccidioidomycosis), and *Pneumocystis carinii.*

51. What are the prodromal symptoms of herpes zoster (shingles)?

Before the vesicles appear, infected individuals experience headache and malaise. Pain and paresthesia may be felt in the involved dermatomes. If the involved dermatome is on the anterior chest wall, the pain may be confused with anginal or MI pain.

52. How can the history and physical examination predict if acute pharyngitis in an adult is due to streptococcal infection?

The presence of fever, pharyngeal and tonsillar exudates, and cervical lymphadenopathy are suggestive of streptococcal pharyngitis but can also occur with viral illness.

53. Who should receive measles vaccine?

Adults born after 1956 should receive primary immunization of live measles vaccine if adequate documentation of live virus vaccination or physician-diagnosed measles is unavailable. Adults born after 1956 should be revaccinated if they work in health care fields where exposure to measles is likely, will travel to an endemic area, or are entering a secondary educational institution. College entry or beginning of employment in a medically related field are important times to ensure completion of both vaccine doses. Measles vaccine can be preferably given in the combined form of measles-mumps-rubella (MMR).

ACP Task Force on Adult Immunization: Guide for Adult Immunization, 3rd ed. Philadelphia, American College of Physicians, 1994.

54. What form of polio vaccine should be given to adults?

An injection of inactivated polio vaccine. Adults have a slightly increased risk of developing paralysis from the live-virus oral polio vaccine.

55. What are some frequent causes of meralgia paresthetica?

Meralgia paresthetica is caused by localized entrapment of the lateral femoral cutaneous nerve that produces pain over the anterolateral thigh. It may occur with diabetes mellitus and pregnancy (during the final weeks of gestation) or during sudden weight loss or gain. Tight girdles, gun belts, and other accessories have been implicated.

56. What are the typical symptoms of a migraine headache? Tension headache? Cluster headache?

Typical Headache Symptoms

SYMPTOM	CLUSTER	MIGRAINE	TENSION
Location	Unilateral	Hemicranial	Entire head or bitemporal
Quality of pain	Burning	Throbbing	Pressure-like ache, tightness
Duration	1–2 hrs	2–6 hrs	Days
Frequency	Flurry of frequent attacks for several weeks	Episodic	Daily
Associated symptoms	Ipsilateral sweating, flushing, lacrimation, and rhinorrhea	Prodrome (scotoma, paresthesia, confusion or behavioral changes)	Neck and shoulder ache

57. What are the symptoms of a transient ischemic attack (TIA) in the anterior (carotid) distribution? Posterior (vertebrobasilar) distribution?

ANTERIOR	POSTERIOR
Transient paresis of face and/or arm	Transient global amnesia
Paresthesia	Ataxia
Aphasia	Dysarthria
Amaurosis fugax (sudden loss of vision in eye)	Weakness, dizziness
Homonymous hemianopia	Hearing loss

58. What is the triad of symptoms of Meniere's syndrome?

Paroxysmal vertigo, hearing loss, and tinnitus. It may be accompanied by nausea and vomiting.

59. What are the leading causes of acute impairment or loss of the sense of smell?

Head trauma, especially in children and active young adults, and viral infections, especially in older adults.

60. What are the characteristics of bacterial conjunctivitis? Viral conjunctivitis? Allergic conjunctivitis?

Characteristics of Conjunctivitis

CHARACTERISTIC	BACTERIAL	VIRAL	ALLERGIC
Foreign body sensation	−	±	±
Itching	±	±	++
Tearing	+	++	+
Discharge	Mucopurulent	Mucoid	−
Preauricular adenopathy	−	+	−

61. What is a wrist ganglion? How is it treated?

The ganglion is the most common tumor of the hand and wrist and occurs more frequently in women. The most common site is the dorsum of the wrist between the extensor tendons of the thumb and index finger. Most do not require treatment, but aspiration and/or corticosteroid injection may be useful. If the ganglion recurs after treatment, surgical excision may be necessary.

62. How do you treat a coccygeal fracture?

A coccygeal fracture is treated conservatively with analgesia and use of an inflatable "donut" cushion when sitting. It most often results from a direct blow, usually a fall onto the buttocks.

63. What is Phalen's maneuver? Tinel's sign?

In carpal tunnel syndrome, forced flexion or hyperextension of the wrist (Phalen's maneuver) reproduces the symptoms of pain and paresthesia as well as numbness in the palm and first three or four fingers. In Tinel's sign the symptoms are reproduced when the median nerve is tapped lightly over the wrist.

64. What should be included in the examination of a patient complaining of a "sprained ankle?"
The history should include the details of the injury, particularly whether or not the ankle was inverted or a tearing sensation was felt. The initial exam should check for tenderness along the anterior talofibular ligament (located slightly anterior to the lateral malleolus), fibulocalcaneal ligament (immediately below the lateral malleolus), and the posterior talofibular ligament (posterior to the lateral malleolus). The latter two structures are tender usually only in more severe strains. The degree of swelling should be noted. If ecchymosis is present, there is at least a second-degree injury.

Ankle stability is tested by the anterior drawer sign. With the patient relaxed, the lower leg is grabbed anteriorly, firmly with one hand. The heel and calcaneus are grasped with the other, and the foot is pulled forward. The ankle should be held in 20° flexion. The examiner notes how far the ankle can be moved in comparison to the uninvolved ankle. Foot strength, sensation, and blood flow are noted. An x-ray is needed in almost all strains to check for a fracture.

65. What is a second-degree ankle sprain? How is it treated?
In a second-degree ankle sprain, a portion of a ligament is torn without complete disruption. On exam, there is ecchymosis and slight asymmetry between the involved and uninvolved ankle on the anterior drawer sign. It is treated with elevation, bulky dressing or elastic bandage, and ice packs for 20 minutes every 3–4 hours for 2–3 days. The patient should avoid any weight-bearing and use crutches. He or she can begin plantar- and dorsiflexion exercises after 48 hours. Weight-bearing can be allowed after 5–10 days if the pain and swelling are decreased.

66. Where are the locations of muscle weakness, sensory loss, and reflex absence associated with an L4 root compression?

Associated Findings with Root Compressions

ROOT	DISC	MUSCULAR	SENSORY	REFLEX
L4	L3–4	Leg extensors (quadriceps)	Anterolateral thigh, medial lower leg	Patellar
L5	L4–5	Large toe dorsiflexion (extensor hallucis longus), heel walking (tibialis anterior)	Dorsum of foot	None
S1	L5–S1	Toe walking (gastrocnemius)	Lateral foot and 5th toe	Ankle

67. Which toe fractures should be referred to an orthopedist?
Fractures of the proximal phalanx of the first toe. If a fracture involves the distal phalanx and extends into the interphalangeal joint, this should also be referred.

68. Describe the physical examination findings seen in a patient with a rotator cuff tendinitis.
With rotator cuff tendinitis, there is subacromial tenderness and pain on passive elevation (usually to a certain point). Specific findings include:
- Positive impingement signs
- Rotator cuff and biceps weakness
- Positive supraspinatus test
- Pain with abduction from 70°-to 120° (painful arc)
- May be atrophy of shoulder muscles—compare to opposite side
- May be tender over corocoacromial ligament

Julian MJ, Mathews M: Shoulder injuries. In Mellion MG: The Team Physician's Handbook. Philadelphia, Hanley & Belfus, 1990, p 326.

69. How do you manage a patient with lumbosacral strain?
Patients with acute back strain should remain at strict bedrest on a firm mattress or a hard floor for at least 2 days. If needed, a bed board may be inserted between the mattress and box spring. Controlled physical activity after 2 days of rest will aid in recovery, and prolonged bedrest is discouraged. Ice or dry or moist heat (depending on patient's preference) for 20 minutes 3–4 times a day may be beneficial. NSAIDs are most useful for pain control. If significant muscle spasm is found on physical examination, muscle relaxants such as cyclobenzaprine are useful.

70. What is Reiter's syndrome?
Reiter's syndrome is common in young, white men and produces arthritis of the lower extremities (knees, ankles, small joints of the feet). Accompanying symptoms include urethritis (dysuria with mucopurulent penile discharge) and mild conjunctivitis. There may also be plantar fasciitis (heel pain), diffuse swelling of the toes (sausage digits), shallow painless oral ulcers or penile lesions, and onychodystrophy (crumbling of the nails). The characteristic skin rash is called **keratoderma blennorrhagica** and appears as discrete papules. The illness may develop after an acute, diarrheal illness.

71. What conditions may present as chronic fatigue?

Conditions Causing Chronic Fatigue

Psychologic	Depression, anxiety, somatization disorders
Endocrine-metabolic	Hypothyroidism, diabetes mellitus, apathetic hyperthyroidism of the elderly, pituitary insufficiency, hyperparathyroidism or hypercalcemia of any origin, Addison's disease, chronic renal failure, hepatocellular failure
Pharmacologic	Hypnotics, antihypertensives, antidepressants, tranquilizers, drug abuse and withdrawal
Infectious	Endocarditis, tuberculosis, infectious mononucleosis, hepatitis, parasitic disease, chronic Epstein-Barr virus infection, cytomegalovirus, HIV infection
Neoplastic	Occult malignancy
Hematologic	Severe anemia
Cardiopulmonary	Chronic congestive heart failure, chronic obstructive pulmonary disease
Connective tissue disorders	Rheumatoid arthritis, chronic fatigue syndrome, fibromyalgia
Sleep disturbances	Sleep apnea, esophageal reflux, allergic rhinitis

Goroll AH, May LA, Mulley HG: Primary Care Medicine: Office Evaluation and Management of the Adult Patient, 3rd ed. Philadelphia, J.B. Lippincott, 1995, p 34.

72. To which clinical syndrome does "hayfever" refer?
Seasonal allergic rhinitis, which incidentally is not specifically caused by hay or associated with fever. This perennial rhinitis has symptoms of sneezing, nasal passage obstruction, rhinorrhea, itching, and lacrimation. It is brought on by airborne pollens being trapped in the nasal folds, with digestion of the outer coat by mucosal enzymes and release of protein allergen. There is usually a family history of similar allergic conditions. Vasomotor rhinitis is a kindred symptom complex without a known allergic basis.

73. What is Tietze's syndrome?
A mild inflammation of the costochondral junction that produces localized warmth, swelling, erythema, and pain. The symptoms are reproduced by palpation of the involved area.

74. What are the diagnostic criteria for major depression?
At least 5 of the following symptoms must have been present nearly every day for 2 weeks:
1. Depressed mood most of the day
2. Markedly diminished interest or pleasure in nearly all activities
3. Weight loss or gain (> 5% of body weight in a month) or decrease or increase in appetite
4. Insomnia or hypersomnia

5. Psychomotor agitation or retardation
6. Fatigue or loss of energy
7. Feelings of worthlessness or inappropriate guilt
8. Decreased ability to think or concentrate
9. Recurrent thoughts of death, suicidal ideation, or suicide attempt

American Psychiatric Association: Diagnostic and Statistical Manual of Mental Disorders, 4th ed. Washington, DC, APA, 1994, pp 237.

75. Which medical illnesses can cause depression?

Medical Illnesses Causing a Depressed Mood

Endocrine	Hyperthyroidism, hypothyroidism, Cushing's syndrome, Addison's disease, hypercalcemia, hyperparathyroidism
Rheumatic	Rheumatoid arthritis, systemic lupus erythematosus, fibromyalgia
Neurologic	Temporal lobe epilepsy, chronic hematoma, cerebrovascular accident, multiple sclerosis, frontal lobe tumor, Alzheimer's dementia
Infectious	Hepatitis, infectious mononucleosis
Nutritional	Vitamin B_{12} deficiency
Toxic	Alcoholism, drug withdrawal

76. Which antidepressants are sedating?

Sedative Potency of Antidepressants

DRUG	SEDATION	DRUG	SEDATION
Amitriptyline	Marked	Nefazodone	Mild
Desipramine	Mild	Bupropion	None
Doxepin	Marked	Fluoxetine	None
Imipramine	Moderate	Paroxetine	None
Nortriptyline	Mild	Sertraline	None
Trazodone	Marked	Venlafaxine	Mild

Depression Guideline Panel: Depression in Primary Care: Vol 2. Treatment of Major Depression, Clinical Practice Guideline, Number 5. Rockville, MD, Agency for Health Care Policy and Research, April 1993. [AHCPR publ no. 93–0551.]

77. Which antidepressant causes priapism?
Trazodone (Desyrel).

78. What is agoraphobia? How is it treated?
Agoraphobia is the fear of being in public places. The patient with agoraphobia may live a reclusive life. It is usually first seen in women in their late teens or early 20s and may be associated with panic attacks. During panic attacks, the patient will have at least four of the following symptoms, in addition to apprehension or fear: dyspnea, palpitations, chest discomfort, choking sensation, dizziness, feelings of unreality, paresthesia, hot and cold flashes, sweating, faintness, trembling, or fear of dying or going crazy. Severe agoraphobia is best treated in consultation with a therapist skilled in behavioral therapies such as desensitization. If the patient has panic attacks without the avoidant behavior (panic disorder), a selective-serotonergic reuptake-inhibiting antidepressant (sertraline, paroxetine, or fluoxetine), alprazolam, or imipramine may be useful.

American Psychiatric Association: Diagnostic and Statistical Manual, 4th ed. Washington, DC, APA, 1994.

79. What is the hyperkinetic heart syndrome?
This is a syndrome found in asymptomatic young males who present with increased cardiac output of no discernible cause. They usually seek medical attention because of palpitations, tachy-

cardia, and atypical chest pain. The diagnosis is uncertain and has been variously listed as neurasthenia, anxiety neurosis, DaCosta syndrome, effort syndrome, and soldier's heart.

80. List some of the organic causes of impotence.

Organic Causes of Impotence

Endocrine	Primary testicular failure, hypothalamic disease, diabetes mellitus, acromegaly, adrenal or pituitary adenomas, chromophobe adenoma, hypothyroidism, hyperthyroidism
Urologic	Peyronie's disease, prostatitis, phimosis, priapism
Neurologic	Autonomic peripheral neuropathy (including diabetic), amyotrophic lateral sclerosis, spinal cord tumors or transection, multiple sclerosis, tabes dorsalis
Vascular	Cardiorespiratory, athero-obstructive, aortoiliac disease, aneurysm, arteritis, cardiomyopathy, coronary insufficiency, chronic obstructive pulmonary disease
Hematologic	Hodgkin's disease, leukemia, chronic sickle cell anemia
Toxic	Lead, herbicides, alcohol
Infectious	Genital tuberculosis
Organ failure	Cirrhosis, chronic renal failure
Surgical	Aortoiliac surgery, radical pelvic surgery, postprostatectomy
Medications	Benzodiazepine, antidepressants, major tranquilizers, antihypertensive agents

Gottfried LA, Richie JP: Sexual problems. In Branch WT Jr (ed): Office Practice of Medicine, 2nd ed. Philadelphia, W.B. Saunders, 1987, p 1410.

81. What are some of the early signs and symptoms of anorexia nervosa?

Anorexia nervosa should be suspected in an adolescent female with amenorrhea, weight loss, and a distorted body image (feeling "fat" in the face of emaciation). It can occur in women in their 30s.

82. What are the risk factors for suicide?

1. Male sex
2. Single or widowed marital status
3. Unemployment
4. Social isolation
5. Urban area residence
6. Recent loss of health or surgery
7. History of impulsive behavior or suicide attempts
8. Presence of chronic pain syndrome, major depression, psychosis, alcoholism, substance abuse, organic brain syndrome, or chronic illness
9. Family history of suicide

83. What is an anniversary reaction?

A bereaved patient will frequently experience a depressed mood or somatic symptoms on the anniversary of the death of a close friend or relative. An anniversary reaction can occur after any significant loss, such as job loss, amputation of a limb, or divorce.

84. How do you make the diagnosis of alcoholism?

Alcoholism is persistent, heavy drinking that interferes with the person's health, interpersonal relationships, position in society, or means of livelihood. It is the consequences of drinking that define alcoholism. Internists and family physicians often miss, or choose to ignore, the diagnosis of alcoholism in the patients they treat. Unfortunately, this avoidance behavior interferes with the physician's ability to get at the real cause for some common presenting complaints, such as insomnia, nonspecific GI symptoms, and depression. It also makes the doctor an unwitting accomplice in the patient's destructive behavior.

One rapid, simple, and reliable screening test for alcoholism is the **CAGE test.** A positive answer to at least 2 of the questions warrants an in-depth review of drinking habits.

C—Have you ever felt the need to **cut** down on drinking?
A—Have you ever felt **annoyed** by criticism of your drinking?
G—Have you ever felt **guilty** about your drinking?
E—Have you ever taken a morning **eye-opener?**

Johnson B, Clark W: Alcoholism: A challenging physician-patient encounter. J Gen Intern Med 4:445–452, 1989.

85. How is the nicotine patch used in smoking cessation?

The nicotine patch should be used by patients who have already stopped smoking to maintain smoking cessation. The nicotine patch should not be used for a patient who continues to smoke.

Typically, an initial dose of 14–21 mg/day of nicotine is used, depending on the previous cigarette use. After 4–6 weeks of initial therapy, the dose is decreased and eventually discontinued. Nicotine substitution therapy is usually ineffective unless combined with behavioral therapy.

86. What is the differential diagnosis of chronic cough?

Differential Diagnosis of Chronic Cough

Environmental irritants	Cigarette smoking, pollutants, dusts, lack of humidity
Lower respiratory tract problems	Lung cancer, asthma, COPD, interstitial lung disease, congestive heart failure, pneumonitis, bronchiectasis
Upper respiratory tract problems	Chronic rhinitis, chronic sinusitis, disease of the external auditory canal, pharyngitis
Extrinsic compressions	Adenopathy, malignancy, aortic lesions, aneurysm
GI problems	Reflux esophagitis
Psychogenic factors	—

Adapted from: Goroll AH, et al: Primary Care Medicine: Office Evaluation and Management of the Adult Patient, 3rd ed. Philadelphia, J.B. Lippincott, 1994, p 233.

87. What are the health consequences of smoking?

Smoking is associated with increased morbidity and mortality from COPD, malignancy (including lung cancer), and cardiovascular disease. Smokers also have an increased incidence of recurrent respiratory infections, peptic ulcer disease, cerebrovascular disease, sudden death, death from abdominal aortic aneurysm, and graft occlusion after lower extremity vascular reconstruction. The overall morbidity and mortality among smokers after any type of surgery are also increased.

88. What is the characteristic history of most patients with occupationally related asthma?

The history reveals a cyclical pattern of:
(1) Wellness upon arrival at work
(2) Symptoms appearing toward the end of the shift period
(3) Symptoms increasing in severity for a period of time after departing from the worksite
(4) Symptoms gradually regressing over time away from the worksite.
Holidays and weekends are free from asthma.

89. Describe the findings of acute arterial occlusion?

With acute peripheral arterial occlusion, the patient complains of the sudden onset of severe pain. In some patients there may be a more insidious onset over several hours. The patient may also complain of numbness, paresthesia, and muscle weakness or paralysis. On exam, the involved limb is pale and cold with no pulses distal to the occlusion.

90. How does arterial insufficiency typically present?

The patients are frequently elderly and have a history of smoking. The typical symptoms include pain or muscle tightness in the calf predictably reproduced after a certain amount of exercise. The pain or tightness is relieved by rest. Other symptoms include numbness and paresthesia. With progressive disease, the patient may develop ulcerations of the feet and pain developing at rest. Patients also describe pain awakening them from sleep, relieved by dangling the feet over the bed.

91. What should be included in a foot care plan for a patient with arterial insufficiency?

1. Inspect both feet daily, particularly the soles, for trauma.
2. Wash daily with lukewarm water (test the water temperature with the hand or elbow prior to immersing the feet).
3. Avoid prolonged soaking.
4. Use a moisturizing cream daily.
5. Use an antifungal powder as needed.
6. Place lamb's wool between the toes at areas of pressure.
7. Cut toenails straight across.
8. Wear properly fitting shoes at all times.
9. Treat corns and calluses with physician supervision.
10. Avoid trauma.

92. When would you refer a patient with claudication for surgery?

Patients with rest pain, nonhealing distal ulcers, or early gangrene should be referred for surgical evaluation. Patients with disabling symptoms that interfere with their lifestyle should be referred. Counsel all patients with claudication to stop smoking.

93. What are the physical findings of deep venous thrombosis (DVT)? How sensitive are these findings?

One may find unilateral swelling, warmth, pitting edema, or engorged superficial veins in the involved extremity. The patient may complain of aching pain. The occurrence of DVT, particularly in the postoperative period, may be asymptomatic. The physical findings may be present in as few as 50% of the cases. Although frequently cited as a sign of DVT, Homan's sign (calf pain with forced dorsiflexion) is not useful. There may be a palpable cord.

94. What are the characteristics of an ulcer due to venous stasis disease?

A venous stasis ulcer is usually pigmented with hemosiderin and is located on the medial leg.

95. What is an advanced directive?

An advanced directive is a person's written or oral statement that indicates his or her treatment preferences for end-of-life therapies. A **living will** is an example of an advanced directive. Living wills typically state that a person does not want life-sustaining treatments such as artificial ventilation or resuscitation started or continued if he or she has a terminal illness without effective treatments.

BIBLIOGRAPHY

1. ACP Task Force on Adult Immunization: Guide for Adult Immunization, 3rd ed. Philadelphia, American College of Physicians, 1994.
2. Barker LR, Burton JR, Zieve PD: Principles of Ambulatory Medicine, 4th ed. Baltimore, Williams & Wilkins, 1995.
3. Branch WT Jr: Office Practice of Medicine, 3rd ed. Philadelphia, W.B. Saunders, 1994.
4. Dale DC, Federman DD: Scientific American Medicine. New York, Scientific American Inc., 1994.
5. Goroll AH, May LA, Mulley AC (eds): Primary Care Medicine: Office Evaluation and Management of the Adult Patient, 3rd ed. Philadelphia, J.B. Lippincott, 1995.
6. Mladenovic J: Primary Care Secrets. Philadelphia, Hanley & Belfus, 1995.

17. GERIATRIC CARE

George E. Taffet, M.D.

> *But when old age has silver'd o'er thy head,*
> *When memory fails, and all thy vigour's fled,*
> *Then may'st thou seek the stillness of retreat,*
> *Then hear aloof the human tempest beat,*
> *Then will I greet thee to my woodland cave,*
> *Allay the pangs of age, and smooth thy grave.*
>
> James Grainger (1723–1767)
> *Solitude*

GENERAL TOPICS

1. Two things can increase the maximum lifespan of animals. What are they?

Caloric restriction can increase the maximum lifespan of rodents by over 50%. These animals are fed approx. two-thirds of their ad-lib diet, and proper nutrition is ensured. On this diet, mice will live 4 or more years longer than animals on a normal diet.

The second method of life prolongation will not work for warm-blooded animals. However, in cold-blooded animals, simply **decreasing the environmental temperature** will increase the maximum lifespan.

2. Are there any organs in the human body that normally "fold up shop" as we age?

A few organs appear to have programmed death. The **ovaries** in women seem to have a predetermined rate of follicle production that ends with menopause. The **thymus** is also essentially gone by age 65 in both sexes. The involution of the thymus starts after puberty and is progressive thereafter. The importance of the thymus in maintaining immune function has prompted many to suggest that aging is primarily a loss of immunocompetence.

3. Discuss the three major theories of aging.

1. **Cellular theory:** Proposes that genetic instability (such as accumulated errors in DNA replication) and progressive cellular damage (from both internal and environmental factors) cause the aging process.

2. **Autoimmune theory:** Proposes that aging is the result of progressive "self-destruction" through autoimmune mechanisms. This process may be mediated by genetic, environmental, endocrine, or other factors.

3. **Neuroendocrine theory:** Proposes that changes in the neural and endocrine systems cause aging. These changes may lead to the development of diseases that limit lifespan (cancers, atherosclerotic cardiovascular diseases, etc.).

4. What is the rate at which most organ systems age?

Most changes seen in organ system function in the aged occur as the result of a gradual loss over the course of a person's life. The "1% rule" expresses the generalized rate of decline. Most organ systems lose approx. 1% of their functional capacity per year after age 30.

5. What overall changes in human morphology are associated with aging?

↓ height (stooped posture secondary to ↑ kyphosis)
↓ weight
↑ fat-to-lean body-mass ratio
↓ total body water

6. Name some organ-specific changes in human morphology and function associated with aging.

Organ-specific Changes Associated with Aging

SYSTEM	MORPHOLOGY	FUNCTION
Skin	↑ wrinkling Atrophy of sweat glands	—
Cardiovascular	Elongation and tortuosity of arteries ↓ maximum cardiac output ↑ intimal thickening of arteries ↑ fibrosis of the media of arteries ↓ rate of cardiac hypertrophy Sclerosis of heart valves	↓ maximum cardiac output ↓ heart rate response to stress ↓ compliance of peripheral blood vessels
Kidney	↑ number of abnormal glomeruli	↓ creatinine clearance ↓ renal blood flow ↓ maximum urine osmolarity
Lung	↓ elasticity ↓ cilia activity	↓ vital capacity ↓ maximal O_2 uptake ↓ cough reflex
GI tract	↓ hydrochloric acid ↓ saliva flow ↓ number of taste buds	—
Bones	Osteoarthritis Loss of bone substance	—
Eyes	Arcus senilis ↓ pupil size Growth of lens	↓ accommodation Hyperopia ↓ visual acuity ↓ color perception ↓ depth perception
Hearing	Degenerative changes of the ossicles ↑ obstruction of eustachian tube Atrophy of external auditory meatus Atrophy of cochlear hair cells Loss of auditory neurons	↓ high-frequency perception ↓ pitch discrimination
Immune	—	↓ T-cell function
Nervous	↓ brain weight ↓ cortical cell count	↑ motor response time Slower psychomotor performance ↓ complex learning ↓ hours of sleep ↓ hours of REM sleep
Endocrine	↓ free testosterone ↑ insulin ↑ norepinephrine ↑ parathyroid hormone (PTH) ↑ vasopressin	—

From Kane RL, et al: Essentials of Clinical Geriatrics, 2nd ed. New York, McGraw-Hill, 1989, p 7, with permission.

7. Older people often complain of dry mouth (xerostomia). What happens to the rate of saliva production with increasing age?

As tested using a maximal stimulus (10% citric acid), the production of saliva by the parotid glands decreases little with age in normal elders. In contrast, the submandibular glands appear to decrease their maximum function with increasing age, resulting in a decrease in total saliva production. Many drugs commonly used in the elderly have anticholinergic side effects that result in dry mouth.

Wu AJ, et al: Extended stimulated parotid and submandibular secretion in a healthy young and old population. J Gerontol 50A:M45–M48, 1995.

8. What is the most common "ailment" self-reported in people over age 65 years? How many report it?

Arthritis	53%
Hypertension	42%
Hearing impairments	40%
Heart conditions	34%
Visual impairment	23%

9. What percentage of persons over age 65 are fully independent in activities of daily living (ADLs)?

The ADLs consist of bathing, toileting, dressing, walking, and eating. Despite the prevalent image of dependent, frail old people, >90% of people over age 65 do not require any assistance in performing their ADLs.

10. What changes are seen on a glucose tolerance test in older patients? Why?

Fasting glucose changes very little with increasing age, perhaps 1 mg/dl for each decade over age 30. The impairment in glucose tolerance is much larger. At 1 and 2 hours after the challenge meal (usually 100 gm of glucose), the plasma glucose increases 5–6 mg/dl for each decade above 30. The same impairment is seen with a standard meal. If the normal 30-year-old has a 2-hour postprandial glucose of 140 mg/dl, then the normal 70-year-old might reach 160 or more (diabetic by some criteria). Insulin release is delayed, and its maximum serum concentration is higher in the elderly. Insulin resistance at the tissue level is thought to be a predominant mechanism in the impaired glucose tolerance of the elderly, and this may be explained by increased fat mass in the older person.

Cefalu WT, et al: Contribution of visceral fat mass to the insulin resistance of aging. Metab Clin Exp 44:954–959, 1995.

11. Do men over age 80 still have intercourse?

A recent survey of healthy men aged 80–102 revealed that 63% were having sexual intercourse at least several times a year. For women, the percentage was only 30%. This may be a reflection of the much higher numbers of women alive in these age groups (six women for each man). The point is that the male climacteric (age-related hypogonadal state) is an unusual phenomenon.

12. Why are older people more prone to accidental hypothermia?

More than half of patients hospitalized with accidental hypothermia are over age 65. This is due in part to the impairment in temperature regulation that is seen in normal elderly people. The "thermostat" within the hypothalamus is less responsive to changes in both skin temperature and core temperature in the elderly and therefore signals shivering to begin at a lower temperature. However, shivering in the elderly appears to generate normal amounts of heat. The loss of subcutaneous tissue with aging produces a loss of insulation, leading to more rapid loss or gain of heat. The basal metabolic rate of the older person is lower than in the young, so there is less heat to conserve in the first place. Finally, the older person has a reduced drive to micro-acclimatize (put on warm clothing) when the surroundings are cold. All of these small changes (especially in the presence of impaired cognition or sedative medications) add up to a large risk of accidental hypothermia.

13. How does the body composition change as we age from 25–75? Does gender make a difference?

There is a marked increase in fat mass and corresponding decrease in lean body mass that accompany normal aging in men. For women, the changes are less dramatic, since they have significantly more fat mass throughout life.

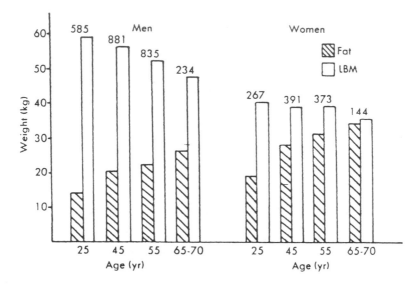

Changes in lean body mass (LBM) and fat content as a function of age in men and women. Number of subjects at each age is shown above bar graphs. (From Conrad KA, Bressler R: Drug Therapy for the Elderly. St. Louis, Mosby, 1982, p 44; with permission.)

14. How do the age-associated changes in body composition affect drug pharmacokinetics?

There is more fat and less muscle (water volume) in which the drug can distribute. Water-soluble drugs may have higher concentrations due to this decreased volume of distribution. Highly fat-soluble drugs may have lower concentrations at effector sites in the elderly. Furthermore, these drugs are stored in body fat, which then acts as a depot when therapy is discontinued, prolonging the time for drugs to "wash out."

15. Hepatic metabolism of drugs has three components that determine handling. What are they and how are they affected by aging?

There are three important determinants of hepatic metabolism of drugs: (1) hepatic blood flow, (2) phase I reactions, and (3) phase II reactions.

Hepatic blood flow decreases with age in both the arterial and portal systems. This decreased delivery makes an important contribution to increasing the half-life of certain agents and narrowing the oral dose/parenteral dose discrepancies for drugs that are heavily metabolized during the "first pass" through the liver.

The liver handles drugs in two general ways: phase I reactions are oxidations and reductions, and phase II reactions are acetylations and glucuronidations. Phase I reactions decrease significantly with age, whereas phase II reactions are well-preserved.

16. What is the strongest risk factor for adverse drug reactions?

There are many risk factors, but the strongest is polypharmacy, the number of drugs to which the patient is exposed. Other predisposing factors are female sex, small body size, hepatic or renal insufficiency, and previous drug reactions. The presence of multiple diseases, altered compliance, and decreased homeostatic mechanisms may also predispose an older person to such reactions.

17. Why are old people more likely to become dehydrated?

Water and salt homeostasis are well-maintained in the healthy elderly in the absence of stress. With stress, however, this may not be the case. The elderly have a decreased thirst drive, and it takes a larger change in plasma osmolarity to stimulate water intake. Even then, the amount of water ingested is less than that in the young and is often less than necessary. The amount of sweat produced is decreased, the threshold temperature for sweating is increased, and the renal losses seem to be more significant. The renal changes with aging are multiple, but most relevant to this question is the impairment of the maximum concentrating ability of the kidneys (1200 mOsm in the young and <800 mOsm in the elderly). Furthermore, the elderly are slower to respond to a water deficit. It takes 24 more hours of water deprivation for the older person to reach maximum urine concentrations.

18. Does sweating change with aging?
Yes. The temperature required to produce sweating in a healthy elderly person sitting in a sauna is 1–2° higher than that in a young person—i.e., the threshold temperature is increased. The maximum sweating rate is lower due to either a decrease in the number of glands and/or a decrease in the maximum production by each gland. The sweat glands of older patients are less responsive to exogenous or endogenous acetylcholine. The decreased function is seen in both eccrine and apocrine sweat glands.

19. How large is the age-associated decrease in hemoglobin seen in healthy men and women?
There is no decrease in hemoglobin in healthy elderly men or women.

20. Is there any benefit to smoking cessation for smokers above age 65?
Yes. The most immediate benefit is to the heart and circulation, where the benefits may be seen almost immediately. FEV_1 decreases at a much faster rate in smokers than in nonsmokers. Although the absolute level of FEV_1 does not improve with cessation of smoking, the rate of decline does. The rate of decrease that occurs in smokers (about 75–100 ml/yr) quickly returns to the rate of decrease seen in nonsmokers (about 25–30 ml/yr).

The elderly smoker is difficult to change, and successful cessation rates for those over 65 are not good. Nevertheless, the elderly smoker has much to gain by stopping.

21. Many old people complain about difficulties sleeping. How many hours of sleep does the average 75-year-old require? Does the requirement change with further aging?
There is considerable controversy in this area, but it is now thought that the number of hours of sleep per 24-hour period changes very little throughout adult life. Older persons seem to increase their daytime sleeping (naps) and decrease their nocturnal sleeping, so the number of hours of sleep at night goes down. There is a large change in the amounts of sleep time spent in the various stages of sleep. Older persons spend more time in stage I (light sleep/sleep-awake transition). There is also an age-associated decrease in stage IV sleep.

22. Sjögren's syndrome is more common than previously thought in older patients. What findings are seen in this syndrome?
Sjögren's syndrome has recently been reported in up to 2% of nursing home residents (predominantly women). This chronic inflammatory disease of unknown etiology primarily involves the lacrimal, salivary, and excretory glands. The symptoms are dry mouth, dry eyes, recurrent salivary pain or swelling, dyspareunia, cough, and dysphagia. In most patients, the ESR is elevated, but because the ESR may be elevated in the healthy elderly, this is nondiagnostic. Antibodies to the Lane SSB antigen are diagnostic. In the elderly population the extraglandular involvement is less frequent than in younger patients with Sjögren's syndrome.

23. How much money is spent on health care costs for each person over 65? How much of this is their own money?
Incredibly in 1985, about $4000 was spent on health care for each elderly person. Even though many of these expenses were covered by private insurance or Medicare, out-of-pocket ex-

penses totaled $1000 for each person that year. One can expect that the total figure per person over 65 has more than doubled since 1985.

24. Is there any evidence for the idea that our lifespan is programmed in our genes?

Yes, there is substantial evidence that our maximum lifespan is primarily genetically determined:

1. There are large differences in maturation and maximum lifespan among species, from days to more than a century.

2. In some short-lived species, breeding has successfully lengthened maximum lifespan about 50% (fruit flies).

3. In almost all species, the female outlives the male.

4. The similarities in aging and life expectancy between monozygotic twins are remarkable and are closer than those between dizygotic twins.

25. An older person under your care is unable to live independently at home. What available resources might you consider before concluding that the person needs a nursing home?

Programs such as Meals on Wheels and Home Health Aides may bring food (usually one hot meal daily) or a person to help with personal needs. Not only can nurses, but also physical therapists and occupational therapists can come into the home. If supervision can be provided by the family during the evening and nighttime hours, then adult day centers or psychiatric day hospitals may be valuable. Finally, never underestimate the informal network of friends that many people have who can check and be helpful.

Elon, R: Outpatient evaluation for nursing home admission. In Yoshikawa T (ed): Ambulatory Geriatric Care. St. Louis, Mosby, 1993, pp 142–148.

CARDIOVASCULAR DISORDERS

26. What maximum heart rate should be expected for a 75-year-old man wishing to start an exercise program? How about a 75-year-old woman?

Data from men in the Baltimore Longitudinal Study who were vigorously screened for the presence of occult coronary artery disease yielded the following regression equation:

$$\text{Max HR} = 208.2 - 0.95 \times (\text{age in yrs})$$

Thus, in a 75-year-old man, the calculation would be:

$$208.2 - 0.95 \times 75 = 137 \text{ bpm}$$

Women usually only attain 85% of this calculated maximal heart rate. Remember that the target heart rate for training is 50% to 85% of the calculated increase that occurs with exercise. If a patient's resting heart rate is 75, the target range for training should be 106–128.

27. What percentage of elderly men with congestive heart failure (CHF) have a normal ejection fraction (EF)?

At least 40% of men over age 75 with CHF have normal EFs as determined by echocardiogram or nuclear ventriculography, a result that is not different from results found in studies that look at all age groups. In older women, it is likely that the percentage is even higher. This is important because the elderly are most likely to have problems with digoxin. Unless there is a clear indication for this agent (such as atrial fibrillation with rapid ventricular response), elderly patients with CHF and normal EFs should not receive digoxin.

Luchi RJ: Clinical Geriatric Cardiology. Edinburgh, Churchill Livingstone, 1989.

28. How great of a decrease in systolic blood pressure (BP) upon standing is considered normal in patients over 75?

One working definition of orthostatic hypotension requires a decrease of systolic BP of >20 mm Hg upon arising. However, decreases of >20 mm Hg have been reported in 20–30% of the community-dwelling elderly. The relative contributions of longstanding hypertension, antihypertensive agents, and age have not yet been clarified. Decreases of >20 mm Hg have little prognostic significance in unselected elders.

Raiha I, et al: Prevalence, predisposing factors and prognostic importance of postural hypotension. Arch Intern Med. 155:930–935, 1995.

29. How does Osler's maneuver affect the diagnosis of hypertension?

BP measurement involves the compression of the brachial artery by pressure applied via a cuff. Patients with heavily calcified arteries have rigid, hard-to-compress arteries but may not have high intra-arterial pressures. If the cuff is pumped above the systolic BP and the brachial or radial arteries are still palpable, this is a positive Osler's maneuver. Using cuff measurements of BP in patients with a positive Osler's maneuver results in a gross overestimate of the actual intra-arterial pressures.

30. Is the presence of a fourth heart sound (S_4) on a cardiac exam in an older person of importance?

Auscultation of an S_4 is very common in older persons and is usually of limited clinical significance. It may be a manifestation of the decreased compliance of the aged heart. However, the presence of an S_3 gallop is not normal and is characteristic of CHF.

31. How many of those over age 70 have significant (75% or higher) coronary artery stenoses at autopsy? How many of those over age 90?

The prevalence of coronary artery disease (CAD) increases with age, but for men the prevalence appears to level off after age 70. Over 50% of all persons over age 70 have at least one arterial site of 75% stenosis at autopsy. By age 90, the prevalence increases to about 70%, women accounting for the increase. By noninvasive testing, the prevalence of CAD is somewhat less but is still above 50% in the elderly.

32. What clues suggest the presence of renovascular hypertension?

Renovascular hypertension is a common secondary cause of hypertension. It should be investigated in the elderly patient with:

1. The sudden development of hypertension (especially systolic and diastolic elevations rather than isolated systolic BP elevation).

2. A history of well-controlled hypertension which suddenly becomes difficult to control.

3. Hypertension in a person who develops acute oliguric renal failure when given an ACE inhibitor.

4. Hypertension in a person who is found to have an abdominal or flank bruit.

5. Known atherosclerotic disease in a person who develops renal insufficiency.

Rosmarin PC: Secondary hypertension. Clin Geriatr Med 5:753–768, 1989.

33. What is the difference between aortic stenosis and aortic sclerosis? Can these be differentiated on physical examination?

Aortic sclerosis is the source of many benign murmurs in patients over 70 years of age. It is due to sclerosis (hardening and fibrosis) of the aortic cusps and is not hemodynamically significant. **Aortic stenosis** is not uncommon in the elderly and is usually due to calcification of a bicuspid valve in the younger elderly patient or degenerative calcification in those older than 75. By definition, there is impedance to flow in aortic stenosis.

Although many physical findings have been reported to distinguish the murmur of aortic stenosis from that of aortic sclerosis, unless the stenosis is severe (producing a thrill or very prolonged ventricular impulse), they are unreliable. It is most prudent to evaluate the patient with echocardiography. For example, the narrowed pulse-pressure characteristic of aortic stenosis in younger people is not often seen in the elderly with the same degree of aortic stenosis. This is probably due to the age-related increase in stiffness of the arterial tree. For the same reason, the "pulsus parvis et tardus" at the carotids also may not be seen in elderly patients with significant aortic stenosis.

Luchi RJ: Clinical Geriatric Cardiology. Edinburgh, Churchill Livingstone, 1989.

34. What is the natural history of an abdominal aortic aneurysm (AAA)? What if it is >6 cm in diameter?

It appears that all AAAs enlarge progressively, but do so at varying rates. The likelihood of a 6-cm AAA lasting 2 years without rupture is <50%. It is this threshold (6 cm in diameter) at which elective surgery is most appropriate and probably should be recommended. Additionally, not only the size but also the rate of growth may provide prognostic information and dictate timing of surgery. Even slow aneurysms that grow rapidly over a 6-month interval require intervention. All AAAs need frequent size evaluation.

35. Are the symptoms of abdominal or low back pain important in patients known to have an abdominal aortic aneurysm?

AAAs tend to rupture, not dissect. Elective aneurysmectomy can be performed with acceptable operative mortality, but emergent surgery is very risky (50% mortality). Hypogastric pain or low back pain in a person known to have an AAA is often due to rapid expansion and may suggest that rupture is occurring or is imminent.

36. How frequently is amyloid protein seen on autopsy in atria of hearts from patients older than 90? What is its significance?

Small amounts of amyloid protein, limited to the atria of the heart, may be seen in 80–90% of autopsy specimens from the very elderly. This protein has not been shown to have pathologic importance, and it is considered a benign age-associated marker. Some researchers consider this amyloid to be similar to the atrial natriuretic peptide.

37. What is the significance of frequent premature ventricular contractions (PVCs) on routine ECG or continuous ambulatory recordings in asymptomatic, healthy men over 65 with no coronary artery disease (CAD)?

None. In older populations rigorously screened for CAD, 80% have PVCs. At least 20% have frequent PVCs (>100 in 24 hours), and 10% may have couplets or other complexity. The presence of these arrhythmias has little impact on prognosis.

Fleg JL, Kennedy HL: Long-term prognostic significance of ambulatory electrocardiographic findings in apparently healthy subjects greater than or equal to 60 years of age. Am J Cardiol, 70:748–751, 1992.

38. Why is atrial fibrillation tolerated hemodynamically by young people but produces heart failure in older persons?

Atrial systole provides relatively little of left ventricular (LV) filling during diastole, and essentially 80% occurs during rapid filling early in diastole. In contrast, left atrial systole provides almost 50% of LV filling in old age. This change in atrial filling fraction occurs in normal elders independent of disease.

Kitzman DW et al: Age-related alterations in Doppler left ventricular filling indices in normal subjects are independent of left ventricular mass, heart rate, contractility, and loading conditions. J Am Coll Cardiol. 18:1243–1250, 1991.

NEUROLOGIC/PSYCHIATRIC DISORDERS

39. Why is it important to distinguish patients with cardiovascular syncope from those with syncope of other causes?

Patients with a cardiovascular etiology (anatomic, myocardial, or electrical) for syncopal episodes have a much higher 1-year mortality (20%) than those with a defined noncardiovascular etiology or those whose etiology is uncertain after workup. This is thought to be due to the underlying cardiovascular diseases for which the syncope serves as a marker (especially aortic stenosis).

40. THA is a drug with activity in Alzheimer's disease (AD). How does it work? What problems are associated with its use?

THA (tetrahydroaminoacridine) is an anticholinesterase. One of the hallmarks of AD is a decrease in the brain levels of the neurotransmitter, acetylcholine. By blocking the enzyme that metabolizes acetylcholine, THA makes more acetylcholine available to the receptors.

Two problems occur with THA. The first is a dose-related hepatotoxicity that appears to be reversible with decreases in the dose. The second is a hypothetical decrease in cognitive function with further increases in THA. This may be due to excessive acetylcholine at the receptor site. The drug does not appear to change the progression of AD and has modest efficacy in most patients.

Soares JC, Gershon S: THA—historical aspects, review of pharmacological properties and therapeutic effects. Dementia 6:225–234, 1995.

41. What is the triad of normal pressure hydrocephalus (NPH)? Why is it important?

The three components of NPH are gait disorders, urinary incontinence, and dementia. This reversible dementia is treated by ventriculoatrial shunting, and a good response is correlated to the presence of all three parts of the triad. The presence of incontinence is unusual early in the course of other dementias, as is the presence of gait abnormalities. When incontinence and gait instability are present in a demented patient, a high level of suspicion of NPH should be raised.

Black PM: Idiopathic normal-pressure hydrocephalus: Results of shunting in 62 patients. Neurosurgery 52:371–377, 1980.

42. Does jaw pain upon chewing have any significance? How about headache with scalp tenderness?

Both of these unusual complaints may be the symptoms of **temporal arteritis.** Both problems are most common in very elderly women. Temporal arteritis may rapidly produce monocular or binocular blindness and needs to be addressed urgently when suspected. Corticosteroids can prevent blindness.

The ESR is usually >50 mm/hr in these patients. However, the definitive diagnosis requires a temporal artery biopsy. This procedure can be performed shortly after the institution of steroid therapy with prednisone, 60 mg/day, in divided doses.

Grob D: Common muscle disorders. In Reichel W (ed): Clinical Aspects of Aging, 2nd ed. Baltimore, Williams & Wilkins, 1989.

43. How common is dementia in people over age 85?

Severe dementia is present in <1% of those over 65 but in > 15% of those over 85. This group (those over 85) is the fastest growing segment of the population. The incidence of dementia is highest in the ninth decade, and it appears to decline thereafter, so that new onset of dementia due to Alzheimer's disease is less common in patients above 90.

Katzman R: Alzheimer's disease. N Engl J Med 314:964–973, 1986.

44. What percentage of dementia is caused by Alzheimer's disease (AD)?

At least 50–60% of patients with dementia have AD or have a component of AD coexisting with another dementing illness, commonly multi-infarct dementia.

45. What are the two ways to make a definite diagnosis of Alzheimer's disease?

Autopsy or brain biopsy. The diagnosis of definite AD requires a clinical history consistent with AD and histopathologic confirmation. However, using a reasonable approach to exclude other causes of dementia should allow a practitioner to be 90% correct when using only clinical findings to make the diagnosis of probable AD.

46. Are any neurologic signs present in patients with dementia?

Focal neurologic findings are a clue that the etiology of the dementia may be multiple infarcts and not Alzheimer's disease. Cranial nerve findings should suggest the presence of chronic meningitis and prompt further investigation, including lumbar puncture.

There is a set of neurologic findings seen in dementia, perhaps because of loss of the inhibitory influences. These include the snout reflex, suck reflex, and glabellar blink. The sensitivity and specificity of these "soft" neurologic signs in identifying patients with dementia are poor relative to those of a mental status exam.

47. How can you differentiate depression from dementia?

This differential may be very difficult. Depression has been called pseudodementia. On the mental status examination, depressed patients frequently answer questions with "I don't know," whereas demented patients try to answer even though their answer may be wrong. Depressed patients often have complaints about memory impairments that are out of proportion to the severity of findings on exam. The routine use of a depression questionnaire, such as the Hamilton Depression Scale, has been suggested, as has neuropsychological testing. If the uncertainty in the diagnosis persists, then a diagnostic/therapeutic trial of a tricyclic antidepressant (with low anticholinergic activity) may be warranted.

Remember, in up to one-third of cases, a demented person will have coexistent depression. These people may improve functionally when their depression is treated, even though the underlying dementia is not affected by the treatment.

Reynolds CF, et al: Bedside differentiation of depressive pseudodementia from dementia. Am J Psychiary 145:1099–1103, 1988.

48. Why is depression common after a stroke?

Depression is said to affect up to 60% of stroke victims. The reasons are uncertain but appear to relate to the physical limitations produced by the stroke. The location of the stroke is also important, as patients with left frontal infarctions have the highest risk of depression. This area of the brain may play a key role in maintenance of mood.

Collie SJ, et al: Depression after stroke. Clin Rehab 1:27–32, 1987.

49. What neurologic findings are abnormal in a young patient and normal in an older one?

The passage of time has many effects on the normal nervous system. On cranial nerve exam, a marked limitation of upward gaze is seen in most elderly persons as well as relatively constricted pupils. There is a slowing of rapid alternations of movement, which is termed dysdiadochokinesia. In the distal extremity, there may be sensory impairments, and ankle jerks may frequently be absent. Abdominal reflexes may also be absent.

50. How can handwriting help in the differential diagnosis of tremor? What can a glass of wine do in this regard?

Essential tremor worsens with intention and usually improves with ethanol. Parkinsonism patients characteristically have **micrographia,** a condition in which the handwriting is very small. The administration of ethanol does not significantly alter the tremor of Parkinson's disease.

51. Who gets tardive dyskinesia? How is it treated?

Tardive dyskinesia usually follows prolonged use of neuroleptic agents. Although older patients seem to be more likely to develop tardive dyskinesia, it is not clear that duration use, the specific agent, or the total dose has any direct relation to the appearance of the involuntary movements. There is little evidence that tardive dyskinesia can be treated with drugs, although in a certain percentage of patients, the movements may disappear, even with the continuation of the neuroleptic agent.

52. Does an asymptomatic carotid bruit imply impending stroke?

No. The risk of a cerebrovascular accident (CVA) without warning transient ischemic attacks (TIAs) is only about 1% in the year following the discovery of a bruit. However, the bruit is a marker of widespread atherosclerosis, and the risk of CVA is elevated. The scenario becomes quite different once the bruit becomes symptomatic with ipsilateral TIAs. At this point, therapy is indicated.

DISORDERS OF THE SENSES

53. Other than cataracts, which changes in the eye occur with normal aging?

There are a multitude of changes in the aging eye other than those leading to cataract formation. The periorbital tissues atrophy. The upper lid may droop, and the lower lid can turn inward or outward. The pupil becomes smaller, and adaptation of the eye to changes in lighting is much slower. The lens loses elasticity, leading to an inability to focus on near items (presbyopia), and the ability to distinguish objects from background is impaired, requiring more contrast between objects.

54. Are changes in hearing part of normal aging?

The most representative loss of auditory function that occurs with aging is in the high-frequency range. The minimum sound appreciated by the older ear is increased (louder). This is sensorineural hearing loss, which is usually noted in middle age and becomes problematic in later life.

A parallel finding is the decrease in speech discrimination. When the patient is given words to both ears simultaneously and then asked about information given to one ear, older patients seem to have a large age-related loss in discriminant function. Because this test is performed with sounds above the auditory threshold, it is thought to be due to a central processing deficit independent of the sensorineural problem.

55. How common are macular degeneration and cataracts in those above 75?

The prevalence of these two eye problems is very high. The Framingham study reported macular degeneration in about 6% of patients aged 65–74 and in 18% of those 75 or older. Cataracts were noted in 13% of those 65–74 and in approx. 40% of patients 75 and older.

56. What are the ophthalmoscopic findings of senile macular degeneration?

There are two types of senile macular degeneration: nonexudative (dry) and exudative (wet). The **nonexudative** type is most common and is characterized by drusen (hyaline excrescences in Bruch's membrane). The underlying changes in the pigmented epithelia can produce geographic atrophy. This disorder produces a slowly progressive central visual loss, though only 10% of patients progress to legal blindness. There is no adequate therapy.

The **exudative** form of senile macular degeneration is accompanied by neovascularization that weeps and bleeds. Laser photocoagulation can be used to slow the progression of visual loss in the exudative type.

57. Are there any types of hearing loss that do not respond to hearing aids?

Though there are still some who do not believe that sensorineural hearing loss will respond to amplification, it appears that both of the common types of age-associated hearing loss, conductive and sensorineural, respond to amplification provided by hearing aids. The third type of communication defect, a central processing problem in which the words are heard but not properly understood, may be made worse by a hearing aid that also amplifies the background sound. These patients need to have extraneous sound reduced for optimal function.

SKIN DISORDERS

58. Are there any risk factors, aside from immobility, that are associated with developing pressure sores (decubitus ulcer)?

The relative contribution of various factors in producing pressure sores is not clear. Some risk factors, in addition to the pressure itself, include hypoalbuminemia, fecal incontinence, immobility, weight loss, hypotension, and fractures. A depressed sensorium increases the risk of pressure sores, as does any other process that impairs the patient's ability to sense and respond to discomfort.

59. Why do pressure sores heal so much slower than similarly sized skin wounds of other types?

Three factors lead to ischemia of the surrounding tissue and slow healing:

1. **Shear forces:** Many pressure sores involve shearing, which occurs because of body position. In addition to producing ischemia by compressing vessels, the shear forces may disrupt the blood supply to the area.

2. **Thrombosis:** At times of low blood flow (or no blood flow), clot may form in the vascu-

lar supply to the area. There is decreased fibrinolytic activity in the area of the ulcer which causes the clot to persist.

3. **Transmission of pressure:** There is a tendency to assume that the skin area that is involved projects cylindrically into the deeper tissues. It appears that the projection is more like a cone, with a narrow skin site of pressure and a much wider, deeper area of ischemia below the surface.

60. How are pressure sores graded?

All of the popular classification systems to grade pressure sores use maximum depth of penetration to measure the severity of the lesion.

Shea's Decubitus Grading System

Grade 1—Decubiti penetrate into the dermis
Grade 2—Decubiti extend into the subcutaneous fat
Grade 3—Decubiti extend into the fascia
Grade 4—Decubiti extend deeper than fascia and are without apparent boundaries

61. Why is the "head-elevated" bed position so likely to produce pressure sores?

The head-elevated position produces shearing forces at the sacrum. The body is pulled by gravity, while friction holds the skin to the sheet, thus producing the shearing force. The patient should not remain in this position for long periods.

62. What are seborrheic keratoses? What treatments are effective for them?

Seborrheic keratoses are benign epidermal lesions frequently seen in the elderly. These hyperpigmented, hyperkeratotic lesions have distinct borders and an irregular, scaly surface. They are light or dark brown, wart-like papules of varying size, generally described as having a "stuck-on" appearance. They are usually multiple and are most commonly found on the trunk. As they enlarge, they darken and develop a greasy scale.

Although they have no malignant potential, because of their dark color they can sometimes be confused with malignant melanoma. These lesions can be treated with curettage, electrodesiccation, liquid nitrogen, and topical glycolic acid.

Kleinsmith DM, Perricone NV: Common skin problems in the elderly. Clin Geriatr Med 5:189–211, 1989.

63. What age-related skin changes produce xerosis?

Rough, dry skin (xerosis) is the reflection of a number of age-related skin changes that facilitate drying of the skin. These include a decrease in sebum secretion and a decrease in eccrine sweat glands. There are also changes in the stratum corneum and epidermal atrophy.

INFECTIONS AND IMMUNITY

64. How frequently do elderly persons with active tuberculosis (TB) have a nonreactive skin test?

In as many as 30% of patients with active TB, the skin test may be negative. The frequency of this situation appears to increase with increasing age. The booster effect (a more powerful reaction seen after a second PPD applied 7–10 days after the first) reveals that many of the patients who are initially negative have active disease. This is a worthwhile procedure for TB in skin-testing most elderly patients.

65. Which age-related changes make the older person more likely to develop pneumonia?

Multiple changes that occur with aging make the older person more likely to develop pneumonia. The most common way for an older person to introduce pathogens into the lungs is aspiration. Older people appear to aspirate more frequently while swallowing and have a poorer cough reflex, thus incompletely clearing the aspirate. Drugs that sedate the patient and allow aspiration to occur are also more frequently administered to the elderly. The organisms that inhabit the oropharynx are usually nonpathogenic in the younger person (with some exceptions), but an increased amount of gram-negative organisms appears in the flora in up to 20% of community-dwelling elderly individuals, as well as almost all nursing home residents.

Changes in the immune system, especially T-cell changes and antibody affinity changes, may also increase the risk of pneumonia. Finally, the increased frequency of influenza leads to an increased frequency of pneumonia.

66. When is antiviral therapy indicated in the treatment of herpes zoster in the immunocompetent elderly?

In general, neither acyclovir nor vidarabine is recommended for immunocompetent elderly patients with uncomplicated shingles because of the expense and potential side effects. For ophthalmic zoster infection, immunocompetent patients should be treated with oral acyclovir. Prednisone is given to many immunocompetent elderly with shingles to prevent postherpetic neuralgia, but its effectiveness is uncertain. Postherpetic neuralgia is 3–5 times more frequent in patients over age 60 years.

67. Are vaccinations useful in preventing illness in the elderly? If so, which illnesses and in which elderly patients?

Influenza, pneumococcal, and tetanus-diphtheria (Td) vaccinations are all recommended for older patients. The **flu** vaccine is about 70% effective in elderly patients and should be given yearly, in the fall, to all people over 65, especially those who live in nursing homes.

The newest **pneumococcal** vaccine includes antigen from 23 serotypes that probably cause 85% of pneumococcal pneumonia. Recommendations suggest that patients over 65 have one lifetime pneumococcal vaccination and that those who received the earlier (14-serotype) vaccine do not need to be immunized again.

Although **tetanus** is still a fairly uncommon disease, the percentage of patients over age 50 has been increasing. These people often have been immunized in the remote past but not recently. The same is true for diphtheria. Booster immunizations with *adult* Td vaccine should be done every 10 years throughout adult life.

68. How is the antibody response to an antigen different in an old person compared to a younger one?

The total amount of antibody produced in response to a challenge (perhaps an immunization) is essentially unchanged with increasing age. The quality of the antibody produced is poorer because the affinity of the antibody for its intended antigen may be less than that produced by a young person. The specificity of the antibody is a function of the T cell that is directing the B-cell response. Many of the functions of the T cell, especially those dependent on interleukin-2, are significantly impaired with increasing age.

UROLOGIC DISORDERS

69. When is a chronic Foley catheter indicated?

There are only a few indications for a chronic indwelling Foley catheter.

- Urinary retention should be treated with chronic catheterization if it produces renal dysfunction, infections, or overflow incontinence, and if it is not treatable with surgery, medications, and intermittent catheterization.
- If incontinent urine is soiling skin wounds, decubitus ulcers, or skin irritations, then the catheter is appropriate while the wound is healing.
- A small group of patients with terminal illnesses or severe debility (a person with severe rheumatoid arthritis in whom any movement is very painful) may require the catheter, and an even smaller group wants the catheter for patient or caregiver convenience.

70. What can be done to decrease the rate of colonization of indwelling urinary catheters?

Almost all indwelling Foley catheters become colonized with bacteria. Irrigation or antibiotic therapy does not eradicate colonization but does produce changes in the flora. For suspected urinary tract infection, it is important to remove the old catheter and sample urine for cultures from the new catheter. Condom catheters, when twisted, kinked, or clogged, have a frequency of infection that is as bad as that of the indwelling catheter. Perhaps the most important point is to evaluate the absolute indication for the catheter and be certain that it is not just for nursing convenience.

71. How frequent is urinary incontinence seen in community-dwelling elderly? In those in nursing homes?

The frequency of insignificant loss of urine is quite common in women of all ages. However, the frequency of urine loss of sufficient magnitude to produce social compromise or health problems is found in 10–30% of community-dwelling elderly, with a lower frequency in men. Surveys of elderly nursing home residents have reported urinary incontinence in 50% of inhabitants. The very high frequency in institutionalized populations is primarily due to their underlying diseases, but it is sometimes the product of physical restraints and medications.

72. What are the four different types of urinary incontinence? What are their distinguishing features and causes?

Urinary incontinence is not a part of normal aging, nor is it caused by aging. However, many of the physiologic consequences of aging can contribute to urinary incontinence.

1. **Stress incontinence:** The involuntary loss of small volumes of urine related to events that cause increased intra-abdominal pressure (coughing, laughing, exercise). It is more common in females (present with laughing in 50% of young females) and increases with aging. Its causes include weakness or laxity of pelvic floor muscles, bladder outlet, or urethral sphincter.

2. **Urge incontinence:** The involuntary loss of larger volumes of urine due to the inability to delay voiding when the sensation of bladder fullness (urge) is perceived. Causes include detrusor motor and/or sensory instability, either alone or in combination with one of the following:

- Local GU conditions such as cystitis, urethritis, tumors, stones, diverticula, and outflow obstruction.
- CNS disorders such as stroke, dementia, parkinsonism, and suprasacral spinal cord injury or disease.

3. **Overflow incontinence:** Involuntary loss of small amounts of urine resulting from mechanical forces on an overdistended bladder or from other effects of urinary retention on bladder and sphincter function. Causes are anatomic obstruction by the prostate, stricture, or cystocele; acontractile bladder associated with diabetes mellitus or spinal cord injury; and neurogenic (detrusor-sphincter dyssynergy) associated with multiple sclerosis and other suprasacral spinal cord injury.

4. **Functional incontinence:** Leakage of urine associated with inability to toilet because of impairment of cognitive and/or physical functioning, psychological unwillingness, or environmental barriers. It is seen in severe dementia and other neurologic disorders as well as psychological factors such as depression, regression, anger, and hostility.

Kane RL, et al: Essentials of Clinical Geriatrics, 2nd ed. New York, McGraw-Hill, 1989, p 151.

73. How are the four types of urinary incontinence treated?

1. **Stress incontinence:** Pelvic floor (Kegel) exercises, α-adrenergic agonists, estrogen, biofeedback, behavioral training, surgical bladder neck suspension.

2. **Urge incontinence:** Bladder relaxants, estrogen (if vaginal atrophy is present), training procedures (e.g., biofeedback, behavioral therapy), surgical removal of obstructing or other irritating pathologic lesions.

3. **Overflow incontinence:** Surgical removal of obstruction, intermittent catheterization (if practical), indwelling catheterization.

4. **Functional incontinence:** Behavioral therapies (e.g., habit training, scheduled toileting),

environmental manipulations, incontinence undergarments and pads, external collection devices, bladder relaxants (selected patients), indwelling catheters (selected patients).

Kane RL, et al: Essentials of Clinical Geriatrics, 2nd ed. New York, McGraw-Hill, 1989 p 168.

74. What are the important causes of acute and reversible urinary incontinence?

Because of the severe physical, psychologic, social, and economic costs of urinary incontinence, it is important to identify reversible cases and render the needed treatment. The causes of acute and reversible forms of urinary incontinence can be remembered by the **DRIP** mnemonic:

D = Delirium

R = Restricted mobility, retention

I = Infection, inflammation, impaction (fecal)

P = Polyuria, pharmaceuticals

Infection and inflammation refer to acute symptomatic urinary tract infection (UTI), atrophic vaginitis, or urethritis. Polyuria may be due to hyperglycemia or volume-expanded states causing excessive nocturia (e.g., CHF, venous insufficiency).

Kane RL, et al: Essentials of Clinical Geriatrics, 2nd ed., New York, McGraw-Hill, 1989, p 149.

75. What are the complications and adverse effects of urinary incontinence?

Physical health	**Social**
Skin breakdown	Stress on family, friends, and caregivers
Recurrent UTIs	Predisposition to institutionalization
Psychological	**Economic**
Isolation and dependency	Supplies (padding, catheters, etc.) and
Depression	laundry
	Labor (nurses, housekeepers)
	Management of complications

Kane RL, et al: Essentials of Clinical Geriatrics, 2nd ed. New York, McGraw-Hill, 1989, p 140.

76. Is single-dose therapy for cystitis as successful in older women as it is in younger women? How long should treatment be continued?

No. Even with the lower bacterial load seen in asymptomatic bacteriuria, single-dose therapy was effective in less than two-thirds of elderly women. It is anticipated that symptomatic UTI would be even less responsive to this treatment regimen. Most experts are currently recommending 7–10 days of antibiotic therapy for uncomplicated UTIs.

77. Among younger persons with UTIs, women outnumber men 8–10 to 1. In those over age 70, men and women are represented equally. Why do the demographics change?

Most of the change in distribution is due to an increase in incidence of UTI in men, with much of the blame on the prostate. Prostatic hypertrophy results in increased residual urine, and the incomplete emptying allows bacteria to grow and produce symptoms. There are changes in the immune system in the bladder, with an increase in bacterial binding to uroepithelial cells in old men. The production of a specific protein (Tamm-Horsfall protein) that binds gram-negative bacteria is decreased with age. Other components of prostatic secretions are antibacterial and their production is decreased with age. Finally, instrumentation and catheterization of the bladder is more common in advanced age and increases the frequency of infections.

Tunkel AR, Kaye D: Urinary tract infections. In Hazzard WR, et al (eds): Principles of Geriatric Medicine and Gerontology, 3rd ed. New York, McGraw-Hill, 1994.

GASTRIC DISORDERS

78. What are the causes of fecal incontinence?

1. Fecal impaction with overflow diarrhea
2. Laxative overuse or abuse

3. Neurologic disorders (dementia, stroke, spinal cord injury)

4. Colorectal disorders (diarrheal illnesses, rectal sphincter damage, neoplastic or inflammatory processes)

79. What are the long-term complications of cascara or henna laxatives?

The most important side effect is degeneration of myoneural chains in the colon. This impairs peristalsis and may set up a vicious cycle in which decreased colonic motility leads to worsened constipation and increased use of laxatives.

80. What are the complications of nasogastric feeding?

In addition to the displeasure that the patient may express, some important complications may result from enteral feedings:

- Aspiration pneumonia
- Trauma to nasal mucosa and/or gastric and esophageal mucosa producing erosions
- Gastric distention due to decreased motility
- Diarrhea due to increased motility or other causes (especially osmotic loading)
- Fluid overload leading to hyponatremia or CHF

81. What are the common causes of lower GI bleeding in an elderly person?

Bleeding from diverticula is the most common cause, followed by bleeding from angiodysplasia. These two conditions makeup 75% of lower GI bleeding. Other causes of blood loss in the elderly are colonic polyps, colon carcinoma, ischemic colitis, and inflammatory bowel disease. Old people can also have hemorrhoids as a cause of bleeding. One study has shown that 30% of the elderly known to have diverticula were bleeding because of another reason. It is therefore unwise to empirically attribute lower GI blood loss to diverticula.

CANCER

82. What is the leading cause of death in women aged 55–74? Women older than 74?

While heart disease is the leading cause of death in men across these age groups, cancer is the number one killer for women aged 55–74. Older women most frequently die of heart disease.

83. Why is it that in men, lung cancer peaks in incidence at age 70 and declines afterwards?

The development of lung cancer is very strongly associated with cigarette use. Above age 70, many of the smokers are dead or have stopped smoking for other reasons. Therefore, the population as a whole has a lower risk of developing lung cancer. For smokers, the risk of lung cancer appears to continue to increase with increasing age.

84. What differences are seen between breast cancers in younger women and older women?

Elderly women are much more likely to have estrogen-receptor-positive breast cancer, implying a malignancy that will be more responsive to hormonal manipulation and possibly slower-growing.

85. What percentage of prostate cancers is confined to the prostate or local pelvis at time of diagnosis?

Only about 30% of prostate cancers are local at time of diagnosis. This means that two-thirds are widespread and incurable at diagnosis. Fortunately, the malignancy is usually responsive to hormonal manipulation, which controls the disease and alleviates symptoms.

86. Are patients with shingles very likely to have an underlying malignancy?

No. Although there probably is a small increase in the chance of cancer in patients with herpes zoster recurrence, it is not large enough to merit evaluation for malignancy in every patient who presents with shingles.

Raggazino MW, et al: Risk of cancer after herpes zoster: A population-based study. N Engl J Med 307:393–397, 1982.

87. When an older person is found to a have a monoclonal gammopathy of undetermined significance (MGUS), what are the chances of developing a related malignancy in the next 10 years?

A monoclonal gammopathy is a monoclonal protein noted on serum protein electrophoresis of <3 g/dl and without associated signs or symptoms of hematologic abnormalities. At 10 years of follow-up, 40% of elderly patients with MGUS are stable, 40% have died from other causes, and 10–20% have myeloma, macroglobulinemia, amyloidosis, or non-Hodgkin's lymphoma.

Kyle RA: Monoclonal gammopathy of undetermined significance. Blood Rev 8:135–141, 1994.

88. What treatments are used for early chronic lymphocytic leukemia (CLL)?

None. At the present time, patients with a normal hemoglobin and platelet count should be monitored frequently for any progression of the disease. Therapy can be useful for more advanced stage CLL, but most elderly die *with* CLL, not *from* it.

89. What group of elderly patients is at risk for osteogenic sarcoma? Is there a marker for malignant conversion?

Although osteogenic sarcoma is usually found in growing adolescents and is quite rare in the elderly, it occurs in one subgroup of elderly patients: patients who have active Paget's disease of the bone. In these patients, there usually is a significant increase in serum alkaline phosphatase heralding the malignancy. Although these tumors develop in <1% of elderly patients with Paget's disease, their prognosis and response to treatment are very poor.

MUSCULOSKELETAL DISORDERS

90. How is Paget's disease of the bone most often diagnosed in the elderly?

It is frequently recognized via multichannel screening of blood. The elevation of alkaline phosphatase in the absence of liver disease is often found to be a marker of the increased bone turnover that is part of Paget's disease. Confirmation is made radiographically. Paget's disease is present in >10% of those over age 80 and is more common in the northern U.S. than in the southern U.S.

91. What are the clinical manifestations of Paget's disease of bone?

Although most patients are symptomatic at diagnosis, in 90% of cases it has a variety of manifestations:

Bone manifestations (commonest):
1. Bone pain in the pelvis, hips, and back
2. Bone deformities due to the remodeling process. Most commonly seen as bowing of the femur and tibia, skull enlargement, and loss of height due to scoliosis and vertebral collapse.
3. Pathologic fractures due to bone remodeling
4. Increased warmth over affected areas of bone due to an increase in vascularity

Cardiovascular manifestations (rare):
1. High cardiac output state with or without CHF
2. Hypertension
3. Exacerbation of ischemic heart disease
4. Cardiomegaly
5. Arterial and valvular calcification

Neurological manifestations (rare):
1. Compression of cranial nerves (most often CN VIII) or blood vessels (causing stroke).
2. Middle ear deafness due to ossification of the stapedius tendon
3. Hydrocephalus due to compression of the foramina of Luschka or Magendie
4. Spinal compression syndromes

Other manifestations:
1. Hypercalcemia and hypercalciuria (with or without renal calculi)
2. Osteogenic sarcoma

92. What are the indications for specific treatment of Paget's disease of bone?

Criteria for Specific Treatment of Paget's Disease

1. Disabling pain not relieved by analgesics or anti-inflammatory medications
2. Progression of skeletal aspects of the disease, as indicated by increasing deformity, head or appendicular bone enlargement, frequent fracture, nonunion of fractures, vertebral compression, or acetabular protrusion
3. Neurologic complications
4. Increasing deafness
5. High-output congestive heart failure
6. Immobilization hypercalcemia, before and after major orthopedic surgery

Lifschitz ML, Harmon CE: Musculoskeletal problems in the elderly. In Schrier RW (ed): Clinical Internal Medicine in the Aged. Philadelphia, W.B. Saunders, 1982, p 193.

93. What treatment modalities are available for Paget's disease of bone?

1. **NSAIDs:** for relief of symptoms

2. **Calcitonin:** Inhibits osteoclast production and activity, which may decrease and improve manifestations of the disease, reverse some of the pathologic changes, and lead to partial normalization of the biochemical markers of the disease. The initial effects are seen in approx. 2 weeks, and therapy reaches maximal effectiveness in 6–12 months. Side effects (which are usually not significant) include nausea, vomiting, facial flushing, and polyuria. Development of resistance due to antibodies against salmon calcitonin may require the use of human calcitonin.

3. **Bisphosphonates:** Causes a slowdown in bone growth and turnover by binding to hydroxyapatite crystals in the bone; blocking their growth and dissolution, and inhibiting osteoclast activity. Bisphosphonates have the advantage of oral administration and are usually given in 6-month courses. Side effects are usually not significant.

4. **Mithramycin:** Although not approved for use in Paget's disease, this cytotoxic antibiotic has been used to suppress the manifestations of the disease in some patients. Remissions of many years' duration have been reported after a single course of therapy. Side effects can be severe and include hepatic, renal, and bone marrow toxicities.

5. **Surgery:** Can be used to increase mobility and joint motion, as well as to relieve nerve compression syndromes. Should be performed after several months of medical therapy to decrease postoperative bleeding and hypercalcemia.

94. What types of falls are most commonly seen in patients with parkinsonism?

Falls are very common in patients with parkinsonism, with the symptoms of bradykinesia, rigidity, gait disturbance, and postural instability contributing to this increased frequency of falls. The typical festinating gait, in which patients appear to be accelerating as if to catch up with their center of gravity, may lead to forward falls. At the time of arising, postural instability may lead to falling backwards. Short steps that do not clear the ground adequately increase the likelihood of tripping over objects.

Johnell O, et al: Fracture risk in patients with parkinsonism: A population-based study of Olmstead County, Minnesota. Age Aging 21:32–38, 1992.

95. List the risk factors for hip fracture.

Since hip fracture is the most severe complication of osteopenia, many of the risk factors are the same for the two conditions.

Risk Factors for Hip Fracture

Female sex	Increasing age
White race	Psychotropic drugs
Thin body habitus	Ethanol use
Hemiplegia	Previous hip fracture
Cigarette smoking	Surgical bilateral oophorectomy
Chronic corticosteroid use	(before natural menopause)
Prior history of falls	

96. How frequently do patients with hip fractures have prior falls?

Hip fractures are very common and one of the most dread sequelae of falling. About 15% of patients with hip fracture report previous falls. Therefore, early intervention in patients who fall may prevent recurrent falls and significantly decrease the number of hip fractures leading to death, disability, or institutionalization.

97. What are premonitory falls? Which diseases are associated with them?

About 5% of falls are premonitory, signaling the presence of a serious systemic illness. These underlying illnesses typically are pneumonia, urinary tract infections, or CHF. However, a fall can be the presenting complaint in an acute myocardial infarction in elderly patients.

98. Why do younger women with osteoporosis who fall suffer Colles' fractures, whereas older women suffer hip fractures?

Colles' fracture is a fracture of the distal radius that occurs when persons fall with outstretched hands to try to catch themselves. With age, the reaction time increases, so that the older person who is falling may not have sufficient time to extend the arm. This leads to trauma absorbed directly by the hip and an increased potential for hip fracture.

99. Besides menopause, what are the other known risk factors for osteoporosis?

There are two types of osteoporosis, postmenopausal and age-related. Risk factors for osteoporosis include:

Female sex	Hemiplegia
White or Oriental race	Psychotropic drugs
Thin body habitus	Cigarette smoking
Increasing age	Ethanol use
Low calcium intake	Chronic corticosteroid use
Surgical bilateral oophorectomy	Multiple pregnancies
(before natural menopause)	Sedentary lifestyle

100. How effective are supplemental estrogens in preventing hip fractures in postmenopausal women?

Very effective, producing a 50% decrease in the incidence of hip fractures. Estrogen replacement retards bone loss and thereby prevents the development of osteoporosis. The most bone mass is conserved if the estrogen replacement is instituted shortly after menopause. However, the evidence that estrogen is not as useful when instituted >5 years after menopause is hypothetical and appears not to be supported by some studies.

101. Does supplemental estrogen produce any adverse effects?

The most well-known of the adverse effects is the 10-fold increase in the incidence of endometrial cancer in women on supplemental estrogen. This risk can be substantially decreased by the addition of supplemental progestins, which lead to cyclical shedding of the endometrium. The estrogen-replacement therapy does appear to increase the risk of gallstones and may promote the development of breast cancer (controversial).

102. What are contractures? How long do they take to develop?

Contractures are the result of fibrosis of periarticular structures and shortening of muscles and tendons. The process can occur within just 7 days if regular full motion of the joint is not maintained. Any reason for immobility of a joint will produce contractures. Because contractures are so difficult to treat once they are present, preventative measures, such as bedside passive range of motion exercises, are very beneficial and should be used in all immobilized patients.

103. What is the importance of a positive antinuclear antibody test (ANA) in an older patient?

There is a 15% frequency of a positive ANA in normal older people. These are usually of low titer (1:16 or less) and, in isolation, are of little clinical significance.

104. Which joints are most commonly involved in osteoarthritis?

The distal interphalangeal (DIP) and proximal interphalangeal (PIP) joints of the hands, the knees, the first carpometacarpal (CMC) joint of the feet, and, less frequently, the hips.

105. Which patients are at increased risk of untoward reactions when vitamin D supplementation is used for prophylaxis against osteoporosis?

Vitamin D supplementation has an unclear role in prevention of osteoporosis, although some physicians do administer this agent for prophylaxis. The groups at risk for untoward reactions to this therapy are those with kidney stones, patients with sarcoidosis, and, if the active form of vitamin D (1,25-dihydroxy vitamin D) is administered, anyone with decreased creatinine clearance.

BIBLIOGRAPHY

1. Beck JC: Geriatrics Review Syllabus: A Core Curriculum in Geriatric Medicine. New York, American Geriatrics Society, 1990.
2. Forciea MA, Lavizzo-Mourey, RJ: Geriatric Secrets. Philadelphia, Hanley & Belfus, 1996.
3. Hazzard WR, et al (eds): Principles of Geriatric Medicine and Gerontology, 3rd ed. New York, McGraw-Hill, 1995.
4. Kane RL, et al: Essentials of Clinical Geriatrics, 3rd ed. New York, McGraw-Hill, 1994.

INDEX

Page numbers in **boldface type** indicate complete chapters.

485

Index